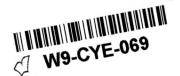

# A Cross Section of Nursing Research

## Journal Articles for Discussion and Evaluation

### Fifth Edition

Roberta J. Peteva

Editor

 **Pyrczak Publishing**
P.O. Box 250430 • Glendale, CA 91225

"Pyrczak Publishing" is an imprint of Fred Pyrczak, Publisher, A California Corporation.

Although the editor and publisher have made every effort to ensure the accuracy and completeness of information contained in this book, we assume no responsibility for errors, inaccuracies, omissions, or any inconsistency herein. Any slights of people, places, or organizations are unintentional.

Project Director: Monica Lopez.

Editorial assistance provided by Cheryl Alcorn, Randall R. Bruce, Jenifer Dill, Karen Disner, Sherwin Ercia, Brenda Koplin, Jack Petit, Erica Simmons, and Sharon Young.

Cover design by Robert Kibler and Larry Nichols.

Printed in the United States of America by Malloy, Inc.

ISBN 1-884585-96-5

# Contents

Level I.

Level II.

*Continued* →

## Quasi-Experimental Research

## Pre-Experimental Research

## Program Evaluation/Process Evaluation

## Qualitative Research

*no level–simply lit. review*

*New to the Fifth Edition

*v*

# Notes

# Introduction

This book is designed for students who are learning how to evaluate published nursing research. The 39 research articles in this collection provide the stimulus material for such a course.

## Selection of the Articles

Several criteria were used in the selection of the articles. The first was that the articles be comprehensible to students taking their first research methods course. Thus, it was necessary that the articles have straightforward research designs and employ only basic statistics.

Second, the articles were to illustrate a wide variety of approaches to research. You will notice in the Contents that the articles represent nine types of research such as True Experimental Research, Program Evaluation/Process Evaluation, Qualitative Research, and so on.

Finally, the articles were to be drawn from a large number of different journals. Because each journal has its own genre as well as criteria for the selection of submissions for publication, students can get a sense of the wide variations in approaches to nursing research only by reading articles from a wide variety of journals.

## How to Use This Book

This collection of research articles can be used for instruction in several ways. Most common is to assign one or two articles for homework at each class meeting. At the next class meeting, the article(s) can be discussed with the instructor, who will lead a discussion of the answers to the questions at the end of each article. Another common use is to make each student responsible for leading the discussion of one or two of the articles after all members of the class have read them for homework.

## About the Questions at the End of Each Article

There are three types of questions at the end of each article. First, there are *Factual Questions*. The answers for these are explicitly stated in the articles. In addition to writing down the answers, students should record the line numbers where they found the answers. The line numbers will facilitate discussions if there are disagreements on what constitutes a correct answer to a question.

Second, there are *Questions for Discussion*. Because these are designed to stimulate classroom discussions, most of the questions ask for students' opinions on various decisions made by the researchers in conducting and writing up their research. In field tests, these questions led to lively classroom discussions. Since professional researchers often debate such issues with each other, students should not be surprised by such debates taking place in their own classrooms.

Third, students are asked to make *Quality Ratings* for each article. This is done by applying 13 fundamental criteria for evaluating research, which are repeated at the end of each article.

## Reading the Statistics in This Book

Students who have taken a statistics class as a prerequisite to their research methods class should feel quite comfortable with the overwhelming majority of statistics found in this collection because articles that contained large numbers of obscure or highly advanced statistics were excluded from this book.

Students who are learning about statistics for the first time in the course in which they are using this book may need some additional help from their instructors. Keep in mind that it is not realistic to expect instructors of a methods class to also teach a full-fledged course in statistical methods. Thus, there may be times when an instructor asks students to concentrate on the researcher's *interpretation* of statistics without getting bogged down in discussions of the theory underlying specific statistics. It is possible to focus on the interpretation instead of specific statistics because almost all researchers describe their results in words as well as numbers.

## The Classification of the Articles

If you examine a number of research methods textbooks, you will probably find that they differ to some extent in their system for classifying various types of research. While some labels such as "true experiment" and "qualitative research" are common to almost all textbooks, others that you find in some textbooks may be more idiosyncratic. In addition, some categories of research overlap. An interesting classroom discussion topic is whether a given article can be classified as more than one type of research.

## About the Fifth Edition

The Fifth Edition contains most of the articles that were in the Fourth Edition. The Fifth Edition also contains 10 additional articles (i.e., article numbers 1, 3, 5, 11, 14, 17, 22, 24, 28, and 39), which provide more variety and keep this volume up-to-date.

## Acknowledgments

I am grateful to Mildred L. Patten, who is the author of a similar collection titled *Educational and Psychological Research: A Cross Section of Journal Articles for Analysis and Evaluation.* Her popular book emphasizes broad issues of interest to both psychologists and educators, while this book emphasizes topics of interest to students preparing for careers as nursing professionals. Some structural elements of Patten's book were employed in this one, such as the inclusion of three types of questions at the end of each article.

I am indebted to the publishers who hold the copyrights to the articles in this book. Without their cooperation, it would not be possible to amass a collection such as you find here.

Roberta J. Peteva

# Article 1

# A Survey of Emotional Difficulties of Nurses Who Care for Oncology Patients

**Fahriye Oflaz, Filiz Arslan, Şenay Uzun, Ayfer Ustunsoz, Elif Yilmazkol, Emine Ünlü**[*]

ABSTRACT. Nurses who care for dying patients are under pressure emotionally because of their beliefs and values about death as well as the emotions and reactions of the patients and their families. This study examines the emotional difficulties of nurses caring for oncology patients in Turkey. The study used a descriptive survey design. The participants were 157 nurses from three medical oncology units in Ankara. Results showed that nurses had difficulty in talking to oncology patients about end-of-life issues and found that caring for dying patients affected their personal lives. This study also showed that the length of nurses' work experience had no effect on their feelings and perceptions toward terminally ill patients. However, the nurses who had more work experience were more likely to report difficulty in talking to patients. Most of the nurses expressed feelings of inadequacy and hopelessness about pain management and treatments.

From *Psychological Reports*, *106*, 119–130. Copyright © 2010 by Psychological Reports. Reprinted with permission.

Of all health care professionals, nurses have the longest and most frequent contact with patients and their families during the terminal phase of disease. While they are giving physical care, they also must
5 deal with the emotional suffering, chronic grief, and anxiety of patients and families related to that anticipated death (Fry, 1998; Sellers & Haag, 1998; Wilkinson, Gambles, & Roberts, 2002; Skilbeck & Payne, 2005; Priest, 2006; Oflaz, 2007). However, many hos-
10 pital nurses, despite being skilled in high technology treatments and care, usually feel unprepared to care for a dying patient (Durham & Weiss, 1997; Konishi & Davis, 1999; Kruijver, Kerkstra, Francke, Bensing, & van de Wiel, 2000; Georgaki, Kalaidopoulou, Li-
15 armakopoulos, & Mystakidou, 2002; Weigel, Parker, Fanning, Reyna, & Gasbarra, 2007). Studies examining the experiences of nurses who give end-of-life care suggest that most nurses feel confident about the physical care but not quite as confident in meeting the psy-
20 chosocial needs of the patients. Nurses appear not to be comfortable talking to those patients about life-and-death issues (Fallowfield & Jenkins, 1999; Ferrell, Vi-

rani, Grant, Coyne, & Uman, 2000; Sumner, 2000; Georgaki et al., 2002; Skilbeck & Payne, 2005). How-
25 ever, during the life-threatening illness experience, patients and their families need a continuing dialogue that can provide information in helping them make decisions (Ferrell et al., 2000; Sumner, 2000). In addition, it seems that patient and family dissatisfaction
30 often revolve around inadequate communication (Lederberg, 1998, Fallowfield, Saul, & Gilligan, 2001).

Nurses are subject to various sources of pressure that make the process of caring for dying patients uncomfortable for them (Buckman, 1992). They are dis-
35 tressed by witnessing unrelieved pain or other symptoms and their continual involvement in the inadequate care of the dying patient (Ferrell et al., 2000; Skilbeck & Payne, 2005; McGrath & Holewa, 2006; Weigel et al., 2007). In addition, nurses' own feelings and per-
40 ceptions about death and dying and loss or experience of cancer in their personal lives also make it harder for them to help patients and families who are struggling to cope with painful situations (Bauer & Barron, 1995; Sellers & Haag, 1998; Ferrell et al., 2000; Sumner,
45 2000; Taylor & Mamier, 2005; Johnston & Smith, 2006). Feelings of inadequacy in coping with problems, fear of confronting death, and the need to distance themselves from pain and suffering (Lederberg, 1998; Shapiro, 2008; Maguire & Pitceathly, 2003) put
50 constraints on nurses' abilities to deliver effective psychological care (Fallowfield & Jenkins, 1999; Van Dover & Bacon, 2001; Perreault, Fothergill-Bourbonnais, & Fiset, 2004; Weigel et al., 2007). That is why it is important for nurses to understand their own feelings
55 and evaluate their own attitudes that are influenced by these processes (Durham & Weiss, 1997).

The vast majority of terminally ill patients in Turkey die in the oncology units of general hospitals. As yet, there are no hospices in Turkey. In addition, death-
60 related issues are generally not discussed with patients and their families because of traditional values and the role ambiguity within health care teams. Everyone wants to protect the patient as much as possible from unpleasantness by avoiding talking about end-of-life

[*]*Address correspondence to*: Fahriye Oflaz, R.N., Ph.D., Gulhane Military Medical Academy School of Nursing, Faculty of Psychiatric Nursing Department, 06018 Etlik-Ankara, Turkey. E-mail: foflaz@yahoo.com or foflaz@gata.edu.tr

65  issues, as Konishi and Davis (1999) reported finding in Japan. While patients and their families are informed about the cancer diagnosis itself, they are not given clear explanations about the course of the disease or its terminal phase. For this reason, nurses are exposed to
70  many questions from patients and their relatives. These nurses usually find themselves in a position between physicians and patients or between patients and their families. However, the perceptions and difficulties of nurses have so far received minimal research attention.
75  For these reasons, the aim of this study is to examine the concerns of nurses who care for oncology patients and the relationship between those concerns and the working experience of nurses. Thus, exploring how nurses experience the care of terminally ill patients
80  may help to improve the quality of the care process itself.

## Method

This descriptive study used a questionnaire survey design and convenience sampling technique. The questionnaires were administered at three teaching hospitals
85  in Ankara, Turkey. One is a general hospital with a large oncology department, and the others are hospitals specializing in oncology patients and include medical and surgical units. These hospitals are both treatment and palliative care hospitals, and usually patients who
90  are in specific illness stages are placed together. The study hospitals are the government hospitals, and the nurses who were employed in these hospitals were assigned to work there. At the medical oncology units of these hospitals, 250 nurses were employed during the
95  study. Permissions for the study were obtained from the scientific committees of the relevant institutions of each hospital.

### Participants

The nurses who were not available to interview in person for reasons such as sick calls and working night
100  shifts were excluded from the study. Thus, the participants in the study were 170 nurses who were available to interview and willing to participate in the study. After giving information about the purpose of the study and obtaining verbal consent, questionnaires were ad-
105  ministered to those nurses who were willing to take part. They were given a week to fill in surveys and then these were collected by the researchers. Thirteen questionnaires were excluded from the data analysis because of inappropriate or irrelevant answers, so 157
110  questionnaires were analyzed.

### Instruments and Data Analysis

The questionnaire consisted of three parts: the first part included details such as age, the educational level of the nurses, and their work experience (in years); the second part measured concerns and feelings about car-
115  ing for dying patients; and the third part assessed nurses' thoughts about pain management and treatments during the terminal phase.

In the questionnaire, the statements about the nurses' concerns and feelings were mainly adapted
120  from the list of feelings in Durham and Weiss's paper (1997, Table 3). Durham and Weiss (1997) emphasized that these statements were prepared to make it easier for nurses to express their emotions. The statements were translated into Turkish by the researchers and
125  administered to 15 nurses to examine the clarity of wording. After completing the revisions, two nurses and one nursing faculty member confirmed the clarity of the items again before the study. Nurses were expected to respond to these statements with "yes" or
130  "no" according to their own experiences. In addition, they were expected to write down their difficulties and thoughts answering the open-ended questions that were related to caring for a terminally ill patient and pain management and treatment.
135  Cronbach's coefficient alpha value of the questionnaire was estimated to test the internal consistency reliability of the survey ($\alpha = .72$). There were four categories of work experience: $\leq 5$ yr.; 6–10 yr.; 11–15 yr.; > 16 yr. All of the statistical analyses were performed
140  with SPSS, Version 13.0, software. Frequencies were shown as $n$ (%) notation. Differences between the categorical variables, such as the number of working years and yes/no answers, were analyzed by the chi-square test. Statistical significance was confirmed at $p < .05$.

## Results

145  The participants' mean age was 35.0 yr. ($SD = 6.2$). Most of the nurses who participated in the study had been working more than 5 yr. ($n = 125$, 79.6%) and half of them ($n = 82$, 52.2%) had graduated from an associate degree program (see Table 1). All nurses
150  were female.

Table 1
*Professional Characteristics of the Nurses*

| Characteristic | $N = 157$ | % |
|---|---|---|
| Years in nursing | | |
| $\leq 5$ yr. | 32 | 20.4 |
| 6–10 yr. | 65 | 41.4 |
| 11–15 yr. | 30 | 19.1 |
| > 16% yr. | 30 | 19.1 |
| Education degrees | | |
| High school diploma | 56 | 35.7 |
| Associate degree, 2 yr. | 82 | 52.2 |
| Bachelor's degree | 19 | 12.1 |

Table 2 shows cancer-related experiences of nurses in their personal lives. Of the nurses, 70.7% ($n = 111$) had at least one relative who had been diagnosed with cancer, 60.5% ($n = 95$) had experienced loss because of
155  cancer, and 82.8% ($n = 130$) had experienced the death of a patient because of cancer. Almost half of the nurses (49.0%, $n = 77$) stated that their personal lives were affected by the loss of their patients and/or because of caring for patients with cancer. Table 3 shows
160  the number and percentages of nurses who responded to the statements and the comparisons of these state-

ments with their years of experience. Most of the nurses (95.5%, $n = 150$) did not want to tell a patient that he or she was in the terminal phase. Seventy-nine
165 percent ($n = 125$) of the nurses agreed with the statement "Being with a terminally ill patient who is dying reminds me that someday I will die too," 75.8% ($n = 119$) reported disturbance about being around a dying patient, and 75.8%, ($n = 119$) described discom-
170 fort while they were talking to a terminally ill patient. However, most of the nurses stated that they could articulate their fear and feelings about death ($n = 123$, 78.3%) and believed that they could describe their own feelings about caring for terminally ill patients
175 ($n = 115$, 73.2%). Approximately one-third of the nurses ($n = 46$, 29.3%) stated that they were afraid of being too attached to dying patients and of not being able to control their feelings. On the other hand, 68.8% ($n = 108$) stated that they could assist a patient to feel
180 comfortable with his or her impending death.

Table 2
*Nurses' Own Experiences Related to Cancer*

| Characteristic | $n$ | % |
|---|---|---|
| Cancer history in the family | | |
| Yes | 111 | 70.7 |
| No | 46 | 29.3 |
| Loss of a close relative because of cancer | | |
| Yes | 95 | 60.5 |
| No | 62 | 39.5 |
| Loss of a patient | | |
| Yes | 130 | 82.8 |
| No | 10 | 6.4 |
| No answer | 17 | 10.8 |
| Being influenced in personal life because of caring for patients with cancer | | |
| Yes | 77 | 49.0 |
| No | 52 | 33.1 |
| No answer | 28 | 17.8 |
| Making mental associations between the patient and the relative with cancer | 31 | 27.9 |

There was a statistically significant difference between groups with different work experience in frequencies of the two possible responses to the statement "I don't think a person should be told his/her condition
185 is incurable or terminal" ($\chi^2 = 9.35$, $p = .025$; V = .50); nurses with the most experience (i.e., more than 16 yr. experience) were more likely to agree ($n = 24$, 80.0%). There was no statistically significant difference between groups with various amounts of work experience
190 in frequencies of agreement with other statements (see Table 3).

Answers given to open-ended questions are shown in Tables 4 and 5. The difficulties expressed by nurses are displayed in Table 4. The question was "What dif-
195 ficulties do you experience in caring for terminally ill patients?" A few nurses stated that they had experienced no problems ($n = 10$, 6.3%) and 29.2% ($n = 46$) stated that they had experienced difficulties in dealing with distress related to the expression of emotions by
200 their patients and their relatives in cases of "denial of

their situation" ($n = 29$, 18.5%), "dissatisfaction" ($n = 7$, 4.5%), and "refusal of treatments" ($n = 10$, 6.4%). These statements were grouped as "distress with emotional expressions of patients and their families" in
205 Table 4. The statements about patients' conditions were grouped as "distress caused by a patient's condition itself" and 26.7% ($n = 42$) of nurses reported difficulties in dealing with distress related to the condition of their patients. These conditions included "the unre-
210 lieved pain and suffering of the patient" ($n = 11$, 7.0%), "sadness at the young age of the patient" ($n = 3$, 1.9%), "anxiety at knowing that the patient will die" ($n = 7$, 4.4%), and "helping the patient to relieve the fear of death" ($n = 21$, 13.4%).
215    Of the nurses, 29.9% ($n = 47$) stated they had difficulties in dealing with distress related to their own feelings (Table 4). These feelings were desperation and incompetence ($n = 5$, 3.2%), sadness and sorrow ($n = 27$, 17.2%), being afraid of facing the patient's ques-
220 tions ($n = 12$, 7.6%), and avoidance of becoming attached to the patient ($n = 3$, 1.9%).

The feelings of nurses toward treatment and pain management are shown in Table 5. Statements such as "There are new methods to relieve the cancer pain of
225 the patient in the terminal stage" or "There are new developments related to pain management" were evaluated as *positive* thoughts including hope ($n = 30$, 19.1%), and statements like "I feel inadequate and desperate," "I am uncomfortable about not being able to
230 relieve cancer pain," "I feel hopeless about cancer pain and management," or "Talking about cancer pain is useless" were evaluated as *negative* thoughts including inadequacy and hopelessness ($n = 95$, 60.5%).

## Discussion

This study showed that nurses were usually uncomfortable with talking to a dying patient, but they stated
235 that they were comfortable with expressing their own feelings. In addition, areas causing distress in nurses were categorized under three headings: distress about the expression of emotions by patients and their families, distress caused by the patient's condition itself,
240 and the nurses' own feelings. Approximately half of them expressed feelings of hopelessness and discomfort about cancer pain and treatments.

In the present study, most of the nurses agreed that
245 they were uncomfortable with talking to a terminally ill patient and, regardless of their experience, they did not want to tell the patient that he was in the terminal phase. These findings support the results of the previous studies related to difficulties that nurses experience
250 (Sumner, 2000; White, Coyne, Urvashi, & Patel, 2001; Thompson, McClement, & Daeninck, 2006; Weigel et al., 2007). By contrast, Zervekh (1994) argued that caring for a dying patient teaches nurses how to talk about death. Nevertheless, "to become engaged and
255 connected with the suffering other, is far from automatic in human nature" (Shapiro, 2008, p. 2) and noted

Table 3
*Comparisons of the Years of Experience and Nurses' Concerns with Terminally Ill Patients*

| Concerns of nurses about terminally ill patients | | Total | | Working years | | | | | | | | $\chi^2$ | $p$ |
|---|---|---|---|---|---|---|---|---|---|---|---|---|---|
| | | | | < 5 | | 6–10 | | 11–15 | | > 16 | | | |
| | | $n$ | % | $n$ | % | $n$ | % | $n$ | % | $n$ | % | | |
| I don't want to inform a patient that he/she is in the terminal phase. | Yes | 150 | 95.5 | 32 | 100.0 | 63 | 96.9 | 28 | 93.3 | 27 | 90.0 | 4.29 | .232 |
| | No | 7 | 4.5 | 0 | 0.0 | 2 | 3.1 | 2 | 6.7 | 3 | 10.0 | | |
| Being with a patient who is dying reminds me that someday I will die too. | Yes | 125 | 79.6 | 25 | 78.1 | 56 | 86.2 | 20 | 66.7 | 24 | 80.0 | 4.85 | .182 |
| | No | 32 | 20.4 | 7 | 21.9 | 9 | 13.8 | 10 | 33.3 | 6 | 20.0 | | |
| I experience a feeling of disturbance whenever I think of being around a dying person. | Yes | 119 | 75.8 | 22 | 68.8 | 47 | 72.3 | 24 | 80.0 | 26 | 86.7 | 3.51 | .318 |
| | No | 38 | 24.2 | 10 | 31.3 | 18 | 27.7 | 6 | 20.0 | 4 | 13.3 | | |
| I don't think death should be discussed in the presence of children. | Yes | 119 | 75.8 | 23 | 71.9 | 52 | 80.0 | 21 | 70.0 | 23 | 76.7 | 1.45 | .692 |
| | No | 38 | 24.2 | 9 | 28.1 | 13 | 20.0 | 9 | 30.0 | 7 | 23.3 | | |
| I feel uncomfortable when I have to talk to a terminally ill patient. | Yes | 119 | 75.8 | 22 | 68.8 | 48 | 73.8 | 24 | 80.0 | 25 | 83.3 | 2.21 | .528 |
| | No | 38 | 24.2 | 10 | 31.3 | 17 | 26.2 | 6 | 20.0 | 5 | 16.7 | | |
| I don't think a person should be told his illness is incurable or terminal. | Yes | 95 | 60.5 | 14 | 43.8 | 41 | 63.1 | 16 | 53.3 | 24 | 80.0 | 9.35 | .025* |
| | No | 62 | 39.5 | 18 | 56.3 | 24 | 36.9 | 14 | 46.7 | 6 | 20.0 | | |
| I don't know what to say to a patient who knows he/she will die. | Yes | 82 | 52.2 | 21 | 65.6 | 48 | 73.8 | 24 | 80.0 | 20 | 66.7 | 2.12 | .546 |
| | No | 75 | 47.8 | 11 | 34.4 | 17 | 26.2 | 6 | 20.0 | 10 | 33.3 | | |
| I am afraid I will get too attached to a dying patient and eventually not be able to control my feelings. | Yes | 46 | 29.3 | 10 | 31.3 | 18 | 27.7 | 10 | 33.3 | 8 | 26.7 | 0.47 | .924 |
| | No | 111 | 70.7 | 22 | 68.8 | 47 | 72.3 | 20 | 66.7 | 22 | 73.3 | | |
| I can articulate my fears and feelings about death. | Yes | 123 | 78.3 | 26 | 81.2 | 52 | 80.0 | 24 | 80.0 | 21 | 70.0 | 1.54 | .672 |
| | No | 34 | 21.7 | 6 | 18.8 | 13 | 20.0 | 6 | 20.0 | 9 | 30.0 | | |
| I can describe my feelings about caring for a dying patient. | Yes | 115 | 73.2 | 26 | 81.2 | 51 | 78.5 | 17 | 56.7 | 21 | 70.0 | 6.31 | .097 |
| | No | 42 | 26.8 | 6 | 18.8 | 14 | 21.5 | 13 | 43.3 | 9 | 30.0 | | |
| I can assist a dying patient to feel more comfortable with his/her impending death. | Yes | 108 | 68.8 | 22 | 68.8 | 43 | 66.2 | 20 | 66.7 | 23 | 76.7 | 1.14 | .767 |
| | No | 49 | 31.2 | 10 | 31.3 | 22 | 33.8 | 10 | 33.3 | 7 | 23.3 | | |
| I can do postmortem procedures competently. | Yes | 119 | 75.8 | 23 | 71.9 | 49 | 75.4 | 22 | 73.3 | 25 | 83.3 | 2.53 | .469 |
| | No | 38 | 24.2 | 9 | 28.1 | 16 | 24.6 | 8 | 26.7 | 5 | 16.7 | | |

*Statistically significant difference in response frequencies by experience.

the option of "staying away" instead. So, one communication issue may be the appearance of a distancing strategy in the nurses as suggested by Maguire and Pitceathly (2003). This situation could negatively affect the individual's ability to establish effective communication. On the other hand, some constraints on giving psychological care such as the priority placed on attending to physical health needs, multiple demands on nurses' time, and the varying expectations of nurses and health care institutions concerning the nurses' role in giving psychological care may prevent nurses from communicating effectively (Sumner, 2000; Van Dover & Bacon, 2001).

In this study, neither years of experience nor level of education appeared to be a factor related to feelings and concerns of nurses who care for terminally ill patients. However, most of the nurses who had more than 16 years of experience stated that they did not want a patient to be told that his condition was terminal. Some studies suggest that nurses with more years of experience are more positive in their attitudes in dealing with terminally ill patients (Kruijver et al., 2000; Thompson et al., 2006; Weigel et al., 2007). In Thompson et al. (2006), nurses stated that they wanted to feel relaxed about subjects such as death but that it is necessary to have experience in caring for dying patients in order to be able to help patients and their families. However, there are also studies showing the opposite result. In the study of White et al. (2001), nurses were not comfortable talking about death with patients and their families, and older nurses emphasized the need for more training. In the current sample, findings showed that the more working experience nurses had, the more discomfort they expressed. This may be explained by avoidance and distance toward patients that nurses build up over the years. This result is also important because in Turkey, the senior nurses usually have the role of teaching the junior nurses how to communicate and how to give psychological care in the units (Fallowfield et al., 2001; Priest, 2006). Thus, the difficulties and experiences of senior nurses merit further research.

Table 4
*Expressed Difficulties Related to Caring for Terminally Ill
Patients (N = 157)*

| | n | % |
|---|---|---|
| Dealing with distress related to emotional expressions of patients and their families | 46 | 29.2 |
| Denial of their situation | 29 | 18.5 |
| Dissatisfaction | 7 | 4.5 |
| Refusal of treatments | 10 | 6.4 |
| Dealing with distress caused by patient's condition | 42 | 26.7 |
| Seeing unrelieved pain and suffering of the patient | 11 | 7.0 |
| Sadness at the young age of the patient | 3 | 1.9 |
| Anxiety at knowing that the patient will die | 7 | 4.4 |
| Helping the patient to relieve the fear of death | 21 | 13.4 |
| Dealing with distress caused by nurses' own feelings | 47 | 29.9 |
| Desperation and incompetence | 5 | 3.2 |
| Sadness and sorrow | 27 | 17.2 |
| Being afraid of facing the patient's questions | 12 | 7.6 |
| Avoiding becoming attached to the patient | 3 | 1.9 |
| Expressed that they experienced no difficulty | 10 | 6.4 |
| No answer | 12 | 7.6 |

Table 5
*Feelings of Nurses Related to Cancer Pain Management and
Treatment (N = 157)*

| | n | % |
|---|---|---|
| Inadequacy and helplessness about pain management and treatment | 95 | 60.5 |
| Feeling hopeful about the developments in treatments | 30 | 19.1 |
| No answer | 32 | 20.4 |

One-third of the nurses expressed the fear of not being able to control their own feelings, but most of them stated that they could nevertheless describe their feelings (Table 3). This result has been understood to mean that nurses were aware of their own feelings and that they could verbalize them when the appropriate environment or conditions were created. On the other hand, to what extent these expressions describe real feelings and to what extent they indicate suppression or avoidance must be assessed by different methods (Sadock & Sadock, 2007).

Approximately half of the nurses stated that they do not know what to say to a patient who knows he will die (Table 3). Also, one-third of them expressed difficulty in dealing with distress related to emotional expressions of patients and families (Table 4). In addition, most of the nurses seemed hopeless about cancer pain management and treatments. McGrath and Holewa (2006) indicated that nurses express difficulty in witnessing the stress of terminally ill patients and their efforts to cope with invasive treatments and technology. Since effective pain management is one of the basic factors in the quality of life of terminally ill patients, the hopelessness of nurses in relation to cancer

pain and treatment has been considered an important issue to deal with. The negative beliefs and expectations of nurses may limit their capacity to cope with the pain and spiritual distress of their patients (Lynch & Abraham, 2002). These feelings can also create unwillingness and cause burnout in nurses (Fallowfield & Jenkins, 1999). Supporting these findings, in Pavlish and Ceronsky (2007), patients found nurses not competent to meet their patients' emotional needs and stated that some nurses were not competent to relieve their pain. For these reasons, obtaining up-to-date information about the treatment of cancer and increasing nurses' confidence in their ability to care for their patients adequately have been considered as important factors in being able to provide effective care.

According to Johnston and Smith (2006), facing a terminal illness is a stressful and frightening experience that affects all aspects of life. Difficulties in end-of-life care can force everyone to question themselves and think about their own lives (Fry, 1998). Caring for cancer patients can also have a serious effect on nurses both personally and professionally. In relation to this, almost half of the nurses in this study stated that their personal lives were affected by caring for a dying patient.

More than half of the nurses in this sample had a relative with cancer or had experienced a loss because of cancer. As Perreault et al. (2004) stated, they may experience feelings of helplessness and lack of ability in relation to these relatives with cancer, and they can transfer these feelings to the process of caring for patients so that these feelings can block the caring relationship. For these reasons, these concerns merit future research and have important implications for hospital administrators in terms of the need for more support for the nursing staff. Skilbeck and Payne (2005) indicated that the support received by the nurses for the terminally ill affects quality of care and patient satisfaction.

*Conclusions*
The findings of this study can be added to the findings of other studies dealing with end-of-life issues and difficulties that are common in nursing practice. Nurses stated that they were not comfortable with talking to patients about their impending death, and almost half of the nurses made statements about their feelings of hopelessness and inadequacy in relation to providing effective treatment and pain management. These findings suggest that nurses who are working with terminally ill patients need to be supported to overcome their own difficulties and feelings to achieve a good quality of care. There is a need for curricula to include end-of-life care issues specifically and death education programs to improve nurses' skills in these areas. In addition, nurses need to be supported by integrated approaches, including ongoing supervision, follow-up courses, and feedback on their performance in the workplace to give more range and depth to their learn-

ing and more opportunity to reflect on their practice
380 (Wilkinson et al., 2002; Maguire & Pitceathly, 2003).

Further research is needed to understand the effects of the difficulties on nurses' personal lives and their reflections on patient care. In this respect, this study is a step toward forming a framework for future studies in
385 this area. Qualitative studies could be more useful in identifying difficulties in giving effective end-of-life care. Although this study is limited to three centers, the large number of participants ensures that it is representative of the concerns of nurses in Turkey.

## References

Bauer, T., & Barron, C. R. (1995). Nursing interventions for spiritual care: Preferences of the community-based elderly. *Journal of Holistic Nursing, 13*, 268–279.

Buckman, R. (1992). *How to break bad news: A guide for health care professionals.* Baltimore, MD: John Hopkins Univer. Press.

Durham, E., & Weiss, L. (1997). How patients die. *American Journal of Nursing, 97*, 41–47.

Fallowfield, L., & Jenkins, V. (1999). Effective communication skills are the key to good cancer care. *European Journal of Cancer, 35*, 1592–1597.

Fallowfield, L., Saul, J., & Gilligan, B. (2001). Teaching senior nurses how to teach communication skills in oncology. *Cancer Nursing, 24*, 185–191.

Ferrell, B., Virani, R., Grant, M., Coyne, P., & Uman, G. (2000). End-of-life care: Nurses speak out. *Nursing, 30*, 54–57.

Fry, S. (1998). Guidelines for making end-of-life decisions. *International Nursing Review, 45*, 143–144.

Georgaki, S., Kalaidopoulou, O., Liarmakopoulos, I., & Mystakidou, K. (2002). Nurses' attitudes toward truthful communication with patients with cancer. *Cancer Nursing, 25*, 436–441.

Johnston, B., & Smith, L. N. (2006). Nurses' and patients' perceptions of expert palliative nursing care. *Journal of Advanced Nursing, 54*, 700–709.

Konishi, E., & Davis, A. J. (1999). Japanese nurses' perceptions about disclosure of information at the patients' end of life. *Nursing and Health Sciences, 1*, 179–187.

Kruijver, I. P. M., Kerkstra, A., Francke, A. L., Bensing, J. M., & van de Wiel, H. B. M. (2000). Evaluation of communication training programmes in nursing care: A review of the literature. *Patient Education and Counseling, 39*, 129–145.

Lederberg, M. S. (1998). Oncology staff stress and related interventions. In J. C. Holland, W. Breitbart, P. B. Jacobsen, M. S. Lederberg, M. Loscalzo, M. J. Massie, & R. McCorkle (Eds.), *Psycho-oncology.* New York: Oxford Univer. Press. 1035–1046.

Lynch, M., & Abraham, J. (2002). Ensuring a good death. *Cancer Practice, 10* (1 suppl.), S33–S38.

Maguire, P., & Pitceathly, C. (2003). Improving the psychological care of cancer patients and their relatives: The role of specialist nurses. *Journal of Psychosomatic Research, 55*, 469–474.

McGrath, P., & Holewa, H. (2006). Missed opportunities: Nursing insights on end-of-life care for hematology patients. *International Journal of Nursing Practice, 12*, 295–301.

Oflaz, F. (2007). Yaşamin son günlerinde hemşirelik bakimi [The end-of-life care]. In N. Akbayrak, A. Akbayrak, G. Ançel, & S. Erkal-İlhan (Eds.), *Hemşirelik bakim planlari [Nursing care plans]* Ankara, Turkey: Alter Publishing. 143–153.

Pavlish, C., & Ceronsky, L. (2007). Oncology nurses' perceptions about palliative care. *Oncology Nursing Forum, 34*, 793–800.

Perreault, A., Fothergill-Bourbonnais, F., & Fiset, V. (2004). The experience of family members caring for a dying loved one. *International Journal of Palliative Nursing, 10*, 133–143.

Priest, H. M. (2006). Helping student nurses to identify and respond to the psychological needs of physically ill patients: Implications for curriculum design. *Nurse Education Today, 26*, 423–429.

Sadock, B. J., & Sadock, V. A. (2007). End of life and palliative care. In H. Aydin & A. Bozkurt (Eds.), *Comprehensive textbook of psychiatry.* Ankara, Turkey: Güneş Kitabevi. 2336–2365. [in Turkish]

Sellers, S. C., & Haag, B. A. (1998). Spiritual nursing interventions. *Journal of Holistic Nursing, 16*, 338–354.

Shapiro, J. (2008). Walking a mile in their patients' shoes: Empathy and othering in medical students' education. *Philosophy, Ethics, and Humanities in Medicine, 3*, 1–11.

Skilbeck, J. K., & Payne, S. (2005). End of life care: A discursive analysis of specialist palliative care nursing. *Journal of Advanced Nursing, 51*, 325–334.

Sumner, H. C. (2000). Recognizing and responding to spiritual distress. *American Journal of Nursing, 98*, 26–31.

Taylor, E. J., & Mamier, I. (2005). Spiritual care nursing: What cancer patients and family caregivers want. *Journal of Advanced Nursing, 49*, 260–267.

Thompson, G., McClement, S., & Daeninck, P (2006). Nurses' perceptions of quality end-of-life care on an acute medical ward. *Journal of Advanced Nursing, 53*, 169–177.

Van Dover, L. J., & Bacon, J. M. (2001). Spiritual care in nursing practice: A close-up view. *Nursing Forum, 36*, 18–28.

Weigel, C., Parker, G., Fanning, L., Reyna, K., & Gasbarra, D. B. (2007). Apprehension among hospital nurses providing end-of-life care. *Journal of Hospice and Palliative Nursing, 9*, 86–91.

White, K. R., Coyne, P. J., Urvashi, B., & Patel, U. B. (2001). Are nurses adequately prepared for end-of-life care? *Journal of Nursing Scholarship, 33*, 147–151.

Wilkinson, S. M., Gambles, M., & Roberts, A. (2002). The essence of cancer care: The impact of training on nurses' ability to communicate effectively. *Journal of Advanced Nursing, 40*, 731–738.

Zervekh, J. (1994). The truth-tellers: How hospice nurses help patients confront death. *American Journal of Nursing, 94*, 31–34.

# Exercise for Article 1

## Factual Questions

1. How many questionnaires were excluded from the data analysis because of inappropriate or irrelevant answers?

2. What was the participants' mean age?

3. What percentage of the nurses did not want to tell a patient that he or she was in the terminal phase?

4. How many nurses expressed that they experienced no difficulties related to caring for terminally ill patients?

5. Besides years of experience, what other factor appeared unrelated to feelings and concerns of nurses who care for terminally ill patients?

6. When caring for terminally ill patients, how many nurses expressed sadness at the young age of the patient?

## Questions for Discussion

7. Using the same methods and under the same conditions, do you think the results would vary greatly if the study were conducted in the United States? Explain. (See lines 83–97.)

8. In your opinion, did the exclusion of nurses who were not available to interview in person affect the results of the study? Explain. (See lines 98–100.)

9. How important was Table 3 in helping you understand the results of the study? Explain. (See Table 3 and lines 299–312.)

10. Do you agree that qualitative studies could be more useful in identifying difficulties in giving effective end-of-life care? Explain. (See lines 385–387.)

11. Do you think that this study has important implications for nursing professionals? (See lines 363–380.)

12. If you were conducting a study on the same topic, what changes in the research methodology, if any, would you make?

## *Quality Ratings*

Directions: Indicate your level of agreement with each of the following statements by circling a number from 5 for strongly agree (SA) to 1 for strongly disagree (SD). If you believe an item is not applicable to this research article, leave it blank. Be prepared to explain your ratings. When responding to criteria A and B, keep in mind that brief titles and abstracts are conventional in published research.

A.  The title of the article is appropriate.

   SA   5   4   3   2   1   SD

B.  The abstract provides an effective overview of the research article.

   SA   5   4   3   2   1   SD

C.  The introduction establishes the importance of the study.

   SA   5   4   3   2   1   SD

D.  The literature review establishes the context for the study.

   SA   5   4   3   2   1   SD

E.  The research purpose, question, or hypothesis is clearly stated.

   SA   5   4   3   2   1   SD

F.  The method of sampling is sound.

   SA   5   4   3   2   1   SD

G.  Relevant demographics (for example, age, gender, and ethnicity) are described.

   SA   5   4   3   2   1   SD

H.  Measurement procedures are adequate.

   SA   5   4   3   2   1   SD

I.  All procedures have been described in sufficient detail to permit a replication of the study.

   SA   5   4   3   2   1   SD

J.  The participants have been adequately protected from potential harm.

   SA   5   4   3   2   1   SD

K.  The results are clearly described.

   SA   5   4   3   2   1   SD

L.  The discussion/conclusion is appropriate.

   SA   5   4   3   2   1   SD

M.  Despite any flaws, the report is worthy of publication.

   SA   5   4   3   2   1   SD

# Article 2

# Post-Anesthesia Care Unit Nurses' Knowledge of Pulse Oximetry

**John P. Harper**, MSN, RN, BC[*]

ABSTRACT. The purpose of this study was to assess post-anesthesia care unit (PACU) nurses' knowledge of pulse oximetry. A convenience sample of 19 nurses completed a 32-item questionnaire that included a 20-item true-false test on pulse oximetry. Overall, nurses demonstrated a knowledge deficit in pulse oximetry. Competency in the use of pulse oximetry is vital to ensure a positive clinical outcome. Nurse educators are responsible for identifying knowledge deficits among staff and implementing strategies to correct these deficits. It is incumbent on nurse educators to provide research-based education on pulse oximetry and opportunities to participate in continuing education.

From *Journal for Nurses in Staff Development, 20,* 177–180. Copyright © 2004 by Lippincott Williams & Wilkins. Reprinted with permission.

Pulse oximetry (SpO$_2$), a measurement of arterial oxygen saturation, has been used for years in the post-anesthesia care unit (PACU) to detect hypoxemia in patients emerging from anesthesia. Consequently,
5 competency in the use of pulse oximetry is vital to ensure a positive clinical outcome. Severinghaus and Astrup (1986) described pulse oximetry as one of the most significant technological advances made in monitoring the well-being and safety of patients during anesthesia, recovery, and critical care. Today, pulse oximetry is used throughout the entire continuum of patient care. The purpose of this study was to assess PACU nurses' knowledge of pulse oximetry.

## Literature Review

Stoneham, Saville, and Wilson (1994) reported on a
15 study that assessed knowledge of pulse oximetry among medical and nursing staff. This study sample consisted of 30 senior house officers and 30 staff nurses employed at a general hospital in the United Kingdom. Questions were asked about the theory behind pulse oximetry, factors affecting readings, "normal" values in various patients, values in hypothetical clinical situations, and what education participants had received. Ninety-seven percent of physicians and nurses did not understand how a pulse oximeter
25 worked and were confused about factors influencing readings. Respondents gave a wide range of acceptable saturation values (e.g., 90–100% for a fit adult). In addition, there were serious errors made in evaluating saturation readings in hypothetical clinical situations.

30 Kruger and Longden (1997) surveyed physicians, nurses, and anesthesia technicians ($N = 203$) at an Australian Base Hospital to assess their knowledge of the principles of pulse oximetry. Less than 50% of participants believed they had adequate education in the use
35 of pulse oximetry. Only 68.5% of the participants correctly stated what the pulse oximeter measures. Answers to questions regarding the principles of pulse oximetry, potential errors, normal ranges, and the physiology of oxygen hemoglobin dissociation varied,
40 but generally reflected limited understanding.

Howell (2002) reported on 50 staff members, consisting of both physicians and nurses, within a large general hospital in the United Kingdom. Participants' responses to a questionnaire and to six clinical scenar-
45 ios on pulse oximetry were analyzed. Overall, there was a deficit in participants' knowledge of pulse oximetry.

There were no studies in the literature that assessed PACU nurses' knowledge of pulse oximetry. An ex-
50 tremely beneficial monitoring tool, pulse oximetry can detect hypoxemia before it is clinically evident. PACU nurses routinely monitor arterial oxygen saturation, using pulse oximetry technology on all patients emerging from anesthesia. Based on the results of previous
55 studies, it is important to assess PACU nurses' understanding of pulse oximetry to ensure continued competence during this critical phase of anesthesia care.

## Research Question

The following research question was addressed: What is the knowledge of PACU nurses regarding the
60 basic concepts and physiology of pulse oximetry?

## Method

### Research Design

A descriptive correlational design was used. This design permitted description of the phenomena of in-

---

[*]*John P. Harper* is a quality monitoring-improvement reviewer and per diem clinical educator, Taylor Hospital, Ridley Park, Pennsylvania.

terest and the relationships among selected variables and knowledge of pulse oximetry.

*Sample and Setting*

65     The target population was PACU nurses working in a four-hospital healthcare system in the Mid-Atlantic region. Nineteen nurses constituted the convenience sample for the study.

*Instrument*

    The data collection instrument was a 32-item
70  investigator-developed questionnaire. Twelve items elicited demographic information; a 20-item true-false test was designed to assess knowledge of pulse oximetry. Content validity was established by having a panel of three critical care and PACU nurse educators
75  review the questionnaire. Minor changes were incorporated in the final version. The questionnaire was pilot tested by two PACU nurses and additional revisions were made to improve clarity.

*Data Collection*

    The study was approved by the Institutional Review
80  Boards at the four hospitals. Data were collected over a 4-week period in June and July 2003. Packets containing a cover letter explaining the study, the questionnaire, and test were distributed to PACU nurses working on the day of data collection. Completion of the
85  questionnaire and test was considered as consent to participate. The respondents were asked not to use any reference materials or discuss test items with their colleagues. Upon completion of the questionnaire and test, the respondents sealed the completed questionnaire and
90  test in a manila envelope and returned it to the investigator.

*Data Analysis*

    Descriptive statistics, including frequencies, were used to describe the sample. Pearson's correlation was used to identify relationships among selected variables
95  and knowledge of pulse oximetry. The true-false test was used to assess knowledge of pulse oximetry and scored electronically.

## Results

    A total of 19 questionnaires were returned. Of the 19 respondents who completed the survey, 88% were
100 female and 12% were male. The age of the respondents ranged from 30 to 55 years, with a mean of $47 \pm 6.9$ years. The highest level of nursing education for 44% of the respondents was a baccalaureate; 28% had an associate's degree; and 17% had a diploma. Eleven
105 percent had a master's degree. The nurses' experience in the PACU ranged from 1.5 to 27 years, with a mean of $9.5 \pm 7.8$ years. Their experience with pulse oximetry ranged from 4 to 28 years, with a mean of $13 \pm 6.2$ years (see Table 1). All regularly worked during the
110 day shift.

    Respondents first learned about pulse oximetry from a colleague (39%), nursing school (33%), in-

service education (22%), or through a journal article/ reference book (6%). Fifty-nine percent indicated that
115 the initial learning session was adequate. Thirty-five percent of respondents reported that they had participated in continuing education on pulse oximetry since their initial learning session.

Table 1
*Demographic Profile of Survey Respondents (N = 19)*

| Variable | Frequency | Percent |
|---|---|---|
| Gender | | |
| Female | 15 | 88 |
| Male | 2 | 12 |
| Highest level of education | | |
| Baccalaureate | 8 | 44.4 |
| Associate's degree | 5 | 27.8 |
| Diploma | 3 | 16.7 |
| Master's | 2 | 11.1 |
| Hours worked per week | | |
| 36–40 | 12 | 66.7 |
| 20–35 | 4 | 22.1 |
| > 40 | 1 | 5.6 |
| < 20 | 1 | 5.6 |

    Test scores ranged from 40 to 75, with a mean of
120 $62 \pm 9.09$ on a scale of 0 to 100. Thirty-two percent of the respondents thought the pulse oximeter measured the absorption of electrical waves by hemoglobin. The pulse oximeter measures the absorption of light by hemoglobin (Grap, 2002).
125     Twenty-one percent of the respondents thought the $SpO_2$ value was the same as the partial pressure of arterial oxygen ($PaO_2$) value on the arterial blood gas (ABG). $SpO_2$ is an estimation of arterial oxygen saturation ($SaO_2$) (Grap, 2002).
130     Eighty-nine percent of respondents thought that for the $SpO_2$, 95% of the data fell within $\pm 1\%$ of the actual arterial oxygen saturation. Actually, the data fell within $\pm 4\%$ of the actual saturation, within a 95% confidence level (Grap, 2002). For example, in a patient
135 with an $SpO_2$ of 90%, 95% of the time the $SaO_2$ value, as measured by the ABG, would be between 86% and 94%.

    Eighty-nine percent of respondents thought the normal $SpO_2$ in adults ranged between 93% and 100%,
140 and 84% thought the normal $SpO_2$ in children ranged between 97% and 100%. The normal $SpO_2$ for both adults and children is 95–100% (Grap, 2002).

    Forty-two percent of respondents thought that $SpO_2$ is a reliable indicator of ventilation status. $SpO_2$ is an
145 indicator of oxygenation, the amount of hemoglobin that is saturated with oxygen. It does not directly measure ventilation (Grap, 2002).

    Only 63% of respondents thought that performance of a probe placed on a finger is generally better than
150 performance of a probe placed at other sites. In addition, only 58% of respondents thought the finger probe might damage skin integrity. Overall, performance of

finger probes is generally found to be better than performance of probes at other sites. Digital injury induced by the oximeter probe has been reported (Grap, 2002).

Thirty-seven percent of respondents thought the finger probe could be used on the same extremity as an arterial line and blood pressure cuff. The probe should be placed on the extremity opposite an arterial line and blood pressure cuff so that pulsatile flow is not interrupted (Grap, 2002).

Forty-two percent of respondents thought a falsely low $SpO_2$ value may occur in smokers. Actually, a falsely high $SpO_2$ value may be obtained from smokers because of the presence of carbon monoxide. The carbon monoxide turns hemoglobin bright red and the pulse oximeter is unable to determine the difference between hemoglobin molecules saturated with oxygen and those carrying carbon monoxide (Howell, 2002).

Only 79% of respondents thought a patient with hypovolemia may have an altered $SpO_2$ value. Oximeter readings are altered in low perfusion states (Howell, 2002).

All respondents thought the $SpO_2$ would decrease in cardiac arrest. The oximeter requires a pulsatile signal and an alarm will sound when the pulse is lost. As a result, there will be no reading displayed (Howell, 2002).

Fifty-three percent of respondents thought obtaining ABGs was the first priority for a sudden fall or sustained trend of falling $SpO_2$ values. With a change in $SpO_2$ values, assessment of the airway and breathing is the first priority (Howell, 2002).

Pearson's correlation was used to identify relationships among selected variables and knowledge of pulse oximetry. There was a positive correlation between level of education and test scores ($r = .25$) and between length of experience with pulse oximetry and test scores ($r = .14$).

### Discussion and Implications

Although measurement of arterial oxygen saturation by pulse oximetry is a standard of care in the PACU (American Society of Perianesthesia Nurses, 2002), it may be taken for granted and considered a simple monitoring technique. Overall, nurses demonstrated a knowledge deficit in pulse oximetry that is comparable to previous studies (Howell, 2002; Kruger & Longden, 1997; Stoneham et al., 1994).

While respondents first learned about pulse oximetry from a colleague (39%), nursing school (33%), in-service education (22%), or through a journal article/reference book (6%), only 59% indicated that the initial learning session was adequate. Thirty-five percent of respondents reported that they had participated in continuing education on pulse oximetry since their initial learning session. Learning about pulse oximetry came from several sources and may reflect different information. The majority of nurses had not partici-

pated in continuing education on pulse oximetry and therefore may lack current knowledge in pulse oximetry. To increase staff awareness of the need for such knowledge, the results of the study were published in the hospitals' *Nursing Research Newsletter* and distributed to all staff throughout the healthcare system.

Nurse educators are responsible for identifying knowledge deficits among staff and implementing strategies to correct these deficits. It is incumbent on nurse educators to provide research-based education on pulse oximetry and opportunities to participate in continuing education. Since nurses initially learn about pulse oximetry from a variety of sources, competency should be validated during orientation and on a regular basis. Competency in the use of pulse oximetry on patients emerging from anesthesia is vital to ensure a positive clinical outcome.

### References

American Society of Perianesthesia Nurses. (2002). *2002 Standards of perianesthesia nursing practice.* Cherry Hill, NJ: American Society of Perianesthesia Nurses.

Grap, M. (2002). Protocols for practice: Pulse oximetry. *Critical Care Nurse, 22,* 69–76.

Howell, M. (2002). Pulse oximetry: An audit of nursing and medical staff understanding. *British Journal of Nursing, 11,* 191–197.

Kruger, P., & Longden, P. (1997). A study of a hospital staff's knowledge of pulse oximetry. *Anesthesia and Intensive Care, 25,* 38–41.

Severinghaus, J., & Astrup, P. (1986). History of blood gas analysis, VI: Oximetry. *Journal of Clinical Monitoring, 2,* 270–288.

Stoneham, M., Saville, G., & Wilson, I. (1994). Knowledge about pulse oximetry among medical and nursing staff. *Lancet, 344,* 1339–1342.

**Acknowledgment**: The author acknowledges the assistance and support of Elizabeth W. Bayley, PhD, RN.

**Address correspondence to**: John P. Harper, 408 Essington Avenue, Essington, PA 19029-1237. E-mail: HarpJP2@aol.com

# Exercise for Article 2

## *Factual Questions*

1. According to the literature review, were there previous studies in the literature that assessed PACU nurses' knowledge of pulse oximetry?

2. Of the 32 items in the data collection instrument, how many were designed to assess knowledge of pulse oximetry?

3. How was content validity established?

4. What was the mean test score?

5. What does a pulse oximeter measure?

6. What was the value of the Pearson correlation coefficient for the relationship between level of education and test scores?

## Questions for Discussion

7. The researcher refers to the sample in this study as a "convenience sample." What is your understanding of the meaning of this term? (See lines 67–68.)

8. The researcher states that the questionnaire was pilot tested by two PACU nurses and additional revisions were made to improve clarity. In your opinion, was this step in the research important? Explain. (See lines 76–78.)

9. The respondents were asked not to use any reference materials or discuss test items with their colleagues. In your opinion, is it likely that all the respondents followed these instructions? Explain. (See lines 86–88.)

10. Although the researcher states that a total of 19 questionnaires were returned, he does not indicate how many questionnaires were distributed. Would this be useful information to know? Explain. (See line 98.)

11. The correlation coefficient for the relationship between length of experience with pulse oximetry and test scores is reported as .14. In your opinion, is this a strong relationship? Explain. (See lines 187–190.)

12. If you were conducting a study on the same topic, what changes in the research methodology, if any, would you make?

## Quality Ratings

Directions: Indicate your level of agreement with each of the following statements by circling a number from 5 for strongly agree (SA) to 1 for strongly disagree (SD). If you believe an item is not applicable to this research article, leave it blank. Be prepared to explain your ratings. When responding to criteria A and B, keep in mind that brief titles and abstracts are conventional in published research.

A. The title of the article is appropriate.

SA   5   4   3   2   1   SD

B. The abstract provides an effective overview of the research article.

SA   5   4   3   2   1   SD

C. The introduction establishes the importance of the study.

SA   5   4   3   2   1   SD

D. The literature review establishes the context for the study.

SA   5   4   3   2   1   SD

E. The research purpose, question, or hypothesis is clearly stated.

SA   5   4   3   2   1   SD

F. The method of sampling is sound.

SA   5   4   3   2   1   SD

G. Relevant demographics (for example, age, gender, and ethnicity) are described.

SA   5   4   3   2   1   SD

H. Measurement procedures are adequate.

SA   5   4   3   2   1   SD

I. All procedures have been described in sufficient detail to permit a replication of the study.

SA   5   4   3   2   1   SD

J. The participants have been adequately protected from potential harm.

SA   5   4   3   2   1   SD

K. The results are clearly described.

SA   5   4   3   2   1   SD

L. The discussion/conclusion is appropriate.

SA   5   4   3   2   1   SD

M. Despite any flaws, the report is worthy of publication.

SA   5   4   3   2   1   SD

# Article 3

# Male and Female Nursing Applicants' Attitudes and Expectations Towards Their Future Careers in Nursing

**Barbara Mullan**, PhD, **Jon Harrison**, RN[*]

ABSTRACT. This paper investigates the assumption that men have a greater opportunity for career success in the nursing profession than women. This study investigates, through the use of a questionnaire, the attitudes and future expectations of male and female individuals attending interviews to enter a preregistration nursing course. The results from the questionnaires were analysed using both descriptive and inferential methods of analysis, and the findings were discussed in relation to the existing research. In only two of the items, significant differences were found between male and female nursing applicants' attitudes and expectations towards their future careers. The results of this study indicate that it is unlikely to be the individual differences between males and females that determine their career progress, and instead it is more likely to be the organisational barriers within the health service or changes in expectations that are continuing to slow the career progress of female nurses. The results from this study have many implications for recruitment to nurse education programmes for men and women within nursing and the health service organisation as a whole.

From *Journal of Research in Nursing, 13*, 527–539. Copyright © 2008 by Sage Publications. Reprinted with permission.

## Introduction

There has been considerable research in nursing into the apparent advantages that men experience (e.g., Evans, 1997; Kleinman, 2004; Williams, 1992). Many reasons are proposed to explain this, including the cul-
5 ture of the institution (Evans, 1997) and managers' beliefs that men are better leaders (Kleinman, 2004). However, the most commonly posited explanation includes working part time (Evans, 1997; Whittock et al., 2002), taking career breaks (Buchan et al., 1989) and
10 having children (Wajcman, 1996). Other research has suggested that it is more to do with the aspirations of females (Skevington & Dawkes, 1988). However, with the exception of the study by Winson (2003), the majority of research in the field has explored the aspira-
15 tions and expectations of qualified and experienced nurses. Indeed, the Winson (2003) study was a retro-

spective study; therefore, nothing is known about the aspirations and expectations of those just about to embark on their nursing careers. Thus, the study outlined
20 in this paper investigates the career intentions and attitudes of male and female individuals who are not qualified nurses, but who are instead applying to train as nurses.

### Literature Review
*Gender and Nursing: Male Success in Nursing*

Much has been written recently about the potential
25 shortfall of nurses that certain Western countries are facing (Trossman, 2003; Whittock & Leonard, 2003). One recommendation is to increase the number of men in the profession (Sochalski, 2002; Trossman, 2003). Men only make up between 5% and 10% of the work-
30 force in the UK, USA, and Canada. For example, in March 2000, only 5.4% of nurses in the USA were male (Trossman, 2003). Although a small percentage, it actually represents a 226% increase in the number of male nurses in the past two decades (Trossman, 2003).
35 There are many reasons suggested for the lack of men in nursing. For example, Poliafico (1998) suggests that peers considered nursing to be unmanly, which was a disincentive for becoming a nurse. Another reason suggested as to why men are not attracted to nursing is
40 the low economic status accorded to nursing (Meadus, 2000).

However, the most commonly proposed reason is that men are less likely to enter female jobs than women are to enter male occupations (Jacobs, 1989,
45 cited in Williams, 1992). Men have always had a role in nursing (Mackintosh, 1997), and furthermore, Evans (1997) suggests that the small number of men currently in the profession occupy a privileged position compared with their female colleagues. In the UK, 9% of
50 nurses are male, but just over half of the UK's top nursing positions are held by males (Wright et al., 1998). Furthermore, men are three times more likely

---
[*] *Barbara Mullan* is coordinator of health psychology, School of Psychology, The University of Sydney, New South Wales, Australia. *Jon Harrison* is senior lecturer, Child Division, University of Central England, Birmingham, UK.

than women to be found in higher grades in nursing (Whittock et al., 2002).

55   This is supported by other research in the UK, which found that men make up around 35% of managerial grades (Gaze, 2003; Hunt, 1991; Leroy, 1983; Nuttall, 1983; Ratcliffe, 1996). A study by Finlayson and Nazroo (1997) found that despite only making up 7%
60   of the nursing workforce in 1995, men were more than twice as likely as women to be an H or an I grade (senior nursing grades in the UK). Studies have also indicated that men are not only overrepresented in the senior posts, they also achieve promotion more quickly
65   than women at all levels of the nursing hierarchy above the initial grade (Nuttall, 1983; Ratcliffe, 1996). The reasons for this overrepresentation are challenged by Villeneuve (1994) in a Canadian literature review that argues that overrepresentation of men at higher grades
70   is due to more men being full-time staff, and further suggests that, in Canada, any differences are negligible. This is partially supported by research in the UK where only 5% of males in nursing work part time compared with 33% of women (Whittock et al., 2002). However,
75   the reasons given to explain this are very different to those of Villeneuve (1994). Whereas Whittock et al. (2002) argue that research exists that shows the equal commitment of female part-timers, they suggest that managers perceive part-time female staff to be less
80   attached to their careers. Furthermore, Evans (1997) believes that male nurses were seen to bring stability to the nursing profession, which had always been seen to be at the mercy of marriage and motherhood, but that this attitude reflected hidden advantages for men and
85   disadvantages for women. In 1998, for example, 65% of all working mothers with children aged under 5 worked part time compared with only 3% of fathers (Labour Force Survey, 1998). Homans (1989) states that there is clear evidence from National Health Ser-
90   vice (NHS) employees at all levels that women balance their own earnings against the costs of childcare, and it is these calculations that sometimes contribute to women opting for part-time jobs in the NHS. Although part-time work can enable the combination of work and
95   family life for many women, Callender (1996) notes that part-time work often attracts poor conditions of employment and limited opportunities for promotion and career development.

Adams (1994) suggests that the disproportionate
100   number of men occupying key decision-making or managerial positions in the NHS has arisen because generally men do not have to make the same sort of choices as those faced by women; that is, family life versus a career. Studies have shown that marriage or
105   cohabitation can have an effect on the female nurses' career progress. For example, Hardy (1986) and Hutt (1985) found that those women who become senior managers are more likely than men to be single and less likely to have children. A more recent study by the
110   NHS Women's Unit (1995) found evidence similar to

these findings. Another study carried out in the UK by the British Institute of Management (cited in Davidson & Burke, 2000) also found that only 58% of women
115   managers are married compared with 93% of male managers, and of these married men and women, male managers are three times more likely to have children than their female colleagues. Research by Wajcman (1996) reports that many female managers consciously
120   choose to centre their lives on their career and "have clearly decided that childlessness is a precondition for a successful managerial career" (p. 620). In addition, it could be assumed that men tend to reach the higher positions because they are more likely to receive sup-
125   port from their partners and are less likely to have their careers restrained by their spouse or family (Kerswell & Booth, 1995). Specifically in nursing, it has been argued that for male nurses, being married is a significant advantage (Evans, 1997). Studies have consis-
130   tently reported that one of the major reasons for women's slower progress in nursing is the number and length of career breaks taken by women, particularly to have children (Buchan et al., 1989). One of the most recent studies indicated that women were 10 times
135   more likely than men to have taken a career break to care for children (Finlayson & Nazroo, 1997).

Other reasons for the success of men in nursing have been proposed. Hardy (1986) suggests that where men tend to make linear career moves up the nursing hierarchy, lateral movement is more a part of the ca-
140   reers of females and is likely to delay upward mobility for an average of 9.4 years. In addition, Hunt (1991) reported that where both linear and lateral career moves were made, males still progressed more quickly than females. Ratcliffe (1996) suggests that the differ-
145   ence in career movement between males and females is not due to "some kind of inherently female trait, but because the structure of the labour market affects men and women differently" (p. 390). Davidson and Cooper (1992) state that "women are confronted by a glass
150   ceiling when it comes to entering positions of power...this glass ceiling is invisible but women experience it as a very real barrier when they vie for promotion to top jobs" (p. 15). According to Finlayson and Nazroo (1997), however, the glass ceiling is "almost
155   certainly a misnomer, as difficulties for women are present at relatively junior positions, for example in the transition from F to G grade" (p. 84). This is in contrast to what Williams (1992) has called the *glass elevator* for men, where men in female dominated areas feel
160   under pressure to advance from clinical/practice areas into more senior administrative areas, leading to even more disparity between the sexes.

Several studies have indicated the possibility that women may be generally less orientated towards a ca-
165   reer, which includes the prospects of promotion and management. A study by Skevington and Dawkes (1988) found that with the exception of those who were about to retire, all the men in the study expressed a

desire for promotion, compared with 53% of women.
This finding is supported by Winson (2003), who explored the career aspirations of men and women at two points in their career: at qualification (asked about retrospectively) and "now" (in their current position of nurse manager or sister/charge nurse). The findings showed that men were much more likely to have high aspirations on entering nursing than women and to continue the desire to obtain promotion.

It has also been suggested that nursing structures opportunities for men independent of their individual desires or motives (Williams, 1992).

Nonetheless, a study by Davies and Rosser (1986) casts doubt on the notion that women are less career orientated than men. The study found no support at all for the notion that men were career minded and women were not. Similar results were found in the study by Finlayson and Nazroo (1997), which clearly reported that women are just as interested in their careers as men but did not expect to be promoted in the near future.

With the exception of the study by Winson (2003), the majority of research in the field has explored the aspirations and expectations of qualified and experienced nurses, and, indeed, Winson's (2003) study was a retrospective study; therefore, nothing is known about the aspirations and expectations of those just about to embark on their nursing careers. Thus, this study intends to investigate the career intentions and attitudes of male and female individuals who are not qualified nurses, but who are instead applying to train as nurses.

## Hypotheses

$HO_1$

There will be no difference between males and females on the importance they place on the 16 aspects of the nursing role considered.

$HO_2$

There will be no difference between males and females on their expected position in 10 years' time.

$HO_3$

There will be no difference between males and females on their ideal position in 10 years' time.

$HO_4$

There will be no relationship between the ideal and expected positions of respondents.

## Methodology

*Design*

The research tool used was a self-administered questionnaire, which was specifically designed for this particular study. The questionnaires were partly designed on the basis of the literature review but also incorporated an established tool by Finlayson and Nazroo (1997). The questionnaire consisted of 16 closed statements measured on a five-point Likert scale ranging from *very important* to *very unimportant*. There were six questions relating to future ambitions and expectations. To complete the questionnaire, there were three questions on demographics; that is, age, gender and entry qualifications.

*Sample*

A nonprobability convenience method of sampling was used in this study. The conveniently available sample was the people undertaking an interview for the nursing degree course at the selected university in three intake years. In total, 600 questionnaires were distributed and 273 questionnaires were returned, of which 239 (87.5%) were from females and 34 (12.5%) were from males, producing an overall response rate of 45.5%.

*Ethical Considerations*

Ethical approval from the university where the research was undertaken was obtained. Participants were informed that their participation was voluntary, the purpose of the research explained, and confidentiality assured to uphold rights pertaining to informed consent and confidentiality.

*Analysis*

The Statistical Package for Social Sciences (SPSS Version 11.5 for Windows, Chicago, Illinois) was used to carry out descriptive and inferential statistical tests on the data obtained from the questionnaires. Descriptive statistics were used to consider the demographic variables of age, gender and socioeconomic class. SPSS proved the data obtained not to be normally distributed, and therefore the nonparametric statistical tests of the Mann-Whitney $U$-test, chi-squared test, and Spearman's correlation were used.

## Results

Using chi-squared test, there were found to be no significant differences between males and females on socioeconomic background or on age.

The inferential statistical test of Mann-Whitney $U$ was carried out on each factor to see if there was a difference between the male and female nursing applicants. It was found that with the $\alpha$-level set at 0.05, there are two significant differences between the male and female nursing applicants (Table 1). These were status of the job and interesting work.

The majority of respondents expected to remain within clinical practice. A larger percentage of females (19.6%) anticipated taking a career break, compared with only 11.8% of males. However, as can be seen in Table 2, this was not significant. Also, there were no other differences between males and females on where they expect to be working 10 years after graduation.

Spearman rho correlations were performed to consider the relationship between respondents' expected and ideal position in 10 years. The results can be found in Table 3. There was a high positive correlation

Table 1
*Results of the Mann-Whitney U-tests Comparing Male and Female Nursing Applicants' Views About Factors Influencing Their Choice of Nursing As a Career*

| Factor | Z | p |
| --- | --- | --- |
| Helping others | −0.806 | 0.42 |
| A job suiting your talents | −0.201 | 0.84 |
| Opportunities to travel | −0.082 | 0.935 |
| Opportunities to take responsibility | −0.155 | 0.877 |
| Opportunities to supervise | −1.083 | 0.279 |
| Security of employment | −1.342 | 0.180 |
| Prospects of promotion | −1.376 | 0.169 |
| Prospects of further training | −1.129 | 0.259 |
| Starting salary | −1.300 | 0.194 |
| Long-term salary prospects | −0.445 | 0.656 |
| Status of the job | −2.088 | 0.037 |
| Interesting work | −2.569 | 0.010 |
| Rewarding work | −0.066 | 0.947 |
| Family member or friend in nursing | −1.133 | 0.257 |
| Structured career | −0.594 | 0.552 |
| Availability of work | −0.159 | 0.874 |

Table 2
*Career Aspirations of Respondents 10 Years After Their Graduation*

| Occupation 10 years after graduation | Female | Male |
| --- | --- | --- |
| Working in clinical practice | 88.7% ($n = 212$) | 91.2% ($n = 31$) |
| Undertaking research, further education | 38.1% ($n = 91$) | 35.3% ($n = 12$) |
| Working abroad as a nurse | 32.2% ($n = 77$) | 29.4% ($n = 10$) |
| In a non-nursing job | 0.01% ($n = 2$) | 0.0% ($n = 0$) |
| Working in nurse education | 15.1% ($n = 36$) | 17.6% ($n = 6$) |
| Having a career break | 19.6% ($n = 47$) | 11.8% ($n = 4$) |
| Do not know | 11.3% ($n = 27$) | 11.8% ($n = 4$) |

between the expected and ideal jobs of both males and females. Using the Mann-Whitney *U*-test, no differences were found between males and females on their expected or ideal positions.

Table 3
*Spearman Correlations of Ideal and Expected Future Positions*

|  | r | n | p |
| --- | --- | --- | --- |
| Males | 0.800 | 31 | 0.01 |
| Females | 0.612 | 197 | 0.01 |

### Discussion

Two significant differences between male and female nursing applicants with regards to their attitudes toward their careers were found. These were "Status of the job" and "Interesting work." In both instances, females found that these factors were more important to them in choosing nursing as a career than males did.

For the other factors, there were no significant differences between males and females. This therefore implies that male and female nursing students have the same attitudes toward their careers. These findings support those of Davies and Rosser (1986) and Finlayson and Nazroo (1997), who both found that there was no difference in the career orientation of female nurses compared with male nurses. It would therefore be feasible to say that on the basis of this study, it is unlikely that male nursing applicants have any career advantage as a result of their greater orientation to career and work.

It has been suggested that it is the organisational barriers encountered within the NHS and not the individual's own career orientations that may determine the success of each individual's career progression (Goss & Brown, 1991; Callender, 1996; Finlayson & Nazroo, 1997). For example, a number of studies have linked women's slower career progression to the number and length of the career breaks taken by the female nurse (Buchan et al., 1989; Finlayson & Nazroo, 1997). Within this present study, the nursing applicants were asked whether they would have a career break within 10 years of their graduation. It can be seen in the results that a much higher percentage of female respondents compared with male respondents indicated that they would have a career break within 10 years of their graduation (19.6% female, 11.8% male). This finding supports those of Buchan et al. (1989) and Finlayson and Nazroo (1997) who found that women were considerably more likely than men to have taken a career break and were also more likely to have taken a longer break. This study has found that there is no significant

15

difference between male and female nursing applicants' attitudes towards their careers, and it has in fact been identified that in some respects, the female respondents are more likely than males to identify the importance of promotional and management opportunities. Assuming that both the male and female respondents complete the degree, they will both have the same nursing qualifications, and, therefore, the only major difference between the two groups within this study is that the female respondents are more likely to take a break in their careers within 10 years of graduation than the male respondents. The questionnaire used in the present study did not ask the respondent whether the career break would be specifically to care for children, but previous studies have indicated that it is more than likely that career breaks are taken for family reasons (Goss & Brown, 1991; Finlayson & Nazroo, 1997). The influence of families has been found to affect the progress of males and females in different ways. It has been found that taking a career break to have and care for a child is often associated with downward occupational mobility, especially amongst women who return to part-time work (Corby, 1991). The current career structures within the NHS are largely unsupportive of the high proportion of individuals who are often unable or sometimes unwilling to work full time. This group of individuals is predominately made up of women, many of whom have family responsibilities. It can therefore be stated that taking a career break to have children and working part time are likely to have great implications for the career progression of women.

In the present study, there were no differences between men and women in the level they expected to have attained 10 years into their career. This contrasts with Skevington and Dawkes (1988) and Winson (2003), who looked specifically at the respondents' desire for promotion and found that a higher proportion of male nurses expressed a desire for promotion. This was supported by Finlayson and Nazroo (1997), who also found that men were more likely than women to have reported that promotion was very important to them when making their decision to do nursing. However, they did find that women did not expect to be promoted in the near future. Hardy (1986) suggested that where differences in career orientations between men and women were identified, this could be a result of their evaluation of both the likelihood and costs of success. One possible explanation may be that having spent time within a health care system, it is feasible that female nurses begin to perceive limited promotional opportunities because they have observed that women are not well represented at senior management levels. It is also possible that personal issues, such as family responsibilities, may also lead to the female nurse having concerns about undertaking the responsibilities and time demands associated with promotion and management, and this, too, may influence her per-

ceptions about future career opportunities. There is some research that suggests that the majority of men also "doubt their efficacy to handle competently the combined demands of job and parenthood" (Bandura, 1997, p. 193). "However, men do not often have to make the decision between career success and family responsibilities, as it is still regarded as acceptable within society for men to escape the difficulties of juggling multiple roles with minimal involvement in housework and childcare" (Bandura, 1997).

Although many previous studies have concentrated on the differences between male and female nurses, this study has actually found that before becoming a registered nurse, it, in fact, seems that there are instead more similarities than differences between potential male and female nurses. The reasons why female nurses are progressing more slowly than their male counterparts may not, as previous studies have concluded, be the result of a difference in attitude towards their careers. The differences in career progression may instead be due to the female's anticipation of disadvantage once they start their work within the NHS, perhaps as a result of the barriers relating to their greater family responsibilities.

The findings of this study therefore suggest that it is not the differences in male and female orientations towards their careers that determine their career progression, but it is instead the organisational barriers encountered within the NHS that are slowing the career progression of female nurses once they become registered. This suggestion is substantiated by past studies such as Goss and Brown (1991) and Finlayson and Nazroo (1997), which have also identified the impact that organisational barriers have on female nurses' careers. The overall findings can be seen to be positive in that the explanations for female nurses' career progression are unlikely to be related to female nurses' lack of career orientation. Instead, the explanations for the slower career progression of females is more likely to be related to the organisational barriers found within the NHS, and it is hoped that these barriers will eventually be eliminated so as to allow gender equality within all positions of the nursing hierarchy. The overall strength of this study has been in emphasising the problems that women face when trying to progress in their careers. The main limitations of the study relate to sampling. Although nonprobability sampling "is less likely than probability sampling to produce accurate and representative samples" (Polit & Hungler, 1999, p. 281), constraints on resources meant that this particular sampling method was the most feasible for this particular study. The number of male respondents is small and may have impacted on the nonsignificance of results. However, these small numbers are representative of both the number of males within nursing and the proportion registered on the programmes in question. Therefore, the results may be more representative than they first appear.

## Conclusion

In general, male and female applicants shared the same goals and aspirations for their future nursing careers. It may be that as female nursing applicants are younger than their qualified counterparts, they have different aspirations, having been born after "women's lib." A more likely explanation lies within the culture of the NHS and needs to be researched further.

## Key Points

The main recommendation therefore is that the NHS should ensure that they take action to reduce and eliminate these barriers (which are causing so many problems for the registered female nurse). To overcome these barriers to women, it is of vital importance that there is an understanding of the ways in which organisational culture impacts on different individual's abilities to contribute in the workplace. Despite the fact that the number of women in paid employment is continuing to rise, many workplaces such as the NHS have not altered their expectations of employees or provided work policies to allow women, and indeed men who choose to share dependent care, to balance work and family responsibilities. For example, the availability of childcare facilities within the NHS remains very poor (Finlayson & Nazroo, 1997) despite the fact that the number of women with children participating in the paid workforce has increased markedly over the recent decades (Equal Opportunities Commission, 1999). This lack of childcare facilities within the NHS is perhaps one of the greatest barriers to women's progression in their careers, and it is therefore recommended that this is one of the greatest areas in need of reform. Other areas that need to be urgently addressed by the NHS relate to the need for increased flexible work practices and also increased part-time work in all nursing specialties and grades within the NHS.

## References

Adams, J (1994) Opportunity 2000. *Nurs Times* **90**: 31–32.

Bandura, A (1997) Self-efficacy: The Exercise of Control. New York: W.H. Freeman.

Buchan, J, Waite, R, Thomas, J (1989) Grade Expectations: Clinical Grading and Nurse Mobility: A Study for the Royal College of Nursing. Brighton, Sussex. Institute of Manpower Studies, University of Sussex.

Callender, C (1996) Women and employment. In: Hallett, C (ed), Women and Social Policy: An Introduction. London: Prentice Hall/Harvester Wheatsheaf.

Corby, S (1991) When two halves make total sense. *Health Service Journal* **101**: 20–21.

Davidson, MJ, Burke, RJ (2000) Women in Management. London: Sage.

Davidson, MJ, Cooper, CL (1992) Shattering the Glass Ceiling: The Woman Manager. London: P.Chapman.

Davies, C, Rosser, J (1986) Processes of Discrimination: A Report on a Study of Women Working in the NHS. London: DHSS.

Evans, J (1997) Men in nursing: Issues of gender segregation and hidden advantage. *J Adv Nurs* **26**: 226–231.

Finlayson, LR, Nazroo, JY (1997) Gender Inequalities in Nursing Careers. London: Policy Studies Institute.

Gaze, H (2003) Man appeal. *Nurs Times* **83**: 24–27.

Goss, S, Brown, H (1991) Equal opportunities for women in the NHS. London: HMSO.

Hardy, L (1986) Career politics: The case of career histories of selected leading male and female nurses in England and Scotland. In: White, R (ed), Political Issues in Nursing: Past, Present and Future. Chichester: Wiley.

Homans, H (1989) Women in the National Health Service: Report of a Case Study into Equal Opportunities in Clinical Chemistry Laboratories. London: HMSO.

Hunt, M (1991) Who flies highest. *Nurs Times* **87**: 29–30.

Hutt, R (1985) Chief Officer Career Profiles: A Study of the Backgrounds, Training and Career Experiences of Regional and District Nursing Officers. Brighton: Institute of Manpower Studies.

Kerswell, J, Booth, J ( 1995) New degree of prejudice. *Nurs Stand* **9**: 46.

Kleinman, CS (2004) Understanding and capitalizing on men's advantages in nursing. *J Nurs Adm* **34**: 78–82.

Labour Force Survey (1998) Labour Force Survey. London: Office for National Statistics.

Leroy, L (1983) Continuity and change: power and gender in nursing. *J Prof Nurs* **2**: 28–36.

Mackintosh, C (1997) A historical study of men in nursing. *J Adv Nurs* **26**: 232–236.

Meadus, RJ (2000) Men in nursing: barriers to recruitment. *Nurs Forum* **35**: 5–12.

NHS Women's Unit (1995) Creative Career Paths in the NHS London: Department of Health.

Nuttall, P (1983) Male takeover or female giveaway. *Nurs Times* **79**: 10–11.

Poliafico, JK (1998) Nursing's gender gap. *RN* **61**: 39–42.

Ratcliffe, P (1996) Gender differences in career progress in nursing: towards a nonessential structural theory. *J Adv Nurs* **23**: 389–395.

Skevington, S, Dawkes, D (1988) Fred Nightingale. *Nurs Times* **84**: 49–51.

Sochalski, J (2002) Trends: nursing shortage redux: turning the corner on an enduring problem: enhanced career ladders, better wages, flexible hours, and a more satisfying workplace would aid in retaining RNs in the nursing workforce. *Health Aff* **21**: 157–163.

Trossman, S (2003) Caring knows no gender: break the stereotype and boost the number of men in nursing. *Nev Rnformation* **12**: 19.

Villeneuve, MJ (1994) Recruiting and retaining men in nursing: a review of the literature. *J Prof Nurs* **10**: 217–228.

Wajcman, J (1996) The domestic basis for a managerial career. *Sociol Rev* **44**: 609–629.

Whittock, M, Edwards, C, McLaren, S. Robinson, O (2002) "The tender trap": Gender, part-time nursing and the effects of "family-friendly" policies on career advancement. *Sociol Health Illn* **24**: 305–326.

Whittock, M, Leonard, L (2003) Stepping outside the stereotype. A pilot study of the motivations and experiences of males in the nursing profession. *J Nurs Manag* **11**: 242–249.

Williams, CL (1992) The glass escalator: hidden advantages for men in the "female" professions. *Soc Probl* **39**: 253–267.

Winson, G (2003) A study of nurse career paths. *Sr Nurse* **12**: 11–19.

Wright, CM, Frew, TJ, Hatcher, D (1998) Social and demographic characteristics of young and mature aged nursing students in Australian Universities. *Nurse Educ Today* **18**: 101–107.

**About the authors**: After completing her undergraduate and master's degrees, *Barbara Mullan* (BA [Hons], MA, PGCE, PhD) worked in the hospitality industry for three years, then completed her PhD in Health Psychology with the Open University while employed as a research assistant in UWIC. Between 1997 and 2005, she was employed by the School of Health Sciences, University of Birmingham, as a lecturer in Health Psychology. Barbara's research during this time included work in aggression and violence, sex education, stereotypes and collaborative work with occupational therapists, nurses, physiotherapists and other psychologists. She moved to the University of Sydney in 2005, where she had responsibility for writing the new Masters in health psychology, which started in March 2007, and she is the coordinator of this program. Email: Barbara@ psych.usyd.edu.au. *Jon Harrison* (RN [child], B Nurs [Hons], PGCert Ed) qualified as a children's nurse at the University of Birmingham, in 2001. He then worked at City Hospital, Birmingham for five years within different paediatric units, including neonatal intensive care, general medicine and A and E. During his final year at City Hospital, he worked as a clinical teacher for the Trust's Practice Development Team. His interest in nurse education brought him to the Faculty of Health at the University of Central England, Birmingham. Jon's main responsibilities as a senior lecturer within the Child Health Division involve the coordination of the "Care of the Acutely Ill Child and Young Person in Hospital" module. He is also seconded by the faculty to coordinate the content design and administration of the faculty's Virtual Learning Environment, Moodle. Email: Jon.Harrison@uce.ac.uk

## Appendix

**Questionnaires**

How important to you were each of the following in choosing to apply for a career in nursing?

| | Very important | Fairly important | Neither | Fairly unimportant | Very unimportant |
|---|---|---|---|---|---|
| 1. Helping others | ☐ | ☐ | ☐ | ☐ | ☐ |
| 2. A job suiting your talents | ☐ | ☐ | ☐ | ☐ | ☐ |
| 3. Opportunities to travel | ☐ | ☐ | ☐ | ☐ | ☐ |
| 4. Opportunities to take responsibility | ☐ | ☐ | ☐ | ☐ | ☐ |
| 5. Opportunities to supervise | ☐ | ☐ | ☐ | ☐ | ☐ |
| 6. Security of employment | ☐ | ☐ | ☐ | ☐ | ☐ |
| 7. Prospects of promotion | ☐ | ☐ | ☐ | ☐ | ☐ |
| 8. Prospects of further training | ☐ | ☐ | ☐ | ☐ | ☐ |
| 9. Starting salary | ☐ | ☐ | ☐ | ☐ | ☐ |
| 10. Long-term salary prospects | ☐ | ☐ | ☐ | ☐ | ☐ |
| 11. Status of the job | ☐ | ☐ | ☐ | ☐ | ☐ |
| 12. Interesting work | ☐ | ☐ | ☐ | ☐ | ☐ |
| 13. Rewarding work | ☐ | ☐ | ☐ | ☐ | ☐ |
| 14. Family member or friend in nursing | ☐ | ☐ | ☐ | ☐ | ☐ |
| 15. Structured career | ☐ | ☐ | ☐ | ☐ | ☐ |
| 16. Availability of work | ☐ | ☐ | ☐ | ☐ | ☐ |

17. Other reasons (please specify)

_____

_____

_____

_____

What do you expect to be doing 10 years from now? If still in nursing, what grade or type of nurse would you expect to be? What grade or type of nurse would you ideally like to be?

(Here is the nursing structure and pay scale used by the NHS. Using this as a guide, please tick one "expected" and one "ideal" box below.)

| Grade | Explanation | Pay scale |
|---|---|---|
| D | New staff nurse | £17,060–£18,830 |
| E | More experienced staff nurse | £18,320–£22,015 |
| F | Junior sister/charge nurse | £20,220–£26,180 |
| G | Senior sister/charge nurse | £23,860–£29,035 |
| H | Senior nurse managing other grades | £26,650–£31,960 |
| I | Clinical specialist (may not be ward based) | £29,515–£34,920 |

| Nursing grade | Expected | Ideal |
|---|---|---|
| D | | |
| E | | |
| F | | |
| G | | |
| H | | |
| I | | |
| Nurse specialist | | |
| Nurse educator | | |
| Nurse practitioner | | |
| Other (please specify) _____ | | |

| In 10 years I will be.... (Please tick either yes or no) | Yes | No |
|---|---|---|
| Working in clinical practice | ☐ | ☐ |
| Undertaking research/further education | ☐ | ☐ |
| Working abroad as a nurse | ☐ | ☐ |
| In a non-nursing job | ☐ | ☐ |
| Having a career break (e.g., for family reasons) | ☐ | ☐ |
| Working in nurse education | ☐ | ☐ |
| Don't know | ☐ | ☐ |

Please Tick

Age: ☐

| Gender | Male | Female |
|---|---|---|
|  |  |  |

How would you define your social class?

| | Social class | Occupation or head of household | |
|---|---|---|---|
| A | Upper middle class | Higher managerial, administrative or professional | ☐ |
| B | Middle class | Intermediate managerial, administrative or professional | ☐ |
| C1 | Lower middle class | Supervisor or clerical and junior | ☐ |
| C2 | Skilled working class | Skilled manual workers | ☐ |
| D | Working class | Semi- and unskilled manual workers | ☐ |
| E | Those at the lowest levels of subsistence | State pensioners, etc. with no other earnings | ☐ |
| | | | ☐ |

# Exercise for Article 3

## Factual Questions

1. What is the third hypothesis?

2. The researchers used Likert scale with how many points?

3. Of the 600 questionnaires that were distributed, how many were returned?

4. What was the overall response rate?

5. Was there a significant difference between males and females on socioeconomic background?

6. Was the difference between males and females on the factor of "interesting work" statistically significant? If yes, at what probability level?

## Questions for Discussion

7. Do you think the topic of research is important to the profession of nursing? Explain.

8. Do you think the "research tool" used in this study is described in sufficient detail? (See lines 215–226.)

9. Is using a nonprobability convenience method of sampling ideal? Explain. (See lines 227–231 and 419–425.)

10. In your opinion, is the material on ethical considerations important? Explain. (See lines 236–241.)

11. Do you agree with the researchers that the small number of male respondents is a limitation of this study? Why? Why not? (See lines 419–431.)

12. If you were to conduct a study on the same topic, what changes in the research methodology, if any, would you make?

## Quality Ratings

Directions: Indicate your level of agreement with each of the following statements by circling a number from 5 for strongly agree (SA) to 1 for strongly disagree (SD). If you believe an item is not applicable to this research article, leave it blank. Be prepared to explain your ratings. When responding to criteria A and B, keep in mind that brief titles and abstracts are conventional in published research.

A.  The title of the article is appropriate.

    SA   5   4   3   2   1   SD

B.  The abstract provides an effective overview of the research article.

    SA   5   4   3   2   1   SD

C.  The introduction establishes the importance of the study.

    SA   5   4   3   2   1   SD

D.  The literature review establishes the context for the study.

    SA   5   4   3   2   1   SD

E.  The research purpose, question, or hypothesis is clearly stated.

    SA   5   4   3   2   1   SD

F.  The method of sampling is sound.

    SA   5   4   3   2   1   SD

G.  Relevant demographics (for example, age, gender, and ethnicity) are described.

    SA   5   4   3   2   1   SD

H.  Measurement procedures are adequate.

    SA   5   4   3   2   1   SD

I.  All procedures have been described in sufficient detail to permit a replication of the study.

    SA   5   4   3   2   1   SD

J.  The participants have been adequately protected from potential harm.

    SA   5   4   3   2   1   SD

K.  The results are clearly described.

    SA   5   4   3   2   1   SD

L.  The discussion/conclusion is appropriate.

    SA   5   4   3   2   1   SD

M.  Despite any flaws, the report is worthy of publication.

    SA   5   4   3   2   1   SD

# Article 4

# Physical Activity Barriers and Program Preferences Among Indigent Internal Medicine Patients With Arthritis

**Hammad A. Bajwa**, MD, **Laura Q. Rogers**, MD, MPH[*]

ABSTRACT. The study purpose was to determine, among indigent arthritis patients, physical activity barriers, program preference frequencies, and demographic associations. A structured interview of 223 indigent, internal medicine clinic patients with self-reported arthritis was administered in a cross-sectional study design. The two most frequently reported barriers included bad health (52%) and pain (51%). The majority preferred to exercise alone (54%), close to home (76%), and in the early morning/evening (83%). The preferred method of receiving exercise information was by video- or audiotape. Frequency of reported barriers was significantly associated with age, ethnicity, and gender; specific program preferences were significantly associated with age and gender only. Exercise programs for indigent patients with arthritis should be home-based with flexible scheduling. Educational material should include both video- and audiotape formats. Future interventions should consider barriers related to poor health and pain while remaining responsive to age, gender, and ethnic differences. Nurses can play a pivotal role in such interventions.

From *Rehabilitation Nursing, 32*, 31–34. Copyright © 2007 by the Association of Rehabilitation Nurses. Reprinted with permission.

Exercise reduces pain (Ettinger et al., 1997; Fransen, McConnell, & Bell, 2003; Kovar et al., 1992; O'Reilly, Muir, & Doherty, 1999; Petrella, 2000; Rejeski, Ettinger, Martin, & Morgan, 1998; Smidt et al., 2005) and disability (Ettinger et al.; Rejeski et al.; O'Reilly et al.; Penninx et al., 2001; Roddy, Zhang, & Doherty, 2005) among patients with arthritis, which is the major cause of disability in the United States (Centers for Disease Control and Prevention, 2001, 2006). Patients with arthritis are less active (Hirata et al., 2006; Hootman, Marcera, Ham, Helmick, & Sniezek, 2003; Shih, Hootman, Kruger, & Helmick, 2006) and enhancing physical activity requires providers to understand the barriers and program preferences reported by this population. Only two studies have evaluated such barriers, and none has evaluated program preferences (Fontaine & Haaz, 2006; Neuberger, Kasal, Smith, Hassanein, & Deviney, 1994). Such information is needed to facilitate the efforts of rehabilitation health professionals to enhance the activity level of patients with arthritis. The study aims were to determine (1) physical activity barriers and program preferences among indigent internal medicine clinic patients with arthritis and (2) the influence of gender, age, and ethnicity on barriers and program preferences.

## Materials and Methods

Adult patients in an academic internal medicine clinic participated in a cross-sectional study. Non-English speaking, acutely ill, demented, or psychotic patients were excluded. Overall response rate was 393 out of 444 (88.5%). Of these, 223 had a self-reported diagnosis of arthritis; results from these 223 patients are reported.

A pilot-tested structured interview was administered by trained research staff. The study was approved by the local institutional review board and informed consent was obtained prior to data collection. Patients were asked how often 18 barriers interfered with exercise (5-point Likert-type scale, 1 = *never* to 5 = *very often*). Program preferences measurement utilized yes/no and multiple-choice questions. Body mass index (BMI) was calculated from self-reported height and weight.

Chi-square and Fisher's exact test were used to test gender and ethnicity differences for barriers and program preferences; age differences were examined with independent $t$ tests and ANOVA. Spearman's correlation was used to test the association between age and each barrier. Likert-scale items were dichotomized (*infrequent* = 1, 2, 3; *frequent* = 4, 5) for descriptive analyses. All Likert-scale categories were used for Spearman's correlations.

## Results

A majority of patients were Caucasian women with fewer than 12 years of education and annual income of

---

[*]*Hammad A. Bajwa* is a rheumatology fellow at the University of Minnesota. *Laura Q. Rogers* is associate professor of medicine at SIU Department of Medicine.

under $20,000 (see Table 1). Patients were older (mean = 53 ± 9.1) and obese (mean BMI = 32 ± 7.7); the majority (78%) perceived their health as fair or poor. Payer status information was available on 125 (56%) of participants. Seventy-five (60%) were self-pay, with 46 (37%) being Medicaid/Medicare and 4 (3%) being other.

Table 1
*Demographic Characteristics of Respondents*

| Characteristic | n (%) |
|---|---|
| Gender | |
| Men | 55 (25) |
| Women | 168 (75) |
| Ethnic group | |
| Caucasian | 146 (65) |
| African American | 77 (35) |
| Level of education | |
| Less than 12 years | 148 (66) |
| 12 years | 56 (25) |
| 13 or more years | 19 (9) |
| Yearly income level | |
| Under $5,000 | 42 (19) |
| $5,000–$9,999 | 97 (44) |
| $10,000–$14,999 | 40 (18) |
| $15,000–$19,999 | 22 (10) |
| Over $20,000 | 10 (4) |
| Missing | 12 (5) |
| Patient perception of health | |
| Excellent | 4 (2) |
| Very good | 12 (5) |
| Good | 33 (15) |
| Fair | 79 (35) |
| Poor | 95 (43) |

*Note.* Mean age = 53 (Range = 24–73, Standard deviation = 9.1)
Mean body mass index = 32 (Range = 16–55, Standard deviation = 7.7)

The most frequently reported barriers included bad health, pain, discouragement, fear of injury, lack of discipline, lack of interest, lack of equipment, and lack of time (Figure 1). Barriers that interfered with exercise in fewer than 10% of respondents included cost, lack of enjoyment, weather, knowledge, lack of company, lack of facilities, lack of transportation, embarrassment, lack of skill, and lack of family support.

Discouragement interfered with exercise more in women than men (19% versus 7%, $p = .039$). When compared with African American patients, Caucasians more frequently reported lack of discipline (32% versus 9%, $p < .001$), time (16% versus 7%, $p = .036$), and fear of injury (17% versus 7%, $p = .027$). Age was negatively correlated with embarrassment ($r = -0.24$, $p < .001$), lack of time ($r = -0.16$, $p = .015$), discouragement ($r = -0.20$, $p = .004$), lack of equipment ($r = -0.15$, $p = .022$), transportation ($r = -0.19$, $p = .004$), pain ($r = -0.18$, $p = .009$), and fear of injury ($r = -0.18$, $p = .007$).

Exercising alone was preferred (54%) and 29% wished to exercise with a family member (Table 2). Only 24% preferred to exercise away from home, and 83% preferred to exercise in the early morning/evening. Almost half of respondents (43%) pre-

ferred to receive exercise information via videotape or audiotape, with 29% preferring written materials or information from another source (class or friend). The four most popular group exercise components included good music, fun exercises, convenient scheduling, and an enthusiastic leader.

Table 2
*Exercise Program Preferences Among Indigent Arthritis Patients*

| Program aspects | n (%) |
|---|---|
| Where would you like to exercise? | |
| Outdoors in neighborhood | 84 (38) |
| Inside apartment or home | 82 (37) |
| Away from home (e.g., community center, work, health spa, YMCA) | 53 (24) |
| When would you like to exercise? | |
| Early morning | 101 (48) |
| During the day | 36 (17) |
| Early evening | 73 (35) |
| With whom would you like to exercise? | |
| By myself | 121 (54) |
| Family member | 65 (29) |
| Another person (e.g., co-worker, friend, exercise class) | 37 (17) |
| How would you like to receive information on how to exercise? | |
| Written (e.g., mail, brochure, book) | 62 (28) |
| Video or audiotape | 96 (43) |
| Other (e.g., class or lecture at recreation center, friend) | 64 (29) |
| Elements that a group exercise program needed to make you want to attend?* | |
| Good music | 156 (85) |
| Fun exercises | 190 (85) |
| Classes at convenient time | 187 (84) |
| Enthusiastic leader | 184 (83) |
| Mats or carpets on the floor | 170 (76) |
| Neighborhood leader | 96 (43) |
| Information on diet or weight control | 166 (74) |
| Videotaped leader | 91 (41) |
| Hard exercise | 69 (31) |

*Participants were asked to check "all that apply"; therefore, some percentages add up to greater than 100%.

More women than men preferred good music (75% versus 57%, $p = 0.01$), fun exercises (89% versus 76%, $p = .012$), mats/carpets (82% versus 62%, $p = .004$), and videotaped leader (45% versus 28%, $p = .029$). No ethnic differences existed in program preferences. Patients preferring exercise in early morning were older than those preferring early evening (mean age 55 versus 50, $p = .001$). Older patients also preferred exercising outdoors near their home (mean age = 55) compared with those preferring their home or another site (mean age = 51; $p = .017$ and 0.047, respectively). Younger patients preferred fun exercises and convenient scheduling (mean age 52 versus 57 for both; $p = .003$ and .005, respectively).

## Discussion

Bad health and pain were major barriers to exercise among indigent internal medicine patients with arthritis. The majority preferred to exercise alone or with a

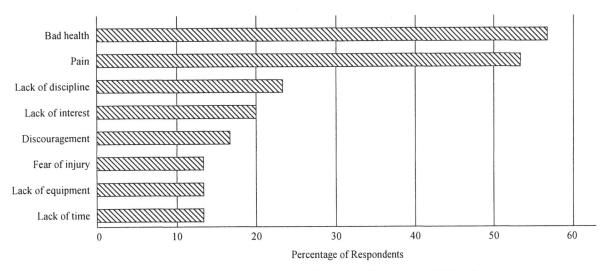

*Figure 1.* Most frequent reported barriers to physical activity among arthritis patients.

family member, close to home, and in the early morning/evening. The preferred method for information dissemination was video- or audiotape. Preferred group exercise components included good music, fun exercises, convenient scheduling, and an enthusiastic leader. Several barriers were significantly associated with age, ethnicity, and gender; and specific program preferences were associated with age and gender only.

Neuberger et al. (1994) studied 100 primarily Caucasian adult outpatients (nonindigent, mean age = 53) with rheumatoid or osteoarthritis, able to undergo bicycle ergometer testing. Major barriers included "exercise was tiring" (57%), "exercise was hard work" (40%), lack of time (33%), inaccessibility to exercise facilities (27%), inconvenient facility schedules (25%), and lack of encouragement by family/friends (25%). Unlike our study, pain and age did not influence barriers, possibly because Neuberger et al. studied a healthier subject population. Consistent with our results, Fontaine and Haaz (2006) reported that joint pain and poor health were associated with reduced levels of physical activity. Ethnicity and gender differences were not examined in either study, and no prior study has evaluated program preferences in patients with arthritis.

Ethnicity influences studied by Masse and Anderson (2003) found that African American women in the lower income group perceived more barriers to physical activity than African American women in the higher income group. A similar difference was not seen for Hispanic women. Differences in specific barriers were not examined. Dergance and colleagues (2003) surveyed elderly Mexican American and European Americans with or without arthritis about physical activity barriers. Mexican Americans reported lack of time as a barrier, and, similar to our findings, European Americans reported lack of discipline. Unlike our results, no ethnic differences existed in fear of injury. Prevalent barriers were similar to those reported by our participants with the exception of pain, which may be due to differences in the study population (i.e., community dwelling rather than clinic based).

Although the use of self-reported diagnosis of arthritis (as opposed to physician and/or radiographic diagnosis) is a possible study limitation, the measure is most likely to have identified patients with clinically symptomatic arthritis (and, hence, clinically significant disease). Sampling for our study was clinic based (not population based), possibly reducing the generalizability of our study results and explaining the frequent reporting of bad health as a barrier. Study strengths include an adequate sample size for evaluating age, gender, and ethnic differences. Also, our study is unique in its focus on an indigent population with minority representation and its examination of specific physical activity barriers and program preferences among arthritis patients.

Future exercise interventions for indigent patients with arthritis should be home based (especially for older patients) with flexible scheduling (allowing differences in age preferences). Educational materials should include video- and audiotape formats. Traditional behavior modification techniques should be included to address barriers such as lack of discipline and discouragement. Furthermore, interventions should consider barriers related to poor health and pain while remaining responsive to age, gender, and ethnic differences in physical activity barriers and program preferences.

## Conclusions

Patients with arthritis are aware of the importance of exercise but lack the necessary information for initiating and maintaining an exercise program (Rosemann et al., 2006). Much-needed exercise interventions in the clinical setting for chronic disease patients such as those with arthritis could be optimized by collaboration between physicians and rehabilitation nurses. Lack of time is the most prevalent physical activity counseling barrier reported by physicians (Walsh, Swangard,

David, & McPhee, 1999). Although it is important for the physician to write a prescription for exercise type, intensity, and duration based on the presence of arthritis and other co-existing and limiting chronic diseases, nurses can play a critical role in assisting the patients with implementing these prescriptions. Nursing professionals can design or adapt available patient educational materials related to exercise, apply basic behavioral modification techniques, and use a self-management approach to helping patients exercise regularly (Blixen, Branstedt, Hammel, & Tilley, 2004; Kinion, Christie, & Villella, 1993; Tulloch, Fortier, & Hogg, in press). They can provide the majority of education and behavior reinforcement through initial and follow-up counseling sessions. They can address barriers to physical activity, discuss relapse prevention, and collaborate with the physician to provide optimal exercise counseling with minimal physician time commitment. Nursing interventions reduce time demands on physicians, yet provide individualized care necessary for physical activity maintenance.

With increasing evidence supporting the benefit of exercise for patients with arthritis, nursing professionals can take a lead role in exercise counseling in an effort to improve quality of healthcare delivery for patients with arthritis. Because of the pivotal role that nurses play in patient care and their clinical knowledge and experience, they are particularly well-suited for helping patients address the health-related barriers reported in our study. The complementary nature of the nurse and physician clinical roles could be used as an opportunity to help patients with arthritis become more active and, in so doing, potentially improve their quality of life.

### References

Blixen, C. E., Branstedt, K. A., Hammel, J. P., & Tilley, B. C. (2004). A pilot study of health education via a nurse-run telephone self-management programme for elderly people with osteoarthritis. *Journal of Telemedicine and Telecare, 10,* 44–49.

Centers for Disease Control and Prevention. (2001). Prevalence of disabilities and associated health conditions among adults: United States, 1999. *Morbidity and Mortality Weekly Report, 50,* 120–125.

Centers for Disease Control and Prevention. (2006). State prevalence of self-reported doctor-diagnosed arthritis and arthritis-attributable activity limitation—United States, 2003. *Morbidity and Mortality Weekly Report, 55,* 477–481.

Dergance, J. M., Calmbach, W. L., Dhanda, R., Miles, T. P., Hazuda, H. P., & Mouton, C. P. (2003). Barriers to and benefits of leisure time physical activity in the elderly: Differences across cultures. *Journal of the American Geriatric Society, 51,* 863–868.

Ettinger, W. H. Jr., Bums, R., Messier, S. P., Applegate, W., Rejeski, W. J., Morgan, T. et al. (1997). A randomized trial comparing aerobic exercise and resistance exercise with a health education program in older adults with knee osteoarthritis. *Journal of the American Medical Association, 277,* 25–31.

Fontaine, K. R., & Haaz, S. (2006). Risk factors for lack of recent exercise in adults with self-reported, professionally diagnosed arthritis. *Journal of Clinical Rheumatology, 12,* 66–69.

Fransen, M., McConnell, S., & Bell, M. (2003). Exercise for osteoarthritis of the hip or knee. *Cochrane Database Systems Review, 3,* CD004286.

Hirata, S., Ono, R., Yamada, M., Takikawa, S., Nishiyama, T., Hasuda, K. et al. (2006). Ambulatory physical activity, disease severity, and employment status in adult women with osteoarthritis of the hip. *Journal of Rheumatology, 33,* 939–945.

Hootman, J. M., Marcera, C. A., Ham, S. A., Helmick, C. G., & Sniezek, J. E. (2003). Physical activity levels among the general US adult population and in adults with and without arthritis. *Arthritis Care and Research, 49,* 129–135.

Kinion, E. S., Christie, N., & Villella, A M. (1993). Promoting activity in the elderly through interdisciplinary linkages. *Nursing Connections, 6,* 19–26.

Kovar, P., Allegrante, J., Mackenzie, C., Peterson, M. G., Gutin, B., & Charlson, M.E. (1992). Supervised fitness walking in patients with osteoarthritis of the knee—a randomized, controlled trial. *Annals of Internal Medicine, 116,* 529–534.

Masse, L. C., & Anderson, C. B. (2003). Ethnic differences among correlates of physical activity in women. *American Journal of Health Promotion, 17,* 357–360.

Neuberger, G. B., Kasal, S., Smith, K. V., Hassanein, R., & Deviney, S. (1994). Determinants of exercise and aerobic fitness in outpatients with arthritis. *Nursing Research, 43,* 11–17.

O'Reilly, S., Muir, K., & Doherty, M. (1999). Effectiveness of home exercise on pain and disability from osteoarthritis of the knee: A randomized controlled trial. *Annals of Rheumatic Diseases, 58,* 15–19.

Penninx, B. W., Messier, S. P., Rejeski, J., Williamson, J. D., DiBari, M., Cavazzini, C., et al. (2001). Physical exercise and the prevention of disability in activities of daily living in older persons with osteoarthritis. *Archives of Internal Medicine, 161,* 2309–2316.

Petrella, R. J. (2000). Is exercise effective treatment for osteoarthritis of the knee? *British Journal of Sports Medicine, 34,* 326–331.

Rejeski, W. J., Ettinger, W. H. Jr., Martin, K., & Morgan, T. (1998). Treating disability in knee osteoarthritis with exercise therapy: A central role for self-efficacy and pain. *Arthritis Care and Research, 11,* 94–101.

Roddy, E., Zhang, W., & Doherty, M. (2005). Aerobic walking or strengthening exercise for osteoarthritis of the knee? A systematic review. *Annals of Rheumatic Disease, 64,* 544–548.

Shih, M., Hootman, J. M., Kruger, J., & Helmick, C. G. (2006). Physical activity in men and women with arthritis, National Health Interview Survey, 2002. *American Journal of Preventive Medicine, 30,* 385–393.

Smidt, N., de Vet, H. C., Bouter, L. M., Dekker, J., Arendzen, J. H., De Bie, R. A., et al. (2005). Effectiveness of exercise therapy: A best-evidence summary of systematic reviews. *Australian Journal of Physiotherapy, 51,* 195.

Tulloch, H., Fortier, M., & Hogg, W. (in press). Physical activity counseling in primary care: Who has and who should be counseling? *Patient Education and Counseling.*

Walsh, J. M., Swangard, D. M., David, T., & McPhee, S. J. (1999). Exercise counseling by primary care physicians in the era of managed care. *American Journal of Preventive Medicine, 16,* 307–313.

**Acknowledgment**: This work was supported by Georgia Affiliate American Heart Association Grant-in-aid.

**Address correspondence to**: Laura Q. Rogers, SIU School of Medicine, Department of Medicine, P.O. Box 19636, Springfield, IL 62794-9636.

# Exercise for Article 4

## *Factual Questions*

1. What four types of patients were excluded from this study?

2. What percentage of the participants were women?

3. "Cost" was cited as a barrier to exercise by what percentage of the participants?

4. What is the value of the correlation coefficient for the relationship between age and embarrassment?

5. Did women *or* men prefer good music? What probability is associated with this difference?

6. The researchers mention two "study strengths." What is the first one they mention?

## Questions for Discussion

7. Is the response rate adequate? Explain. (See lines 29–30.)

8. Is it important to know that informed consent was obtained? Explain. (See lines 34–36.)

9. If you had conducted this study, would you have used self-reported height and weight? Explain. (See lines 40–42.)

10. All the correlation coefficients in lines 74–80 have negative signs. What is your understanding of the meaning of a negative correlation?

11. Do you agree with the researchers that the use of self-reported diagnosis of arthritis is a possible study limitation? Explain. (See lines 150–155.)

12. Do you think that this study has important implications for nursing professionals? (See lines 191–215.)

## Quality Ratings

Directions: Indicate your level of agreement with each of the following statements by circling a number from 5 for strongly agree (SA) to 1 for strongly disagree (SD). If you believe an item is not applicable to this research article, leave it blank. Be prepared to explain your ratings. When responding to criteria A and B, keep in mind that brief titles and abstracts are conventional in published research.

A.  The title of the article is appropriate.

    SA   5   4   3   2   1   SD

B.  The abstract provides an effective overview of the research article.

    SA   5   4   3   2   1   SD

C.  The introduction establishes the importance of the study.

    SA   5   4   3   2   1   SD

D.  The literature review establishes the context for the study.

    SA   5   4   3   2   1   SD

E.  The research purpose, question, or hypothesis is clearly stated.

    SA   5   4   3   2   1   SD

F.  The method of sampling is sound.

    SA   5   4   3   2   1   SD

G.  Relevant demographics (for example, age, gender, and ethnicity) are described.

    SA   5   4   3   2   1   SD

H.  Measurement procedures are adequate.

    SA   5   4   3   2   1   SD

I.  All procedures have been described in sufficient detail to permit a replication of the study.

    SA   5   4   3   2   1   SD

J.  The participants have been adequately protected from potential harm.

    SA   5   4   3   2   1   SD

K.  The results are clearly described.

    SA   5   4   3   2   1   SD

L.  The discussion/conclusion is appropriate.

    SA   5   4   3   2   1   SD

M.  Despite any flaws, the report is worthy of publication.

    SA   5   4   3   2   1   SD

# Article 5

# Tobacco Intervention Attitudes and Practices Among Certified Registered Nurse Anesthetists

**Chad S. Houghton**, MS, CRNA, **Anthony W. Marcukaitis**, MS, CRNA,
**Mary E. Shirk Marienau**, MS, CRNA, **Michael Hooten**, MD,
**Susanna R. Stevens**, MS, **David O. Warner**, MD[*]

## ABSTRACT

*Background*: The period before surgery represents an opportunity for perioperative nurses, including certified registered nurse anesthetists (CRNAs), to address the tobacco use of their patients.

*Objective*: To assess the current practices and attitudes of CRNAs toward tobacco interventions.

*Methods*: A survey assessing current attitudes, practices and beliefs, and respondent demographics was mailed to 1,000 practicing CRNAs randomly selected from the membership of the American Association of Nurse Anesthetists, with one follow-up reminder. Summary statistics of survey responses were prepared.

*Results*: The response rate was 44% (*N* = 439). Almost all respondents (92%) reported routinely asking their patients if they smoke cigarettes, and the majority felt that it was their responsibility to advise their patients to quit smoking. However, most do not routinely do so. Identified barriers to intervention included a lack of time to intervene and a lack of training. Interest in learning more about tobacco interventions was high, with strong majorities willing to take an extra 5 minutes preoperatively to intervene and to refer patients to other intervention services.

*Discussion*: These results can inform efforts to promote tobacco use interventions in surgical patients by CRNAs. Increasing the frequency and effectiveness of tobacco use interventions provided by CRNAs would benefit not only immediate perioperative outcomes, but also the long-term health of surgical patients who take advantage of the surgical episode to initiate long-term tobacco abstinence.

From *Nursing Research*, *57*, 123–129. Copyright © 2008 by Lippincott Williams & Wilkins. Reprinted with permission.

Cigarette smoking is a risk factor for perioperative morbidity, including pulmonary, cardiovascular, and wound-related complications (Warner, 2006). Preoperative abstinence from cigarettes can reduce these
5 risks, although the duration of abstinence necessary for benefit is in most instances unknown (Warner, 2005a). Recent data suggest that the scheduling of surgery can also represent a *teachable moment* for smoking cessation (Warner, 2005b), involving events that motivate
10 individuals to adopt health behaviors that reduce risk (McBride, Emmons, & Lipkus, 2003). Patients undergoing surgery spontaneously quit smoking at rates higher than the general population, especially those undergoing more extensive surgery for diseases clearly
15 related to smoking (Rigotti, McKool, & Shiffman, 1994). It is possible that clinicians who provide perioperative care could exploit this teachable moment to provide tobacco use interventions that could further increase the rate of postoperative abstinence, with ben-
20 efit not only to immediate postoperative outcomes, but also to long-term health (Warner, 2005c).

According to the U.S. Public Health Service Guideline on Tobacco Use and Dependence, it is strongly recommended that all tobacco users who come into
25 contact with the healthcare system be identified and that all healthcare providers "...should strongly advise every patient who smokes to quit because evidence shows that [such] advice to quit smoking increases abstinence rates" (Fiore et al., 2000). Unfortunately, it
30 was found in a prior study that some providers of surgical services, such as anesthesiologists and surgeons, seldom follow this recommendation, with very few providing any assistance to their patients to stop smoking (Warner, Sarr, Offord, & Dale, 2004). Evidence
35 shows that nurses can deliver effective tobacco cessation interventions (Wewers, Sarna, & Rice, 2006) and can play an important national role in the treatment of tobacco dependence (Sarna & Bialous, 2006). However, there may be differences in tobacco cessation
40 intervention by nursing specialty (Rice & Stead, 2006), and there is little information regarding the specific practices and attitudes of certified registered nurse anesthetists (CRNAs) regarding tobacco use interven-

[*]*Chad S. Houghton* is a student nurse anesthetist. *Anthony W. Marcukaitis* is a student nurse anesthetist. *Mary E. Shirk Marienau* is assistant professor of anesthesiology. *Michael Hooten* is assistant professor of anesthesiology. *Susanna R. Stevens* is a data analyst. *David O. Warner* is professor of anesthesiology, departments of anesthesiology and health sciences research, the Anesthesia Clinical Research Unit, and the Nicotine Research Center, Mayo Clinic, Rochester, Minnesota.

tions. Given their important role as providers of anesthesia services in the United States (involved in the provision of approximately 25 million anesthetics annually), effective intervention delivered by CRNAs could have a significant impact (Fallacaro & Ruiz-Law, 2004). To begin exploring this possibility, it is first necessary to ascertain the current practices and attitudes of these practitioners.

The purpose of the study was to examine the self-reported practices and attitudes of CRNAs regarding cigarette smoking cessation interventions in the perioperative period, utilizing a mailed survey.

## Methods

This study was approved by the Mayo Foundation Institutional Review Board. A list of members (approximately 30,000) was generated by the American Association of Nurse Anesthetists. Questionnaires were mailed to 1,000 of these members by the Survey Research Center at Mayo Clinic Rochester, selecting every 30th name in this alphabetical list to receive a survey. Survey packets included a cover letter, the survey instrument, and a postage-paid return envelope. Responses were anonymous. A follow-up postcard was sent out 2 weeks after the original mailing. The postcard served as a note of thanks for participating and a reminder to complete surveys that might not have been returned.

### Questionnaire Items

Questionnaire items were similar to those of the prior survey of surgeons and anesthesiologists (Warner, Sarr et al., 2004), adapted as appropriate to the CRNA audience using expert input from anesthesia providers. Forty-two items were included and are presented verbatim in the data tables in this article.

*Current Practices.* These items related to the current practices of these CRNAs regarding tobacco use interventions according to the 5As approach of the U.S. Public Health Service Guideline on Tobacco Use and Dependence recommendations (Fiore et al., 2000), including the frequency that each element was applied in practice, using a 4-point scale ranging from *never* or *rarely* to *almost always* (> 75% of the time).

*Attitudes and Beliefs.* These items were used to query the attitudes toward and beliefs regarding tobacco use interventions. Items were related to the general categories of (a) perceptions of risks and benefits of perioperative smoking abstinence, (b) perceptions of CRNA responsibility for intervention, (c) knowledge of issues associated with intervention, (d) perceptions of intervention barriers, and (e) interest in learning more about intervention methods. A 5-point Likert scale was used to assess agreement with statements, including an option for *don't know.*

*Demographics.* These items included information regarding practice environment, access to patients preoperatively and postoperatively, and personal characteristics.

### Statistical Methods

Summary statistics of responses were prepared, and these represent the primary focus of this article.

## Results

A total of 443 surveys were returned, for a response rate of 44%. Four surveys were excluded from analysis because the respondents currently were not administering anesthesia. The demographics of the respondents are presented in Table 1. Only 3% of the respondents reported daily smoking, and 28% described themselves as former smokers. Regarding opportunities for interventions, only 16% of respondents reported that they frequently or always see their patients preoperatively prior to the day of surgery and 29% frequently or always see them postoperatively. Thus, the most consistent opportunity to intervene would appear to be preoperatively on the day of surgery.

Table 1
*Respondent Demographics*

| Characteristic | CRNAs (% N = 439) |
|---|---|
| Practice environment[a] | |
| Private practice, solo | 12 |
| Private practice, group | 60 |
| Academic institution | 18 |
| Other | 13 |
| Practice setting | |
| Urban | 46 |
| Suburban | 31 |
| Rural | 23 |
| Patient mix | |
| Primarily inpatients | 5 |
| Primarily outpatients | 42 |
| Even mix of inpatients/outpatients | 54 |
| See patients preoperatively prior to the day of surgery | |
| Never or rarely | 63 |
| Sometimes | 20 |
| Frequently | 7 |
| Almost always | 9 |
| See hospitalized patients postoperatively | |
| Never or rarely | 32 |
| Sometimes | 39 |
| Frequently | 16 |
| Almost always | 13 |
| Years in practice since completion of training | |
| 5 years or less | 21 |
| 6 to 10 years | 16 |
| 11 to 20 years | 23 |
| 21 years or more | 39 |
| Age (years) | |
| 21 to 30 | 4 |
| 31 to 40 | 20 |
| 41 to 50 | 38 |
| 51 to 60 | 30 |
| 61 or older | 9 |
| Gender | |
| Male | 40 |
| Female | 60 |
| Cigarette smoking status | |
| Never smoked | 69 |
| Former smoker | 28 |
| Current smoker | 1 |

*Note.*[a] Respondents could indicate more than one practice environment; thus, percentages do not sum to 100.

Table 2
*Attitudes and Beliefs—Risks/Benefits and Responsibility (N = 439 Surveys)*

| Question | Strongly agree (%) | Agree (%) | Neutral (%) | Disagree (%) | Strongly disagree (%) | Don't know (%) | Blank (%) |
|---|---|---|---|---|---|---|---|
| Risks/benefits | | | | | | | |
| In general, quitting smoking for 6 months or longer before surgery will significantly reduce the rate of postoperative complications. | 57 | 37 | 2 | 1 | < 1 | 1 | 2 |
| In general, quitting smoking for 1 to 30 days before surgery will significantly reduce the rate of postoperative complications. | 21 | 37 | 18 | 17 | 3 | 2 | 2 |
| All patients should refrain from smoking for as long as possible before and after surgery. | 62 | 28 | 5 | 2 | 1 | < 1 | 1 |
| Responsibility | | | | | | | |
| It is none of my business if a patient chooses to smoke. | 2 | 10 | 19 | 37 | 30 | 0 | 2 |
| It is part of my responsibility as an anesthetist to advise my patients to quit smoking. | 21 | 44 | 19 | 8 | 2 | 1 | 3 |
| It is part of my responsibility as an anesthetist to make sure that patients get the help they need to quit smoking. | 4 | 18 | 43 | 26 | 3 | 2 | 4 |
| The perioperative period is a good time to get patients to permanently stop smoking. | 10 | 41 | 15 | 23 | 8 | 1 | 2 |

*Note.* Questions adapted from Warner, Sarr et al. (2004).

Awareness of the detrimental effects of smoking on postoperative outcomes is widespread (Table 2), with a strong majority of respondents agreeing that patients should refrain from smoking. Sixty-five percent of the respondents agreed or strongly agreed that it was part of their responsibility to advise their patients to quit, but only 22% felt that it was part of their responsibility to ensure that their patients get help.

Regarding barriers to intervention, 34% of the respondents felt that smoking interventions at any time were not very effective (Table 3). Only 30% felt that they knew how to help their patients get the help they needed to quit. There was considerable uncertainty regarding intervention components, such as nicotine replacement therapy. Only 24% of respondents disagreed that they did not have time to intervene (i.e., most felt that lack of time was a barrier to intervention).

Regarding current practices, almost all respondents ask their patients if they smoke (Table 4). Over half (53%) report either frequently or always advising their patients to quit, but only 15% frequently or always provide any further assistance, and essentially no one provides further follow-up. Respondents also indicated their interest in learning about related interventions (Table 5).

**Discussion**

Nurses have an important role to play in tobacco cessation efforts (Rice & Stead, 2006; Sarna & Bialous, 2006). This survey provides a sampling of current practices and attitudes regarding tobacco use interventions among CRNAs in active clinical practice. The results are consistent with the results of a prior survey of other surgical providers (surgeons and anesthesiologists) (Warner, Sarr et al., 2004) and a prior brief survey of CRNAs (published during the conduct of this study; Yankie et al., 2006) and demonstrate both challenges and opportunities for increasing the role of CRNAs in providing tobacco interventions.

As a part of a comprehensive national response in the United States to the tobacco epidemic, current recommendations urge that all contacts with the healthcare system be utilized by providers to provide at least brief interventions to encourage abstinence from smoking (Fiore et al., 2000). There have been concerted efforts to implement these recommendations in primary care practices, with mixed results. The challenge is to design and disseminate effective interventions that can be applied in busy practices. Little attention has been paid specifically to surgical patients, who provide unique challenges and opportunities (Warner, 2005a, 2005b, 2006). Because approximately 50 million patients undergo surgery in the United States annually (Hall & Lawrence, 1998), effective interventions applied to the population could have a real impact. In addition, surgery represents a teachable moment for tobacco use behavior as surgical patients, especially those requiring more extensive surgical procedures, demonstrate a higher rate of spontaneous quitting than observed in the general population; that is, surgery itself (even in the absence of intervention) represents a potent stimulus to quit (Crouse & Hagaman, 1991; France, Glasgow, & Marcus, 2001; Warner, Patten, Ames, Offord, &

Table 3
*Attitudes and Beliefs—Knowledge and Perceptions of Barriers (N = 439 Surveys)*

| Question | Strongly agree (%) | Agree (%) | Neutral (%) | Disagree (%) | Strongly disagree (%) | Don't know (%) | NA (%) | Blank (%) |
|---|---|---|---|---|---|---|---|---|
| **Knowledge regarding interventions** | | | | | | | | |
| Nicotine replacement therapies such as nicotine gum or patches are safe for patients to use during surgery. | 3 | 26 | 18 | 22 | 5 | 23 | | 3 |
| Nicotine replacement therapies such as nicotine gum or patches are safe for patients to use after surgery. | 7 | 50 | 16 | 5 | < 1 | 20 | | 1 |
| Nicotine patches require a prescription. | 3 | 31 | 5 | 27 | 9 | 22 | | 3 |
| There are effective non-nicotine medications to help patients quit smoking. | 4 | 33 | 18 | 5 | < 1 | 37 | | 2 |
| In my surgical patients who smoke cigarettes, symptoms of nicotine withdrawal during hospitalization are a significant problem for them if they do not smoke postoperatively. | 5 | 27 | 17 | 8 | 2 | 34 | 5 | 2 |
| Reimbursement is available for tobacco use intervention in my patients. | 2 | 4 | 10 | 12 | 7 | 60 | 3 | 2 |
| I don't know how to counsel my patients about how to quit smoking. | 8 | 38 | 19 | 29 | 4 | 0 | 1 | 1 |
| I know how to help my patients get the help they need to quit smoking. | 4 | 26 | 20 | 36 | 5 | 6 | < 1 | 3 |
| | | | | | | | | |
| **Perception of barriers** | | | | | | | | |
| In general, efforts at any time (not just around the time of surgery) to help people quit smoking just aren't very effective. | 3 | 31 | 20 | 35 | 4 | 5 | | 2 |
| I shouldn't talk to patients preoperatively about smoking because they may already be nervous and upset about the surgery. | 2 | 12 | 14 | 55 | 15 | 0 | < 1 | 1 |
| I only see a patient for a few minutes preoperatively, and any advice I give to stop smoking won't be effective. | 8 | 37 | 15 | 34 | 3 | 1 | < 1 | 1 |
| I don't have time to counsel my patients about how to quit smoking. | 14 | 43 | 16 | 21 | 3 | < 1 | 1 | 2 |

*Note.* Questions adapted from Warner, Sarr et al. (2004). NA = not applicable.

Schroeder, 2004; Warner, Patten, Ames, Offord, & Schroeder, 2005).

A prior survey of anesthesiologists and surgeons (Warner, Sarr et al., 2004) revealed that, in large part, 180 opportunities to intervene are not being exploited currently. The results of the current survey of CRNAs, which employed a similar methodology, are very similar to the prior survey of anesthesiologists and surgeons, especially when the results from anesthesiolo-185 gists and CRNAs are compared. Our results are also consistent with a recently published brief survey of 271 CRNAs that were queried regarding whether they provided smoking cessation counseling (Yankie et al., 2006). However, direct comparisons with this latter 190 study are not possible because, unlike our study, it did not provide a detailed survey of CRNA attitudes and beliefs, nor did it distinguish among the frequencies with which various components of smoking cessation counseling services are provided. Most healthcare pro-195 fessionals are now aware of the deleterious consequences of cigarette smoking, and the respondents in

this survey are no exception. Although most practitioners ask patients if they smoke, fewer advise them to quit, and very few provide them with any assistance to 200 do so. The two primary barriers to intervention were knowledge and time. Reflecting the fact that very few surgical providers have received any training in tobacco intervention (Warner, Sarr et al., 2004), there were misconceptions regarding the use of effective aids 205 to quitting, such as nicotine replacement therapy, and there was low self-efficacy regarding skills needed to provide help to their patients. Given the demands of busy clinical practices, it is not surprising that survey respondents felt that a lack to time to intervene was a 210 significant barrier.

The current recommendation for brief intervention by healthcare providers suggests a five-step approach, codified as the *5As*: *Ask* about tobacco use at every visit, *Advise* tobacco users to quit, *Assess* their willing-215 ness to quit, *Assist* them in quitting, and *Arrange* for follow-up contact (Fiore et al., 2000). Although the first two *As* are relatively easy to implement, the last

Table 4
*Current Practices (N = 439 responses)*

| | Never or rarely (%) | Sometimes (less than 25% of the time) (%) | Frequently (25% to 75% of the time) (%) | Almost always (over 75% of the time) (%) |
|---|---|---|---|---|
| The following questions deal with your interactions with patients. | | | | |
| How often do you: | | | | |
| Ask your patients if they smoke cigarettes? | 1 | 1 | 6 | 92 |
| Ask your patients if they smoke cigars or a pipe? | 26 | 18 | 15 | 42 |
| Ask your patients if they use snuff or chewing tobacco? | 44 | 22 | 12 | 23 |
| Advise your patients about the health risks of tobacco use? | 17 | 33 | 29 | 21 |
| Advise your patients who use tobacco to quit? | 18 | 30 | 26 | 27 |
| Counsel your patients who use tobacco about how to quit? | 59 | 26 | 10 | 5 |
| Provide resources to your patients who use tobacco to help them quit, such as medications, prescriptions for medications, educational materials, or referral for nicotine dependence treatment? | 81 | 13 | 3 | 2 |
| Follow up with your patients afterwards to address any difficulties with quitting? | 95 | 5 | 0 | < 1 |
| Follow up with your patients afterwards to collect quitting outcome information? | 97 | 2 | 0 | < 1 |

*Note.* Questions adapted from Warner, Sarr et al. (2004).

three require both time and training. An alternative approach is to simplify this strategy to Ask, Advise, and Refer to other intervention services (Schroeder, 2005). One service that has gained popularity recently in the United States is tobacco *quitlines*, which provide interventions via telephone or Internet (Zhu et al., 2002). These services can include multiple telephone counseling sessions and the provision of nicotine replacement therapy and are efficacious in promoting sustained abstinence when applied to populations (Zhu et al., 2002). Quitline services are now available throughout the United States. This approach is potentially quite applicable to CRNA practice as practitioners could easily ask, advise, and provide information regarding the quitline services available in their setting. Indeed, given our results indicating limited patient contact and limited self-efficacy regarding intervention skills, this may be one of the few practical means for them to intervene most effectively as the quitlines can provide the expert extended counseling that promotes success and can deal with important issues such as relapse prevention.

The primary limitation of this study is related to the survey methodology. To maintain anonymity, a targeted strategy was not used for survey nonrespondents, and less than half of the mailed surveys were returned. However, the response rate exceeded the prior survey of anesthesiologists and surgeons (Warner, Sarr et al., 2004). Response bias is likely, such that those practitioners most interested in tobacco control issues would be most likely to return the surveys. Thus, these results may overestimate the actual level of interest in these topics within the general population of CRNAs. We also cannot exclude the possibility of recall bias by respondents in regard to their actual tobacco intervention practices. For example, in primary care practices, the intervention rate recorded by observers is considerably lower than that self-reported by practitioners (Thorndike, Rigotti, Stafford, & Singer, 1998). Thus, our results may overestimate the actual intervention rates in the clinical practice of CRNAs. Ideally, interventions by CRNAs would be only one component of a comprehensive approach to tobacco interventions in surgical patients, an approach that would include other members of the perioperative team (e.g., surgeons and other perioperative nurses) and available resources to provide follow-up care such as telephone quitlines.

In summary, this survey demonstrated that, similar to a prior survey of other surgical providers, there are both challenges to and opportunities for tobacco use interventions by CRNAs in surgical patients who smoke. These results can inform efforts to encourage tobacco use interventions in surgical patients by CRNAs. The potential reach of interventions provided by these professionals is great. It is encouraging that many respondents expressed interest in learning more about how to intervene. Nonetheless, interventions must be designed to account for the realities of clinical practice, taking into account the survey results that time is very limited and that the only consistent time that CRNAs have patient contact is preoperatively on the day of surgery. Considerable evidence shows that even brief interventions may be efficacious (Fiore et al., 2000; Wewers et al., 2006), and our earlier publication suggests how this can be accomplished in the surgical setting (Warner, 2005b). Increasing the frequency and effectiveness of tobacco use interventions provided by CRNAs would benefit not only immediate

Table 5
*Interest in Learning About Interventions (N = 439 Surveys)*

| Question | Strongly agree (%) | Agree (%) | Neutral (%) | Disagree (%) | Strongly disagree (%) | Don't know (%) | NA (%) | Blank (%) |
|---|---|---|---|---|---|---|---|---|
| If I could effectively intervene, I would be willing to spend an extra five minutes preoperatively helping a patient who smokes to quit. | 17 | 54 | 13 | 10 | 1 | 2 | 1 | 2 |
| I would refer a patient who smokes to an effective intervention service available in my practice setting if it did not require extra time on my part. | 23 | 55 | 10 | 6 | 1 | 2 | 1 | 1 |
| I would be interested in learning more about how to help my patients quit smoking. | 9 | 41 | 28 | 16 | 1 | 3 | | 2 |
| I would attend a workshop on tobacco intervention held as part of a national meeting. | 8 | 34 | 24 | 23 | 5 | 5 | | 2 |
| I would attend a workshop on tobacco intervention if offered locally. | 9 | 34 | 24 | 19 | 4 | 8 | | 2 |

*Note.* Questions adapted from Warner, Sarr et al. (2004). NA = not applicable.

perioperative outcomes, but also the long-term health of surgical patients who take advantage of the surgical episode to initiate long-term tobacco abstinence.

Experience has shown that the introduction of tobacco interventions into clinical practice is not an easy task, and clearly, further research is required to develop, validate, and disseminate approaches that are appropriate for nurses in the perioperative setting (Sarna & Bialous, 2006). Because surgical patients receive care from multiple nurses in the perioperative team, interventions developed for CRNAs may have a wide applicability to other nurses who provide perioperative care.

### References

Crouse, J. R., 3rd, & Hagaman, A. P. (1991). Smoking cessation in relation to cardiac procedures. *American Journal of Epidemiology, 134,* 699–703.

Fallacaro, M. D., & Ruiz-Law, T. (2004). Distribution of U.S. anesthesia providers and services. *AANA Journal, 72,* 9–14.

Fiore, M. C., Bailey, W. C., Cohen, S. J., Dorfman, S. F., Goldstein, M. G., Gritz, E. R., et al. (2000). *Treating tobacco use and dependence. Clinical practice guideline.* Rockville, MD: U.S. Department of Health and Human Services Public Health Service.

France, E. K., Glasgow, R. E., & Marcus, A. C. (2001). Smoking cessation interventions among hospitalized patients: What have we learned? *Preventive Medicine, 32,* 376–388.

Hall, M. J., & Lawrence, L. (1998). Ambulatory surgery in the United States, 1996. *Advance Data, 300,* 1–16.

McBride, C. M., Emmons, K. M., & Lipkus, I. M. (2003). Understanding the potential of teachable moments: The case of smoking cessation. *Health Education Research, 18,* 156–170.

Rice, V. H., & Stead, L. (2006). Nursing intervention and smoking cessation: Meta-analysis update. *Heart & Lung, 35,* 147–163.

Rigotti, N. A., McKool, K. M., & Shiffman, S. (1994). Predictors of smoking cessation after coronary artery bypass graft surgery. Results of a randomized trial with 5-year follow-up. *Annals of Internal Medicine, 120,* 287–293.

Sarna, L., & Bialous, S. A. (2006). Strategic directions for nursing research in tobacco dependence. *Nursing Research, 55,* S1–S9.

Schroeder, S. A. (2005). What to do with a patient who smokes. *JAMA, 294,* 482–487.

Thorndike, A. N., Rigotti, N. A., Stafford, R. S., & Singer, D. E. (1998). National patterns in the treatment of smokers by physicians. *JAMA, 279,* 604–608.

Warner, D. O. (2005a). Preoperative smoking cessation: How long is long enough? *Anesthesiology, 102,* 883–884.

Warner, D. O. (2005b). Helping surgical patients quit smoking: Why, when, and how. *Anesthesia and Analgesia, 101,* 481–487.

Warner, D. O. (2005c). Preoperative smoking cessation: The role of the primary care provider. *Mayo Clinic Proceedings, 80,* 252–258.

Warner, D. O. (2006). Perioperative abstinence from cigarettes: Physiologic and clinical consequences. *Anesthesiology, 104,* 356–367.

Warner, D. O., Patten, C. A., Ames, S. C., Offord, K., & Schroeder, D. (2004). Smoking behavior and perceived stress in cigarette smokers undergoing elective surgery. *Anesthesiology, 100,* 1125–1137.

Warner, D. O., Patten, C. A., Ames, S. C., Offord, K. P., & Schroeder, D. R. (2005). Effect of nicotine replacement therapy on stress and smoking behavior in surgical patients. *Anesthesiology, 102,* 1138–1146.

Warner, D. O., Sarr, M. G., Offord, K. P., & Dale, L. C. (2004). Anesthesiologists, general surgeons, and tobacco interventions in the perioperative period. *Anesthesia and Analgesia, 99,* 1766–1773.

Wewers, M. E., Sarna, L., & Rice, V. H. (2006). Nursing research and treatment of tobacco dependence: State of the science. *Nursing Research, 55,* S11–S15.

Yankie, V. M., Price, H. M., Nanfito, E. R., Jasinski, D. M., Crowell, N. A., & Heath, J. (2006). Providing smoking cessation counseling: A national survey among nurse anesthetists. *Critical Care Nursing Clinics of North America, 18,* 123–129, xiv.

Zhu, S. H., Anderson, C. M., Tedeschi, G. J., Rosbrook, B., Johnson, C. E., Byrd, M., et al. (2002). Evidence of real-world effectiveness of a telephone quitline for smokers. *New England Journal of Medicine, 347,* 1087–1093.

**Address correspondence to:** David O. Warner, M.D., Departments of Anesthesiology and Health Sciences Research, the Anesthesia Clinical Research Unit, and the Nicotine Research Center, Mayo Clinic, 200 First Street SW, Rochester, MN 55905. E-mail: warner.david@mayo.edu

# Exercise for Article 5

## *Factual Questions*

1. Questionnaires were mailed to how many individuals?

2. When was a follow-up postcard mailed?

3. How many surveys were returned?

4. Why do the percentages for "Practice environment" in Table 1 sum to more than 100%?

5. Are the results consistent with those of a prior survey?

6. Would a "recall bias" overestimate *or* underestimate the actual intervention rates?

## *Questions for Discussion*

7. The Abstract at the beginning of this article has subheadings (e.g., Background, Objective). Would you recommend the use of subheadings to other researchers who are writing abstracts? Explain.

8. Do you think it was a good idea to keep the responses anonymous? Explain. (See line 65.)

9. The 42 items are presented verbatim in the tables in this report. Does seeing the individual items help you understand this study? Explain.

10. If you had planned this study, would you have expected a response rate of 44%? Explain. (See lines 101–102.)

11. Do you think the study was limited by the possibility of a "response bias"? (See lines 246–250.)

12. Do you think the topic of this research should be explored further in future studies? Explain.

## *Quality Ratings*

Directions: Indicate your level of agreement with each of the following statements by circling a number from 5 for strongly agree (SA) to 1 for strongly disagree (SD). If you believe an item is not applicable to this research article, leave it blank. Be prepared to explain your ratings. When responding to criteria A and B, keep in mind that brief titles and abstracts are conventional in published research.

A. The title of the article is appropriate.

SA   5   4   3   2   1   SD

B. The abstract provides an effective overview of the research article.

SA   5   4   3   2   1   SD

C. The introduction establishes the importance of the study.

SA   5   4   3   2   1   SD

D. The literature review establishes the context for the study.

SA   5   4   3   2   1   SD

E. The research purpose, question, or hypothesis is clearly stated.

SA   5   4   3   2   1   SD

F. The method of sampling is sound.

SA   5   4   3   2   1   SD

G. Relevant demographics (for example, age, gender, and ethnicity) are described.

SA   5   4   3   2   1   SD

H. Measurement procedures are adequate.

SA   5   4   3   2   1   SD

I. All procedures have been described in sufficient detail to permit a replication of the study.

SA   5   4   3   2   1   SD

J. The participants have been adequately protected from potential harm.

SA   5   4   3   2   1   SD

K. The results are clearly described.

SA   5   4   3   2   1   SD

L. The discussion/conclusion is appropriate.

SA   5   4   3   2   1   SD

M. Despite any flaws, the report is worthy of publication.

SA   5   4   3   2   1   SD

# Article 6

# Ethics Content in Community Health Nursing Textbooks

ABSTRACT. Nurses learn ethics content and ethical decision-making strategies through textbooks, basic curricula, continuing education, and professional experience. The author describes an ethics content analysis of community health nursing textbooks, offers suggestions for the improvement of ethics content for textbooks, and raises awareness of the need for more emphasis on public health ethics in nursing and public health professional education.

From *Nurse Educator, 25,* 186–194. Copyright © 2000 by Lippincott Williams & Wilkins. Reprinted with permission.

Recent calls for public health ethics educational improvements[1-3] have tended to be directed primarily toward graduate-level public health educational programs (Master's of Public Health from Schools of Public Health) and often are specifically directed toward epidemiology training programs. Many professionals working in the field of public health, however, are not in either of these categories yet have needs for ethics education and skills in ethical decision making. This article examines public health ethics education for public health nurses, the single largest professional group working in public health, accounting for 23% of the nation's public health work force.[4]

Public health nursing is defined as "the practice of promoting and protecting the health of populations using knowledge from nursing, social, and public health sciences."[5] Services provided by public health nurses are conducted in collaboration with communities, employers, families, and individuals and include ongoing health assessment, coordinated interventions, and care management.[5] Public health nurses can be found in all levels of the official public health system, as well as in nongovernmental community health organizations. The term *community health nursing* is also used to refer to nursing specialties in public health and other community health settings. The terms are used synonymously in this article.

Ethical conduct for all nurses is guided by a professional code of ethics first adopted by the American Nurses Association (ANA) in 1950 and updated periodically since that time, with the most recent version published in 1985.[6] The code offers universal moral principles that prescribe and justify nursing actions that include respect for persons, autonomy, beneficence, nonmaleficence, veracity, confidentiality, fidelity, and justice.[6] The ANA Code for Nurses, while offering a traditional biomedical ethics perspective relevant to nurses in positions of providing health care to individuals, is limited in its guidance for nurses concerned with population-based services. Fowler, in a recent call for revision of the Code, criticizes the current version for giving "too little attention to the social conditions that foster disease, injury, and illness, nationally and worldwide."[7] Increased attention to these issues would be helpful in moving toward inclusion of needed guidance in addressing ethical issues arising in the provision of services to aggregates.

The ANA has adopted a position statement on human rights that describes the relationship between ethics and human rights.[8] This document defines three responsibilities for nurses: 1) delivery of nursing care that meets the needs of the individual and is consistent with their goals; 2) social action and reform to increase the availability of nursing care and to facilitate access to needed health care for all; and 3) patient education and advocacy to ensure that individuals are aware of all options and their consequences and can make informed choices about health care.[8] A second, logical source for ethics guidance for public health nurses would be the American Public Health Association. However, this association of public health professionals has not adopted a code of ethics for public health workers.

Public health nurses learn about ethics in nursing school curricula, through nursing textbooks, in advanced or continuing education in public health or social sciences, and through professional and personal experience. The adequacy of these methods in providing the information and decision-making skills that are needed by nurses working in public health settings can be questioned. As noted, the biomedical perspective alone is inadequate for addressing ethical issues in public health, yet this is clearly the dominant perspective reflected in the Code for Nurses.

[*]*Susan J. Zahner* is a doctoral candidate at the School of Public Health, University of California, Berkeley.

Table 1
*Inclusion and Exclusion Criteria*

| "Public Health Nursing" and "Community Health Nursing" in title | Not specialty-specific (such as maternity or home health) |
| --- | --- |
| | Not a "reader" type of text |
| | Not supervision or management focused |
| | Not history focused |
| | Not focused solely on technical procedures |

75 Two research studies have been conducted on this issue. Aroskar[9] reported that community health nurses turn to colleagues, supervisors, administrators, friends, and family as helpers in dealing with ethical problems, with none identifying formal ethics courses as being a 80 helpful guide. Folmar et al.[10] reported that nurses working in public health settings indicated confidence in their ability to identify ethical problems but less confidence in their ability to resolve ethical conflicts or dilemmas. Formal instruction in ethics was reported by 85 greater than 50% of the nurses surveyed by Aroskar and only 38% of those studied by Folmar et al.[9,10] These data indicate that public health nurses have not uniformly received education in ethics, nor have they found formal education helpful in resolving ethical 90 issues in practice. Clearly, ethics education must be improved to facilitate the resolution of ethical problems facing nurses working in communities.

How can ethics education for public health nurses be improved in the future? To answer this question, it 95 is helpful to reflect on what has constituted ethics education in the past. A thorough review of all ethics-related curricula in nursing education and continuing education programs was beyond the scope of this article. A critical examination of the ethics content of one 100 venue of education for public health nurses, the public health nursing textbook, is presented here. Four research questions were posed:

1. What content on ethics is included in public health nursing textbooks?
105 2. What ethical theories have formed the basis for ethics education for public health nurses through public health nursing textbooks?
3. Has the ethics content or theoretical base changed over time?
110 4. How could the ethics content of textbooks be changed to improve public health ethics education for public health nurses?

A priori, it was expected that a biomedical perspective would dominate the ethics content of the texts and 115 that the more recent texts would be more likely to include a wider range of perspectives useful in addressing public health challenges.

**Study Methods**

A systematic search for relevant textbooks was conducted using a computerized academic library system 120 tem at a large, western United States university. The search terms *public health nursing* and *community*

*health nursing* were used to identify texts specific to the nursing specialty area. The search was limited to books published in the English language. The initial 125 search yielded 529 citations. This list was narrowed to 93 citations through the application of inclusion and exclusion criteria listed in Table 1 and through the elimination of duplicate citations. A two-stage sampling procedure was used to narrow the list of texts. 130 First, a convenience sample based on location at two nearby university libraries or in the author's personal collection was used. Next, a random sample of the texts within each twentieth century decade was used to achieve a sample that included 50% of the texts identi- 135 fied in each decade. This procedure resulted in the final sample of 48 textbooks reviewed for this analysis. On examination of the 48 texts, four were found to not meet the inclusion/exclusion criteria. In summary, 44 community health and public health nursing textbooks 140 were included in this analysis (Table 2).

A data extraction form was designed and systematically used in reviewing each text. First, the text index was checked to identify listings for ethics-related content. Terms including "ethics," "values," "morals," and 145 "philosophy" were noted. Next, the table of contents was examined for chapters with any of the above terms in the title. The content thus identified was then examined for evidence of underlying ethical theory (utilitarian, deontology, human rights, and distributive justice) 150 and for general content and approach. Evidence of the underlying theoretical framework was judged by explicit discussion of the theory and, more often, through content that implied the underlying theoretical base.

A utilitarian base was identified when content re- 155 flected concepts of maximizing good outcomes for the whole population over the individual. A deontology base was identified when text content reflected duty to alleviate suffering of individuals, duty to respect individual values, and issues of informed consent. Human 160 rights as a theoretical base was noted when the content included reference to inviolable rights of humans and the right to health. A distributive justice framework was identified when content addressed the distribution of resources and equity in access to health care. These 165 four theoretical approaches are most useful in understanding and resolving ethical problems in public health[1] and should be addressed in any adequate discussion of ethics and public health.

---

[1] Lecture by Dr. Jodi Halpern, UC Berkeley, Public Health Ethics: Research and Practice course, January 27, 1999.

Table 2
*Ethics Content of Public Health Nursing and Community Health Nursing Textbooks*

| Author | Year | Index | Chapter | Theoretical bases | | | | Primary focus/content |
| | | | | Utilitarian | Duty | Human rights | Distributive justice | |
|---|---|---|---|---|---|---|---|---|
| Gardner (13) | 1916 | | | | ✓ | | ✓ | Noninterference with religious views<br>Observance of professional etiquette<br>Service for those unable to pay |
| Gardner (14) | 1924 | | | | ✓ | | ✓ | Same as above |
| Bryan (15) | 1935 | ✓ | ✓ | ✓ | ✓ | ✓ | | Individual subservient to universal good<br>Respect for privacy, individual values<br>Sacred value of human life |
| Gardner (33) | 1936 | | | | ✓ | ✓ | ✓ | Observe professional ethics<br>Provide service without distinction for race, creed, or color<br>Service available without regard for ability to pay |
| NOPHN (34) | 1939 | ✓ | | | ✓ | | | Duty to physician |
| Gilbert (35) | 1940 | | | | | | | No ethics content |
| Grant (36) | 1942 | | | | | | | No ethics content |
| Rue (16) | 1944 | ✓ | | | ✓ | ✓ | | Duty to physician<br>Worth of human beings and interest in welfare of mankind |
| Waterman (37) | 1944 | | | | | | | No ethics content |
| Freeman (38) | 1950 | | | | ✓ | | ✓ | Respect right to self-determination<br>Make basic services available to all |
| Freeman (39) | 1957 | | | | | | | No ethics content |
| Freeman (40) | 1963 | | | | | | | No ethics content |
| Kallins (41) | 1967 | | | | | | | No ethics content |
| Freeman (42) | 1970 | | | | | ✓ | | Subordination of professional desires to human needs of group being served<br>Maximum self-determination for recipients of care |
| Tinkham and Voorhies (43) | 1972 | | | | ✓ | | | Respect for individual values |
| Lesser et al. (44) | 1975 | | | | | | | No ethics content |
| Benson and McDevitt (45) | 1976 | | | | | | | No ethics content |
| Leahy et al. (46) | 1977 | | | | ✓ | | | Worth and dignity of individual |
| Archer and Fleshman (18) | 1979 | | | | ✓ | | | Informed consent in research settings<br>Respect for patient values |
| Fromer (17) | 1979 | ✓ | ✓ | | ✓ | | | Informed consent<br>Respect for individual values<br>Content on biomedical ethics theories and dilemmas<br>Discussed Code for Nurses (1977)<br>Patient's Bill of Rights |
| Clemen-Stone et al. (47) | 1981 | | | | ✓ | | | Working with families with different values |
| Freeman and Heinrich (48) | 1981 | | | | | ✓ | | Alludes to human rights movement and importance for the future of health services |
| Helvie (19) | 1981 | ✓ | ✓ | | ✓ | | | Code for Nurses<br>Respect for client values<br>Informed consent in decision making |
| Jarvis (49) | 1981 | | | | | | | No ethics content |
| Spradley (50) | 1981 | | | | | | | No ethics content |

*Continued*

Table 2

*Ethics Content of Public Health Nursing and Community Health Nursing Textbooks*

| Author | Year | Index | Chapter | Theoretical bases | | | | Primary focus/content |
|---|---|---|---|---|---|---|---|---|
| | | | | Utilitarian | Duty | Human rights | Distributive justice | |
| Leahy et al. (51) | 1982 | ✓ | | | ✓ | | | Code for Nurses<br>Informed consent |
| Fromer (20) | 1983 | ✓ | ✓ | | ✓ | ✓ | | Biomedical ethics perspective<br>Informed consent in research settings<br>History of Nuremberg Code<br>Raises many questions about ethical issues (e.g., euthanasia, genetic cloning, organ transplants) |
| Burgess and Ragland (21) | 1983 | ✓ | ✓ | ✓ | ✓ | | ✓ | Describes utilitarian and justice (Rawls) theory<br>Steps in ethical decision making<br>Case examples |
| Stanhope and Lancaster (11) | 1984 | ✓ | ✓ | ✓ | ✓ | ✓ | ✓ | Conflict between individual and aggregate focus of community health<br>Code for Nurses, duty of veracity, confidentiality<br>Right to health as a natural human good<br>Discussed theories of justice |
| Jarvis (52) | 1985 | | | | | | | No ethics content |
| Spradley (22) | 1985 | ✓ | ✓ | | ✓ | | ✓ | Values, values clarification, value systems<br>Equity in access to health care<br>Values clarification exercises |
| Clemen-Stone et al. (53) | 1987 | ✓ | | | ✓ | ✓ | ✓ | Code for Nurses, role of ethics committees<br>Decisions on use of resources as ethical issues |
| Turner and Chavigny (54) | 1988 | | | | | | | No ethics content (epidemiology-focused text) |
| McMurray (29) | 1990 | | | | | | | No ethics content (Note: Australian text) |
| Bullough and Bullough (55) | 1990 | ✓ | | | | | | Brief mention of ethics in relation to women's right to work and occupation health hazards |
| Clemen-Stone et al. (56) | 1991 | ✓ | | | ✓ | | | Ethical approaches in decision making<br>Role of ethics committees<br>Code for Nurses |
| Cookfair (23) | 1991 | ✓ | ✓ | ✓ | ✓ | ✓ | | Discusses ethical theories (utilitarian, deontology)<br>Discusses human rights as claims recognized by law<br>Code for Nurses<br>Model for ethical analysis |
| Helvie (25) | 1991 | ✓ | | | ✓ | | | Code for Nurses<br>Values clarification<br>Ethical decision-making framework |
| Clark (24) | 1992 | ✓ | ✓ | ✓ | ✓ | | ✓ | Discusses ethical theories (utilitarian, deontology, libertarianism)<br>Codes of ethics<br>Egalitarian perspectives on distribution of resources<br>Ethical decision-making framework |

Table 2
*Ethics Content of Public Health Nursing and Community Health Nursing Textbooks*

| | | | | Theoretical bases | | | | |
|---|---|---|---|---|---|---|---|---|
| Author | Year | Index | Chapter | Utilitarian | Duty | Human rights | Distributive justice | Primary focus/content |
| Stanhope and Lancaster (12) | 1992 | | ✓ | ✓ | ✓ | ✓ | ✓ | Discusses ethical theories, principles, rules<br>Professional codes of ethics<br>Resolving ethical problems framework<br>Right to health as a basic human right |
| Anderson and MacFarlane (27) | 1996 | ✓ | ✓ | | ✓ | | | Ethics of advocacy and formation of partnerships with community<br>Respect for client freedom of choice |
| Spradley and Allender (26) | 1996 | ✓ | ✓ | | ✓ | | ✓ | Fundamental ethical principles<br>Basic human values<br>Access to health care according to benefit or needs<br>Ethical decision-making framework |
| Hertenstein-McKinnon (57) | 1997 | ✓ | ✓ | | ✓ | | | Addresses autonomy, respect, self-determination<br>Professional accountability<br>Case studies with study questions |
| Clemen-Stone et al. (28) | 1998 | ✓ | | | ✓ | | | Ethical principles<br>Professional ethical responsibilities |

## Study Results

The findings of the review are summarized in Table 2 by decade of publication. The table includes notation of the presence of a reference to ethics in the text index, the presence of a chapter devoted to ethics, reference to one of four major ethical theoretical bases, and comments reflecting the content. The text publication dates in this sample ranged from 1916 to 1998, with 24 (55%) of the texts published since 1980. Ethics was noted in the indices of 20 (45%) texts overall and 16 (67%) of the texts published since 1980. Separate chapters on ethics were found in 13 (30%) of the texts and in 11 (46%) texts published since 1980.

The ethics content of each text was assessed with regard to explicit or implicit reference to any or all of four common ethical theories: utilitarianism, deontology or duty based, human rights, and distributive justice. The dominant theoretical framework identified in this sample of textbooks was deontologic and was apparent in 28 texts (64%). Although common in public health literature, a utilitarian perspective was relatively rare in these textbooks ($n = 6$, 14%). Human rights and distributive justice theories were noted in 10 (23%) and 11 (25%) of the texts, respectively. The ethics content of the texts changed over time. More recent texts were more likely to include chapters on ethics and also addressed more theoretical perspectives. However, the texts published in the 1930s included a broader range of theoretical perspectives on average than any other decade. Only two texts, both by the same authors, Stanhope and Lancaster (1984,[11] 1992[12]), included all four theoretical perspectives.

Table 2 includes short comments on the content found in each text. Early texts touched on ethics with regard to "professional etiquette" or the obligation to respect the physician. For example, Gardner (1916)[13] stated that public health nurses "...should never criticise, by word or unspoken action, any member of the medical profession."[13] Respect for individual values was also emphasized in one of Gardner's nine principles for public health nurses, which stated "...that there should be no interference with the religious views of the patient."[14] A strong emphasis on the responsibility of the nurse to provide services regardless of the ability to pay was also identified in these texts.

The first text to include a full chapter on ethics was Edith Bryan's "The Art of Public Health Nursing," published in 1935.[15] This chapter reflects for the first time a utilitarian perspective, explaining that the nurse "...always looks on her work with a thought of evaluation from the standpoint of the greatest good to the greatest number, for the future as well as the present."[15] Respect for privacy, for individual values, and for the importance of doing no harm were strongly emphasized. A human rights perspective was noted in discussion of the "sacred value of human life" and "persons may be deprived of their freedom for the sake of preserving the life or well-being of their fellows."[15] Also of interest in this text was discussion of concepts supportive of eugenics, reflecting the popular movement of the time. Bryan wrote, "Not only must life be preserved, but it must be saved and protected on the high level of efficiency and well-being, and more recently comes the concept that it should not be created without the promise of a certain perfection. We have gone be-

yond the idea of a bare life to a fuller concept of the possibility of life with full development and fruition,
235 unhindered by physical or mental handicaps."[15]

The eight texts in this sample published in the next three decades included little content on ethics. References to ethical concepts were identified in just two of
240 these texts, predominantly reflecting a duty-based theoretical perspective. A human rights approach also might be implied in Rue's words: "Values in public health nursing are incomplete and shallow unless the nurse has a sincere feeling for the worth of the human being and an honest and far-reaching interest in the
245 welfare of mankind."[16]

With the exception of Margot Joan Fromer's 1979 text,[17] the ethics content of textbooks written in the decade of the 1970s was sparse. Of interest was the first mention of the concept of informed consent, in a
250 research setting in Archer and Fleshman (1979),[18] and in a lengthy discussion using Katz criteria in Fromer (1979).[17,18] The Fromer (1979) text was the first to include significant content on the range of ethical problems that face professionals working in health care
255 (genetic counseling, euthanasia, organ transplantation, fetal research, etc.), perhaps reflecting the tremendous growth in technology occurring at the time. This text was the first to describe the Tuskegee experiment and discuss the ethical issues it raised. The Code for
260 Nurses, the official code of ethics for professional nurses created by the ANA and discussed previously, was also first discussed in this text, despite having been initially published in 1950.[19]

The textbooks from the 1980s varied considerably
265 in their ethics content, with equal numbers of texts (*n* = 4) including no ethics-related content and including a full chapter on ethics. Duty-based theory and biomedical ethics approaches dominated the content in most of these texts. Case scenarios as a teaching tool were first
270 used by Helvie (1981).[19] The second edition text by Fromer (1983)[20] noted distinctions between professional codes of behavior and ethics by writing, "Although most codes make a concerted effort to include only behavior that is ethical, one must never accept
275 these codes at face value. They are not *necessarily* ethically correct. Ethics is a process of search and discovery rather than a behavioral indoctrination."[20] The first text to describe an ethical decision-making process was Burgess and Ragland (1983).[21] Four steps were
280 described for an ethical inquiry: 1) clarification of facts; 2) discussion of decision-making options; 3) implementation of options selected; and 4) acceptance of the consequences of action and case examples are used to educate readers on the use of the inquiry process.[21]
285 Stanhope and Lancaster (1984),[11] in a chapter written by Sara T. Fry, a nurse and philosopher, were the first authors to include a thorough discussion of ethical theory (utilitarian, deontology, natural law), ethical principles (autonomy, beneficence, justice), and ethical
290 rules (informed consent, veracity, protect privacy) and

to apply them to community health nursing examples.[11] This text was the first to include information about the Universal Declaration of Human Rights of the United Nations Assembly as a strong statement of the positive
295 right to health as well as the negative right to be protected from harm.[11] The tension for public health nurses between the utilitarian "public health ethic" perspective ("net benefit to population groups over possible health harms") and the duty-based protection
300 from harm was described in this way: "This emphasis does not align with the highly individualistic emphasis of the Code for Nurses."[11] The Spradley (1985)[22] text includes a chapter, also written by Sara T. Fry, focused on values and values clarification.[22] Values and ethics
305 are connected: "Ethics necessarily involves making evaluative judgments. Moving from the judgment that we *can* do something to the judgment that we ought to do something involves incorporating a set of norms— of judgments of value, right, duties, and responsibili-
310 ties."[22]

The texts of the 1990s show continued growth of the nursing profession and increasing sophistication about the importance and impact of ethics in public health nursing practice. Over half of the texts sampled
315 included separate chapters on ethics (*N* = 6, 55%), and only one text included no ethics content. A number of the texts included models or frameworks for use in ethical decision making. Cookfair (1991)[23] described a six-step model for ethical analysis from the work of
320 Curtin and Flaherty (1982) and used case studies to illustrate the use of the framework.[23] Clark (1992)[24] also described a six-step model that included diagnosis of the ethical dilemma, diagnosis of underlying value conflicts, assessment of priority of values, selection of
325 a course of action, implementation, and evaluation of the action.[24] Two texts used a framework by Thompson and Thompson (1981) to identify and clarify values as part of ethical decision making.[25,26] Stanhope and Lancaster (1992)[12] presented a framework from philoso-
330 pher Andy Jameton for resolving ethics problems. As with the earlier edition of this text, Stanhope and Lancaster (1992) also offered the most thorough presentation of ethics theory, principles, and rules of any of the most recent texts reviewed. Anderson and MacFarlane
335 (1996)[27] added a different dimension to the discussion of ethics and community health nursing with their advocacy perspective: "An ethic of advocacy calls for the formation of partnerships between professionals and community members in order to enhance community
340 self-determination."[27] The most recently published text in the sample, Clemen-Stone et al. (1998),[28] offered little ethics content but offered a new term—"care-based ethics"—that seemed to describe the traditional deontologic approach and was focused on the nurse-
345 client relationship and the moral obligations of professionals to promote well-being of clients.[28]

## Discussion

Although this sample of texts included almost half of the relevant texts available in the academic library system used, it may not be fully representative of all community health/public health nursing textbooks. It included only texts written in English and, with one exception, published in the United States.[29] Ethics content of nursing textbooks is a limited way of examining ethics education available to public health nurses. Nursing ethics texts, course curricula, continuing education courses, and journal articles are additional means for nurses to receive education about ethics and public health. It is also possible that important ethics-related content was missed during data extraction.

Despite the limitations of the approach, answers to the research questions established a priori were possible. This sample of community health and public health nursing textbooks included ethics content, described above, from all four major theoretical frameworks important in public health and biomedical ethics traditions, but, as expected, focused most heavily on content reflective of the duty-based, health-care provider tradition. The ethics content in the texts changed over time in three ways: 1) the amount of ethics information presented increased; 2) a broader scope of perspectives was presented; and 3) the focus on methods or frameworks for ethical decision-making processes increased. Overall, the lack of ethics content in many of the texts was disappointing. Of all the texts in the sample, the 1992 Stanhope and Lancaster[12] text offered the most thorough and useful discussion of ethics and community health nursing. No text provided a good discussion of public health ethics as an issue distinct from biomedical and professional ethics.

## Recommendations for Improvement

Community or public health nursing textbooks educate nursing students on the processes and procedures of nursing in community and public health settings. These texts also serve as references for nurses already practicing in these specialty fields. A number of recommendations related to the ethics content of public health nursing textbooks can be made that would improve the usefulness of the texts to both undergraduate nursing students and for continuing education in the field. First, emphasis should be given to ethical theory and perspectives useful for understanding and resolving ethical problems that arise in public health settings regarding the protection of welfare of the aggregate as well as protection of the welfare of the individual. Both traditional biomedical ethics and public health ethics should be described and the differences between them made clear. Public health nurses face conflicting issues of individual and population welfare with other public health professionals as members of collaborative teams in communities as well as in their daily practice as individual public health nurses and as individual members of society. At a minimum, the ethical theories and perspectives that should be addressed in such a discussion include utilitarianism, deontology, human rights, and distributive justice. The origins and history of these perspectives as well as how they inform current ethical debates in nursing and in public health should be addressed.

Second, a systematic ethical decision-making process should be described and used in discussion of examples of "real life" ethical problems that include both individual and aggregate welfare issues. The process used should be a step-by-step approach that is easy to remember and to follow in an individual decision-making situation as well as with a group of decision-makers. A number of case studies should be included that illustrate the use of the ethical decision-making process by individual community health nurses as well as by teams of public health professionals.

Third, an ideal text would include a number of case studies with discussion questions that could be used by individual students in thinking through ethical problems or by groups of students in classroom discussions. Discussion and interaction between students and with professionals in the field would facilitate learning conceptual ethical content and decision-making skills.

Fourth, community health and public health nursing textbooks should include information about ANA's Code for Nursing, because this professional code provides a set of guidelines applicable to all nurses. An ideal text would also interpret these guidelines with reference to issues faced in public health and community-based settings.

Fifth, because most community health nursing faculty are not highly educated in ethics and philosophy, a text that included a rich "more references" section or a "teacher's guide" would be helpful. Such sections would include more detailed information on the ethical theories and suggestions on ways to present the information to facilitate active learning.

Sixth, public health nursing texts should include information relevant to the ethical conduct of public health and nursing research. This is important from at least two perspectives: First, nurses working in community settings are often in positions to observe the impact of research on individuals and populations being studied and have responsibilities for protection of such vulnerable populations from unethical research practices. Second, nurses will have increasing opportunities for participation and collaboration in research projects as more research is planned and conducted in community settings.

Seventh, future texts should include discussion of ethical issues arising in emergent technologies such as genetic testing and computerized data banks as well as in evolving organizational approaches such as managed care and welfare reform. Students should be able to take away from these texts new knowledge of ethical approaches and decision-making processes as well as a sense of confidence regarding how to approach the

460 resolution of the many future ethical dilemmas that will inevitably arise.

Finally, community health and public health nursing textbooks in the future should include more emphasis on our ethical responsibilities to advocate policies
465 that promote human rights and social justice. Kathleen Chafey calls for "...a community-based practice ethic that can address the just allocation of scarce resources, universal access to health care, and benevolent public policy governing the distribution of social goods."[30]
470 Chafey also recommends an ethic that is socially just and benevolent that promotes healthy communities, described by the World Health Organization as communities with clean and safe physical environments, that have sustainable ecosystems, satisfy basic human
475 needs, optimal levels of accessible, quality public health and illness care, lifelong educational opportunities, and diversified, vital economies.[30] Educating public health nurses in the ethics of social justice will help in societal efforts to achieve optimal population health.

## Conclusion

480 This article examined and made recommendations for improvements in only one limited route for ethics education, the public health nursing textbook. An assessment of ethics curricula in nursing schools as well as the availability of continuing education opportuni-
485 ties in public health ethics would be needed to make more complete recommendations for the improvement of ethics education for public health nurses. Such a survey of ethics education in schools of public health (an avenue for graduate education for many public
490 health nurses) indicated limited required courses and elective offerings in public health ethics.[31] Ethics education in the past for public health nurses has generally been limited in scope and based on the individually focused, traditional biomedical/deontologic approach.
495 This analysis leads one to suspect that nurses educated before 1980 were unlikely to receive education on ethics. It also seems possible from this analysis that even nurses educated in the 1990s may have been exposed to textbooks lacking in ethics content in general and al-
500 most certainly lacking content specific to public health ethics.

The future of ethics education for public health nurses seems more promising with recent calls for revisions of the professional code of ethics, more emphasis
505 on human rights by the professional nursing association, a general trend toward more thorough discussions of ethics included in more recent textbooks, and recently published recommendations for education in public health ethics for public health professionals.
510 However, a lack of awareness of the importance of public health ethics education continues, as evidenced by the lack of mention of ethics in a recently proposed core curriculum for public health workers.[32] Improvements in public health ethics education for all public
515 health professionals are urgently needed to assure that

the knowledge and tools are readily available to address the ever more challenging ethical issues of the future.

## References

1. Coughlin SS. Model curricula in public health ethics. *Am J Prev Med.* 1996;12:247–251.
2. Rossignol A, Goodmonson S. Are ethical topics in epidemiology included in the graduate epidemiology curricula? *Am J Epidemiol.* 1995;142:1265–1268.
3. Coughlin S, Etheredge G. On the need for ethics curricula in epidemiology. *Epidemiology.* 1995;6:566–567.
4. Stevens R. A study of public health nursing directors in state health departments. *Public Health Nursing.* 1995;12:432–435.
5. APHA Public Health Nursing Section. *The Definition and Role of Public Health Nursing—A Statement of the APHA Public Health Nursing Section.* Washington, D.C.: American Public Health Association, Public Health Nursing Section; 1996.
6. ANA. Code for Nurses with Interpretive Statements. Washington, D.C.: American Nurses Publishing; 1985.
7. Fowler M. Ethics: Relic or Resource? The Code for Nurses. *Am J Nurs.* 1999;99(3):56–57.
8. ANA. *Ethics and Human Rights.* Kansas City, MO: American Nurses Association; 1991.
9. Aroskar MA. Community health nurses—their most significant ethical decision-making problems. *Nurs Clin North Am.* 1989;24:967–975.
10. Folmar J, Coughlin SS, Bessinger R, Sacknoff D. Ethics in public health practice: a survey of public health nurses in southern Louisiana. *Public Health Nurs.* 1997;14:156–160.
11. Stanhope M, Lancaster J. *Community Health Nursing Process and Practice for Promoting Health.* St. Louis: CV Mosby Company; 1984.
12. Stanhope M, Lancaster J. *Community Health Nursing Process and Practice for Promoting Health.* 3rd ed. St. Louis: Mosby Year Book; 1992.
13. Gardner MS. *Public Health Nursing.* New York: The MacMillan Company; 1916.
14. Gardner MS. *Public Health Nursing.* 2nd ed. New York: The MacMillan Company; 1924.
15. Bryan ES. *The Art of Public Health Nursing.* Philadelphia: WB Saunders Company; 1935.
16. Rue CB. *The Public Health Nurse in the Community.* Philadelphia: WB Saunders Company; 1944.
17. Fromer M. *Community Health Care and the Nursing Process.* St. Louis: The CV Mosby Company; 1979.
18. Archer S, Fleshman R. *Community Health Nursing: Patterns and Practice.* North Scituate, MA: Duxbury Press; 1979.
19. Helvie C. *Community Health Nursing Theory and Process.* Philadelphia: Harper and Row, Publishers; 1981.
20. Fromer M. *Community Health Care and the Nursing Process.* 2nd ed. St. Louis: CV Mosby Company; 1983.
21. Burgess W, Ragland E. *Community Health Nursing: Philosophy, Process, Practice.* 1983.
22. Spradley B. *Community Health Nursing: Concepts and Practice.* Boston: Little, Brown, and Company; 1985.
23. Cookfair J. *Nursing Process and Practice in the Community.* St. Louis: Mosby Year Book; 1991.
24. Clark M. *Nursing in the Community.* Norwalk, CT: Appleton and Lange; 1992.
25. Helvie C. *Community Health Nursing Theory and Practice.* New York: Springer Publishing Company; 1991.
26. Spradley B, Allender J. *Community Health Nursing: Concepts and Practice.* Philadelphia: Lippincott; 1996.
27. Anderson E, McFarlane J. *Community as Partner: Theory and Practice in Nursing.* 2nd ed. Philadelphia: Lippincott; 1996.
28. Clemen-Stone S, McGuire S, Eigsti D. *Comprehensive Community Health Nursing: Family, Aggregate, and Community Practice.* St. Louis: Mosby; 1998.
29. McMurray A. *Community Health Nursing: Primary Care in Practice.* Melbourne: Churchill Livingston; 1990.
30. Chafey K. Caring is not enough: ethical paradigms for community-based care. In: Spradley B, Allender J, eds. *Readings in Community Health Nursing.* 5th ed. Philadelphia: Lippincott; 1997:211–220.
31. Coughlin SS, Katz WH, Mattison DR. Ethics instruction at schools of public health in the United States. *Am J Public Health.* 1999;89:768–770.
32. Gebbie KM. The Public Health Workforce: Key to Public Health Infrastructure. *Am J Public Health.* 1999;89:660–661.
33. Gardner M. *Public Health Nursing.* New York: The MacMillan Company; 1936.
34. Nursing NOPHN. *Manual of Public Health Nursing.* 3rd ed. New York: The MacMillan Company; 1939.
35. Gilbert R. *The Public Health Nurse and Her Patient.* New York: The Commonwealth Fund; 1940.

36. Grant A. *Nursing: A Community Health Service.* Philadelphia: WB Saunders; 1942.
37. Waterman T. *Nursing for Community Health.* Philadelphia: FA Davis Company; 1944.
38. Freeman R. *Public Health Nursing Practice.* Philadelphia: WB Saunders Company; 1950.
39. Freeman R. *Public Health Nursing Practice.* Philadelphia: WB Saunders Company; 1957.
40. Freeman R. *Public Health Nursing Practice.* 3rd ed. Philadelphia: WB Saunders Company; 1963.
41. Kallins E. *Textbook of Public Health Nursing.* St. Louis: CV Mosby Company; 1967.
42. Freeman R. *Community Health Nursing Practice.* Philadelphia: WB Saunders Company; 1970.
43. Tinkham C, Voorhies E. *Community Health Nursing: Evolution and Process.* New York: Appleton Century Crofts; 1972.
44. Leeser I, Tuchalski C, Carotenuto R. *Community Health Nursing.* Flushing, NY: Medical Examination Publishing Company; 1975.
45. Benson E, McDevitt J. *Community Health and Nursing Practice.* Englewood Cliffs, NJ: Prentice-Hall Inc.; 1976.
46. Leahy K, Cobb M, Jones M. *Community Health Nursing.* 3rd ed. New York: McGraw-Hill Book Company; 1977.
47. Clemen-Stone S, Eigsti D, McGuire S. *Comprehensive Family and Community Health Nursing.* New York: McGraw-Hill Book Company; 1981.
48. Freeman R, Heinrich J. *Community Health Nursing Practice.* 2nd ed. Philadelphia: WB Saunders Company; 1981.
49. Jarvis L. *Community Health Nursing: Keeping the Public Healthy.* Philadelphia: FA Davis Company; 1981.
50. Spradley B. *Community Health Nursing Concepts and Practice.* Boston: Little Brown and Company; 1981.
51. Leahy K, Cobb M, Jones M. *Community Health Nursing.* 4th ed. New York: McGraw-Hill Book Company; 1982.
52. Jarvis L. *Community Health Nursing: Keeping the Public Healthy.* 2nd ed. Philadelphia: FA Davis Company; 1985.
53. Clemen-Stone S, Eigsti D, McGuire S. *Comprehensive Family and Community Health.* New York: McGraw-Hill Book Company; 1987.
54. Turner J, Chavigny K. *Community Health Nursing: An Epidemiologic Perspective Through the Nursing Process.* Philadelphia: JB Lippincott Company; 1988.
55. Bullough B, Bullough V. *Nursing in the Community.* St. Louis: CV Mosby Company; 1990.
56. Clemen-Stone S, Eigsti D, McGuire S. *Comprehensive Family and Community Health Nursing.* 3rd ed. St. Louis: CV Mosby Year Book; 1991.
57. Hertenstein-McKinnon T. *Community Health Nursing: A Case Study Approach.* Philadelphia: Lippincott; 1997.

**Acknowledgments**: This article was originally prepared for "Public Health Ethics: Research and Practice," a graduate course at the University of California, Berkeley, School of Public Health. The author thanks Dr. Patricia Buffler, Dr. Jodi Halpern, and Dr. Thomasine Kushner for the class content and their support and encouragement in this analysis.

# Exercise for Article 6

## *Factual Questions*

1. According to the researcher, what is the dominant perspective in the Code for Nurses?

2. What search terms were used to identify texts specific in the nursing specialty area of interest to the researcher?

3. When examining a text, what did the researcher check first to identify ethics-related content?

4. The researcher states that a utilitarian perspective was relatively rare in the textbooks that were studied. According to the researcher, is this perspective uncommon in public health literature?

5. The researcher reports that only two texts, both by the same authors, included all four theoretical perspectives. What are the authors' names?

6. How many of the texts of the 1990s included separate chapters on ethics?

7. According to the researcher, an "ideal text" would include what?

## *Questions for Discussion*

8. The researcher mentions a two-stage sampling procedure. The first stage used a "convenience sample." What is your understanding of the meaning of this term? (See lines 130–132.)

9. An important concern in evaluating research reports is whether the researcher has described her or his research methods in sufficient detail to permit a replication of the study. Do you think that the methods used in this study are described in sufficient detail? Do you think that a replication by another researcher would be useful? Explain.

10. Do you think that the historical perspective obtained by analyzing textbooks published as early as 1916 is useful in helping you understand the issues examined and the results of this study? (See, for example, the first entry in Table 2.) Explain.

11. An inherent weakness of content analysis of written material is that the results describe only what selected authors (in this case, textbook authors) say and, presumably, believe. It cannot tell us what practicing public health nurses know and believe. Despite this weakness, do you think the content analysis presented in this article provides useful information? In general, do you think that content analysis is a useful research approach for examining important issues in nursing? Explain.

12. The researcher makes eight recommendations for improvement in the section of her report called "Recommendations for Improvement." Do you agree with all the recommendations? Do you think that some are more important than others? Explain.

## *Quality Ratings*

Directions: Indicate your level of agreement with each of the following statements by circling a number from 5 for strongly agree (SA) to 1 for strongly disagree (SD). If you believe an item is not applicable to this research article, leave it blank. Be prepared to explain your ratings. When responding to criteria A and B, keep in mind that brief titles and abstracts are conventional in published research.

A.   The title of the article is appropriate.

   SA   5   4   3   2   1   SD

B.   The abstract provides an effective overview of the research article.

   SA   5   4   3   2   1   SD

C.   The introduction establishes the importance of the study.

   SA   5   4   3   2   1   SD

D.   The literature review establishes the context for the study.

   SA   5   4   3   2   1   SD

E.   The research purpose, question, or hypothesis is clearly stated.

   SA   5   4   3   2   1   SD

F.   The method of sampling is sound.

   SA   5   4   3   2   1   SD

G.   Relevant demographics (for example, age, gender, and ethnicity) are described.

   SA   5   4   3   2   1   SD

H.   Measurement procedures are adequate.

   SA   5   4   3   2   1   SD

I.   All procedures have been described in sufficient detail to permit a replication of the study.

   SA   5   4   3   2   1   SD

J.   The participants have been adequately protected from potential harm.

   SA   5   4   3   2   1   SD

K.   The results are clearly described.

   SA   5   4   3   2   1   SD

L.   The discussion/conclusion is appropriate.

   SA   5   4   3   2   1   SD

M.   Despite any flaws, the report is worthy of publication.

   SA   5   4   3   2   1   SD

# Article 7

# Buried Alive: The Presence of Nursing on Hospital Web Sites

**Alice R. Boyington**, RN, PhD, **Cheryl B. Jones**, RN, PhD, FAAN, **Dianna L. Wilson**, RN, MSN[*]

### ABSTRACT

*Background*: Increasingly, hospitals are using sites on the World Wide Web (Web) to market their services and products and to advertise employment opportunities. These Web sites are a potential resource for information on the hospitals' nursing care and nurses' impact on patient outcomes.

*Objective*: The aim of this study was to explore the presence of nursing—accessible and visible data on nurses, nursing practice, or nursing care—on hospital Web sites.

*Methods*: A random sample of 50 hospital Web sites from the *U.S. News and World Report's* 2003 list of America's best hospitals was examined. A tool developed to capture the characteristics that denote a presence of nursing was used to examine hospital Web sites.

*Results*: All 50 sites had at least two occurrences of visible data in the form of pictures, graphics, or text that related to nurses, nursing care, or nursing practice. However, nurse-related content on these hospital Web sites was minimally to somewhat present and was frequently located on pages deep within the site.

*Discussion*: The presence of nursing on hospital Web sites could represent the importance of nursing, nursing practice, or nursing care for patients entering hospital systems. Instead, nursing content on hospital Web sites primarily focuses on nursing employment.

From *Nursing Research*, 55, 103–109. Copyright © 2006 by Lippincott Williams & Wilkins. Reprinted with permission.

The portrayal of nurses in traditional forms of media has been well-documented. Historically, the importance of nurses and their contributions have been underplayed in the entertainment media (Kalisch & Kalisch, 1982, 1986). References to nurses and their roles in healthcare delivery have been virtually omitted in the print media (Sigma Theta Tau International, 1997). Following the healthcare quality initiative launched in 1996 by the Institute of Medicine, the nursing shortage and the impact on the quality of care have been emphasized through the mass communications media; consumers have been reminded that decreased levels of nurse staffing can have a negative impact on the quality of care and patient safety (Aiken, Clarke, Cheung, Sloane, & Silber, 2003; Kovner, Jones, Zhan, Gergen, & Basu, 2002; Needleman, Buerhaus, Mattke, Stewart, & Zelevinsky, 2002; Page, 2004). Although the public has been informed through the media about the problems or failures of the nursing profession, often, the many accomplishments of nurses are not shown (Gordon, 2005).

A newer type of communications media, the World Wide Web (Web) on the Internet, is popular in the United States and is used throughout the healthcare industry. For instance, Johnson & Johnson developed a Web site (www.discovernursing.com) as part of its advertising program, "The Campaign for Nursing's Future." The site contains in-depth information on nursing education and careers and targets the recruitment of potential candidates into the profession. Countless Web sites offer health and medical information, and healthcare consumers increasingly visit those sites (Fox & Fallows, 2003).

The popularity of the Web among healthcare consumers has not gone unnoticed by hospital marketing professionals. More and more hospitals are using the Web as a marketing tool to promote their healthcare products, services, and employment opportunities (Fell & Shepherd, 2001; Sanchez, 2000; Sanchez & Maier-Donati, 1999). Hospital Web sites have been analyzed with respect to content and purpose. For example, Sanchez and Maier-Donati (1999) derived descriptive categories of hospital Web site characteristics from reviews of the literature and Web sites to guide site evaluation and recommendations for site content. Zingmond, Lim, Etter, and Carlisle (2001) reported that hospitals were using the Web for marketing care that emphasized wellness, health information, and quality of services and that promoted their affiliated physicians. Other researchers included indicators of quality of care in their evaluation of Web sites (Kind, Wheeler, Robinson, & Cabana, 2004). Fell and Shepherd (2001) reported on specific online marketing ac-

[*]*Alice R. Boyington* is associate professor, School of Nursing, University of North Carolina at Chapel Hill. *Cheryl B. Jones* is associate professor, School of Nursing, University of North Carolina at Chapel Hill. *Dianna L. Wilson* is staff nurse, Alamance Regional Medical Center, Burlington, North Carolina.

tivities such as employee recruitment. Although it is unknown whether a nursing product was marketed on any of the hospital Web sites in the above studies, the published reports have not mentioned nurses or nursing care.

The lack of nurse-related findings in the above reports support the observations of Gordon (2005) and Carty, Coughlin, Kasoff, and Sullivan (2000) that nurses (but not physicians) are invisible on hospital Web sites. Medicine is the focus of advertising that highlights descriptions of physician accomplishments and pictures of physicians providing care to patients. A lack of a presence of nursing on hospital Web sites may be one of the standard industry practices that undervalue nurses' knowledge and skills and that underestimate contributions by nurses to hospitals and to patient care (Weinberg, 2003).

Although the low visibility of nurses and nursing care on hospital Web sites is apparent from casual observation, quantitative data to document this invisibility and promote changes in the current focus on medical care and physicians are not found. The absence of messages about the contributions, qualifications, and accomplishments of nurses on hospital Web sites may subtly but negatively influence the public's perception of care that they can expect to receive in hospitals. Omission of positive messages about nurses and their work on hospital Web sites also hinders efforts to attract people available and qualified to work in hospitals and individuals who might want to enter the nursing profession. The most damaging effect of this omission is the subliminal message that misleads the public by failing to recognize nurses as important members of the healthcare team who are responsible for overseeing most of the care patients will receive.

The purpose of the study was to determine (a) whether there is a presence of nursing, (b) the accessibility (based on site depth of the nurse-related content) of the presence of nursing, and (c) the characteristics of the presence of nursing on U.S. hospital Web sites. Literature from healthcare marketing (Fell & Shepherd, 2001; Sanchez, 2000; Sanchez & Maier-Donati, 1999), information science (Atzeni, Merialdo, & Sindoni, 2002; Morkes & Nielsen, 1997; Pirouz, 1997), and nursing science (Kalisch & Kalisch, 1982, 1986; Sigma Theta Tau International, 1997) were used to guide the study.

## Methods

*Sample*

A descriptive design was used to explore Web sites for hospitals and medical centers[1] ranked in 2003 by the *U.S. News and World Report*. This ranking of "America's Best Hospitals" is reported annually in their print and Web media so that hospitals can use that

---

[1] The term "hospitals" will denote both hospitals and medical centers.

ranking to market services. This ranking is more likely to be used by healthcare consumers than, for example, the lesser known "HCIA-Sachs Institute 100 Top Hospitals" or "Solucient's 100 Top Hospitals."

The 2003 online publication of the rankings (*U.S. News and World Report*, 2003) included Web site addresses for all 203 of the ranked hospitals in 17 specialties. Seventeen of the 203 hospitals appeared on an "Honor Roll" that denoted leadership and high-quality care in six or more medical specialties. The sample (*N* = 50) for this study included all 17 hospitals on the "Honor Roll" and an additional 33 selected from the remaining 186 hospitals using an electronic random number generator. A statistician was consulted to verify the number of hospitals needed and the selection process; the sample represented 25% of the total population of hospitals on the list and was deemed sufficient for the study. Each of the hospital Web sites in the sample was accessed via the link provided on the *U.S. News and World Report* Web site.

*Development and Use of the Study Checklist*

The development of the Presence of Nursing: Hospital Web Site Checklist included in-depth preliminary work to identify and categorize nurse-related content on hospital Web sites. Forty hospitals ranked on the *U.S. News and World Report* Web site in 2002 were reviewed, and a list of characteristics relevant to the nursing profession was compiled. The research team, composed of members with expertise in current nursing practice, healthcare systems, healthcare informatics, and the communications media, reviewed this initial list of characteristics.

As a pilot test, the research team used the checklist to examine four hospital Web sites selected from hospitals in the 2002 list. Items to capture the geographical location and type of each hospital were added to the checklist because of this pilot session. The final list of 75 characteristics was organized into five major categories (Table 1), facilitating the flow of the review of hospital Web sites: (a) hospital Web site home page (13 characteristics); (b) nursing organization (17 characteristics); (c) nursing employment, recruitment, and retention (19 characteristics); (d) nursing education and research (18 characteristics); and (e) nursing news (8 characteristics). Each category included an *other* item to capture nurse-related characteristics not on the checklist. This categorical list was formatted in tabular form for purposes of data collection; one column was designated for placement of a checkmark to indicate that the characteristic was present on the Web site.

During the checklist development phase of the study, the research team created a scale to rate the total number of characteristics (range = 0–75) found on hospital Web sites: (a) absent = *no characteristics*, (b) minimally present = *1–15 characteristics*, (c) somewhat present = *16–37 characteristics*, (d) moderately present = *38–59 characteristics*, and (e) very present = *60–75 characteristics*.

Table 1
*Categories and Examples of Characteristics from Presence of Nursing Hospital Web Site Checklist*

| Category | Characteristic |
|---|---|
| Hospital Web site home page | Direct link to nursing Web site on home page |
| | Nursing link under health professions |
| | Recognition of nursing care on hospital Web site |
| Nursing organization | Identification of nursing leaders or administrators |
| | Mission or vision of nursing department |
| | Nurse-to-patient ratios or nurse-staffing |
| Nursing employment, recruitment, and retention | List of positions |
| | Job descriptions |
| | Programs for new graduate nurses (preceptorship, nurse internship, or residency) |
| Nursing education and research | Descriptions of continuing education programs |
| | Nursing research center or department or program |
| | Emphasis on importance of nursing research |
| Nursing news | Online nursing newsletter |
| | Professional awards or recognition |
| | Educational achievements |

*Note.* For more information about the checklist, please contact the authors.

A second scale was developed to measure the accessibility of the presence of nursing on the hospital Web sites. Accessibility was defined according to the site depth of the nurse-related content and was based on the number of pages the user had to click through to get to that content (Pirouz, 1997). Because Web content placed deep within a site is considered to be invisible (Gil, n.d.), this definition of accessibility was used to determine the visibility of nurse-related content on hospital Web sites. The categories to denote accessibility and visibility of nurse-related content were the following: (a) absent = *having to click through six or more pages*, (b) minimally accessible = *having to click through five pages*, (c) somewhat accessible = *having to click through four pages*, (d) moderately accessible = *having to click through three pages*, and (e) very accessible = *having to click through one or two pages*.

Items in the investigator-developed checklist were selected based on the review of literature in healthcare marketing, information science, and nursing science. An iterative process was used in the development and pilot testing of the checklist to categorize nurse-related content on hospital Web sites. Although no reliability and validity tests were conducted, the varied expertise of the research team members was used to verify the face validity of the checklist.

*Data Collection*

Three members of the research team used the study checklist to evaluate the first five Web sites in the selected sample ($N = 50$), and findings were compared to promote a consistent evaluation of sites. All discrepancies in data collection were discussed to reach 100% consensus and to establish a plan for consistently reviewing the study Web sites. The remaining 45 hospital Web sites were accessed and evaluated. The time period for the data collection was kept to a minimum to decrease the influence of any site changes and updates. The checklist data were entered into a Microsoft Excel database.

*Analysis*

Data were analyzed using descriptive statistics to determine whether there was a presence of nursing on the hospital Web sites. Frequencies and other descriptive statistics were used to describe the demographic characteristics of the hospitals, the proportion of hospital Web sites with a presence of nursing, the accessibility of nursing information on the hospital Web sites, and the distribution of the individual characteristics reflecting the presence of nursing.

**Findings**

All hospital Web sites in the sample ($N = 50$) were available using the links on the Web version of the "America's Best Hospitals 2003" (*U.S. News and World Report*, 2003). The hospitals with these Web sites were located throughout the United States: 12 hospitals (24%) were in the North Atlantic region, 6 (12%) were in the South Atlantic region, 14 (28%) were in the North Central region, 7 (14%) were in the South Central region, and 11 (22%) were in the Pacific and Mountain region. Of 50 hospitals, 47 (94%) were academic institutions, 2 (4%) were nonacademic, and 1 was unidentifiable.

All 50 Web sites had at least two occurrences of visible data in the form of pictures, graphics, or text that related to nurses, nursing care, or nursing practice. From the possible 75 characteristics on the checklist, the number identified for the 50 sites ranged from 2 to 42 ($M = 18.2$; $SD = 10.56$). Twenty-three (46%) sites had minimal nursing presence (1–15 characteristics), 23 (46%) had somewhat of a presence (16–37 characteristics), 4 (8%) had a moderate presence (38–59 characteristics), and no site achieved a rating of very present (60–75 characteristics).

The rating of accessibility of the presence of nursing reflected the number of pages that the reviewer had to click through to get to a characteristic of the presence of nursing (Table 2). The presence of nursing on 11 (22%) sites was rated as invisible, and only 1 (2%) site displayed a presence that was very accessible.

Descriptive information for the categories of characteristics assessed on the 50 hospital Web sites is presented in Table 3. All but one hospital Web site had some nursing information in the nursing employment, recruitment, and retention category. The category with the fewest nurse-related characteristics present on hospital Web sites was nursing news, invisible on most (68%) sites. No themes or additions to the checklist were revealed in the items listed as *other*. Details of the characteristics within the five categories follow.

Table 2
*Accessibility of the Presence of Nursing on Hospital Web Sites (n = 50)*

| Accessibility of nursing presence | n | % |
|---|---|---|
| Absent (≥6 clicks) | 11 | 22 |
| Minimally accessible (5 clicks) | 16 | 32 |
| Somewhat accessible (4 clicks) | 11 | 22 |
| Moderately accessible (3 clicks) | 11 | 22 |
| Very accessible (1–2 clicks) | 1 | 2 |

*Note.* The accessibility of the presence of nursing on these hospital Web sites was measured by the number of pages the user had to click through to find the nurse-related content.

Table 3
*Descriptive Information on Nursing Presence on 50 Hospital Web Sites*

| Number of characteristics per category | Hospital Web sites n (%) | Characteristics observed per category M (SD) |
|---|---|---|
| Hospital Web site home page | | 3.34 (2.18) |
| 0 | 4 (8) | |
| 1–3 | 26 (52) | |
| 4–6 | 15 (30) | |
| 7–9 | 5 (10) | |
| 10–12 | 0 | |
| 13 | 0 | |
| Nursing organization | | 2.24 (2.44) |
| 0 | 17 (34) | |
| 1–3 | 17 (34) | |
| 4–6 | 14 (28) | |
| 7–9 | 2 (4) | |
| 10–12 | 0 | |
| 13–15 | 0 | |
| 16–17 | 0 | |
| Nursing employment, recruitment, and retention | | 8.22 (3.35) |
| 0 | 1 (2) | |
| 1–3 | 4 (8) | |
| 4–6 | 10 (20) | |
| 7–9 | 18 (36) | |
| 10–12 | 12 (24) | |
| 13–15 | 5 (10) | |
| 16–18 | 0 | |
| 19 | 0 | |
| Nursing education and research | | 3.08 (3.37) |
| 0 | 14 (28) | |
| 1–3 | 18 (36) | |
| 4–6 | 9 (18) | |
| 7–9 | 5 (10) | |
| 10–12 | 4 (8) | |
| 13–15 | 0 | |
| 16–18 | 0 | |
| Nursing news | | 1.22 (2.34) |
| 0 | 34 (68) | |
| 1–3 | 9 (18) | |
| 4–6 | 2 (4) | |
| 7–8 | 5 (10) | |

### Hospital Web Site Home Page

A hospital home page was considered to be the Web page that served as an entry to the remaining pages on the site. Most Web sites (*n* = 44, 88%) had an internal search engine on the hospital home page. The search engine allowed a site visitor to look for specific information on pages throughout the site. Using *nurse* and *nursing* as key search words disclosed nurse-related content on 24 (48%) sites, but on many sites, several links had to be followed to locate nurse-related content. Magnet status, the highest level of recognition awarded by the American Nurses Credentialing Center to nursing services in the United States and international healthcare communities, was acknowledged with a Magnet symbol on only five (10%) home pages, although 15 of the 50 (30%) hospitals had been granted this prestigious award, as was noted on pages deeper in the site. Six hospital Web site home pages (12%) included testimonials from patients regarding the quality of nursing care as they perceived it. On five (10%) of the home pages, quality nursing care was identified as an important aspect of services provided.

### Nursing Organization

Nurse leaders or administrators in the organization were identified on 10 (20%) hospital Web sites. A nursing philosophy was stated on 11 (22%) hospital Web sites, information on the missions or visions of their nursing departments was provided on 9 (18%), and a nursing slogan or phrase was displayed on 7 (14%). Although nursing departments are typically organized by specialty areas, and job vacancies may be organized and advertised accordingly, a description of specialty areas was shown on only 15 (30%) sites. At least one message from a staff nurse describing nursing practice within the organization was found on 19 (38%) sites.

### Nursing Employment, Recruitment, and Retention

Information on how to apply for vacant positions in nursing was given on 44 (88%) sites, job vacancies with a direct link to employment opportunities for nurses were listed on 43 (86%), and a prospective nurse could complete an online employment application on 40 (80%). Employee benefits were listed on 42 (84%) sites. Innovative scheduling options other than the traditional 8- and 12-hr shifts were described on 11 (22%) sites. Recognition of clinical expertise, such as a clinical ladders program, was present on 11 (22%) sites, and some form of nurse retention program was identified on 6 (12%) sites.

Information on a summer internship/externship program for nursing students who are about to enter their senior year of study was given on 23 (46%) sites. Details on the programs indicated that nursing students worked under the supervision of a nurse within the organization, practiced skills learned in their nursing program, learned about the real world of nursing in practice, and began an acculturation into the organization.

A flexible work schedule that allowed nursing stu-
305   dents to attend classes and work at the hospital was
described on one Web site.

*Nursing Education and Research*

A link to a college or school of nursing affiliated
with the organization was present on 17 (34%) sites,
although a collaboration between nursing services and
310   a college or school of nursing on projects or research
that might indicate endeavors to study and improve
nursing practice was identified on only 4 (8%). Nursing
research endeavors had very little visibility; a nursing
research center or department was listed on 10 (20%)
315   sites, but none described research programs or initiatives.

*Nursing News*

A way to communicate information on the achievements of nurses, such as an online nursing newsletter
or a list of current nurse-related events, was present on
320   only six (12%) of the sites. Professional awards were
published on 12 (24%) sites, and educational achievements were noted on 6 (12%) sites.

## Limitations

One limitation is that hospital Web sites not on the
list of "America's Best Hospitals 2003" (*U.S. News
325   and World Report*, 2003) or not in the sample used
from this list could produce different results. A potential bias in sample selection exists because 94% of the
hospitals were academic health centers. The instrument
to evaluate the presence of nursing on the hospital Web
330   sites was developed specifically for this project and
may not contain an exhaustive list of characteristics.
The data also were collected and analyzed primarily by
a single investigator and are thus subject to bias. However, attempts were made to overcome this limitation
335   by defining the characteristics clearly, using specific
criteria for evaluation and comparing the reviews of
three researchers on five randomly selected sites. As
with any research, potential bias exists when subjective
data are interpreted.

## Discussion

340   In this study, hospital Web sites varied greatly in
content and appearance, as did the presence of nursing
on those sites. Although all Web sites studied had at
least two characteristics denoting a presence of nursing, the nurse-related content was not located easily.
345   This result is consistent with the Woodhull study
(Sigma Theta Tau International, 1997) that reported
minimal nurse-related content in print publications.
Although perhaps unintentional, the unstated message
revealed by findings in this study of hospital Web sites
350   is that the nursing profession is not important, nurses
do not play an important role in the delivery of services, and in turn, the nursing profession does not warrant space on hospital Web sites.

Further data analysis of this sample of hospital Web
355   sites revealed that the presence of nursing, often located several pages deep within the site, is somewhat
difficult to access and may be invisible to site visitors.
Content located deep within a Web site is deemed invisible (Gil, n.d.) and is not indexed in the major exter-
360   nal search engines (Spink, Jansen, Wolfram, & Saracevic, 2002). Thus, Web users who desire specific information on nursing services in hospitals may have
minimal search yields and have little patience with
searching the Web further.

365   Visitors to hospital Web site home pages, both prospective patients and potential nurse applicants, may
have difficulty locating the information they seek. Users of the Web are known to scan pages, pick out individual words, or conduct a keyword search (Morkes &
370   Nielsen, 1997) to fulfill their information need. Users
move on to another site if they do not retrieve what
they want efficiently. Thus, the empty search results on
the terms *nurse* or *nursing* that were evident on more
than half of the hospital Web sites in this sample could
375   be a barrier to locating relevant information.

The primary reason patients are admitted to healthcare facilities is to receive care that they cannot receive
elsewhere. Given that nurses are generally the largest
group of healthcare professionals within most hospitals
380   and they provide hands-on care to patients during most
hospital admissions (Jones & Lusk, 2002), it follows
that prospective patients may seek specific information
on nursing care to better inform decisions on care delivery. The small number of hospital Web sites in the
385   current study that described characteristics of the nursing organization reveals that prospective patients cannot obtain information on nurse leaders, areas with
specialty nurses, nurse-to-patient ratios, staff skill mix,
or advanced practice nurses. This lack of information
390   perpetuates the view of Gordon (2005) that the public
has a poor understanding of the complexity of nursing
care and its influence on patient outcomes and further
supports that information that would enlighten the public on the crucial service it receives from nurses is ba-
395   sically absent from information on hospital Web sites
(Gordon).

Interestingly, today's healthcare consumers are becoming more selective in choosing a hospital and are
seeking information on the quality of agencies and care
400   providers. Yet only one-third of the 15 hospitals in this
sample that had achieved the Magnet status for excellence in nursing elected to place the Magnet symbol on
the hospital home page. If information such as Magnet
status is buried within a Web site, site visitors may not
405   be aware of this recognition of nursing excellence.

All sites had some nurse recruitment content, and
by far, the one category where hospitals excelled was
by providing information on nurse employment opportunities. Surprisingly, only 27 (54%) sites provided job
410   descriptions with information on requirements for education, experience, and skills, which may communicate

that nurses are interchangeable at the agency. Less information was provided on innovative retention strategies. The omission of detailed employment information is a missed opportunity for hospitals to display information that would attract nurses to the agency and perhaps attract individuals into the profession.

Exploration of characteristics of nursing education and research revealed that very few hospital Web sites contained any information on collaborative activities between nursing services in the agencies and schools or colleges of nursing. Such relationships may attract nurses who wish to advance their formal education.

Also, very few sites showcased the organization's nurses. For example, in very few instances were nurses recognized for professional awards or educational achievements. Inclusion of this information would inform nurses about the successes of others, make them feel valuable when their achievements are acknowledged publicly, and communicate to others outside the organization that nurses are supported and valued.

The overall finding that hospital Web sites lack a strong presence of nursing is consistent with the literature (Gordon, 2005; Sigma Theta Tau International, 1997). Hospital marketers have not focused on nurses or nursing care on Web sites but have focused on medicine and employee recruitment (Fell & Shepherd, 2001; Sanchez, 2000; Zingmond et al., 2001). Hospital marketers could collaborate with nurses to ensure the presence of nursing on the Web sites.

Thus, implications for practice center on the involvement of nurses on hospital committees charged with Web site development. Similarly, nurse leaders should collaborate with hospital marketers and Web site developers to ensure that sites promote the nursing profession. Examples of information on nursing on hospital Web sites that should be included are the role of nurses in quality improvement initiatives, specialty areas of care and nurse-patient ratios in these areas, achievements of nursing staff, results of nursing research, and collaborations between nurses and professionals from other disciplines as team members in care delivery. Putting this information on the Web will communicate the important role that nurses play in care delivery, that nurses are valued, and that they are essential members of the healthcare team.

Although nurse-related characteristics were used to denote the presence of nursing in this study, the characteristics that are appropriate and beneficial on hospital Web sites are largely unknown. Further study is needed to determine the important characteristics that should be present on hospital Web sites, including those that are relevant to nursing. This might involve an examination of the checklist developed for this study to verify validity, ensuring that all relevant characteristics and information are captured. In addition, research could show whether the five categories of characteristics and individual characteristics of presence should be weighted in terms of the importance or quality. Finally, studies with larger and more current samples would contribute to advancing our knowledge of the evolving presence of nursing found in this newer form of communication medium by U.S. hospitals.

In keeping with previous research, the lack of visible data in the form of pictures, graphics, or text related to nurses, nursing care, or nursing practice in all communications media must be recognized as a serious concern (Sigma Theta Tau International, 1997). The professional standards upon which nurses base their practice, instead of being advertised, remain unstated, which contributes to the public's lack of comprehension of nurses. This omission sends a message to the public that nurses are not valued as critical members of the healthcare team or as major contributors to hospital services. Hospital Web sites can be used to inform the public of the important role that nurses play in patient outcomes and the role that their collaboration with other disciplines plays to make comprehensive care possible. Because of publicizing the roles and contributions of nurses on hospital Web sites, the nursing profession could attain a visible presence.

## References

Aiken, L. H., Clarke, S. P., Cheung, R. B., Sloane, D. M., & Silber, J. H. (2003). Educational levels of hospital nurses and surgical patient mortality. *Journal of the American Medical Association, 290,* 1617–1623.

Atzeni, P., Merialdo, P., & Sindoni, G. (2002). Web site evaluation: Methodology and case study [Electronic version]. *Lecture Notes in Computer Science, 2465,* 253–263.

Carty, B., Coughlin, C., Kasoff, J., & Sullivan, B. (2000). Where is the nursing presence on the medical center's Web site? *The Journal of Nursing Administration, 30,* 569–570.

Fell, D., & Shepherd, C. D. (2001). Hospitals and the Web: A maturing relationship [Electronic version]. *Marketing Health Services, 21,* 36–38.

Fox, S., & Fallows, D. (2003). *Internet health resources.* Retrieved February 15, 2005, from http://www.pewinternet.org/pdfs/PIP_Health_Report_July_2003.pdf

Gil, P. (n.d.). 2 Layers of visibility, 4 layers of specialization. In *Tutorial: The layers of the World Wide Web.* Retrieved February 19, 2005, from http://netforbeginners.about.com/cs/invisibleweb/a/web_four_layers.htm

Gordon, S. (2005). *Nursing against the odds: How health care cost cutting, media stereotypes, and medical hubris undermine nurses and patient care.* Ithaca, NY: Cornell University Press.

Jones, C. B., & Lusk, S. L. (2002). Incorporating health services research into nursing doctoral programs. *Nursing Outlook, 50,* 225–231.

Kalisch, P. A., & Kalisch, B. J. (1982). Nurses on prime-time television. [Electronic version]. *The American Journal of Nursing, 82,* 264–270.

Kalisch, P. A., & Kalisch, B. J. (1986). A comparative analysis of nurse and physician characters in the entertainment media. [Electronic version]. *Journal of Advanced Nursing, 11,* 179–195.

Kind, T., Wheeler, K. L., Robinson, B., & Cabana, M. D. (2004). Do the leading children's hospitals have quality Web sites? A description of children's hospital Web sites [Electronic version]. *Journal of Medical Internet Research, 6,* e20.

Kovner, C., Jones, C., Zhan, C., Gergen, P. J., & Basu, J. (2002). Nurse staffing and postsurgical adverse events: An analysis of administrative data from a sample of U.S. hospitals, 1990–1996. *Health Services Research, 37,* 611–629.

Morkes, J., & Nielsen, J. (1997). *Concise, SCANNABLE, and objective: How to write for the Web.* Retrieved February 19, 2005, from http://www.useit.com/papers/webwriting/writing.html

Needleman, J., Buerhaus, P., Mattke, S., Stewart, M., & Zelevinsky, K. (2002). Nurse-staffing levels and the quality of care in hospitals. *The New England Journal of Medicine, 346,* 1715–1722.

Page, A. (2004). *Keeping patients safe: Transforming the work environment of nurses.* Committee on the Work Environment for Nurses and Patient Safety. Washington, DC: National Academy Press.

Pirouz, R. (1997). *Click Here. Web Communication Design.* Indianapolis, IN: New Riders.

Sanchez, P. M. (2000). The potential of hospital Web site marketing. *Health Marketing Quarterly, 18,* 45–57.

Sanchez, P. M., & Maier-Donati, P. (1999). Hospital Web site marketing: Analysis, issues, and trends. *Journal of Hospital Marketing, 13*, 87–103.

Sigma Theta Tau International (1997). *The Woodhull study on nursing and the future: Health care's invisible partner (final report).* Indianapolis, IN: Center Nursing Press Sigma Theta Tau International.

Spink, A., Jansen, B. J., Wolfram, D., & Saracevic, T. (2002). From e-sex to e-commerce: Web search changes. *IEEE Computer, 35*, 107–109.

*U.S. News and World Report* (2003). America's best hospitals 2003. Retrieved December 15, 2003, from http://www.usnews.com/usnrew/nycu/health/hosptl/directory/hosp_alph.htm

Weinberg, D. B. (2003). *Code green: Money-driven hospitals and the dismantling of nursing.* Ithaca, NY: Cornell University Press.

Zingmond, D. S., Lim, Y. W., Ettner, S. L., & Carlisle, D. M. (2001). Information superhighway or billboards by the roadside? An analysis of hospital Web sites [Electronic version]. *The Western Journal of Medicine, 175*, 385–391.

**Address correspondence to**: Alice R. Boyington, RN, PhD, School of Nursing, CB 7460, University of North Carolina at Chapel Hill, Chapel Hill, NC 27599-7460. E-mail: ddboying@email.unc.edu

# Exercise for Article 7

## Factual Questions

1. The sample of hospitals for this study represented what percentage of the total population of hospitals?

2. A pilot test was conducted using how many hospital Web sites?

3. How did the researchers define "accessibility"?

4. All 50 sites had at least two occurrences of "visible data." This type of data was in what form?

5. According to the researchers, in what one category did the hospital Web sites "excel"?

6. The researchers explicitly state what implication?

## Questions for Discussion

7. Is it important to know that the additional 17 hospitals were selected at random? Explain. (See lines 115–119.)

8. A sample of the 75 characteristics is shown in Table 1. Is the sample sufficient? Would it help to see all 75? (See lines 141–149 and Table 1.)

9. In your opinion, how important is "accessibility"? (See lines 163–179.)

10. The researchers mention "face validity." What is your understanding of the meaning of this term? (See lines 186–188.)

11. Overall, how helpful are Tables 2 and 3 in giving you an overview of the results of this study? Would the results be as clear without the tables? Explain.

12. In your opinion, how important is the limitation described in lines 323–328?

## Quality Ratings

Directions: Indicate your level of agreement with each of the following statements by circling a number from 5 for strongly agree (SA) to 1 for strongly disagree (SD). If you believe an item is not applicable to this research article, leave it blank. Be prepared to explain your ratings. When responding to criteria A and B, keep in mind that brief titles and abstracts are conventional in published research.

A. The title of the article is appropriate.

    SA   5   4   3   2   1   SD

B. The abstract provides an effective overview of the research article.

    SA   5   4   3   2   1   SD

C. The introduction establishes the importance of the study.

    SA   5   4   3   2   1   SD

D. The literature review establishes the context for the study.

    SA   5   4   3   2   1   SD

E. The research purpose, question, or hypothesis is clearly stated.

    SA   5   4   3   2   1   SD

F. The method of sampling is sound.

    SA   5   4   3   2   1   SD

G. Relevant demographics (for example, age, gender, and ethnicity) are described.

    SA   5   4   3   2   1   SD

H. Measurement procedures are adequate.

    SA   5   4   3   2   1   SD

I. All procedures have been described in sufficient detail to permit a replication of the study.

    SA   5   4   3   2   1   SD

J. The participants have been adequately protected from potential harm.

    SA   5   4   3   2   1   SD

K. The results are clearly described.

    SA   5   4   3   2   1   SD

L.  The discussion/conclusion is appropriate.

SA   5   4   3   2   1   SD

M.  Despite any flaws, the report is worthy of publica-tion.

SA   5   4   3   2   1   SD

# Article 8

# Relationships of Assertiveness, Depression, and Social Support Among Older Nursing Home Residents

**Daniel L. Segal**, PhD[*]

ABSTRACT. This study assessed the relationships of assertiveness, depression, and social support among nursing home residents. The sample included 50 older nursing home residents (mean age = 75 years; 75% female; 92% Caucasian). There was a significant correlation between assertiveness and depression ($r = -.33$), but the correlations between social support and depression ($r = -.15$) and between social support and assertiveness ($r = -.03$) were small and nonsignificant. The correlation between overall physical health (a subjective self-rating) and depression was strong and negative ($r = -.50$), with lower levels of health associated with higher depression. An implication of this study is that an intervention for depression among nursing home residents that is targeted at increasing assertiveness and bolstering health status may be more effective than the one that solely targets social support.

From *Behavior Modification*, 29, 689–695. Copyright © 2005 by Sage Publications. Reprinted with permission.

Most older adults prefer and are successful at "aging in place"—that is, maintaining their independence in their own home. For the frailest and most debilitated older adults, however, nursing home placement is of-
5 tentimes necessary. About 5% of older adults live in a nursing home at any point in time, a figure that has remained stable since the early 1970s (National Center for Health Statistics, 2002). Depression is one of the most prevalent and serious psychological problems
10 among nursing home residents. About 15% to 50% of residents suffer from diagnosable depression (see review by Streim & Katz, 1996).

Social support is also an important factor in mental health among nursing home residents, and psychosocial
15 interventions often seek to bolster the resident's level of supportive relationships.

Assertiveness training plays an important role in traditional behavioral therapy with adults, and it has been recommended as a treatment component among
20 older adults with diverse psychological problems as well (Gambrill, 1986). Assertiveness may be defined as the ability to express one's thoughts, feelings, beliefs, and rights in an open, honest, and appropriate way. A key component of assertiveness is that the communica-
25 tion does not violate the rights of others, as is the case in aggressive communications. It is logical that nursing home residents with good assertiveness skills would more often get what they want and need. Having basic needs met is a natural goal of all people, and failure to
30 do so could lead to depression or other psychological problems. Personal control has long been noted to improve mental health among nursing home residents (see Langer & Rodin, 1976), and assertiveness training would likely help residents express more clearly their
35 desires and needs.

Two studies have examined links between assertiveness, depression, and social support among older adult groups. Among 69 community-dwelling older adults, Kogan, Van Hasselt, Hersen, and Kabacoff
40 (1995) found that those who are less assertive and have less social support are at increased risk for depression. Among 100 visually impaired older adults, Hersen et al. (1995) reported that higher levels of social support and assertiveness were associated with lower levels of
45 depression. Assertiveness may rightly be an important skill among nursing home residents because workers at the institutional setting may not be as attuned to the emotional needs of a passive resident and the workers may respond poorly to the aggressive and acting-out
50 resident. However, little is known about the nature and impact of assertiveness in long-term care settings. The purpose of this study, therefore, was to assess relationships of assertiveness, social support, and depression among nursing home residents, thus extending the lit-
55 erature to a unique population.

## Method

Participants were recruited at several local nursing homes. Staff identified potential volunteers who were ostensibly free of cognitive impairment. Participants

[*]*Daniel L. Segal* received his PhD in clinical psychology from the University of Miami in 1992. He is an associate professor in the Department of Psychology at the University of Colorado at Colorado Springs. His research interests include diagnostic and assessment issues in geropsychology, suicide prevention and aging, bereavement, and personality disorders across the lifespan.

completed anonymously the following self-report measures: Wolpe-Lazarus Assertiveness Scale (WLAS) (Wolpe & Lazarus, 1966), Geriatric Depression Scale (GDS) (Yesavage et al., 1983), and the Social Support List of Interactions (SSL12-I) (Kempen & van Eijk, 1995). The WLAS consists of 30 yes/no items and measures levels of assertive behavior. Scores can range from 0 to 30, with higher scores reflecting higher levels of assertiveness. The GDS includes 30 yes/no items and evaluates depressive symptoms specifically among older adults. Scores can range from 0 to 30, with higher scores indicating higher levels of depression. The SSL12-I is a 12-item measure of received social support that has good psychometric properties among community-dwelling older adults. Respondents indicate on a 4-point scale the extent to which they received a specific type of support from a member of their primary social network (1 = seldom or never, 2 = now and then, 3 = regularly, 4 = very often). Scores can range from 12 to 48 with higher scores corresponding to higher levels of support. The sample included 50 older adult residents (mean age = 74.9 years, $SD$ = 11.9, age range = 50–96 years; 75% female; 92% Caucasian).

## Results and Discussion

The mean WLAS was 18.1 ($SD$ = 4.1), the mean GDS was 9.0 ($SD$ = 5.5), and the mean SSL12-I was 29.2 ($SD$ = 7.3). The correlation between the WLAS and GDS was moderate and negative ($r = -.33$, $p < .05$), with lower levels of assertiveness associated with higher depression. The correlation between the SSL12-I and GDS was small and nonsignificant ($r = -.15$, ns), indicating a slight negative relationship between overall support and depression. Similarly, the correlation between the SSL12-I and WLAS was small and nonsignificant ($r = -.03$, ns), indicating almost no relationship between overall support and assertiveness. Next, correlations between a subjective self-rating of overall physical health status (0–100 scale, higher scores indicating better health) and the WLAS, GDS, and SSL12-I were calculated. As expected, the correlation between physical health and GDS was strong and negative ($r = -.50$, $p < .01$), with poorer health associated with higher depression. The correlation between health and WLAS was positive in direction but small and nonsignificant ($r = .17$, ns), indicating little relationship between health and assertiveness. Similarly, the correlation between health and SSL12-I was also small and nonsignificant ($r = -.02$, ns), indicating no relationship between health and overall support. The slight relationship between health and assertiveness is an encouraging sign because it suggests that assertiveness (which is primarily achieved through effective verbalizations) is not limited to only the least physically impaired nursing home residents. Finally, gender differences on all dependent measures were examined (independent $t$ tests) and no significant differences were found (all $ps$ > .05).

Notably, the mean assertion and depression scores among nursing home residents are consistent with means on identical measures in community-dwelling older adults (assertion $M$ = 19.1; depression $M$ = 7.9; Kogan et al., 1995) and visually impaired older adults (assertion $M$ = 18.3; depression $M$ = 10.4; Hersen et al., 1995), suggesting that the higher-functioning group of nursing home residents are no more depressed and no less assertive than other samples of older persons. Regarding social support, our nursing home sample appeared to show somewhat higher levels of overall support than community older adults in the normative sample ($N$ = 5,279, $M$ = 25.5) in the SSL12-I validation study (Kempen & van Eijk, 1995). This may possibly be due to the nature of institutional living and the large numbers of support staff and health care personnel.

The correlational results regarding the moderate negative association between assertion and depression are consistent with data from community-dwelling older adults ($r = -.36$; Kogan et al., 1995) and visually impaired older adults ($r = -.29$; Hersen et al., 1995), suggesting a pervasive relationship among the variables in diverse older adult samples and extending the findings to nursing home residents. Contrary to the literature, the relationship between social support and depression among nursing home residents was weaker than the one reported in community-dwelling older adults ($r = -.50$; Kogan et al., 1995) and visually impaired older adults ($r = -.48$; Hersen et al., 1995). The relationship between assertiveness and overall support in this study was almost nonexistent, also contrary to earlier reports in which the relationship was moderate and positive in direction. Our results are consistent with prior research showing no gender differences among older adults in assertiveness, depression, and social support using similar assessment tools (Hersen et al., 1995; Kogan et al., 1995). This study also suggests a strong negative relationship between health status and depression among nursing home residents. An implication of this study is that an intervention for depression among nursing home residents that is targeted at increasing assertiveness and bolstering health status may be more effective than the one that solely targets social support.

Several limitations are offered concerning this study. First, the sample size was modest and the sample was almost exclusively Caucasian. Future studies with more diverse nursing home residents would add to the knowledge base in this area. All measures were self-report, and future studies with structured interviews and behavioral assessments would be stronger. We are also concerned somewhat about the extent to which the WLAS is content-valid for older adults. Notably, a measure of assertive behavior competence has been developed specifically for use with community-

dwelling older adults (Northrop & Edelstein, 1998), and this measure appears to be a good choice for future research in the area. A final limitation was that partici-
175 pants were likely the highest-functioning of residents because they were required to be able to complete the measures independently and were selected out if there was any overt cognitive impairment (although no formal screening for cognitive impairment was done),
180 thus limiting generalizability to more frail nursing home residents. Cognitive screening should be done in future studies. Nonetheless, results of this study suggest a potentially important relationship between assertiveness and depression among nursing home residents.
185     Finally, it is imperative to highlight that there are many types of interventions to combat depression among nursing home residents: behavioral interventions to increase exercise, participation in social activities, and other pleasurable activities; cognitive inter-
190 ventions to reduce depressogenic thoughts; and pharmacotherapy, to name a few. (The interested reader is referred to Molinari, 2000, for a comprehensive description of psychological issues and interventions unique to long-term care settings.) The present data
195 suggest that training in assertiveness may be yet one additional option for psychosocial intervention in nursing homes. A controlled outcome study is warranted in which intensive assertiveness training is compared to a control group of nursing home residents who do not
200 receive such training. Only with such a study can cause-and-effect statements be made about the role that assertiveness skills training may play in the reduction of depressive symptoms among nursing home residents.

### References

Gambrill, E. B. (1986). Social skills training with the elderly. In C. R. Hollin & P. Trower (Eds.), *Handbook of social skills training: Applications across the lifespan* (pp. 211–238). New York: Pergamon.

Hersen, M., Kabacoff, R. L., Van Hasselt, V. B., Null, J. A., Ryan, C. F., Melton, M. A., et al. (1995). Assertiveness, depression, and social support in older visually impaired adults. *Journal of Visual Impairment and Blindness, 7*, 524–530.

Kempen, G. I. J. M., & van Eijk, L. M. (1995). The psychometric properties of the SSL12-I, a short scale for measuring social support in the elderly. *Social Indicators Research, 35*, 303–312.

Kogan, S. E., Van Hasselt, B. V., Hersen, M., & Kabacoff, I. R. (1995). Relationship of depression, assertiveness, and social support in community-dwelling older adults. *Journal of Clinical Geropsychology, 1*, 157–163.

Langer, E. J., & Rodin, J. (1976). The effects of choice and enhanced personal responsibility for the aged: A field experiment in an institutional setting. *Journal of Personality and Social Psychology, 34*, 191–198.

Molinari, V. (Ed.). (2000). *Professional psychology in long-term care: A comprehensive guide.* New York: Hatherleigh.

National Center for Health Statistics. (2002). *Health, United States, 2002.* Hyattsville, MD: Author.

Northrop, L. M. E., & Edelstein, B. A. (1998). An assertive-behavior competence inventory for older adults. *Journal of Clinical Geropsychology, 4*, 315–331.

Streim, J. E., & Katz, I. R. (1996). Clinical psychiatry in the nursing home. In E. W. Busse & D. G. Blazer (Eds.), *Textbook of geriatric psychiatry* (2nd ed., pp. 413–432). Washington, DC: American Psychiatric Press.

Wolpe, J., & Lazarus, A. A. (1966). *Behavior therapy techniques.* New York: Pergamon.

Yesavage, J. A., Brink, T. L., Rose, T. L., Lum, O., Huang, V., Adey, M., et al. (1983). Development and validation of a geriatric depression screening scale: A preliminary report. *Journal of Psychiatric Research, 17*, 314–317.

**Acknowledgment**: The author thanks Jessica Corcoran, MA, for assistance with data collection and data entry.

# Exercise for Article 8

## Factual Questions

1. Were the participants cognitively impaired?

2. Was the mean score for the participants on the GDS near the highest possible score on this instrument? Explain.

3. What is the value of the correlation coefficient for the relationship between the WLAS and the GDS?

4. Was the relationship between SSL12-I and GDS strong?

5. Was the correlation coefficient for the relationship between SSL12-I and GDS statistically significant?

6. Was the relationship between physical health and GDS a direct relationship *or* an inverse relationship?

## Questions for Discussion

7. The researcher obtained participants from "several" nursing homes. Is this better than obtaining them from a single nursing home? Explain. (See lines 56–57.)

8. The researcher characterizes the *r* of −.33 in line 86 as "moderate." Do you agree with this characterization? Explain.

9. In lines 85–107, the researcher reports the values of six correlation coefficients. Which one of these indicates the strongest relationship? Explain the basis for your choice.

10. In lines 85–107, the researcher reports the values of six correlation coefficients. Which one of these indicates the weakest relationship? Explain the basis for your choice.

11. For the *r* of −.50 in line 100, the researcher indicates that "*p* < .01." What is your understanding of the meaning of the symbol "*p*"? What is your understanding of ".01"?

12. Do you agree with the researcher that a different type of study is needed in order to determine the role of assertiveness skills training in the reduction of depressive symptoms? Explain. (See lines 197–204.)

## Quality Ratings

Directions: Indicate your level of agreement with each of the following statements by circling a number from 5 for strongly agree (SA) to 1 for strongly disagree (SD). If you believe an item is not applicable to this research article, leave it blank. Be prepared to explain your ratings. When responding to criteria A and B, keep in mind that brief titles and abstracts are conventional in published research.

A.   The title of the article is appropriate.

SA   5   4   3   2   1   SD

B.   The abstract provides an effective overview of the research article.

SA   5   4   3   2   1   SD

C.   The introduction establishes the importance of the study.

SA   5   4   3   2   1   SD

D.   The literature review establishes the context for the study.

SA   5   4   3   2   1   SD

E.   The research purpose, question, or hypothesis is clearly stated.

SA   5   4   3   2   1   SD

F.   The method of sampling is sound.

SA   5   4   3   2   1   SD

G.   Relevant demographics (for example, age, gender, and ethnicity) are described.

SA   5   4   3   2   1   SD

H.   Measurement procedures are adequate.

SA   5   4   3   2   1   SD

I.   All procedures have been described in sufficient detail to permit a replication of the study.

SA   5   4   3   2   1   SD

J.   The participants have been adequately protected from potential harm.

SA   5   4   3   2   1   SD

K.   The results are clearly described.

SA   5   4   3   2   1   SD

L.   The discussion/conclusion is appropriate.

SA   5   4   3   2   1   SD

M.   Despite any flaws, the report is worthy of publication.

SA   5   4   3   2   1   SD

# Article 9

# Extending Work Environment Research Into Home Health Settings

**Linda Flynn**, PhD, RN[*]

ABSTRACT. Organizational attributes in work environments that support nursing practice are theoretically associated with superior nurse and patient outcomes, and lower frequencies of adverse events. This study explored associations between organizational support for nursing practice in home health care agencies and (a) the frequency of nurse-reported adverse events, (b) nurse-assessed quality of care, (c) nurse job satisfaction, and (d) nurses' intentions to leave their employing agency. Data were collected from a sample of 137 registered nurses employed as home health staff nurses in the United States and analyzed using descriptive techniques and bivariate correlation. As anticipated, organizational support for nursing was negatively associated with nurse-reported adverse patient events and intent to leave, and positively associated with nurse-assessed quality of care and job satisfaction. These findings may be helpful to nursing administrators who seek to create work environments in home health agencies that maximize patient outcomes and nurse satisfaction.

From *Western Journal of Nursing Research, 29,* 200–212. Copyright © 2007 by Sage Publications. Reprinted with permission.

A large body of literature indicates that the presence of a set of organizational attributes of the nursing work environment, highly valued by hospital-based staff nurses as important to the support of their professional practice, are associated with positive inpatient outcomes and lower rates of adverse events, including mortality (Aiken, Havens, & Sloane, 2000). Although recent studies have demonstrated that this same set of supportive work environment attributes is similarly valued by staff nurses who practice in the rapidly expanding arena of home health care, few studies have investigated the associations between these supportive attributes and home care outcomes. Using survey methodology, the current study is among the first to explore associations between organizational attributes that support nursing practice, as indicative of a supportive work environment, and nurse-reported adverse patient events in home health care.

According to sociological theories of organizations and professions, organizational attributes in health care settings that support clinical practice—such as decentralization of authority, managerial support, interdisciplinary collaboration, continuity of care, effective communication channels, and adequate resources—are essential to the ability of clinicians, such as nurses, to identify and respond to fluctuating patient conditions. Thus, by supporting clinical surveillance and response, these organizational attributes contribute to high-quality patient care. Theorists further propose that health care organizations that exhibit these supportive attributes will experience higher rates of positive patient outcomes, fewer adverse patient events, and higher levels of job satisfaction and retention among clinical staff (Flood & Scott, 1987; Freidson, 1970; Peters & McKeon, 1998; Shortell & Kaluzny, 1988; Strauss, 1975).

During the past two decades, a large body of literature has been amassed providing empirical support for these propositions. Measured by the Nursing Work Index–Revised (NWI-R; Aiken & Patrician, 2000), attributes of the nursing work environment that support professional practice have been linked to higher levels of job satisfaction, lower rates of burnout, lower rates of needlestick injuries, and lower rates of injury-related disability among hospital-based staff nurses (Aiken, Clarke, & Sloane, 2002; Aiken & Sloane, 1997; Clarke, Sloane, & Aiken, 2002; Laschinger, Almost, & Ther-Hodes, 2003; O'Brien-Pallas et al., 2004; Tigert & Laschinger, 2004). The presence of these supportive work environment attributes has also been associated with a higher level of quality inpatient care, fewer adverse events, lower mortality, and higher levels of satisfaction with care among hospitalized patients (Aiken, Sloane, & Lake, 1997; Aiken, Sloane, Lake, Sochalski, & Weber, 1999; Aiken, Smith, & Lake, 1994; Boyle, 2004; Estabrooks, Midodzi, Cummings, Ricker, & Giovannetti, 2005; Flynn & Aiken, 2002; Vahey, Aiken, Sloane, Clarke, & Vargas, 2004).

From these theoretical and empirical foundations, a conceptual model of nursing organization and outcomes was developed (Aiken, Lake, Sochalski, & Sloane, 1997) and later refined (Aiken, Clarke, & Sloane, 2002). The model conceptualizes *organiza-*

[*]*Linda Flynn* is an assistant professor at The New Jersey Collaborating Center for Nursing, College of Nursing, Rutgers, State University of New Jersey, at Newark.

*tional support* for nursing practice and nurse staffing levels, indicated by nurse-to-patient ratios, as related but distinct variables (Figure 1). *Organizational support for nursing practice*, defined as a set of core attributes of a supportive work environment that are modifiable through managerial decisions, includes those organizational attributes pertaining to (a) resource adequacy, (b) nurse autonomy, (c) nurse control of practice environment, and (d) facilitation of collegial nurse-physician relationships. According to the conceptual model, nurses provide clinical surveillance and early detection of adverse patient events and attempt to modify processes of care based on these assessments. The model further indicates that higher organizational support for nursing practice directly influences and enhances the processes and quality of care, promoting superior nurse and patient outcomes (Aiken, Clarke, & Sloane, 2002).

The research regarding supportive organizational attributes and outcomes has been conducted predominantly in hospitals. Although the empirical literature regarding supportive organizational attributes has guided efforts of hospital nursing administrators to create work environments that promote positive outcomes and prevent adverse events, administrators in the rapidly growing practice area of home health care have had little evidence to guide similar endeavors. This is unfortunate, as nursing leaders in home health care increasingly recognize the need to implement evidence-based initiatives within their agencies that support nursing practice, enhance nurse retention, promote quality patient care, and maximize positive patient outcomes (Ellenbecker & Cushman, 2001; Shaughnessy et al., 2002; Smith-Stoner, 2004). Prompted by recent federal initiatives that monitor the degree to which several selected patient outcomes are achieved, home care administrators are particularly interested in promoting patients' safe self-administration of medications, the effective management of acute and chronic pain, the prevention of unplanned hospitalizations, and the ability of patients to be maintained safely in the community on discharge from home health care services (Centers for Medicare and Medicaid Services [CMS], 2005; Shaughnessy et al., 2002).

Although recent studies (Flynn, Carryer, & Budge, 2005; Flynn & Deatrick, 2003) indicate that home care staff nurses similarly value the same set of supportive work environment attributes that are valued by hospital-based staff nurses, relationships between supportive work environments and positive staff and patient outcomes as proposed by sociological theories of organizations and professions (Flood & Scott, 1987; Freidson, 1970; Shortell & Kaluzny, 1988; Strauss, 1975), and as depicted by the nursing organization and outcomes model (Aiken, Clarke, & Sloane, 2002), have rarely been tested in home health care.

## Purpose of the Study

The purpose of the current study was to preliminarily explore a subset of relationships depicted by the nursing organization and outcomes model. Associations between organizational support for nursing practice, as an indicator of a supportive work environment, in home health care agencies and (a) nurse-assessed quality of care; (b) adverse patient outcomes, such as nurse-reported frequencies of patient-administered medication errors, uncontrolled acute or chronic pain, unplanned hospitalization, and lack of preparation of patient or family member to manage care at time of discharge; (c) nurse job satisfaction; and (d) nurses' intentions to leave were investigated.

## Operational Definitions

Consistent with the model of nursing organization and outcomes, *a supportive nursing work environment* was operationally defined as a score on the Organizational Support for Nursing subscale of the Nursing Work Index–Revised (Aiken, Clarke, & Sloane, 2002); higher scores indicate a more supportive work environment. A score on a 4-point rating scale operationally defined *job satisfaction* and *nurses' assessment of the quality of care* provided by their home care agency. The frequencies of (a) patient-administered medication errors, (b) uncontrolled acute or chronic pain, (c) unplanned hospitalization while receiving home health services, and (d) patient and/or family's lack of preparation to manage care at the time of discharge from home health care services were also operationally defined as scores on 4-point rating scales. The intent to leave an employing home health agency was operationally defined by a response to an item that elicited the respondents' intentions to resign from their current home health care agency within the next 12 months.

## Design

The current study utilized a descriptive, correlational design. A modified Dillman (2000) survey method was used for data collection.

## Sample

To obtain a sample of registered nurses (RNs) currently employed in home health staff nurse positions, 645 names were randomly selected to receive a mailed research packet from a list of subscribers to a prominent journal for home health care nurses. All 645 of the randomly selected subscribers resided in the United States. A total of 25 surveys were returned by the post office as undeliverable. Of the 620 delivered surveys, a response rate of 52.4% produced surveys from 325 nurse respondents. Among these respondents, 68 indicated that they no longer practiced in home health care, and an additional 120 indicated that although they worked in home health care, they were not employed in staff RN positions. Thus, the sample for the current study consisted of 137 RNs, employed as home health staff nurses, from 38 states. A total of 59% of respon-

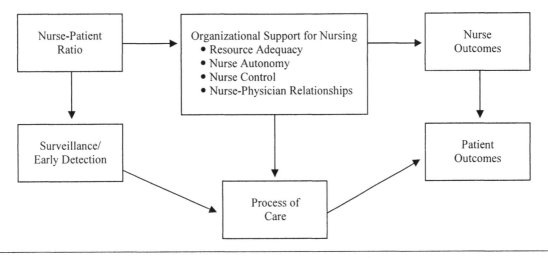

*Figure 1.* Aiken, Clarke, and Sloane (2002). Hospital staffing, organization, and quality of care: Cross-national findings. International Journal for Quality in Health Care, 14(1), 5 and 13. By permission of Oxford University Press.

dents worked full-time, 25% worked part-time, and 16% worked on a per-diem basis. Other demographic characteristics are presented in Table 1.

Table 1
*Sample Characteristics (N = 137)*

| Variable | M | SD |
|---|---|---|
| Age | 50.35 | 9.29 |
| Years at employing agency | 9.92 | 7.67 |

| | n | % |
|---|---|---|
| Gender | | |
| Female | 134 | 97.8 |
| Male | 3 | 2.2 |
| Race | | |
| White | 121 | 88.3 |
| African American | 6 | 4.4 |
| Hispanic | 2 | 1.5 |
| Asian/Pacific Islander | 4 | 2.9 |
| Native American | 2 | 1.5 |
| Not reported | 2 | 1.5 |
| Nursing education | | |
| Diploma | 17 | 12.4 |
| Associate degree | 44 | 32.1 |
| BSN | 53 | 38.7 |
| MSN or higher | 22 | 16.1 |
| Not reported | 1 | 0.7 |

*Note.* BSN = bachelor of science in nursing; MSN = master of science in nursing.

## Method

A key methodological feature of previous hospital-based work environment research has been the use of nurse surveys as a source of data regarding organizational attributes (Aiken, Clarke, & Sloane, 2002; Aiken, Clarke, Sloane, Sochalski, & Silber, 2002) and nurse-reported patient outcomes (Sochalski, 2001, 2004). Staff RNs have been identified as reliable informants regarding organizational attributes and patient outcomes because of their close proximity to patients and their familiarity with the organizational features present in their work environment. Therefore, extending work environment research into home health care,

the current study surveyed staff RNs using the same survey items and measures that have been demonstrated reliable and valid in previous hospital-based research (Aiken, Clarke, Sloane, & Sochalski, 2001; Aiken, Clarke, Sloane, Sochalski, Busse et al., 2001; Sochalski, 2001, 2004).

To ensure that rights of participants were protected, the study protocol was reviewed and approved by the university's Institutional Review Board prior to data collection. Selected subscribers to a home health care nursing journal received a research packet, mailed to their home, which contained a cover letter and survey. In accordance with a modified Dillman (2000) survey method, a reminder postcard was mailed 1 week after the packet was sent, a repeat survey was sent to nonrespondents 2 weeks after the initial survey mailing, and a final reminder postcard was sent to the remaining nonrespondents 4 weeks after the initial survey mailing.

### Measures

The Organizational Support for Nursing subscale, a 9-item subset of the NWI-R, was used to measure the organization's support for nursing practice, defined as a set of core attributes of a supportive work environment that are modifiable through managerial decision-making (Aiken, Clarke, & Sloane, 2002). The Organizational Support for Nursing subscale contains items measuring the presence of modifiable organizational features, influenced by administrative decisions, including (a) resource adequacy, (b) nurse autonomy, (c) nurse control over the practice environment, and (d) nurse-physician relationships. Nurses were asked to rate the degree to which each item on the subscale is present in their current home health care agency; they were not requested to identify their employing home health agency by name or location. Using a summative rating scale ranging from 1 (*strongly disagree* the attribute is present) to 4 (*strongly agree* the attribute is

Table 2
*Descriptive Statistics and Correlation Coefficients of Organization Support and Study Variables (N = 137)*

| Variable | Minimum | Maximum | M | SD | Pearson Correlation |
|---|---|---|---|---|---|
| Job satisfaction | 1 | 4 | 2.87 | .96 | .31*** |
| Care quality | 1 | 4 | 3.37 | .65 | .49*** |
| Medication errors | 1 | 4 | 2.36 | .76 | −.22** |
| Uncontrolled pain | 1 | 4 | 2.41 | .84 | −.30*** |
| Unprepared at discharge | 1 | 4 | 2.28 | .95 | −.35*** |
| Hospitalization | 1 | 4 | 2.90 | .68 | −.13 |

**$p < .01$, ***$p < .001$ (2-tailed).

225 present), possible scores range from 9 to 36. Higher scores indicate a higher organizational support for nursing practice. The validity of the subscale was demonstrated in samples of hospital-based nurses (Aiken & Patrician, 2000), and in samples of U.S. home care and
230 district nurses in New Zealand (Flynn, 2003; Flynn, Carryer, & Budge, 2005; Flynn & Deatrick, 2003). An internal consistency reliability of .91 was observed in a sample of 10,319 hospital-based nurses. In the current study, the internal consistency reliability coefficient
235 was .84 in the sample of home care RNs.

The survey also included items, found to be reliable in previous research, that elicit nurses' responses regarding the frequency of adverse patient events (Aiken, Clarke, Sloane, & Sochalski, 2001; Sochalski, 2001,
240 2004). For the current study, some of these items underwent minor changes in wording to reflect home care practice. The adverse events selected for the current study are prevalent among care patients sensitive to organizational support, and their reduction has been
245 identified by the Centers for Medicare and Medicaid (CMS) as important quality indicators in home health care practice (CMS, 2005; Shaughnessy et al., 2002). Home care staff nurses were instructed to rate on a 4-point scale, from 1 (*never*) to 4 (*frequently*), how often
250 these events occurred to patients in their caseload during the past year.

As a measure of job satisfaction, a single item asked nurses to rate the level of satisfaction with their job on a 4-point scale ranging from 1 (*very dissatisfied*)
255 to 4 (*very satisfied*). Similarly, a single item with a 4-point rating scale ranging from 1 (*poor*) to 4 (*excellent*) measured nurses' assessment of the quality of care delivered by their home health care agency. Nurses' intent to leave was measured by an item asking respon-
260 dents to indicate if they do or do not have plans to leave their home health agency within the next 12 months. These global items, which in the current study substituted the word *home health care agency* for *hospital*, have been repeatedly used as measures among
265 hospital-based nurses and have consistently correlated with theoretically relevant variables (Aiken, Clarke, & Sloane, 2002; Aiken, Clarke, Sloane, Sochalski, Busse et al., 2001; Sochalski, 2001, 2004).

*Analysis of Data*
Correlation coefficients were determined between

270 organizational support and (a) quality of care, (b) reported frequency of each adverse event, and (c) nurse job satisfaction. A logistic regression model estimated the effects of organizational support and job satisfaction on nurses' intent to leave. The demographic vari-
275 ables of level of nursing education and age have been identified in theoretical models as key individual nurse characteristics that may influence intent to leave (Ellenbecker, 2004; Lake, 1998). To control for these individual characteristics, the demographic variables of
280 age and nursing education were included in the regression model.

**Findings**
Descriptive information for study variables and bivariate correlation coefficients between organizational support and study variables are presented in Ta-
285 ble 2. The mean organizational support score and standard deviation for this sample, $M = 25.94$ ($SD = 4.98$), were slightly higher than those published for hospitals on the same measure, which ranged from $M = 21.6$ ($SD = 1.8$) to $M = 23.0$ ($SD = .9$), across 303 international
290 hospitals (Aiken, Clarke, & Sloane, 2002). As anticipated, organizational support for nursing, as an indicator of a supportive work environment, was positively correlated with job satisfaction and nurse-assessed quality of care, and negatively correlated with reported
295 frequencies of patient-administered medication errors, uncontrolled acute or chronic pain, and the inability of patients and/or family members to manage care on discharge from home health care services. Results indicated no significant correlation between organizational
300 support and the frequency of unplanned hospitalization.

Regarding nurses' intentions to leave their agency, logistic regression was used to estimate the effects of organizational support and job satisfaction on nurses' intentions to leave, controlling for the demographic
305 variables of age and nursing education. Among the two demographic variables, only nurses' *level of education*, defined as the highest nursing degree obtained, was significantly associated with intent to leave, in that nurses with a baccalaureate degree were significantly
310 less likely to indicate an intent to leave than nurses with a master's degree or higher, odds ratio (OR) = .086 (.008, .963), $p = .047$. Although job satisfaction had no significant effect on intent to leave, organizational support was a significant predictor of nurses'

315 intentions to leave their agency, OR = .792 (.692, .907), *p* = .001. The odds of intent to leave decreased as the score on the Organizational Support for Nursing subscale increased, indicating that higher organizational support for nursing was associated with lower

320 odds on nurses' intentions to leave their employing agency. To interpret this association within a context of nurse retention, for every 1-point increase on the Organizational Support for Nursing subscale, the odds of nurses not planning to leave their agency increased by

325 26%, OR = 1.26 (1.10, 1.44), *p* = .001.

## Discussion

Hospital-based work environment research has made significant contributions to the health services and nursing literatures regarding the impact of organizational attributes on nurses and patients. The current

330 study is among the first to extend this line of inquiry into the home health care practice setting. Findings from the current study are consistent with the nursing organization and outcomes model (Aiken, Clarke, & Sloane, 2002) and indicate that the presence of attrib-

335 utes in nurses' work environments that reflect organizational support for nursing practice is associated with higher levels of nurse-reported quality of care, fewer nurse-reported adverse patient events, higher nurse job satisfaction, and lower odds of nurses' intentions to

340 leave their employer.

Home health care administrators should carefully consider such findings. Throughout recent years, efforts to control costs have resulted in widespread organizational changes among some home health care

345 agencies, including reductions in support services, disruptions in continuity of patient assignments, limitations in nurses' influence over practice decisions, and reductions in the number of middle-management positions that consequently limit nurses' managerial sup-

350 port (Narayan, 1999; Smith, Maloy, & Hawkins, 2000; Smith-Stoner, 2004). It is ironic to note that many of these managerial-induced changes adversely affect those organizational attributes that provide support for nursing practice, and that were associated in the current

355 study with fewer adverse events.

Study results also indicate that the presence of agency attributes reflecting organizational support for nursing are associated with higher levels of nurse job satisfaction, and reduced odds on nurses' intentions to

360 leave their employing home health agency. These findings may prove helpful to nursing administrators in home health care agencies that are becoming increasingly challenged by a shortfall of nursing staff. Estimates indicate that by 2020, the demand for home care

365 nurses will reach a peak in that the number of RNs needed for home care practice will be twice the number needed in 2000. Unfortunately, this peak demand for home care nurses will occur at a time when the United States will have an estimated shortfall of one million

370 nurses across practice sectors. Many home care agen-

cies are already experiencing difficulty recruiting and retaining nurses, as evidenced by rising attrition and vacancy rates nationwide (Humphrey, 2005; U.S. General Accounting Office, 2001). Results from the current

375 study indicate the implementation and maintenance of agency attributes that support nursing practice may increase nurse retention. Consequently, administrative initiatives undertaken in home health agencies to ensure adequate support services for clinical staff, access

380 to competent and supportive managers, continuity of patient assignments, and facilitation of interdisciplinary collaboration appear to be worth the investment in light of the potential benefits.

No relationship was found in the current study be-

385 tween organizational support and nurse-reported frequencies of unplanned hospitalizations. This relationship can be further explored in subsequent larger studies linking work environment attributes with patient-level data.

390 Some limitations of the current study should be noted. Although nurses are considered reliable informants regarding their patients' experiences and conditions, individual nurses' reports regarding the frequency of adverse events may be inaccurate or biased.

395 A second limitation is that the relatively small sample size limits analytic power. Third, because the study was not designed to obtain responses from multiple nurses employed in identifiable agencies, aggregation of measures to the organizational level was not possi-

400 ble. To prevent these limitations, subsequent larger and more comprehensive studies can be designed that sample large numbers of nurses from each agency, aggregate responses to the organizational level, and link organizational-level estimates of study variables with

405 risk-adjusted, patient-level outcome data.

Despite the limitations, the current study provides preliminary evidence for the relationships between attributes of the nursing work environment that reflect organizational support for nursing and nurses' reports

410 regarding the frequencies of adverse patient events in home health care. By creating work environments that support nursing practice, the home health care sector may make significant strides toward achieving two important aims—retaining a nursing workforce suffi-

415 cient in size to meet the growing demand, and reducing adverse events among the vulnerable recipients of home health care services.

## References

Aiken, L. H., Clarke, S. P., & Sloane, D. M. (2002). Hospital staffing, organization, and quality of care: Cross-national findings. *International Journal for Quality in Health Care, 4*, 5–13.

Aiken, L. H., Clarke, S. P., Sloane, D. M., & Sochalski, J. A. (2001). An international perspective on hospital nurses' work environments: The case for reform. *Policy, Politics, & Nursing Practice, 2*, 255–263.

Aiken, L. H., Clarke, S. P., Sloane, D. M., Sochalski, J. A., Busse, R., Clarke, H., et al. (2001). Nurses' reports on hospital care in five countries. *Health Affairs, 20*, 43–53.

Aiken, L. H., Clarke, S. P., Sloane, D. M., Sochalski, J., & Silber, J. H. (2002). Hospital nurse staffing and patient mortality, nurse burnout, and job dissatisfaction. *Journal of the American Medical Association, 288*, 1987–1993.

Aiken, L. H., Havens, D. S., & Sloane, D. M. (2000). The Magnet Nursing Services Recognition Program: A comparison of two groups of Magnet hospitals. *American Journal of Nursing, 100,* 26–36.

Aiken, L. H., Lake, E. T., Sochalski, J., & Sloane, D. M. (1997). Design of an outcomes study of the organization of hospital AIDS care. *Research in the Sociology of Health Care, 14,* 3–26.

Aiken, L. H., & Patrician, P. (2000). Measuring organizational attributes of hospitals: The revised Nursing Work Index. *Nursing Research, 49,* 146–153.

Aiken, L. H., & Sloane, D. M. (1997). Effects of organizational innovations in AIDS care on burnout among urban hospital nurses. *Work and Occupations, 24,* 453–477.

Aiken, L. H., Sloane, D. M., & Lake, E. T. (1997). Satisfaction with inpatient acquired immunodeficiency syndrome care. *Medical Care, 35,* 948–962.

Aiken, L. H., Sloane, D. M., Lake, E. T., Sochalski, J. A., & Weber, A. L. (1999). Organization and outcomes of inpatient AIDS care. *Medical Care, 37,* 760–772.

Aiken, L. H., Smith, H. L., & Lake, E. T. (1994). Lower Medicare mortality among a set of hospitals known for good nursing care. *Medical Care, 32,* 771–787.

Boyle, S. M. (2004). Nursing unit characteristics and patient outcomes. *Nursing Economics, 22,* 111–123.

Centers for Medicare and Medicaid Services. (2005). Home health compare. Retrieved October 14, 2005, from www.cms.hhs.gov/quality/hhqi/september2005Revisons.pdf

Clarke, S. P., Sloane, D. M., & Aiken, L. H. (2002). Effects of hospital staffing and organizational climate on needlestick injuries to nurses. *American Journal of Public Health, 92,* 1115–1119.

Dillman, D. A. (2000). *Mail and Internet surveys: The tailored design method.* New York: John Wiley.

Ellenbecker, C. H. (2004). A theoretical model of job retention for home health care nurses. *Journal of Advanced Nursing, 47,* 303–310.

Ellenbecker, C., & Cushman, M. J. (2001, July). The nursing shortage: A home care agency perspective. *Caring, 20,* 28–32.

Estabrooks, C. A., Midodzi, W. K., Cummings, G. G., Ricker, K. L., & Giovannetti, P. (2005). The impact of hospital nursing characteristics on 30-day mortality. *Nursing Research, 54,* 74–84.

Flood, A. B., & Scott, W. R. (1987). *Hospital structure and performance.* Baltimore: Johns Hopkins University Press.

Flynn, L. (2003). Agency characteristics most valued by home care nurses: Findings of a nationwide survey. *Home Healthcare Nurse, 21,* 812–817.

Flynn, L., & Aiken, L. H. (2002). Does international nurse recruitment influence practice values in U.S. hospitals? *Journal of Nursing Scholarship, 34,* 67–73.

Flynn, L., Carryer, J., & Budge, C. (2005). Organizational attributes valued by hospital, home care, and district nurses in the United States and New Zealand. *Journal of Nursing Scholarship, 37,* 67–72.

Flynn, L., & Deatrick, J. A. (2003). Home care nurses' descriptions of important agency attributes. *Journal of Nursing Scholarship, 35,* 385–390.

Freidson, E. (1970). *Profession of medicine.* New York: Dodd, Mead.

Humphrey, C. (2005). Exciting new research on recruitment and retention. *Home Healthcare Nurse, 23,* 347.

Lake, E. T. (1998). Advances in understanding and predicting nurse turnover. *Research in the Sociology of Health Care, 15,* 147–171.

Laschinger, H. K., Almost, J., & Ther-Hodes, D. (2003). Workplace empowerment and magnet hospital characteristics: Making the link. *Journal of Nursing Administration, 33,* 410–422.

Narayan, M. C. (1999). Survey highlights the concerns of home healthcare nurses. *Home Healthcare Nurse, 17,* 57.

O'Brien-Pallas, L., Shamian, J., Thomson, D., Alksnis, C., Koehoorn, M., Kerr, M., et al. (2004). Work related disability in Canadian nurses. *Journal of Nursing Scholarship, 36,* 352–357.

Peters, D. A., & McKeon, T. (1998). *Transforming home care: Quality, cost, and data management.* Gaithersburg, MD: Aspen.

Shaughnessy, P. W., Hittle, D. F., Crisler, K. S., Powell, M. C., Richard, A. A., Kramer, A. M., et al. (2002). Improving patient outcomes of home health care: Findings from two demonstration trials of outcome-based quality improvement. *Journal of the American Geriatrics Society, 50,* 1354–1364.

Shortell, S. M., & Kaluzny, A. D. (Eds.). (1988). *Health care management: A text in organizational theory and behavior.* New York: John Wiley.

Smith, B. M., Maloy, K. A., & Hawkins, D. J. (2000). An examination of Medicare home health services. *Care Management Journals, 2,* 238–247.

Smith-Stoner, M. (2004). Home care nurses' perceptions of agency and supervisory characteristics: Working in the rain. *Home Healthcare Nurse, 22,* 536–546.

Sochalski, J. A. (2001). Quality of care, nurse staffing, and patient outcomes. *Policy, Politics, and Nursing Practice, 2,* 9–18.

Sochalski, J. A. (2004). Is more better? The relationship between nurse staffing and the quality of nursing care in hospitals. *Medical Care, 42*(2 Supp), 1167–1172.

Strauss, A. (1975). *Professions, work and careers.* New Brunswick, NJ: Transaction Books.

Tigert, J. A., & Laschinger, H. K. S. (2004). Critical care nurses' perceptions of workplace empowerment, magnet hospital attributes, and mental health. *Dynamics, 15,* 19–23.

U.S. General Accounting Office. (2001, July). *Nursing workforce: Emerging nursing shortages due to multiple factors* (GAO-01-944). Retrieved October 17, 2005, from www.gao.gov/new.items/d011944.pdf

Vahey, D. C., Aiken, L. H., Sloane, D. M., Clarke, S. P., & Vargas, D. (2004). Nurse burnout and patient satisfaction. *Medical Care, 42*(2, Suppl. II), 57–66.

**Acknowledgment:** This study was funded by a research grant from Rutgers College of Nursing.

# Exercise for Article 9

## *Factual Questions*

1. How was "a supportive nursing work environment" operationally defined by the researcher?

2. The samples from this study were from how many states?

3. When was the repeat survey sent to nonrespondents?

4. What is the value of the Pearson correlation coefficient for the relationship between job satisfaction and organizational support? Is it statistically significant?

5. Which one of the study variables had the strongest relationship with organizational support as indicated by the Pearson correlation coefficients?

6. Was there a significant correlation between organizational support and frequency of unplanned hospitalization?

## *Questions for Discussion*

7. Is it important to know that the names were drawn at random? Explain. (See lines 157–161.)

8. In your opinion, is the response rate of 52.4% a sufficiently high rate? Explain. (See lines 164–166.)

9. Are you surprised that the researcher conducted four mailings (a survey, a postcard, a repeat survey, and a final postcard)? Explain. (See lines 197–206.)

10. Would you characterize the Pearson correlation coefficient of −.22 in Table 2 as representing a very strong relationship? Explain.

11. Table 2 contains both positive and negative values of Pearson correlation coefficients. What is your understanding of the difference in meaning between positive and negative values?

12. In your opinion, does this study show that organizational support *causes* job satisfaction? Explain.

## Quality Ratings

Directions: Indicate your level of agreement with each of the following statements by circling a number from 5 for strongly agree (SA) to 1 for strongly disagree (SD). If you believe an item is not applicable to this research article, leave it blank. Be prepared to explain your ratings. When responding to criteria A and B, keep in mind that brief titles and abstracts are conventional in published research.

A.   The title of the article is appropriate.

SA   5   4   3   2   1   SD

B. ′  The abstract provides an effective overview of the research article.

SA   5   4   3   2   1   SD

C.   The introduction establishes the importance of the study.

SA   5   4   3   2   1   SD

D.   The literature review establishes the context for the study.

SA   5   4   3   2   1   SD

E.   The research purpose, question, or hypothesis is clearly stated.

SA   5   4   3   2   1   SD

F.   The method of sampling is sound.

SA   5   4   3   2   1   SD

G.   Relevant demographics (for example, age, gender, and ethnicity) are described.

SA   5   4   3   2   1   SD

H.   Measurement procedures are adequate.

SA   5   4   3   2   1   SD

I.   All procedures have been described in sufficient detail to permit a replication of the study.

SA   5   4   3   2   1   SD

J.   The participants have been adequately protected from potential harm.

SA   5   4   3   2   1   SD

K.   The results are clearly described.

SA   5   4   3   2   1   SD

L.   The discussion/conclusion is appropriate.

SA   5   4   3   2   1   SD

M.  Despite any flaws, the report is worthy of publication.

SA   5   4   3   2   1   SD

# Article 10

# Parent Behavior and Child Distress During Urethral Catheterization

**Charmaine Kleiber**, PhD(C), RN, CPNP, **Ann Marie McCarthy**, PhD, RN, PNP[*]

### ABSTRACT

*Issues and Purpose*: Researchers need a clear understanding of the natural behaviors parents use to help their children cope. This study describes the relationships between naturally occurring parent behaviors and child distress behaviors during urethral catheterization.

*Design and Methods*: In this descriptive study, researchers videotaped the behaviors of parent-child interactions during urethral catheterization.

*Results*: Parents used distraction to maintain calm behavior during the first part of the procedure and used more reassurance when the children started to become distressed. Seven of the nine children displayed calm behavior at least half the time following distraction. Parental reassurance did not decrease distress behavior in most children.

*Practice Implications*: Early implementation of developmentally appropriate nursing interventions to decrease child distress is imperative. Parents may need specific instruction and practice to continue the use of distraction throughout procedures, even when the child is upset.

From *JSPN: Journal of the Society of Pediatric Nurses*, 4, 95–104. Copyright © 1999 by Nursecom, Inc. and the Society of Pediatric Nurses. Reprinted with permission.

Parents are frequently with their children during painful medical procedures, but many of them state they do not know what to say or do to help their children cope with the pain (Bauchner, Vinci, & Waring, 1989; Merritt, Sargent, & Osborn, 1990; Schepp, 1991). Although there is a great deal of interest in teaching parents and children to use cognitive-behavioral techniques (distraction, imagery, deep breathing, relaxation) to modify behavioral distress, few researchers have examined the relationships between specific naturally occurring parental behaviors and children's responses. Before interventions are implemented to modify parental behavior, researchers should have a clear understanding of the natural behaviors that parents use during painful procedures and the effects of those behaviors on children. Without that information, development of sound interventions cannot proceed in a scientific manner.

A few research groups have examined the relationships between naturally occurring parent behaviors and child distress and coping behaviors during procedures, but differences in the categories of behavior chosen for study and differences in analytic methods make it difficult to synthesize the results. Another issue is that most researchers have chosen children with cancer as the sample population. It may not be appropriate to generalize the behaviors of parents of children with cancer to parents of children with different health problems. It can be argued that parents of children with cancer are under greater emotional stress—the potential death of the child. The threat of death may influence how parents behave around their children during stressful situations. In investigating the effects of parental behavior on child behavior, it is important to include groups of children that do not have life-threatening illnesses.

A unique aspect of this study was that the children were undergoing urethral catheterization. Children undergoing this procedure were chosen for this study because these children typically do not have life-threatening conditions, yet they must undergo procedures that are frightening, uncomfortable, and take more than a minute or two to complete. There is evidence that catheterization of the bladder, a common medical procedure, is uncomfortable for children. In a study of children between the ages of 3 to 5 years who had the procedure, Merritt, Ornstein, and Spicker (1994) reported the mean observed distress score was 2.38 on the 5-point Observed Scale of Behavioral Distress (OSBD), and the mean pain rating was 64.78 on the 100-point Oucher pain scale. This indicates that children experience a moderate amount of distress and pain during the procedure. Indeed, for many years recommended practice for urethral catheterization has included the instillation of an anesthetic lubricant into the urethra to decrease discomfort (Chrispin, 1968; Gray, 1996).

---

[*]*Charmaine Kleiber* is an advanced practice nurse, University of Iowa Hospitals and Clinics. *Ann Marie McCarthy* is associate professor, College of Nursing, University of Iowa, Iowa City, Iowa.

The purpose of this pilot study was to investigate the relationships between naturally occurring parent behaviors and child distress behavior during urethral catheterization. This work adds to the developing research base on the relationships between the naturally occurring behaviors of parents and children during painful procedures. This information is crucial to the development of interventions to assist children and their parents in coping with painful procedures.

*Background*

Some parental behaviors that might be viewed intuitively as helping the child cope with a painful procedure, such as giving reassurance or information, have been found to be linked with increased child distress (Blount et al., 1989; Dahlquist, Power, Cox, & Fernbach, 1994; Manne et al., 1992). More needs to be learned about the effects of naturally occurring parental behaviors on children in stressful situations. Because the focus of this study is the relationship between parental behaviors and child distress, the literature review is limited to studies in that area.

Three groups of researchers have investigated the relationships between specific naturally occurring parental and child behaviors during painful procedures. Blount et al. (1989) audiotaped 23 children, ages 5 to 13 years, with cancer who were having a bone marrow aspiration and/or lumbar puncture. Verbalizations made by parents and children during the procedure were coded using the Child-Adult Medical Procedure Interaction Scale (CAMPIS), which consists of 12 adult-to-child vocal behaviors and 15 child vocal behaviors. Sackett's lag analysis was used to investigate the impact of particular vocalized behaviors on other behaviors. Thus, the impact of child behavior on adult behaviors was analyzed as well as the impact of adult behavior on child behavior. Conditional probabilities and behavioral chains, with each discrete behavior as the criterion starting the chain, were constructed. Major findings were that reassuring comments, apology, empathy, criticism, or giving control to the child by adults occurred before child distress behaviors ($p < .0001$ for each finding).

The timing of adult behaviors was the focus of a second analysis by Blount, Sturges, and Powers (1990). The relationship between adult and child behaviors was separated into phases of pre-, during, and postprocedure. The major findings were that child distress increased from preprocedure to during procedure, and remained high postprocedure. Adults used more distraction in the preprocedural phase and more commands to relax during the procedure. One limitation of these studies is that the temporal relationship—how much time elapsed—between adult and child behaviors is unknown. Another limitation is that the CAMPIS tool relies only on vocalizations audible on a tape recorder as indicators of distress in children.

Jacobsen et al. (1990) described the relationship between observed parental behavior and child distress during venipuncture in 3- to 10-year-old children ($N = 70$) with cancer using a tool developed by the researchers (Procedure Behavior Rating Scale–Venipuncture Version [PBRS–VV]). Analysis of variance revealed that children were more distressed if their parents used the behaviors of bargaining ($p = .001$), explaining ($p = .002$), or distracting ($p = .04$). Because the level of analysis did not allow for a temporal relationship, it was not possible to determine whether one behavior followed another.

To determine temporal relationships between behaviors, Manne et al. (1992) conducted a follow-up study, assessing the behaviors of 43 parent/child dyads. The children were cancer patients, ages 3 to 9 years, undergoing venipuncture. The researchers used an observational scale adapted from the CAMPIS and PBRS–VV that consisted of three child behavior categories and six adult behavior categories. An important difference between the behavioral observation tool used in this study and the CAMPIS tool used in the Blount study is that behaviors were defined using both visually observed and auditory categories. Another difference is that for parent behavior, the category "explanation" was added to the tool, and "reassurance" was deleted. The researchers used sequential analysis to assess the temporal relationships between parent and child behaviors. Behaviors had to occur within 5 seconds of each other to be counted as a sequence. Probable expectancies were calculated for all possible pairs of child and adult behavior categories. The results were that children used more coping behaviors when adults used distraction, and children exhibited fewer coping behaviors when adults used explanation, commands to use coping, praise, criticism, or giving control to the child. The only adult behavior that had beneficial results on both child coping and distress was distraction. All other adult behaviors decreased the likelihood that children would engage in coping behaviors.

Dahlquist et al. (1994) observed 66 children with cancer between the ages of 2 and 17 years during bone marrow aspiration. Child behavioral distress was measured with the Observed Scale of Behavioral Distress (OSBD) (Jay, Ozolins, Elliott, & Caldwell, 1983), which consists of 11 verbal, vocal, and motor distress behaviors that are assigned intensity weights. Parent-child interactions were recorded using the Dyadic Pre-Stressor Interaction Scale (DPIS) (Bush, Melamed, Sheras, & Greenbaum, 1986). Parent behaviors in this scale are informing, distracting, reassuring, ignoring, restraining, and agitation; child behaviors are attachment, distress, exploration, and prosocial behaviors. Pearson product-moment correlations were computed between parent and child DPIS behaviors and OSBD scores. For younger children (ages 2 to 7 years), "preprocedural" OSBD distress scores were positively correlated with parental reassurance ($r = .48$), and "dur-

170  ing-procedure" distress was positively related to parental restraining of the child ($r = .50$). For the older children, ages 8 to 17 years, none of the adult behaviors significantly correlated with distress scores in the "pre-
175  procedural" phase, but "during-procedure" OSBD distress scores were positively correlated with parental reassurance ($r = .40$) and parental information giving ($r = .34$). Although this study found age- and phase-specific relationships between the parental behaviors "reassuring" and "informing" and child distress, the
180  use of correlation to describe relationships between adult and child behaviors does not establish a temporal link (e.g., information about the timing of the behaviors).

In summary, the relationships between child dis-
185  tress behavior and parent behaviors are unclear. Although several researchers have taught parents to use behavioral strategies successfully, such as distraction, to decrease their children's distress during painful procedures (Blount et al., 1992; Broome, Lillis, McGahee,
190  & Bates, 1992; Jay & Elliott, 1990; Manne et al., 1990; Vessey, Carlson, & McGill, 1994), it is imperative that such interventions be based on a clear understanding of the interaction between parent and child behaviors.

The purpose of this study was to continue to inves-
195  tigate the relationship between naturally occurring parental behavior and child distress behaviors during a specific medical procedure: urethral catheterization. The specific research questions addressed in this study were:

200  1.  What behaviors do parents display during the urethral catheterization of their children?
2.  To what extent do children display distress behaviors during urethral catheterization?
3.  What are the relationships between parent behav-
205     ior and child distress behavior during urethral catheterization? Specifically:
   (a)  What is the child's behavioral response to parent behaviors?
   (b)  What is the parent's behavioral response to
210        child distress behavior?

## Methods

Behavioral analysis of videotaped procedures was used in this descriptive study of naturally occurring parent-child interactions during urethral catheterization.

### Setting

215  The setting was the urology clinic at a large tertiary-care Midwestern hospital. There was no program of cognitive-behavioral therapy to assist families with stress or pain during procedures in this clinic. Parents were given the option to be with their children during
220  the procedure, but parents were not coached in what to say or do to help their children.

### Subjects

Subjects were children undergoing urethral cathe-

terization for diagnostic tests and the parents who were present during the procedure. Inclusion criteria were
225  that the parents and children understood English and the children were between the ages of 3 and 7 years. The age of the children in this study was thus limited because it has been shown that young children are most likely to display distress behavior during medical pro-
230  cedures. The children were developmentally normal and had no known abnormality in perineal sensation.

Twelve children and their parents were approached to participate in this study. Two children declined. Ten children (eight girls, two boys) and their parents were
235  recruited. The mean age was 4.6 years (range 3.2–6.9 years), and the average number of previous urinary catheterizations the children had experienced was 5.8 (range 3–10). All the children were under follow-up for recurrent urinary tract infections. Seven of the children
240  were accompanied by a mother, two were accompanied by a father, and one child had both parents present through the procedure.

### Data Collection

Demographic and historical data were collected from each family, including information on the child's
245  age, sex, and history of previous catheterizations or other painful or uncomfortable procedures.

Behaviors recorded on the videotapes were coded using a behavior coding scheme (Table 1) developed by the investigators based on behavioral descriptors in
250  the Child Adult Medical Procedure Scale–Revised (CAMPIS–R) (Blount et al., 1990) and the Observed Scale of Behavioral Distress–Revised (OSBD) (Jay et al., 1983). Concurrent validity of the CAMPIS–R has been reported with significant correlations between
255  CAMPIS–R parent behavioral categories and child behavioral distress as measured by the OSBD and the Behavioral Approach–Avoidance and Distress Scale. Parental behaviors comprised only verbalizations, including distraction, reassurance, information giving,
260  praise, and command to use a coping strategy. Verbalizations that did not fall into those categories were labeled "other." Child distress behaviors included vocalizations ranging from whimper to scream, and the motor behaviors of physical fighting including kicking or
265  hitting. These behaviors were chosen because they indicate a higher level of distress than a frown or holding the body rigidly. Coding for child behavior was simply the presence or absence of any behavioral distress.

### Procedure

Approval for the study was obtained from the Insti-
270  tutional Review Board. Families in the urology clinic waiting room were approached by the principal investigator prior to their clinic visit to discuss the study and obtain informed consent from the parent and verbal assent from the child. If families agreed to participate,
275  demographic data were collected and the investigator escorted the family to the procedure room.

Table 1
*Definitions of Parent and Child Behaviors*

**Parent behaviors**

**Distraction**
Nonprocedure-related talk to child. Talk about the child's pets, school, activity, questions unrelated to the child's illness. Jokes or humorous statements made to the child.

**Information**
Procedure-related talk, including giving explanation, information. Any statement denoting what is about to occur, including washing, insertion of medical instrument. "This is going to feel cold." "You'll feel a little pressure."

**Reassurance**
Comments directed to the child with the intent to reassure or ease tension. "It's OK." "I'm almost through." "We're hurrying." "It's almost over."

**Command to use coping strategy**
Commands that required the child to participate in some coping behavior, such as, "Take a deep breath." "Relax." "Squeeze my hand." "Breathe in and out."

**Praise**
Statements referring to the child's past, present, or future behavior that is positive and shows approval. "You are doing great." "That's right." "Good job," and "Good girl."

**Other**
Talk directed to adults in the room; commands to the child to engage in some procedure-related activity (e.g., "Bring your legs up like a frog.").

**Child behaviors**

**Distress behavior**
Crying, screaming, whimpering, fighting, verbal noncompliance or verbal resistance, verbal pain, or verbal fear.

The sterile catheterization was performed by the urology clinic nurses using standard care procedures. The child was placed on the exam table with the parent
280 positioned at the head. The child's perineal area was washed with a soap solution, rinsed, and then a small amount of sterile lidocaine anesthetic lubricant was instilled into the urethra with a prefilled smooth-tipped syringe (see Gray, 1996, p. 308, for a description of
285 lidocaine lubricant use with urinary catheterization). After waiting a few minutes for the anesthetic to take effect, more of the lubricant was instilled. After waiting again for a few minutes, a Foley catheter (6 or 8 Fr.) was inserted.
290 The nurses informed the children about the sensations they would be feeling as each step of the procedure progressed. The investigator focused the video camera on the faces of the child and parent throughout the procedure. Videotaping started when the child was
295 placed on the exam table in the treatment room and continued until the clinic nurse indicated that the catheter was in place and secured with tape.

*Data Analysis*

The audio portion of each videotape was transcribed to allow written, auditory, and visual data to be
300 used for coding the behaviors. Prior to analysis, two practice tapes were used to train the investigators in the coding system and to establish interrater agreement.
First, all parent behaviors were coded. A parent behavior began with a parent's verbalization and ended

305 when the parent paused, allowing for the child to respond. Then, each child behavior following every parent behavior was coded as either indicative of distress or not. Table 2 gives an example of a sequence of parent and child behaviors. In this example, there are four
310 parent behaviors immediately following four child behaviors (1–2, 3–4, 5–6, 7–8). The mother used reassurance once, which was followed by child distress (1–2), and distraction three times, once followed by child distress (3–4) and twice followed by no distress (5–6,
315 7–8). Analyzing this passage for the parent's behavioral response to child distress, one needs to look at the child behaviors first. There are three child behaviors immediately followed by parent behavior (2–3, 4–5, 6–7). The child was distressed twice (2–3, 4–5) and calm
320 once (6–7). The parent used distraction after each of the child's behaviors.

Table 2
*Example of a Sequence of Parent and Child Behaviors*

1. Mother (*softly*): "Shh. Hush now, it's OK." (**Reassurance**)
2. Child (*crying*). (**Distress**)
3. Mother: "Can you tell me where we are going to lunch today?" (**Distraction**)
4. Child (*whimpering*). (**Distress**)
5. Mother: "Tell me what your favorite pizza place is." (**Distraction**)
6. Child (*frowning but quiet*). (**No distress**)
7. Mother: "Should we have pizza with pepperoni or sausage on it?" (**Distraction**)
8. Child: "No sausage. Just cheese pizza." (**No distress**)

The videotapes were coded to 100% agreement by the two investigators. Disagreements were resolved by discussing the likely intent of parent behaviors. Some-
325 times the parent's tone of voice and the pattern of parent-child interaction had to be taken into consideration in categorizing verbalizations. For example, the "shhh" sound was used by parents to communicate different things. Some parents used it as a soft, sooth-
330 ing reassurance, but others appeared to use it as a command to be quiet. Each verbalization made by the parents was classified as distraction, reassurance, information giving, command to use coping strategy, praise, or "other." Nonverbal parent behaviors, such as
335 stroking the child's head, were not coded. The presence or absence of child distress just prior to and immediately following each parent behavior was documented.
Because of the small sample size, the binomial sign test was chosen to determine the relationship between
340 child distress and parent behaviors. The unit of analysis was "subject" rather than "behavior across subjects" in order to meet the assumption of independence. Two sets of analyses were conducted: how parents respond to children and how children respond to parents. Fre-
345 quencies of parent behavior and child behavior just prior to and immediately following each parent behavior were tallied and percentages calculated for each parent/child dyad. For each parent/child dyad, the relationship between child distress and parent behavior was

350 given a positive sign if distress occurred more than 50% of the time, and a negative sign if distress occurred less than 50% of the time. For example, referring to the behavioral sequence in Table 2, the mother's distraction behavior was preceded by child
355 distress two of three times. Because the child was distressed more than half of the time prior to distraction, the dyad would receive a positive sign for "child distress present prior to parent distraction." The mother's distraction was followed by child distress one out of
360 three times. Because the child displayed distress less than 50% of the time immediately following the parent's distraction, the dyad would receive a negative score for "child distress present following parent distraction."

## Results

365 Data were collected on 10 parent/child dyads. One videotape was not usable because the parent did not say anything and stood still during the entire procedure. For the remaining nine videotapes, the catheterization procedures lasted an average of eight minutes from the
370 time the child was placed on the exam table to the time the catheter was taped in place.

*Research Question 1: What behaviors do parents display during the urinary catheterization of their children?*

Totals of 684 parent behaviors were coded and are described in Table 3. The most commonly used behaviors were distraction (33%) and reassurance (23%);
375 however, there was a wide range in usage among the nine parents in this sample. Distraction was used from 8 to 89 times (mean = 25), and reassurance was used from 1 to 41 times (mean = 17.3) during the catheterization procedures. Information giving, praise, and
380 commands to use coping strategies were used infrequently on average (means = 6.6, 5.4, and 5.4, respectively).

Table 3
*Description of 684 Parent Behaviors (N = 9)*

| Behavior | Frequency for total sample | Percentage of total behaviors | Mean frequency | Range of frequency |
|---|---|---|---|---|
| Distraction | 225 | 33% | 25.0 | 8–89 |
| Reassurance | 156 | 23% | 17.3 | 1–41 |
| Information | 60 | 9% | 6.6 | 1–19 |
| Praise | 49 | 7% | 5.4 | 0–11 |
| Command to cope | 49 | 7% | 5.4 | 0–26 |
| Other | 145 | 21% | 16.0 | 5–26 |

*Research Question 2: To what extent do children display distress behaviors during urinary catheterization?*

On average, the children displayed distress behavior following 41% of all coded parent behaviors. The
385 range of distress behavior, however, was striking. One child did not display any distress behavior; another child displayed only one mild distress behavior. Four children were more calm than distressed following parent behavior. Two children displayed more distress
390 behavior than calm behavior, and one child screamed and cried throughout the entire procedure regardless of her parent's efforts to calm her.

In this descriptive study, analysis of distress behavior was done for the whole procedure rather than by
395 "phase" of procedure. In analyzing the tapes, several "invasive" aspects to this procedure appeared: the washing of the perineum, the instillation of anesthetic jelly, and the insertion of the catheter. The beginning of each aspect of the procedure was surmised from the
400 nurse verbalizations on the videotape. A trend was evident in that seven children showed signs of discomfort (crying out; whining; saying, "It stings.") during the washing part of the procedure, and eight of the nine children screamed suddenly and loudly during the time
405 that the catheter was passed through the urethra. It appeared that most children were uncomfortable during washing and anesthetic application, and experienced sudden pain during the catheter insertion.

*Research Question 3: What is the child's behavioral response to parent behaviors? What is the parent's behavioral response to child distress behavior?*

Table 4 shows the number of children who were
410 distressed immediately before and immediately after the parent behaviors of distraction, information giving, and reassurance. These parent behaviors were chosen for analysis because they were used by all the parents in the study and were the most frequently used parent
415 behaviors.

Table 4
*Time-Sensitive Relationships Between Parent Behaviors and Child Distress Behavior*

| | Child distress behavior | |
|---|---|---|
| | **BEFORE** the parent behavior | **AFTER** the parent behavior |
| | # of children showing distress (Sign test) | # of children showing distress (Sign test) |
| Distraction | 3 of 9 (p = .5) | 2 of 8[a] (p = .28) |
| Reassurance | 6 of 9 (p = .5) | 5 of 9 (p = 1.0) |
| Information giving | 4 of 9 (p = 1.0) | 6 of 9 (p = .5) |

[a]One child displayed equal numbers of distress and nondistress behaviors following parent distraction.

None of the relationships between parent and child behavior reached statistical significance, which is not surprising considering the small sample size. However, trends in the data are evident. Parents tended to use
420 distraction to maintain calm behavior in the child. Six of the nine parents initiated distraction during calm behavior. Seven of the nine children displayed calm behavior at least half the time following distraction.

Six of the nine children displayed distress before
425 the parents used reassurance, and five children continued to show distress following reassurance. Parents

tended to use reassurance later in the procedure, when the child was distressed. Six parents followed the pattern of using distraction first (when the child was calm
430 during the beginning of the procedure), reassurance when the child started to become upset, and returned to using distraction when the child calmed down again.

Information was offered infrequently by the parents and often was meant to reinforce information given by
435 the nurse, such as "The soap will feel cold." The children's behavior was mixed prior to and after receiving information.

Praise generally was offered at the end of the procedure. Eight parents told their children they did a
440 good job during the procedure. Five parents gave praise when the children were calm, whereas two praised their children most frequently when they were still upset but winding down. One parent gave praise once when the child was upset and once when the child was calm.

445 Commands to cope were made by six parents. Although commands were used infrequently, it appeared that general instructions such as "just relax" had no noticeable effect on these young children. The children seemed more able to follow directive commands such
450 as "take a deep breath" and "squeeze my hand."

## Discussion

Parents tended to use distraction during times when the children were not distressed. When the children were presented with distraction by their parents, six of the nine children continued to remain calm, while two
455 children tended to display distress, and one child displayed an equal number of calm and distress behaviors. The results of this study support the findings of Blount et al. (1990) that parents tend to use more distraction during the early part of the procedure, and the findings
460 of Manne et al. (1992) that children tend not to show distress behavior following parent use of distraction.

Parents tended to use reassurance when the children became distressed, typically later in the procedure. This finding supports observations reported by two other
465 research groups (Blount et al., 1990; Dahlquist et al., 1994) that child distress and reassurance are related. However, where other researchers have speculated that reassurance might evoke distress in the child, we suggest a different explanation: Child distress may evoke
470 parent reassurance. This was evident in the pattern seen with parents using distraction initially, using reassurance when children start to show distress, and then going back to using distraction when the children were less distressed. Perhaps parents feel the need to acknowledge their children's discomfort by using reas-
475 suring comments like "it's OK" or "I know." Five of the nine children continued to be distressed after parental reassurance, but the children's level of distress did not escalate (e.g., from whining to crying) following
480 reassurance. Although reassurance did not decrease distress behavior in most children, it did not seem to be a distress-promoting behavior.

Information was offered infrequently by parents in this study and often was used to reinforce sensory
485 preparation by the nurse. The children's behavior prior to and following information was mixed. This does not support the conclusions of other researchers (Jacobsen et al., 1990; Manne et al., 1992) that information or explanation is linked with increased child distress.

490 The major limitation of this study is its small sample size. Although trends in patterns of behavior are evident, larger studies are needed to validate these findings. Another limitation is possible differences between male and female catheterizations. This study included
495 two boys and eight girls, so comparisons of gender differences were not possible.

In summary, the pattern of parent behavior that emerged in this study was that parents used distraction to maintain calm behavior during the first part of the
500 procedure when nothing painful was happening. When children had a marked behavior change indicative of more intense discomfort, however, some parents abandoned distraction and started using reassurance. This finding, in conjunction with previous research, has
505 implications for researchers and clinicians. In a meta-analysis of 16 studies representing a total sample of 491 young children, Kleiber and Harper (1999) found that distraction had a positive effect on children's distress behavior during medical procedures. Additionally,
510 there is evidence that child distress is influenced by distraction during both the anticipatory and the invasive phases of medical procedures. Blount et al. (1990) reported that directing the child to use coping strategies was associated with decreased child distress during the
515 painful part of bone marrow aspiration. Manne et al. (1992) found that parent use of distraction had a significantly positive effect on child coping during the preparation, insertion, and completion phases of venipuncture. The results of the current study suggest
520 that parents may need specific instruction and practice to continue the use of distraction or imagery throughout procedures.

Many children with urinary problems undergo repeated catheterizations. Future research should investi-
525 gate children's behavioral responses during their first catheterization experience. In this study, children already had experienced between 3 and 10 urinary catheterizations. Other studies have found that the child's previous negative experience with procedures is a po-
530 tent predictor of future distress (Dahlquist et al., 1986; Pate, Blount, Cohen, & Smith, 1996). Thus, for pediatric urology patients, early implementation of developmentally appropriate nursing interventions to decrease child distress is imperative. These interventions may
535 include strategies for the child, the adults involved in the procedure, or both.

## Conclusions

There is a broad variability in parents' behaviors and in children's distress behavior during urinary catheterization. As a group, children showed distress behavior after 41% of parent behaviors during the procedure. A pattern of parent behavior emerged in this study: Parents used distraction to maintain calm behavior during the first part of the procedure and used more reassurance when the children started to become distressed.

*How Do I Apply These Findings to Nursing Practice?*

To develop scientifically sound interventions, researchers and clinicians should have a clear understanding of the natural behaviors that parents use during medical procedures and the effects of those behaviors on children. This study suggests that parents tend to use distraction early in the procedure to maintain calm behavior and reassurance when the child becomes distressed. Because previous research indicates that distraction can decrease child distress behaviors during both the preparatory and invasive phases of medical procedures, parents may need assistance in using distraction throughout the procedure, even when the child is upset.

Other researchers have identified a relationship between parent use of reassurance and child behavioral distress. This study suggests that child distress behavior triggers parent use of reassurance. Although reassuring comments such as "it's OK" and "almost through, just a little longer" did not seem to decrease children's distress behavior, reassurance might have an unrecognized psychological effect on children. Perhaps reassurance lets children know their parents have not abandoned them, and that their "upset" is acknowledged. Further research is needed to clarify how parents' use of distraction and reassurance influences children during medical procedures.

### References

Bauchner, H., Vinci, R., & Waring, C. (1989). Pediatric procedures: Do parents want to watch? *Pediatrics, 84,* 907–909.

Blount, R. L., Bachanas, P. J., Powers, S. W., Cotter, M. C., Franklin, A., Chaplin, W., Mayfield, J., Henderson, M., & Blount, S. D. (1992). Training children to cope and parents to coach them during routine immunizations: Effects on child, parent, and staff behaviors. *Behavior Therapy, 23,* 689–705.

Blount, R. L., Corbin, S. M., Sturges, J. W., Wolfe, V. V., Prater, J. M., & James, L. D. (1989). The relationship between adult's behavior and child coping and distress during BMA/LP procedures: A sequential analysis. *Behavior Therapy, 20,* 585–601.

Blount, R. L., Sturges, J. W., & Powers, S. W. (1990). Analysis of child and adult behavioral variations by phase of medical procedure. *Behavior Therapy, 21,* 33–48.

Broome, M. E., Lillis, P., McGahee, T. W., & Bates, T. (1992). The use of distraction and imagery with children during painful procedures. *Oncology Nursing Forum, 19,* 499–502.

Bush, J. P., Melamed, B. G., Sheras, P. L., & Greenbaum, P. L. (1986). Mother-child patterns of coping with anticipatory medical distress. *Health Psychology, 5,* 137–157.

Chrispin, A. (1968). Radiological investigations. In D.I. Williams (Ed.), *Paediatric urology* (pp. 531–543). New York: Appleton-Century-Crofts.

Dahlquist, L. M., Gil, K. M., Armstrong, F. D., DeLawyer, D. D., Greene P., & Wuori, D. (1986). Preparing children for medical examinations: The importance of previous medical experience. *Health Psychology, 5,* 249–259.

Dahlquist, L. M., Power, T. G., Cox, C. N., & Fernbach, D. J. (1994). Parenting and children distress during cancer procedures: A multi-dimensional assessment. *Children's Health Care, 23,* 149–166.

Gray, M. (1996). Atraumatic urethral catheterization of children. *Pediatric Nursing, 22,* 306–310.

Jacobsen, P. B., Manne, S. L., Gorfinkle, K., Schorr, O., Rapkin, B., & Redd, W. (1990). Analysis of child and parent behavior during painful medical procedures. *Health Psychology, 9,* 559–576.

Jay, S. M., & Elliott, C. H. (1990). A stress inoculation program for parents whose children are undergoing painful medical procedures. *Journal of Consulting and Clinical Psychology, 58,* 799–804.

Jay, S. M., Ozolins, M., Elliott, C. H., & Caldwell, S. (1983). Assessment of children's distress during painful medical procedures. *Health Psychology, 2,* 133–147.

Kleiber, C., & Harper, D. (1999). Effects of distraction on children's pain and distress during medical procedures: A meta-analysis. *Nursing Research, 48,* 44–49.

Manne, S. L., Bakeman, R., Jacobsen, P. B., Gorfinkle, K., Bernstein, D., & Redd, W. (1992). Adult–child interaction during invasive medical procedures. *Health Psychology, 11,* 241–249.

Manne, S. L., Redd, W. H., Jacobsen, P. B., Gorfinkle, K., Schorr, O., & Rapkin, B. (1990). Behavioral intervention to reduce child and parent distress during venipuncture. *Journal of Consulting and Clinical Psychology, 58,* 565–572.

Merritt, K. A., Ornstein, P. A., & Spicker, B. (1994). Children's memory for a salient medical procedure: Implications for testimony. *Pediatrics, 94,* 17–23.

Merritt, K.A., Sargent, J.R., & Osborn, L.M. (1990). Attitudes regarding parental presence during medical procedures. *American Journal of Diseases in Children, 144,* 270–271.

Pate, J. T., Blount, R. L., Cohen, L. L., & Smith, A. J. (1996). Childhood medical experience and temperament as predictors of adult functioning in medical situations. *Children's Health Care, 25,* 281–298.

Schepp, K. G. (1991). Factors influencing the coping effort of mothers of hospitalized children. *Nursing Research, 40,* 42–46.

Vessey, J. A., Carlson, K. L., & McGill, J. (1994). Use of distraction with children during an acute pain experience. *Nursing Research, 43,* 369–372.

**Acknowledgments:** The authors wish to thank Bonnie Wagner, RN; Lisa Gerard, RN; and the staff of the UIHC Urology Clinic for their support of this research. This study was funded by a grant from the Society of Pediatric Nurses.

**Address correspondence to:** charmaine.kleiber@uiowa.edu, with a copy to the editor: roxie.foster@uchsc.edu

# Exercise for Article 10

## *Factual Questions*

1. Why were children undergoing urethral catheterization chosen for this study?

2. Why was this study limited to children between the ages of 3 and 7 years?

3. On what did the investigator focus the video camera?

4. When coding the videotapes, what percentage of agreement was reached by the two investigators?

5. On average, the catheterization procedures lasted how many minutes?

6. Were any of the relationships between parent and child behavior statistically significant?

7. The researchers note that one limitation of the study is the small sample size. What is the other limitation that is explicitly mentioned?

## Questions for Discussion

8. The researchers refer to their study as a "pilot study." Do you agree with this classification? Why? Why not? (See line 57.)

9. What is your opinion on the researchers' decision to exclude the children's nonverbal behaviors such as frowning or holding the body rigidly? (See lines 265–267.)

10. What is your opinion on the researchers' decision to exclude parents' nonverbal behaviors such as stroking their child's head? (See lines 334–335.)

11. The children in this study had already experienced between 3 and 10 urinary catheterizations. Is this a limitation of the study? Explain. (See lines 235–238.)

12. If you were to conduct another study on the same topic, what changes in the research methodology, if any, would you make?

## Quality Ratings

Directions: Indicate your level of agreement with each of the following statements by circling a number from 5 for strongly agree (SA) to 1 for strongly disagree (SD). If you believe an item is not applicable to this research article, leave it blank. Be prepared to explain your ratings. When responding to criteria A and B, keep in mind that brief titles and abstracts are conventional in published research.

A. The title of the article is appropriate.

SA 5 4 3 2 1 SD

B. The abstract provides an effective overview of the research article.

SA 5 4 3 2 1 SD

C. The introduction establishes the importance of the study.

SA 5 4 3 2 1 SD

D. The literature review establishes the context for the study.

SA 5 4 3 2 1 SD

E. The research purpose, question, or hypothesis is clearly stated.

SA 5 4 3 2 1 SD

F. The method of sampling is sound.

SA 5 4 3 2 1 SD

G. Relevant demographics (for example, age, gender, and ethnicity) are described.

SA 5 4 3 2 1 SD

H. Measurement procedures are adequate.

SA 5 4 3 2 1 SD

I. All procedures have been described in sufficient detail to permit a replication of the study.

SA 5 4 3 2 1 SD

J. The participants have been adequately protected from potential harm.

SA 5 4 3 2 1 SD

K. The results are clearly described.

SA 5 4 3 2 1 SD

L. The discussion/conclusion is appropriate.

SA 5 4 3 2 1 SD

M. Despite any flaws, the report is worthy of publication.

SA 5 4 3 2 1 SD

# Article 11

# Skin-to-Skin Contact After Cesarean Delivery: An Experimental Study

**Silvia Gouchon**, MSc, RN, **Dario Gregori**, PhD, **Amabile Picotto**, RN,
**Giovanna Patrucco**, MD, **Marco Nangeroni**, MD, **Paola Di Giulio**, MSc, RN[*]

### ABSTRACT

*Background*: The effectiveness of skin-to-skin contact (SSC) after vaginal delivery has been shown. After cesarean births, SSC is not done for practical and medical safety reasons because it is believed that infants may suffer mild hypothermia.

*Objective*: The aim of this study was to compare mothers' and newborns' temperatures after cesarean delivery when SSC was practiced (naked baby except for a small diaper, covered with a blanket, prone on the mother's chest) with those when routine care was practiced (dressed, in the bassinet or in the mother's bed) in the 2 hours beginning when the mother returned from the operating room.

*Methods*: An experimental, noninferiority adaptive trial was designed with four levels of analysis: 34 pairs of mothers and newborns, after elective cesarean delivery, were randomized to SSC ($n = 17$) or routine care ($n = 17$). Temporal artery temperature was taken with an infrared ray thermometer at half-hour intervals.

*Results*: Compared with newborns who received routine care, SSC cesarean-delivered newborns were not at risk for hypothermia. The mean temperatures of both groups were almost identical: after 30 min, 36.1°C for both groups (±0.4°C for SSCs and ±0.5°C for the controls), and after 120 min, 36.2°C ± 0.3°C for SSCs versus 36.4°C ± 0.7°C for the controls (no significant differences). Time from delivery to the mothers' return to their room was 51 ± 10 min. The SSC newborns attached to the breast earlier (nine SSC newborns and four controls after 30 min) were breast-fed (exclusively or prevalently) at discharge (13 SSCs and 11 controls) and at 3 months (11 SSCs and 8 controls), and the SSC mothers expressed high levels of satisfaction with the intervention.

*Discussion*: Cesarean-delivered newborns who experienced SSC within 1 hour of delivery are not at risk for hypothermia.

From *Nursing Research*, 59, 78–84. Copyright © 2010 by Lippincott Williams & Wilkins. Reprinted with permission.

Skin-to-skin contact (SSC) is the positioning of the naked baby prone on the mother's bare chest, immediately or in the very first hours after birth (Moore, Anderson, & Bergman, 2007). A Cochrane Collaboration systematic review (Moore et al., 2007) showed the efficacy of SSC on the baby's thermoregulation (Bergman, Linley, & Fawcus, 2004; Chiu, Anderson, & Burkhammer, 2005; Fransson, Karlsson, & Nilsson, 2005), breast-feeding (Carfoot, Williamson, & Dickson, 2003; Jonas, Wiklund, Nissen, Ransjö-Arvidson, & Uvnäs-Moberg, 2007; Moore et al., 2007), bonding (Feldman, Eidelman, Sirota, & Weller, 2002; Klaus et al., 1972; McClellan & Cabianca, 1980; Tessier et al., 1998), and development and, overall, on the general well-being of mothers and infants. No negative effects were observed on respiratory control and thermoregulation (Bohnhorst, Heyne, Peter, & Poets, 2001). The World Health Organization (WHO) guide on kangaroo mothers' care (Gruppo di Studio Della SIN, 2006; WHO, 2003) recommends SSC for all newborns, irrespective of context, weight, gestational age, and clinical conditions.

Skin-to-skin contact is well known and implemented widely in full-term infants born by vaginal delivery (WHO, 1997), but major obstacles persist after cesarean births (Erlandsson, Dsilna, Fagerberg, & Christensson, 2007), for practical and safety reasons. The main difficulty in promoting SSC, also in vaginally delivered children (Chiu et al., 2005), is the potential for hypothermia: a skin temperature of 36°C–36.4°C is defined as mild hypothermia (WHO, 1997). Hypothermia occurs throughout the world and in all climates, and it is more common than expected. Heat loss increases with air movement, and a baby risks getting cold even at a room temperature of 30°C if there is a draft (WHO, 1997).

The main data on hypothermia derive from studies on preterm infants: Bergman et al. (2004) showed that for infants having a birth weight between 1,200 and

[*]*Silvia Gouchon* is a nursing coordinator, Research and Education Unit, Ospedali Riuniti, Pinerolo, Italy. *Dario Gregori* is statistician and associate professor, Department of Public Health and Microbiology, Turin University, Turin, Italy. *Amabile Picotto* is a nursing coordinator, Mother and Child Department; *Giovanna Patrucco* is a pediatrician and former head of the Neonatology Unit; and *Marco Nangeroni* is a pediatrician, head of the Neonatology Unit, Ospedali Riuniti, Pinerolo, Italy. *Paola Di Giulio* is an associate professor, Department of Public Health and Microbiology, Turin University, Turin, Italy.

40 2,199 g exposed to SSC, the risk of hypothermia is significantly reduced compared with conventional incubator care; all SSC participants were stable in the 6th hour compared with 6/13 incubator infants.

Extended periods of cold stress may cause harmful 45 side effects such as increased oxygen consumption, and this can lead to acidosis and hypoglycemia, a fall in blood pressure, decreased plasma volume and cardiac output, and increased peripheral resistances (Knobel & Holditch-Davis, 2007). Hypothermia also may cause 50 coagulation defects, delayed readjustment from fetal to newborn circulation (McCall, Alderdice, Halliday, Jenkins, & Vohra, 2008). After birth, there is a rise in the newborn's temperature due to the increase in metabolic rate (Christensson et al., 1992), but most cooling 55 occurs in the first 10–20 minutes after birth (WHO, 1997).

Babies delivered via cesarean are at higher risk for hypothermia because of (a) the low temperature of the operating room, (b) the mothers themselves, or (c) the 60 locoregional anesthesia (Hui et al., 2006; Peillon, Dounas, Lebonhomme, & Guittard, 2002; Saito, Sessler, Fujita, Ooi, & Jeffrey, 1998); (d) the redistribution of body heat from core to periphery (Horn et al., 2002), with a typical decrease in core temperature of 0.5°C– 65 1°C (Arkiliç, Akça, Taguchi, Sessler, & Kurz, 2000); and (e) the newborn, especially in the first 90 minutes, compared with full-term vaginally delivered newborns. Infants delivered by cesarean section are exposed to drugs that may affect thermoregulation, and the sym- 70 pathoadrenal system is not mobilized to the same extent as in vaginally delivered infants (Christensson et al., 1993). Only two trials on SSC were found to have included cesarean-delivered healthy infants, assessing mothers' perception of their babies after SSC in the 75 first 12 hours after delivery (McClellan & Cabianca, 1980) and the effect of SSC with the father on crying and prefeeding behavior (Erlandsson et al., 2007). Cesarean-delivered babies generally are not included in studies; therefore, scarce information exists on the ef- 80 fect of SSC on this population. In addition, due to the increasing number of cesarean births, the Cochrane review recommends further research on SSC after cesarean delivery (Moore et al., 2007).

The aim of this study was to assess the safety of 85 early SSC after cesarean delivery on newborns' temperature in the 2 hr after the mothers return from the operating room. Secondary end points were the assessment of the benefits of SSC on first attachment to breast, minutes postbirth of first attachment, crying, 90 breast-feeding at discharge and after 3 months, and maternal satisfaction with SSC. The hypothesis was that there would be no differences in temperature variations between infants exposed to SSC or to usual care.

## Methods

This study was conducted in the Mother and Child 95 Department of Pinerolo Hospital (Turin, Italy), which averages 1,200 deliveries per year. In 2006, out of 1,098 deliveries, 309 (28.1%) were cesarean sections. There were 55.6% exclusively breast-fed infants at discharge after cesarean births and 66.2% for sponta- 100 neous vaginal deliveries.

A design described by O'Brien and Fleming (1979) was used in this noninferiority adaptive trial that began on February 13 and ended early in August 2007. The maximum number of patients needed was established, 105 but sequential levels for analysis were designed (Bauer, 1989) to identify any risk of hypothermia promptly. Four levels for analysis were planned (O'Brien & Fleming, 1979). The mother-newborn pairs were randomized to SSC or to routine care. Italian women 110 scheduled for elective cesarean delivery with locoregional anaesthesia were recruited from the maternity ward of Pinerolo Hospital. Only cesarean births with full-term newborns were eligible (38–42 weeks gestation, 1- and 5-min Apgar scores $\geq$ 7, weight > 115 2,500 kg).

A meeting was held with 13 nurses and health care personnel involved in the study to discuss the protocol and train for data collection, including the use of scales.

### Sample

120 A maximum of 68 women-newborn pairs per arm was calculated to give 80% power at the 5% significance level to show a mean difference of temperature more than 0.1°C. This value was agreed on after a consensus meeting with the neonatologists of the ward and 125 based on the results obtained from a pilot study (data not published) on 21 newborns in which the standard deviation of temperatures was 0.4°C. According to the adaptive design, four interim analyses were planned, after 17 pairs per arm. After each step, the null hy- 130 pothesis can be rejected at increasing levels of significance (depending on the α function employed) or accepted with a Student's $t$ test for paired samples. The protocol was approved by the local ethical committee.

### Randomization

If women met the inclusion criteria, they were ap- 135 proached at around 36–37 weeks, at their scheduled checkup, the week before their elective delivery. They were informed about the study, verbally and with an information sheet, and were asked to sign an informed consent form. Mothers were then randomized using 140 opaque, sealed envelopes, each containing the next allocation, from a computer-generated randomization list. Confidentiality was guaranteed.

The day of surgery, the nurse opened the envelope. When the baby was back from the operating room, the 145 father or the closest relative was then informed of the group allocation (routine care or SSC). The mother was informed when she returned to her room.

### Interventions

After the umbilical cord had been cut and a general

assessment of the newborn and the Apgar score were
150 completed, infants of both groups were dried, wrapped
in a towel, handed to their mother for a brief contact,
and transported to the neonatal ward in an incubator.
The staff pediatric nurse (with the father or a relative)
inspected the infant, bathed and dried it, and weighed
155 it. Average time elapsed from birth to the newborn's
arrival to the room was $51 \pm 10$ min. After surgery, the
mothers were transported to the obstetrical ward.

Newborns assigned to routine care were bathed,
dried, and dressed and held by the father or put in the
160 radiant warmer if there were no relatives or considered
hypothermic; then, if not contraindicated, the infant
was taken to the mother's room when she returned. The
mother was instructed on how to breast-feed and, during the 2-hr observation time, could choose whether to
165 keep the baby in her bed, in a crib next to the bed, or in
the neonatal center. She could choose whether to
breast-feed or not.

The newborns assigned to SSC received the same
treatment, but they were not dressed; they were fitted
170 with a disposable diaper and a cap and wrapped in a
warm cloth. When the mother was back in her room,
the newborn was placed on the mother's skin, between
her breasts, and left covered with the cloth, the bed
sheet, and blanket for a maximum of 2 hr. During this
175 time, the mother was instructed on how to breast-feed.

No changes in practices occurred during the time of
the study.

*Skin Temperature.* Skin temperature in both groups
was taken at arrival from the operating room, after the
180 bath, when the mother returned to the room, and every
half hour for 2 hr, with an infrared ray thermometer on
the forehead (THERMOFOCUS, 01500 series, Tecni-
med, Varese, Italy) that measures the temperature
without skin contact. This technique provides reliable
185 results (Martin & Kline, 2004; Matsukawa, Ozaki,
Nishiyama, Imamura, & Kumazawa, 2000). The same
model was used for the mother's and room temperature. Three dedicated thermometers were used for
mothers and newborns.
190 *Breast-Feeding.* The nurses measured the effectiveness of the first breast-feeding session with the Infant Breast-feeding Assessment Tool (IBAT; Matthews, 1988). Measures were readiness to feed, rooting
(at the touch of the nipple to cheek, the baby opens his
195 or her mouth and tries to grasp the nipple), sucking,
and latching onto the breast. Each behavior is assessed
on a 3-point Likert scale, with a possible total score
ranging from 0 to 12. The mother's satisfaction for
breast-feeding does not add to the score. The mothers
200 could choose when to start breast-feeding and for how
long; time to first attachment was measured. The first
attachment was effective if the score was $\geq 8$.

*Exclusive Breast-Feeding at Discharge.* Data were
collected from clinical and nursing records. Breast-
205 feeding was considered exclusive if only mother's milk
had been offered in the last 24 hr before discharge

(WHO, 1998). After 3 months, women were contacted
by telephone to collect information on feeding in the
first 3 months.
210 *Satisfaction.* Mothers and fathers in the SSC group
were asked to complete together a questionnaire with
seven close-ended questions on a 5-point Likert scale
(from *not at all* to *complete agreement*). The questionnaire is used to assess the mothers' perceptions of dif-
215 ficulties, negative effect on father, positive effect on
mother-baby interaction and discomfort, the father's
feeling of exclusion and the effect on his attachment,
improvement of the relationship with the baby, and
willingness to continue SSC at home or to recommend
220 it to other mothers.

*Data Analysis*

Data were analyzed on an intention-to-treat basis.
Means, mean differences, and standard deviations were
calculated and statistical analysis was done using Student's $t$ test for paired samples, according to the adap-
225 tive design protocol, after the first 17 pairs per group.

**Results**

From February to August 2007, out of 170 cesarean
births, 96 women (56%) had an elective cesarean delivery. Fifty-five women were not contacted because of
organizational difficulties, unavailability of nurses, or
230 lack of time ($n = 25$) or because they did not attend the
hospital clinic for preadmission check-up and blood
tests ($n = 30$) and therefore could not be asked for consent before delivery. Of the 41 women contacted, 2 did
not consent to the study and 3 had an unscheduled ce-
235 sarean section (Figure 1). Of the 36 randomized wom-
en, 1 woman in the SSC group withdrew consent and 1
woman in the control group was sedated and therefore
excluded. Data are presented on 34 mother-child couples (17 SSC and 17 controls). The mothers' and new-
240 borns' main characteristics are presented in Table 1.

The main indication to elective cesarean delivery
was a previous cesarean (10 SSC newborns, 8 controls)
or a breech presentation (5 in both groups). The two
groups were comparable; no intrapartum complications
245 occurred and no newborns needed resuscitation support. Only 1 woman in the control group had hypoten-
sion during surgery, but her blood pressure had returned to normal when she went back to her room. No
woman required morphine during or after locoregional
250 anesthesia.

The two groups also were comparable for general
conditions (Table 2). The SSC newborns, in the time
between their arrival from the operating room and the
mothers' return to the room, had a slightly smaller but
255 not statistically significant drop in temperature ($M = 0.2$, $SD = 0.6$) than the controls ($M = 0.4$, $SD = 0.5$).

In both groups, 13 newborns were held by their fathers and 3 were put under a radiant warmer; 1 SSC
was put in the crib, and for 1 in the routine group, the
260 information was missing. Mean time between delivery

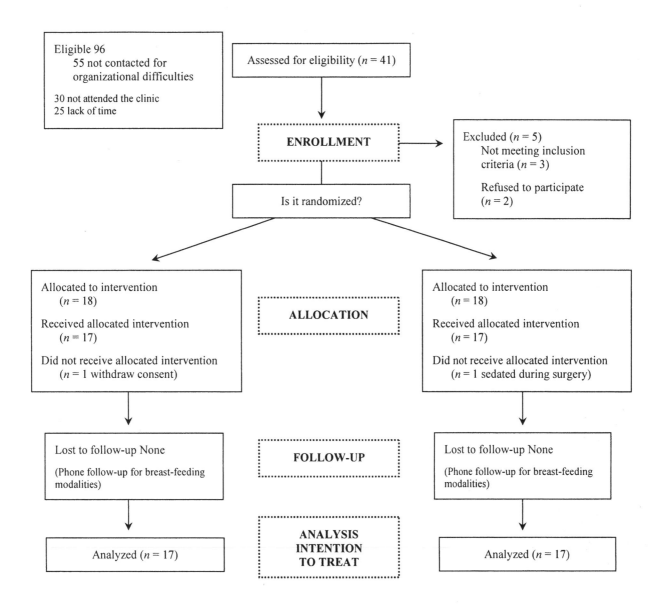

*Figure 1.* Flow of participants.

and bathing was 23 ± 15 min for the SSC group and 20 ± 7 min for controls. Mean time from delivery to the mother's return to her room was 51 ± 10 min in both groups. Only 1 of the 17 women assigned to SSC re-
265 fused it. After the first 30 min, 12 women were sustaining SSC and 10 women after 60, 90, and 120 min. Mean duration of SSC was 82.9 ± 45.9 min (range, 32–215 min).

*Temperature*

There were no differences in newborns' mean tem-
270 peratures at each interval. When the babies were held by the father before the mother's arrival, the mean temperature drop was from 36.0°C to 35.0°C for SSCs and from 36.3°C to 35.9°C for controls. Except for 3 SSC newborns and 2 controls, the temperatures of the
275 babies and the mothers rose (Table 3). The reduction in

temperature after 120 min was 0.2°C, 0.2°C, and 0.1°C in the 3 SSC newborns and 0.5°C and 0.3°C in the 2 controls.

*First Attachment to the Breast and Breast-Feeding at Discharge*

The average time that elapsed from the mother's re-
280 turn before the baby was attached to the breast was 22 ± 8 min in the SSC group and 43 ± 67 min in the controls. The first suckling was effective in both groups (IBAT mean scores: 9.2 ± 3.8 for SSC and 8.2 ± 3.2 for controls).

285 During the first half hour, 9 SSC newborns and 4 controls were breast-fed. Seven SSC newborns and 2 controls were breast-fed for at least 1 hr during the first 2 hr. Five SSC newborns and 7 controls did not start breast-feeding.

*Routine care* (handwritten)

Table 1
*Main Characteristics of Mothers and Newborns*

| | Skin to skin (n = 17) | | Controls (n = 17) | |
|---|---|---|---|---|
| | n | % | n | % |
| Mothers | | | | |
| Age, M (SD), years | 35 (5) | | 33 (5) | |
| Gestation, M (SD), weeks | 38.6 (0.5) | | 38.6 (0.5) | |
| Education | | | | |
| Elementary school | 7 | 41 | 5 | 29 |
| High school | 5 | 29 | 8 | 47 |
| University degree | 5 | 29 | 4 | 29 |
| Primigravidae | 2 | 12 | 6 | 35 |
| Previous breastfeeding | 11 | 69 | 9 | 82 |
| Complications during delivery | 0 | | 1 | |
| Ice bag at arrival from operating room | 15 | | 14 | |
| Newborns | | | | |
| Males | 8 | | 10 | |
| Birthweight, M (SD), g | 3,409 (390) | | 3,305 (290) | |
| 1-min Apgar score, M (SD) | 9 (0.3) | | 9.3 (0.6) | |
| 5-min Apgar score, M (SD) | 10 (0) | | 9.9 (0.3) | |

*Note.* Differences not statistically significant.

*dependent* (handwritten)

Table 2
*Temperatures (°C) of Mothers, Newborns, and Rooms*

*independent* (handwritten)

| | Skin to skin (n = 17) | | Controls (n = 17) | |
|---|---|---|---|---|
| | M | SD | M | SD |
| Mothers' temperature | | | | |
| Before surgery | 36.6 | 0.5 | 36.6 | 0.5 |
| After surgery | 36.5 | 0.6 | 36.5 | 0.6 |
| When holding the baby | 35.2 | 0.4 | 35.5 | 0.4 |
| Newborns' temperature | | | | |
| On arrival from operating room | 36.0 | 0.5 | 36.3 | 0.2 |
| After bathing | 35.9 | 0.7 | 36.2 | 1.4 |
| When given to the mother to hold | 35.9 | 0.4 | 35.9 | 0.4 |
| Room temperature | | | | |
| Operating room | 22.0 | 0.9 | 21.8 | 1.0 |
| Room where the newborn was bathed | 25.7 | 1.6 | 26.4 | 1.4 |
| Mother's room | 23.7 | 1.8 | 24.8 | 2.2 |

*Note.* Differences not statistically significant.

Table 3
*Temperatures (°C) at Different Intervals*

| | Skin to skin | | | | Controls | | | |
|---|---|---|---|---|---|---|---|---|
| | Newborns | | Mothers | | Newborns | | Mothers | |
| | M | SD | M | SD | M | SD | M | SD |
| Mothers' arrival from operating room | 35.9 | 0.4 | 35.2 | 0.4 | 35.9 | 0.4 | 35.5 | 0.5 |
| After 30 min | 36.1 | 0.5 | 35.4 | 0.4 | 36.1 | 0.4 | 35.8 | 0.5 |
| After 60 min | 36.2 | 0.4 | 35.6 | 0.4 | 36.3 | 0.5 | 35.9 | 0.6 |
| After 90 min | 36.1 | 0.4 | 35.8 | 0.4 | 36.3 | 0.6 | 36.3 | 0.6 |
| After 120 min | 36.2 | 0.3 | 36 | 0.4 | 36.4 | 0.7 | 36.3 | 0.6 |

*Note.* Differences not statistically significant.

290   More controls than SSC newborns were held by relatives (1 SSC and 5 controls at 60 min; 2 SSCs and 8 controls after 120 min). After 90 min, 1 SSC infant was put under a radiant warmer (the newborn's temperature was 36.6°C, but the mother's temperature was low, 295 35.3°C, and she was feeling cold); one control was put under a warmer after 120 min at the mother's request (the baby's temperature was 36.4°C, the mother's was 36.6°C).

At discharge, 13 SSC (9 exclusive, 4 prevalent) newborns and 11 (9 exclusive, 2 prevalent) controls were breast-fed. When contacted by telephone after 3 months, 11 SSC (8 exclusive, 3 prevalent) women and 8 (5 exclusive, 3 prevalent) controls were breast-feeding: SSC, 63 ± 38.8 days, and controls, 48 ± 34.9 days.

*Satisfaction*

Twelve SSC women (5 did not complete the questionnaire) were very satisfied and convinced that SSC contributed to the feeling of closeness to the child (very much/completely); 10 stated that it improved the relationship with the child (very much/completely). Only 1 father felt excluded, but this feeling was not shared by the others (9 couples answered not at all, 2 just a little).

None of the women experienced uneasiness with SSC; 7 were convinced that it significantly improved breast-feeding (very much/completely). Only 2 did not perceive any benefit. Eleven women would suggest SSC to a friend and 8 would continue it at home. The mothers confirmed that the experience elicited positive feelings such as love, tenderness, and touch and limited the feeling of "tearing (stretching/ripping)" that some associated with cesarean delivery.

## Discussion

The results support the use of SSC in cesarean deliveries and indicate that it was not associated with a drop in temperature. This study extends to cesarean births the findings of previous studies on newborns' skin temperature during SSC. The smaller temperature drop in the SSC newborns than in controls before the mother's arrival may be due to the cap worn by SSC newborns that prevented heat dispersion (McCall et al., 2008). After the mother's arrival, no differences were observed between groups. Some differences in data collection mean that results cannot be compared with those in other studies. As noted by Carfoot et al. (2003), in other studies (Christensson et al., 1992), controls were separated from their mothers and kept in an incubator or in the nursery, whereas in this study, rooming-in was offered, and in both groups, a nurse helped with breast-feeding. Therefore, it is harder to find differences.

Techniques for recording temperatures were also different: axillary, intrascapular, and foot temperature, recorded with three electronic digital thermometers every 5 min after delivery (Christensson et al., 1992, 1993), or axillary temperature 5–14 and 90 min after delivery with a digital thermometer (Christensson et al., 1993), before SSC, and immediately and 2 hr after (Bohnhorst et al., 2001), with continuous recording (Fransson et al., 2005). In this study, temporal arterial temperature was taken with an infrared thermometer on the forehead, to reduce interference in the mother-child relationship.

Unlike in other studies, where SSC newborns showed better performance than did controls (8.7 ± 2.1 vs. 6.3 ± 2.6; *p* < .02; Moore & Anderson, 2007), in the current study, both groups suckled well. The lack of difference might be due to the close monitoring in both groups (every half hour, the temperature was taken and breast-feeding advice was provided if needed). Results observed are better than those observed in routine care; in fact, most newborns (70.6%) in the current study center, whether delivered vaginally or by cesarean section, are breast-fed within 2 hr while the percentage rose to 88.2% in both study groups. In this study, only two newborns in each group were not breast-fed within 2 hr. The SSC vaginally delivered newborns started breast-feeding sooner than the controls, as reported in other studies (Moore & Anderson, 2007). At discharge, 13 (76%) SSC babies and 11 (64.7%) controls were being breast-fed exclusively (in routine care overall, 66.6% of newborns by vaginal and cesarean deliveries are breast-fed), and the number was still higher in the SSC group 1, 2, and 3 months after delivery. This is supported by a systematic review (Anderson et al., 2007; Moore et al., 2007) on vaginally delivered newborns confirming the effectiveness of SSC on breast-feeding at 1–4 months (odds ratio = 1.82, 95% confidence interval = 1.08 to 3.07; Moore et al., 2007). These results are not confirmed in other studies (Moore & Anderson, 2007) on account of the small population.

This study confirms the feasibility of SSC after cesarean deliveries both from the organizational and the mothers' perspective. This study was organized in a public hospital on a volunteer basis and did not require extra personnel or an increase in resources, showing that the inclusion of SSC after a cesarean section can be easily adopted. The mothers' level of satisfaction was very high (the mothers who did not answer the questionnaire did practice SSC for at least 1 hr). The mean duration of SSC was 1 hr and 39 min, as in the study by Moore and Anderson (2007).

A limitation of the study is that operating rooms are not usually close to the obstetrics department, so SSC is not always possible immediately after delivery. This was the case in this study, so that, on average, 51 min had elapsed before the mothers were back in their rooms, and metabolic adaptation of the newborn may have occurred already (Christensson et al., 1992). Another limitation is the fact that the IBAT questionnaire is not validated in Italian. The results of this study can be extended to women exposed to locoregional but not to general anesthesia.

It is not possible to say whether SSC performed immediately after the delivery is equally safe, neither if it is feasible from the organizational point of view. Further multicenter studies would be required, which would also account for the variability in delivery and ward practices.

## Conclusions

Cesarean-delivered newborns exposed to SSC within 1 hr from delivery are not at risk for hypothermia.

410 The results show the feasibility of SSC (still not practiced widely in Italy after cesarean deliveries). The WHO recommendations highlight the importance of helping mothers start early breast-feeding after delivery, because early SSC was related to suckling imme-
415 diately after delivery, even for cesarean deliveries (WHO, 1998). The results of this study show that SSC can be performed safely in cesarean deliveries because it does not increase the risk of hypothermia.

## References

Arkiliç, C. F., Akça, O., Taguchi, A., Sessler, D. I., & Kurz, A. (2000). Temperature monitoring and management during neuraxial anesthesia: An observational study. *Anesthesia and Analgesia, 91*(3), 662–666.

Bauer, P. (1989). Multistage testing with adaptive designs. *Biometrie und Informatik in Medizin und Biologie, 20,* 130–148.

Bergman, N. J., Linley, L. L., & Fawcus, S. R. (2004). Randomized controlled trial of skin-to-skin contact from birth versus conventional incubator for physiological stabilization in 1200- to 2199-gram newborns. *Acta Paediatrica, 93*(6), 779–785.

Bohnhorst, B., Heyne, T., Peter, C. S., & Poets, C. F. (2001). Skin-to-skin (kangaroo) care, respiratory control, and thermoregulation. *Journal of Pediatrics, 138*(2), 193–197.

Carfoot, S., Williamson, P., & Dickson, R. (2003). A systematic review of randomised controlled trials evaluating the effect of mother/baby skin-to-skin care on successful breastfeeding. *Midwifery, 19*(2), 148–155.

Chiu, S. H., Anderson, G. C., & Burkhammer, M. D. (2005). Newborn temperature during skin-to-skin breastfeeding in couplets having breastfeeding difficulties. *Birth, 32*(2), 115–121.

Christensson, K., Siles, C., Cabrera, T., Belaustequi, A., de la Fuente, P., Lagercrantz, H., et al. (1993). Lower body temperatures in infants delivered by cesarean section than in vaginally delivered infants. *Acta Paediatrica, 82*(2), 128–131.

Christensson, K., Siles, C., Moreno, L., Belaustequi, A., de la Fuente, P., Lagercrantz, H., et al. (1992). Temperature, metabolic adaptation and crying in healthy full-term newborns cared for skin-to-skin or in a cot. *Acta Paediatrica, 81*(6–7), 488–493.

Erlandsson, K., Dsilna, A., Fagerberg, I., & Christensson, K. (2007). Skin-to-skin care with the father after cesarean birth and its effect on newborn crying and prefeeding behavior. *Birth, 34*(2), 105–114.

Feldman, R., Eidelman, A. I., Sirota, L., & Weller, A. (2002). Comparison of skin-to-skin (kangaroo) and traditional care: Parenting outcomes and preterm, infant development. *Pediatrics, 110*(1 Pt. 1), 16–26.

Fransson, A. L., Karlsson, H., & Nilsson, K. (2005). Temperature variation in newborn babies: Importance of physical contact with the mother. *Archives of Disease in Childhood. Fetal and Neonatal Edition, 90*(6), F500–F504.

Gruppo di Studio Della SIN, Sulla Care in Neonatologia. (2006). Kangaroo mother care: Una guida pratica [Italian ed.]. *Acta Neonatologica & Pediatrica, 20*(1), 5–39.

Horn, E. P., Schroeder, F., Gottschalk, A., Sessler, D. I., Hiltmeyer, N., Standi, T., et al. (2002). Active warming during cesarean delivery. *Anaesthesia and Analgesia, 94*(2), 409–414.

Hui, C. K., Huang, C. H., Lin, C. J., Lau, H. P., Chan, W. H., & Yeh, H. M. (2006). A randomised double-blind controlled study evaluating the hypothermic effect of 150 $\mu$g morphine during spinal anaesthesia for caesarean section. *Anaesthesia, 61*(1), 29–31.

Jonas, W., Wiklund, I., Nissen, E., Ransjö-Arvidson, A. B., & Uvnäs-Moberg, K. (2007). Newborn skin temperature two days postpartum during breastfeeding related to different labour ward practices. *Early Human Development, 83*(1), 55–62.

Klaus, M. H., Jerauld, R., Kreger, N. C., McAlpine, F., Steffa, M., & Kennel, J. H. (1972). Maternal attachment: Importance of the first post-partum days. *New England Journal of Medicine, 286*(9), 460–463.

Knobel, R., & Holditch-Davis, D. (2007). Thermoregulation and heat loss prevention after birth and during neonatal intensive-care unit stabilization of extremely low-birthweight infants. *Journal of Obstetric, Gynecologic, and Neonatal Nursing, 36*(3), 280–287.

Martin, S. A., & Kline, A. (2004). Can there be a standard for temperature measurement in the pediatric intensive care unit? *AACN Clinical Issues, 15*(2), 254–266.

Matsukawa, T., Ozaki, M., Nishiyama, T., Imamura, M., & Kumazawa, T. (2000). Comparison of infrared thermometer with thermocouple for monitoring skin temperature. *Critical Care Medicine, 28*(2), 532–536.

Matthews, M. K. (1988). Developing an instrument to assess infant breastfeeding behaviour in the early neonatal period. *Midwifery, 4*(4), 154–165.

McClellan, M. S., & Cabianca, W. A. (1980). Effects of early mother-infant contact following cesarean birth. *Obstetrics and Gynecology, 56*(1), 52–55.

McCall, E. M., Alderdice, F. A., Halliday, H. L., Jenkins, J. G., & Vohra, S. (2008). Interventions to prevent hypothermia at birth in preterm and/or low birthweight infants. *Cochrane Database Systematic Reviews.* Issue 1. doi: 10.1002/14651858.CD004210.pub3.

Moore, E. R., & Anderson, G. C. (2007). Randomized controlled trial of very early mother-infant skin-to-skin contact and breast-feeding status. *Journal of Midwifery & Women's Health, 52*(2), 116–125.

Moore, E. R., Anderson, G. C., & Bergman, N. (2007). Early skin-to-skin contact for mothers and their healthy newborn infants [review]. *Cochrane Database of Systematic Reviews.* Issue 3. doi: 10.1002/14651858. CD003519.pub2.

O'Brien, P. C., & Fleming, T. R. (1979). A multiple testing procedure for clinical trials. *Biometrics, 35*(3), 549–556.

Peillon, P., Dounas, M., Lebonhomme, J. J., & Guittard, Y. (2002). Hypothermie sévère au décours de césariennes sous rachianesthésie [Severe hypothermia associated with caesarean section under spinal anaesthesia]. *Annales Françaises d'Anesthésie et de Réanimation, 21*(4), 299–302.

Saito, T., Sessler, D. I., Fujita, K., Ooi, Y., & Jeffrey, R. (1998). Thermoregulatory effects of spinal and epidural anesthesia during cesarean delivery. *Regional Anesthesia and Pain Medicine, 23*(4), 418–423.

Tessier, R., Cristo, M., Velez, S., Giron, M., de Calume, Z. F., Ruiz-Palaez, J. G., et al. (1998). Kangaroo mother care and the bonding hypothesis. *Pediatrics, 102*(2), e17.

World Health Organization, Department of Reproductive Health and Research. (2003). *Kangaroo mother care: A practical guide.* Geneva, Switzerland. Retrieved May 9, 2009, from http://whqlibdoc.who.int/publications/2003/9241590351.pdf

World Health Organization, Division of Child Health and Development. (1998). *Evidence for the ten steps to successful breastfeeding.* Geneva, Switzerland. Retrieved May 8, 2009, from http://whqlibdoc.who.int/publications/2004/9241591544_eng.pdf

World Health Organization, Maternal and Newborn Health, Safe Motherhood Unit of Reproductive Health. (1997). *Thermal protection of the newborn: A practical guide.* Geneva, Switzerland. Retrieved May 8, 2009, from http://whqlibdoc.who.int/hq/1997/WHO_RHT_MSM_97.2.pdf

**Acknowledgments:** This study was made possible thanks to the support of the coordinator, the director, and a consultant of neonatology; the health care workers (pediatric nurses, nurses' aides, midwives); and the nursing students and mothers who agreed to participate.

**Address correspondence to:** Paola Di Giulio, MSc, RN, Department of Public Health and Microbiology, Turin University, Turin, Italy 10100. E-mail: paola.digiulio@unito.it

# Exercise for Article 11

## *Factual Questions*

1. Was randomization used in this study?

2. Did the mothers *or* the researchers choose when to start breastfeeding?

3. Breastfeeding was considered exclusive only if what condition had been met?

4. How many women in the SSC group withdrew consent?

5. What was the mean age of the mothers in the control group?

6. Did the researchers conclude that SSC can be performed safely in cesarean deliveries?

## Questions for Discussion

7. This research article is classified as true experimental research. Do you agree with this classification? Explain.

8. Are the two treatment conditions described in sufficient detail? Explain. (See lines 158–175.)

9. Is the measurement of satisfaction described in sufficient detail? Explain. (See lines 210–220.)

10. Is it important to know how many women did not consent to the study? Explain. (See lines 233–234.)

11. How helpful is Figure 1 in helping you understand the design of this study? Explain. (See Figure 1.)

12. Do you think this topic warrants further investigation in future studies? Why? Why not?

## Quality Ratings

Directions: Indicate your level of agreement with each of the following statements by circling a number from 5 for strongly agree (SA) to 1 for strongly disagree (SD). If you believe an item is not applicable to this research article, leave it blank. Be prepared to explain your ratings. When responding to criteria A and B, keep in mind that brief titles and abstracts are conventional in published research.

A. The title of the article is appropriate.

SA   5   4   3   2   1   SD

B. The abstract provides an effective overview of the research article.

SA   5   4   3   2   1   SD

C. The introduction establishes the importance of the study.

SA   5   4   3   2   1   SD

D. The literature review establishes the context for the study.

SA   5   4   3   2   1   SD

E. The research purpose, question, or hypothesis is clearly stated.

SA   5   4   3   2   1   SD

F. The method of sampling is sound.

SA   5   4   3   2   1   SD

G. Relevant demographics (for example, age, gender, and ethnicity) are described.

SA   5   4   3   2   1   SD

H. Measurement procedures are adequate.

SA   5   4   3   2   1   SD

I. All procedures have been described in sufficient detail to permit a replication of the study.

SA   5   4   3   2   1   SD

J. The participants have been adequately protected from potential harm.

SA   5   4   3   2   1   SD

K. The results are clearly described.

SA   5   4   3   2   1   SD

L. The discussion/conclusion is appropriate.

SA   5   4   3   2   1   SD

M. Despite any flaws, the report is worthy of publication.

SA   5   4   3   2   1   SD

# Article 12

## Life Review Therapy As an Intervention to Manage Depression and Enhance Life Satisfaction in Individuals With Right Hemisphere Cerebral Vascular Accidents

**Marsha Courville Davis**, PhD, RN, CRRN, LPC, NCC[*]

ABSTRACT. This pilot study sought to determine if the use of Life Review Therapy would result in lower levels of depression and higher degrees of life satisfaction in individuals with right hemisphere cerebral vascular accidents (CVAs). Fourteen subjects in a Southern rehabilitation center were randomly assigned to either an experimental or control group. The experimental group received three one-hour sessions of Life Review Therapy and the control group viewed three one-hour sessions of neutral video with a follow-up discussion. Following the third session of each group, subjects were administered the Zung Scale for Depression and the Life Satisfaction Index–Form Z. A one-way ANOVA revealed a significantly lower level of depression ($p < .01$) and a significantly higher degree of life satisfaction ($p < .01$) in the Life Review Therapy group.

From *Issues in Mental Health Nursing*, 25, 503–515. Copyright ©
2004 by Taylor and Francis, Inc. Reprinted with permission.

Cerebral Vascular Accident (CVA) is a leading cause of adult disability affecting approximately 750,000 people per year in the United States (Williams, Jaing, Matchar, & Samsa, 1999). Depression is the
5 most commonly reported psychiatric diagnosis in individuals who have experienced a CVA. Rates of post-stroke depression have ranged from 25% to 60% (Andersen, Vestergaard, Ingemann-Nielsen, & Lauritzen, 1995; Astrom, Adolfsson, & Asplund, 1993; Hermann,
10 Black, Lawrence, Szekely, & Szalai, 1998; Paolucci, Antonucci, Pratesi, Traballesi, Grasso, & Lubich, 1999).

Life review therapy is a treatment strategy defined as "the process of facilitation of the life review experi-
15 ence or mental process of reviewing one's life" (Butler, 1963, p. 66). Butler postulated that the life review is a natural process experienced by the elderly, by younger persons for whom death is imminent, and by those experiencing a crisis or a transition. It is a process of re-
20 membering and mentally reviewing life histories and addressing unsettled conflicts. Life review therapy may be one alternative nonpharmacological strategy to improve the quality of life in the CVA patient population.

No known existing studies of using life review
25 therapy for a crisis such as a CVA were found in the review of the literature. Additionally, the empirical studies on life review therapy are limited and show inconsistent results. Because of the limited nature of the empirical studies and the lack of research on life
30 review therapy with patients in crisis and the high incidence of CVA in the United States, this research study sought to add to the body of knowledge of life review therapy as well as that of psychological adjustment to CVA. The purpose of the study, therefore, was to de-
35 termine if life review therapy could produce lower levels of depression and higher levels of life satisfaction among individuals with CVA.

### Rationale

The adjustment process is individual for each person. Difficulties with adjustment have, therefore, his-
40 torically been treated as they arise. If it could be determined that life review therapy could produce lower levels of depression and higher levels of life satisfaction in the CVA population, thereby facilitating adjustment, the life review process could be initiated with
45 this population in crisis and allow the patient an opportunity to be more quickly involved in the business of learning to proceed with his or her life.

### Review of the Literature

*Theoretical Framework*

Butler's (1963) Life Review was the framework for this study. According to Butler, life review helps the
50 patient to maintain self-esteem, reaffirm a sense of identity, reduce feelings of loss and isolation, and emphasize the positive aspects of one's life. The theorist points out that life review is not merely reminiscence— the art or process of recalling the past—but it is a pur-
55 posive process leading to personality reintegration. The

---

[*] *Marsha Courville Davis* is former associate professor of nursing at Southeastern Louisiana University.

function of the life review is to allow for an opening of the personality so that it is free to evolve and change in response to the experiences of life.

*Life Review Process*

Haight (1991) published a 30-year literature search on the subject of life review/reminiscence. Haight concluded that there was a rapidly growing interest in the subject and called for more well-designed research. Merriam (1993) argued that the life review process may not be a universal one, experienced by all people as they enter old age, as Butler (1963) had postulated. Kropf and Greene (1993) concluded that undergoing the life review process helped parents who care for developmentally disabled family members gain a stronger sense of control over their lives. Waters (1990) reported on methods of facilitation of the life review by mental health counselors. O'Connor (1994) identified salient themes in the life review of frail elderly men and women in London. Peachey (1992) offered a set of life review questions. Muntz and White (1989) concluded that there was no evidence that the life satisfaction, psychological well-being, or depression scores of high-risk mentally competent older adults were affected significantly by the life review. Froehlich and Nelson (1986) explored affective meanings of life review through activities and discussions in groups. They perceived life review as "powerful" (p. 32) and encouraged the use of activities to facilitate the life review. Sherman (1987) conducted a study to determine whether social support and a sense of well-being among the elderly could be developed using reminiscence groups. Both experimental groups in his study increased in life satisfaction and self-concept.

Giltinan (1990) explored the effect of life review and discussion on the self-actualization process in elderly women. A self-actualization measure was administered prior to six life review sessions for the experimental group and to a comparison group that received no treatment. No significant differences between groups were shown in self-actualization at posttest. Haight (1992) studied the long-term effects of the structured life review process in a group of 52 homebound elderly clients. Subjects tested one year post-treatment revealed little change on (a) life satisfaction, (b) psychological well-being, (c) depression, or (d) activities of daily living. Stevens-Ratchford (1993) investigated the effects of life review and reminiscence on self-esteem and depression in older adults. Results showed no significant effects on self-esteem and depression scores using a life review reminiscence treatment. Molinari, Cully, Kendjelic, and Kunik (2001) studied reminiscence in older psychiatric patients as it related to attachment and personality in an effort to explain the apparent efficacy of life review treatment. The findings revealed higher scores on the teach/inform reminiscence function for securely attached patients. Extroversion and conversation reminiscence were found to be related, as was the personality factor of openness with identity and problem solving.

*Adjustment to CVA*

Paolucci, Antonucci, Pratesi, Traballesi, Grasso, and Lubich (1999) studied post-stroke depression and its role in rehabilitation. Results revealed depression occurring in 27% of the population of 470 patients, with female patients showing more depression than males. The authors recommended that antidepressant therapy be initiated as soon as possible, preferring serotonergic drugs over the tricyclics because of side effects and safety factors.

The meaning of stroke in elderly women was investigated by Hilton (2002). Themes of transformation and transition were identified. The elderly women revealed they were unable to "become themselves again as they had known themselves to be" (Hilton, 2002, p. 23). In adjusting to transformation, the women were able to identify new roles and coping strategies as well as accept the realities of their new limitations. With regard to identification of themes of meaning of stroke, the elderly women identified changes as a result of the stroke, developed new strategies to overcome obstacles, mourned losses, and were able to resolve issues that arose. The women experienced uncertainty and regret, reduction of autonomy, and despair, isolation, and frustration.

Self-care self-efficacy as it related to quality of life after stroke was explored by Robinson-Smith (2002). The research revealed that patients with higher self-care self-efficacy reported fewer depression symptoms. Motivation of patients to develop strategies to enhance their quality of life, especially as it related to independence, was recommended.

Rochette and Desrosiers (2002) investigated coping strategies post-stroke. Coping strategies were not found to change over time, and women were found to use more coping strategies than men, despite the fact that in this study the women were not more depressed than the men. The researchers argued that the level of actualization of those experiencing a stroke may affect the type of coping strategies used, with more positive coping strategies chosen by those with a higher level of self-actualization. Employing more positive coping strategies may facilitate adaptation, according to the authors.

Psychological well-being three years after severe stroke was studied by Lofgren, Gustafson, and Nyberg (1998). Results revealed that 64% of the study participants showed high or middlerange scores for psychological well-being. A strong association between psychological well-being and depression also was found, with lower levels of depression in those subjects with high psychological well-being.

## Method

### Research Design

A posttest-only control-group design was used in the study. This design was chosen due to the short period of time that generally existed between attempting pretest and posttest. The researcher sought to guard
170 against effects of a pretest (Polit, Beck, & Hungler, 2001). Using a table of computer-generated random numbers, the researcher randomly assigned subjects to the experimental or alternative treatment. At the end of the last session for the subjects assigned to each treat-
175 ment, posttest measures of the dependent variables were administered by the researcher.

### Sample

Participants were recruited through referral from their physician or designated staff members at the rehabilitation center where the study was conducted. Cri-
180 teria for inclusion in the study included: (a) no previous history of CVA, (b) onset of CVA within 6 months at the time of the study, (c) no other acute medical or psychiatric/psychological complications since the occurrence of the CVA, and (d) ability to verbally com-
185 municate.

### Setting

The sessions were conducted by the researcher in a physical rehabilitation center in the USA in the evening, after the completion of the evening meal. The same room was used to administer the Life Review
190 treatment and alternative treatment.

### Procedure

A consent form was developed and approved by the Institutional Review Board (IRB) of the rehabilitation center. The proposal for the study was reviewed by the IRB and permission for the study to begin was given.
195 In order to identify a sample for this study, the researcher distributed the list of criteria for inclusion in the study to designated staff members who were responsible for generating referrals, insofar as the researcher was not an employee and had no access to
200 medical records. The staff members were to screen all new CVA admissions and then refer possible participants to the researcher. The researcher made contact with at least one staff member responsible for screening the new admissions on a weekly basis, even if no
205 referrals were received, to encourage continued interest in the study. As referrals were received and consent given, the researcher randomly assigned the participants to either the experimental or the control treatment using a computer-generated table of random numbers.
210 The researcher flipped a coin and determined that the elements designated as "1" would be the experimental group, leaving the element designated as "0" for the control group. There was no restriction in the random assignment such as blocking or stratification. Be-
215 cause the lengths of stays in rehabilitation centers at the time of this study were shorter than they had been pre-

viously, and the possibility of early discharge existed, the sessions began the following weekday of the referral and were conducted on consecutive days as often as
220 possible.

Materials utilized in the study were Haight's Life Review and Experiencing Form (Haight, 1982), as well as three video recordings on the subjects of food safety, fire safety, and telephone courtesy. The video re-
225 cordings were chosen due to their neutral but informative content and entertaining nature, as well as for their appropriate length of approximately 35 minutes for each video. Questions to stimulate discussion following each video also were developed.
230 Each of the participants in the experimental treatment received three individually administered one-hour sessions of life review therapy using Haight's (1982) Life Review and Experiencing Form. This instrument is composed of 68 items that cover childhood, adoles-
235 cence, family and home, adulthood, and a summary. During the first session, childhood items were reviewed (through the fifth adolescence question). The childhood items included such questions as earliest memory of life and memories of brothers or sisters.
240 The first five adolescence questions reviewed items such as earliest teenage memories and school activity. Session two presented the remainder of adolescence questions as well as family and home questions and concluded with adulthood question number five. Ex-
245 amples of the last adolescence items included questions about hardships and first love.

The family and home section reviewed such memories as relationships and atmosphere of the home. The first five adult items included memories such as impor-
250 tance of religion and work experience. In session three, adulthood and summary questions were reviewed. The final adulthood questions involved memories about significant relationships, marriage, and difficulties of adult years. The summary questions elicited such
255 thoughts as what the person would change or leave unchanged and main satisfactions of the person's life.

For the control treatment, each participant spent the same amount of time individually with the researcher in an alternative activity. Each participant viewed three
260 videos, one each during three one-hour sessions. Following each of the videos, the researcher asked the participant a number of predetermined questions regarding the content of the video, and engaged in a discussion of the video with the participant. There was no
265 therapeutic intent in this activity.

Following the third session of each participant in both treatments, the researcher administered the Zung Scale for Depression (ZSD; Zung, 1967) and the Life Satisfaction Index–Form Z (LSI–Z; Wood, Wylie, &
270 Schaeffer, 1969). Due to vision problems associated with CVAs, the researcher read the inventories to each participant.

*Instruments*

Two instruments were used in this study—the Zung Scale for Depression (ZSD) and the Life Satisfaction Index–Form Z (LSI–Z). Following review of other possible instruments and a pilot study, these were chosen due to their simplicity and the 10-minute length of time for administration, considering the fatigue factor of the participants.

The ZSD is a Likert scale instrument composed of 20 items, each coded one, two, three, or four for none or little of the time, some of the time, good part of the time, or most or all of the time. If a participant chooses most or all of the time for the item, "I feel downhearted, blue and sad," he or she would score four points on that item, for instance. The total points are then computed for each participant, yielding the depression score.

There are only minimal data available concerning the reliability of the ZSD, either internal or temporal. No reliability correlations could be found. However, validity of the instrument is well documented. Numerous studies have demonstrated the ZSD to reliably distinguish between normal and clinically depressed individuals. Scores on the ZSD, according to Keyser and Sweetland (1985), correlated highly with scores on the Hamilton Rating Scale, Beck Depression Inventory (.79), Costello-Comrey Depression Scale (.74), and Depression Scale of the Multiple Affect Adjective Check List (.57).

The Life Satisfaction Index was designed to measure life satisfaction and is composed of 13 agree or disagree statements. Each of the statements is coded either two or zero for agree, or two or zero for disagree. The items coded as two are those indicative of high life satisfaction. The participant marks either one of the choices, and the total score is then computed. A high life satisfaction is based upon a high score, with the highest score possible of 26. Wood et al. (1969) reported a split-half reliability coefficient of .79. Wood et al. (1969) also reported a correlation of .57 between the LSI–Z and the clinically based Life Satisfaction Ratings Instrument. The correlation is considered weak evidence, however, for the convergent validity of the LSI–Z. Baiyewu and Jegede (1992) reported an internal consistency value of zero following administration of the LSI–Z to 945 Nigerians, age 60 and over. Factor composition analysis revealed that LSI–Z scores correlated significantly with items on self-assessed health, loneliness, and sex. Items that measured social contact did not correlate at a significant level.

*Null Hypotheses*

**Hypothesis 1**: There will be no statistically significant difference in the mean scores of the Zung Scale for Depression (Zung, 1967) between the individuals who were administered life review therapy and the individuals who viewed the videos.

**Hypothesis 2**: There will be no statistically significant difference in the mean scores of the Life Satisfaction Index–Form Z (Wood, Wylie, & Schaefer, 1969) between the individuals who were administered life review therapy and the individuals who viewed the videos.

*Data Analysis*

The hypotheses were tested using a one-way analysis of variance (ANOVA). The scores on each of the instruments were compared from experimental group to control group to determine if there was a significant difference. An alpha level of .05 was set for statistical significance.

## Results and Discussion

*Results*

The first hypothesis was tested using the scores from the ZSD from the experimental and control groups in a one-way ANOVA. The ANOVA revealed a significant difference between groups $F(1,12) = 22.46$ $p < .01$. The mean of the experimental group posttest score ($M = 31.9$, $SD = 3.24$) was lower than that of the control group ($M = 44.6$, $SD = 5.68$). Therefore, the first null hypothesis was rejected.

The second hypothesis was tested using the scores from the LSI–Z from the experimental and control groups in a one-way ANOVA. The ANOVA revealed a significant difference between groups $F(2,12) = 14.98$, $p < .01$. The mean scores of the experimental group ($M = 24.3$, $SD = 3.24$) were found to be significantly higher than the control group ($M = 20.3$, $SD = 5.68$). The second null hypothesis was rejected.

Eighteen individuals had originally agreed to participate in the study. Two participants who had been assigned to the control treatment withdrew from the study during the data collection phase. Additionally, the researcher eliminated data from two other individuals, one from the experimental group and one from the control group. The latter participants were withdrawn from the study because it was determined that they subsequently did not meet the criteria for inclusion. The participant from the control group expressed to the researcher that she had given inaccurate answers on the posttest because for religious reasons she did not want to give negative answers. The participant in the experimental group began to cry during the last session, sharing that he had recently been diagnosed with prostate cancer and that his wife of 46 years had died within the last month.

The remaining 14 individuals ranged in age from 45 to 87, with a mean age of 68. There were three females and four males in the experimental group as well as in the control group. The mean age of the control group was 67.5; 68.5 was the mean age of the experimental group. All participants were Caucasian, although two of the original 18 were African American. Eleven were married, one was divorced, and two were widows.

*Discussion*

This exploratory pilot study is the first to examine Life Review as a treatment to manage depression and increase life satisfaction in individuals who have ex-
385 perienced CVAs. The study involved a small sample (*n* = 14) due to the restrictive nature of the criteria for admission to the study. Three years were required to obtain the small sample, possibly due to the restrictive inclusion criteria. The researcher was receiving refer-
390 rals on an extremely irregular basis and decided after three years to accept the sample size of 14.

Experiencing a CVA is considered to be a major life crisis, changing an individual's and his or her family's life. Butler (1963) postulated that the life review
395 process occurs at times of crisis; this process can be facilitated psychodynamically, either individually or in groups. In this study, facilitation of the life review demonstrated at < .01 level of significance a difference between experimental and control groups with regard
400 to higher degree of life satisfaction and lower levels of depression.

Lower levels of depression and higher degrees of life satisfaction with the life review process with individuals who have experienced a CVA could also mean
405 that life review therapy could be beneficial in assisting the participants in the adjustment process related to their CVA, thereby helping them to overcome the life crisis of a CVA.

Previous data-based and theoretical studies on the
410 life review process have yielded conflicting results. Muntz and White (1989) and Stevens-Ratchford (1993) revealed no significant effects using the life review. The longitudinal study of Haight (1992) is most consistent with the present study, demonstrating no increases
415 in depression nor decreases in self-esteem one-year post-life-review treatment and significant gains in life satisfaction and psychological well-being eight weeks post-life-review treatment.

*Limitations*

There were several limitations of the study.

420 1. The sample size was only 14. The high acuity level of admitted patients at the time of the study may have been a significant factor as well as the restrictive inclusion criteria.
2. The researcher administered the treatment and al-
425 ternative treatments to individuals in the experimental and control group as well as administering the instruments. Experimenter bias may have occurred.
3. The participants had interaction with other health-
430 care providers and family members, which could have influenced responses on the posttest.
4. Family dynamics that may have influenced depression and life satisfaction could have been present unbeknownst to the researcher.
435 5. The cultural composition of the sample was Caucasian. African Americans and Asian Americans,

however, were considered for the study but did not meet inclusion criteria. This final sample may pose a problem with generalizability.

440 Even though there were limitations, the results of this pilot study add to the growing body of literature supporting the need for nonpharmacological interventions for this population. As one subject stated, "Now I don't feel like I'm just a person with a left arm and leg
445 that don't work. I realize that I am still a valuable person with a lot to offer people around me."

*Implications*

Current research utilizing life review therapy is inconsistent with regard to therapeutic efficacy but does lead one to assume that there may be value to the inter-
450 vention. This intervention could be implemented by nurses in rehabilitation settings as well as in home health settings with CVA patients. When working with patients having depressive or other mental disorders, it is recommended that a qualified practitioner be avail-
455 able in the event that follow-up counseling is needed to address sensitive issues.

The researcher cautiously interprets the results due to the small sample size. However, the results of this study have theoretical implications in that this study
460 addressed the issue of the process of the life review occurring during time of crisis. The findings of the study support the psychodynamic theory of life review and crisis. Because this study demonstrated significantly lower levels of depression and a higher degree
465 of life satisfaction, the researcher very cautiously concludes that the participants in the experimental group may possibly be better able to meet the crisis of a right hemisphere CVA. Further research with a larger sample size is recommended.

## References

Anderson, G., Vestergaard, K., Ingemann-Nielsen, M., & Lauritzen, L. (1995). Risk factors for post-stroke depression. *Acta Psychiatrica Scandinavica, 92,* 193–198.

Astrom, M., Adolfsson, R., & Asplund, K. (1993). Major depression in stroke patients: A three-year longitudinal study. *Stroke, 24,* 976–982.

Baiyewu, O., & Jegede, O. (1992). Life satisfaction in elderly Nigerians: Reliability and factor composition of the Life Satisfaction Index–Z. *Age and Aging, 21,* 256.

Butler, R. (1963). The life review: An interpretation of reminiscence in the aged. *Psychiatry, 26,* 65–76.

Froehlich, J., & Nelson, D. (1986). Affective meanings of life review through activities and discussion. *American Journal of Occupational Therapy, 40,* 27–33.

Giltinan, J. (1990). Using life review to facilitate self-actualization in elderly women. *Gerontology and Geriatrics Education, 10,* 75–83.

Haight, B. (1982). *Haight's life review and experiencing form.* Unpublished instrument. Medical University of South Carolina, Charleston, SC.

Haight, B. (1991). Reminiscing: The state of the art as a basis for practice. *International Journal of Aging and Human Development, 33,* 1–32.

Haight, B. (1992). Long-term effects of a structured life review process. *Journal of Gerontology, 47,* 312–315.

Hermann, N., Black, S. E., Lawrence, J., Szekely, C., & Szalai, J. P. (1998). The Sunnybrook stroke study of depressive symptoms and functional outcome. *Stroke, 29,* 618–624.

Hilton, E. (2002). The meaning of stroke in elderly women. *Journal of Gerontological Nursing, 28,* 19–26.

Keyser, D. J., & Sweetland, R. C. (Eds.). (1985). *Test critiques* (vol. 3). Kansas City, MO: Westport.

Kropf, N., & Greene, R. (1993). Life review with families who care for developmentally disabled members: A model. *Journal of Gerontological Social Work, 2,* 25–39.

Lofgren, B., Gustafson, Y., & Nyberg, L. (1998). Psychological well-being three years after severe stroke. *Stroke, 30,* 567–572.

Merriam, S. (1993). Butler's life review: How universal is it? *International Journal of Aging and Human Development, 37,* 163–175.

Molinari, Y., Cully, J., Kendjelic, E., & Kunik, M. (2001). Reminiscence and its relationship to attachment and personality in gero-psychiatric patients. *International Journal of Aging and Human Development, 52,* 173–184.

Muntz, M., & White, J. (1989). The use of a structured life review process as a therapeutic nursing intervention with institutionalized older adults. Unpublished manuscript.

O'Connor, P. (1994). Salient themes in the life review of a sample of frail elderly respondents in London. *Gerontologist, 24,* 224–230.

Paolucci, S., Antonucci, G., Pratesi, L., Traballesi, M., Grasso, M., & Lubich, S. (1999). Post stroke depression and its role in rehabilitation patients. *Archives of Physical Medicine and Rehabilitation, 80,* 985–990.

Peachey, N. (1992). Helping the elderly person resolve integrity versus despair. *Perspectives in Psychiatric Care, 28,* 29–30.

Polit, D. P., Beck, C. T., & Hungler. B. P. (2001). *Essentials of Nursing Research.* Philadelphia: Lippincott.

Robinson-Smith, G. (2002). Self-efficacy and quality of life after stroke. *Journal of Neuroscience Nursing, 34,* 91–98.

Rochette, A., & Desrosiers, J. (2002). Coping with the consequences of a stroke. *International Journal of Rehabilitation Research, 25,* 17–24.

Sherman, E. (1987). Reminiscence groups for community elderly. *Gerontologist, 7,* 569–572.

Stevens-Ratchford, R. (1993). The effect of life review reminiscence activities on depression and self-esteem in older adults. *American Journal of Occupational Therapy, 47,* 413–430.

Waters, E. (1990). The life review: Strategies for working with individual and groups. *Journal of Mental Health Counseling, 12,* 270–278.

Williams, G. R., Jaing, J. G., Matchar, D. B., & Samsa, G. P. (1999). Incidence and occurrence of total (first-ever and recurrent) stroke. *Stroke, 30,* 2523–2528.

Wood, V., Wylie, M. L., & Schaefer, B. (1969). An analysis of a short self-report measure of life satisfaction: Correlation with rater judgments. *Journal of Gerontology, 24,* 465–469.

Zung, W. (1967). A self-rating depression scale. *Archives of General Psychiatry, 12,* 63–70.

**Address correspondence to**: Marsha Courville Davis, 801 Harmony Lane, Mandeville, LA 70471. E-mail: litlnurs@bellsouth.net

# Exercise for Article 12

## *Factual Questions*

1. What is the explicitly stated purpose of the study?

2. What method was used to assign subjects to the experimental or alternative treatments?

3. Participants were recruited through referral from whom?

4. Each of the participants in the experimental treatment received three individually administered sessions of life review therapy. How long did each session last?

5. Did members of the control group engage in activities with the researcher?

6. Of the original 18 individuals who had originally agreed to participate in the study, how many completed the study?

7. Were both null hypotheses rejected?

## *Questions for Discussion*

8. How important is the "Theoretical Framework" presented in lines 48–58 in helping you understand the study?

9. The researcher did not administer pretests. In your opinion, is this a flaw in the research methodology? Explain. (See lines 166–169.)

10. In lines 191–194, the researcher states that "A consent form was developed and approved by the Institutional Review Board (IRB) of the rehabilitation center. The proposal for the study was reviewed by the IRB and permission for the study to begin was given." In your opinion, is it important for researchers to make such statements in their research reports? Explain.

11. The Life Review Therapy administered to participants in the experimental group is described in lines 230–256. In your opinion, is it described in sufficient detail? Explain. While answering this question, keep in mind that the researcher has provided references where a consumer of research can obtain additional information on this type of therapy.

12. Is it important to know that scores on the ZSD correlated highly with scores on other measures of depression such as the Beck Depression Inventory? Explain. (See lines 295–300.)

13. Do you agree with the researcher that this study is an "exploratory pilot study"? Why? Why not? (See lines 382–385.)

14. This research article is classified as an example of "True Experimental Research" in the table of contents for this book. Do you agree with this classification? Explain.

## *Quality Ratings*

Directions: Indicate your level of agreement with each of the following statements by circling a number from 5 for strongly agree (SA) to 1 for strongly disagree (SD). If you believe an item is not applicable to this research article, leave it blank. Be prepared to explain your ratings. When responding to criteria A and B, keep in mind that brief titles and abstracts are conventional in published research.

A. The title of the article is appropriate.

SA   5   4   3   2   1   SD

B.  The abstract provides an effective overview of the
research article.

SA   5   4   3   2   1   SD

C.  The introduction establishes the importance of the
study.

SA   5   4   3   2   1   SD

D.  The literature review establishes the context for
the study.

SA   5   4   3   2   1   SD

E.  The research purpose, question, or hypothesis is
clearly stated.

SA   5   4   3   2   1   SD

F.  The method of sampling is sound.

SA   5   4   3   2   1   SD

G.  Relevant demographics (for example, age, gender,
and ethnicity) are described.

SA   5   4   3   2   1   SD

H.  Measurement procedures are adequate.

SA   5   4   3   2   1   SD

I.  All procedures have been described in sufficient
detail to permit a replication of the study.

SA   5   4   3   2   1   SD

J.  The participants have been adequately protected
from potential harm.

SA   5   4   3   2   1   SD

K.  The results are clearly described.

SA   5   4   3   2   1   SD

L.  The discussion/conclusion is appropriate.

SA   5   4   3   2   1   SD

M.  Despite any flaws, the report is worthy of publication.

SA   5   4   3   2   1   SD

# Article 13

# An Intervention Study to Enhance Medication Compliance in Community-Dwelling Elderly Individuals

**Terry T. Fulmer**, PhD, RN, FAAN, **Penny Hollander Feldman**, PhD, **Tae Sook Kim**, RN, MSN, **Barbara Carty**, EdD, RN, **Mark Beers**, MD, **Maria Molina**, MD, **Margaret Putnam**, BA[*]

## ABSTRACT

*Objective*: To determine whether daily videotelephone or regular telephone reminders would increase the proportion of prescribed cardiac medications taken in a sample of elderly individuals who have congestive heart failure (CHF).

*Methods*: The authors recruited community-dwelling individuals age 65 and older who had the primary or secondary diagnosis of CHF into a randomized controlled trial of reminder calls designed to enhance medication compliance. There were three arms: a control group that received usual care; a group that received regular daily telephone call reminders; and a group that received daily videotelephone call reminders. Compliance was defined as the percent of therapeutic coverage as recorded by Medication Event Monitoring System (MEMS) caps. Subjects were recruited from two sources: a large urban home health care agency and a large urban ambulatory clinic of a major teaching hospital. Baseline and postintervention MOS 36-Item Short-Form Health Survey (SF-36) scores and Minnesota Living with Heart Failure (MLHF) scores were obtained.

*Results*: There was a significant time effect during the course of the study from baseline to postintervention ($F[2,34] = 4.08$, $p < .05$). Over time the elderly individuals who were called, either by telephone or videotelephone, showed enhanced medication compliance relative to the control group. There was a trend, but no significant difference between the two intervention groups. Both SF-36 and MLHF scores improved from baseline to postintervention for all groups. There was no significant change in the SF-36 scores for the sample, but there was a significant change for the MLHF scores ($p < .001$). The control group had a significant falloff in the medication compliance rate during the course of the study, dropping from 81% to 57%.

*Conclusions*: Telephone interventions are effective in enhancing medication compliance and may prove more cost effective than clinic visits or preparation of prepoured pill boxes in the home. Technologic advances which enable clinicians to monitor and enhance patient medication compliance may reduce costly and distressing hospitalization for elderly individuals with CHF.

From *Journal of Gerontological Nursing*, 25, 6–14. Copyright © 1999 by SLACK Incorporated. Reprinted with permission.

Medication compliance is a critical element in the successful management of treatable diseases and symptoms. Noncompliance poses a serious health risk to those who are unable or unwilling to take their medications as prescribed, and certain populations may be at increased risk for the complications resulting from poor adherence to a medication regimen. Elderly individuals who live at home are such a population. It has been well documented that the compliance rate, in general, for elderly individuals taking medications is problematic (Cargill, 1992; Kruse et al., 1992; Salzman, 1995).

Estimates of noncompliance in the geriatric population vary from study to study, depending in part on the definition used and the method of measurement. Kruse et al. (1992) used the microprocessor-based Medication Event Monitoring System (MEMS) (Cramer, Mattson, Prevey, Scheyer, & Ouellette, 1989; Kruse & Weber, 1990) to measure compliance, which was defined as the percentage of prescribed doses taken. The reliability and validity of the MEMS for measuring compliance has been addressed (DeGeest, Dunbar-Jacob, & Vanhaeckel, 1998) in a hypertension study where interviews were conducted to compare patient reports of compliance versus the MEMS data, and superior specificity and reliability were documented. Based on a sample of 18 independently living elderly patients discharged from the hospital, they reported patient-specific noncompliance rates ranging from 0% to 76%, with a mean of 31% in the third week after discharge (DeGeest et al., 1998). Fineman and DeFelice (1992) measured compliance by administering a 20-question survey instrument to elderly individuals attending senior citizen centers. Using this self-report method, they found 15% of their sample to be noncompliant with a prescribed medication regimen (Fineman & DeFelice, 1992).

[*]*Terry T. Fulmer* is professor, Division of Nursing, New York University, New York, New York. *Tae Sook Kim* is research doctoral fellow, Division of Nursing, New York University, New York, New York. *Barbara Carty* is clinical associate professor, Division of Nursing, New York University, New York, New York. *Penny Hollander Feldman* is director, Center for Home Care Policy and Research of the Visiting Nurse Service, New York, New York. *Margaret Putnam* is project coordinator, Center for Home Care Policy and Research of the Visiting Nurse Service, New York, New York. *Mark Beers* is associate editor, *Merck Manuals* and Senior Director Geriatrics, Merck and Company, West Point, Pennsylvania. *Maria Molina* is intern, Elmhurst General Hospital, Elmhurst, New York.

Regardless of the exact range or percentage of coverage one accepts as the true reflection of medication noncompliance, practitioners agree that the health risks associated with poor adherence warrant serious experimentation with strategies designed to improve compliance rates. This article reports one such experiment: a randomized trial aimed at testing two interventions for enhancing medication compliance among elderly patients with congestive heart failure (CHF). The purpose of the study was to determine whether daily videotelephone or regular telephone reminders would increase the proportion of prescribed cardiac medications taken by these patients. The authors anticipated that the modest commitment of time required for a daily call to each elderly individual would yield a significant improvement in compliance.

### Factors Affecting Medication Compliance

Researchers have studied a variety of factors posited to affect medication compliance among elderly individuals. Patient-related factors include: knowledge and understanding of the medication regimen and its purpose (Fineman & DeFelice, 1992; Fitten, Coleman, Siembieda, Yu, & Ganzell, 1995; Klein, German, McPhee, Smith, & Levine, 1982; Wolfe & Schirm, 1992); cognitive functioning (Isaac & Tamblyn, 1993); age; and depressive symptomatology (Spiers & Kutzik, 1995). Overall, researchers have not found a significant relationship between knowledge and compliance behaviors in elderly individuals. In contrast, elderly individuals, ages, cognitive abilities, and levels of depression have been found to be significant predictors of compliance (Isaac & Tamblyn, 1993; Spiers & Kutzik, 1995).

Other factors posited to affect medication compliance are associated with the medication regimen per se. These include the number of medications, the number of pills, the complexity of the drug regimen, and the packaging of the prescribed medication. Evidence on these factors is mixed. Isaac and Tamblyn (1993) found no relationship between medication compliance and the number of medications, number of pills, or complexity of the regimen. On the other hand, in a randomized study of medication dosing and packaging alternatives, Murray, Birt, Manatunga, and Darnell (1993) found evidence to suggest that simplifying complex drug regimens to twice-daily administration with unit-of-use packages may improve medication compliance rates.

### Strategies for Enhancing Compliance

Strategies for improving compliance can be categorized into three groups: enabling, consequence, and stimulant (McKinney, Munroe, & Wright, 1992). Enabling strategies are intended to equip patients to be compliant. Such strategies include counseling patients, providing patient education, simplifying the medication regimen, increasing access to medical care and prescription sources, and prescribing less costly therapies. Consequence strategies are aimed at reinforcing compliant behavior. Instructing patients to maintain records of pill-taking and rewarding them for acceptable compliance levels is an example of this approach. Stimulant strategies are intended to prompt pill taking. Examples of tested approaches include tailoring doses to daily rituals, placing reminder cards in prominent places in patients' homes, visiting the patients' homes to reinforce compliance, having spouses or friends remind patients to take their medications, and using special drug packaging to organize and prompt dose-taking.

The results of studies using enabling strategies are mixed, suggesting that neither patient education nor increased knowledge of medications per se necessarily leads to improved compliance. Wolfe and Schirm (1992) investigated the effect of medication counseling by a nurse on elderly individuals' medication knowledge and compliance behaviors and found no significant compliance differences between patients who received medication counseling and those who did not. Cargill (1992) tested the relative impact of a 20-minute teaching session, including a review of medication times, compared to a similar 20-minute teaching session followed by a 1-week to 2-week follow-up telephone call in which a nurse reviewed the medication regimen with the patients. Those patients who received a telephone call in addition to the teaching session showed a significantly greater improvement in medication-taking behavior ($F = .31$, $p < .01$). The patients in the teaching group who did not receive a telephone call demonstrated only a weak and insignificant increase in pill percentage compliance. The findings of the Cargill (1992) study suggest that a stimulant intervention (e.g., a follow-up telephone call) added to an enabling strategy may enhance home medication-taking behaviors.

Because of advanced technology, several electronic aids currently are available to support stimulant strategies designed to increase medication compliance. Examples are computer-generated reminder charts (Raynor, Booth, & Blenkinsopp, 1993); electronic medication compliance aids (McKinney et al., 1992); and MEMS (Lee et al., 1996; Matsuyama, Mason, & Jue, 1993). The latter have been described extensively in the literature, with excellent validity and with multiple methods of understanding the adherence based on the method of calculation (Rohay, Dunbar-Jacobs, Sereika, Kwoh, & Burke, 1998). McKinney et al. (1992) investigated the impact of an electronic medication compliance aid on long-term blood pressure control in ambulant patients residing in a retirement community or attending a primary care center. Patients were assigned randomly to one of two groups: an experimental group that received antihypertensive medication in vials fit with an electronic timepiece cap; and a control group that received antihypertensive medication in vials fit with standard caps. Patients in the experimental group received one timepiece cap for each drug prescribed. Blood pressure was recorded at the

150 outset of the study and monitored periodically during the subsequent 12 weeks. Subjects using the timepiece cap showed an average compliance rate of 95.1%, an average decrease in systolic pressure of 7.6 mm Hg ($p < .01$), and an average decrease in diastolic pressure of
155 8.8 mm Hg ($p < .01$). Subjects in the control group had an average compliance rate of only 78% and a decrease of only 2.8 mm Hg and .2 mm Hg in systolic and diastolic pressures, respectively.

Raynor et al. (1993) studied the effect of computer-
160 generated reminder charts on patients' compliance with drug regimens after discharge from the hospital. Patients were assigned randomly to four groups: Group A received brief counseling from a nurse (usual care); Group B received the counseling from a nurse, plus a
165 reminder chart; Group C received structured counseling from a pharmacist; Group D received structured counseling from a pharmacist, plus a reminder chart. Of those patients who received the reminder chart, 83% correctly described their dose regimen, compared with
170 47% of those without the chart ($p < .001$). Raynor et al. (1993) concluded that an automatically generated individualized reminder chart could be a practical and cost-effective aid to compliance.

The study described in this article also used advanced
175 technology to support a stimulant strategy. It was designed to test the effectiveness of videotelephone reminders—compared to regular telephone calls or usual care—in improving medication compliance among a home-based elderly population with a chronic
180 illness. Medication Event Monitoring System (MEMS) caps (Aprex Corporation, Fremont, California)—computerized medication caps placed on a participant's medication bottles—were employed as the means for measuring compliance. Based on the stimulant strategy
185 literature (McKinney et al., 1992), both auditory and visual stimulation were selected as prompts to determine any differences. The Medical Outcome Survey 36-Item Short-Form Health Survey (SF-36) (Ware & Sherbourne, 1992) was selected to determine if quality-
190 of-life scores would be affected by adherence. The Minnesota Living with Heart Failure (MLHF) Questionnaire (Rector, Kubo, & Cohn, 1987) was used to understand specific symptoms of the disease related to medication compliance. It was hypothesized that im-
195 proved medication compliance would improve both SF-36 and MLHF scores.

## Methods

The authors recruited community-dwelling individuals age 65 and older who had the primary or secondary diagnosis of CHF to participate in a randomized
200 controlled study of reminder calls designed to enhance medication compliance. The study consisted of three arms: a control group receiving usual care ($n = 18$); a group that received daily telephone calls ($n = 15$); and a group that received daily videotelephone calls ($n =
205$ 17). The rationale for varying the prompt mode (video-telephone versus telephone) came from a clinical belief that elderly individuals would do better and improve medication-taking behavior with a video (i.e., face-to-face simulation) rather than through a telephone inter-
210 vention alone. Compliance was defined as the percent of therapeutic coverage (proportion of prescribed medication doses taken) as recorded by the MEMS caps.

### Subject Recruitment

Subjects were referred from two sources: a large urban home health care agency and a large urban am-
215 bulatory care clinic of a major teaching hospital. Institutional review board (IRB) approval was obtained for each site. Inclusion criteria were:

- Current patient of the Visiting Nurse Service (VNS)
220 of New York or Columbia Presbyterian Medical Center (CPMC).
- Primary or secondary diagnosis of CHF, age 65 or older.
- Resident of Manhattan.
225 - No prepour medications order (i.e., medications were not dispensed via unit of use packages such as daily or weekly dosing dispensers).
- Use of an angiotensin-converting enzyme (ACE) inhibitor, calcium channel blocker, or beta-blocker.
230 - Fluency in English or Spanish.
- Mini Mental-Status Examination (MMSE) (Folstein, Folstein, & McHugh, 1975) score of 20 or better.
- Experience in using a telephone.
235 - Home equipped with a telephone and a modular telephone jack.
- Home not in a high-crime building requiring a security guard to accompany research interviewer.

At VNS, eligible subjects were identified through
240 an automated flag implemented via the agency's management information system. At CPMC, eligible subjects were identified by the use of a medical logic module in the CPMC informatics network. Both methods had IRB approval. After referral, subjects were
245 either asked in person by the nurse or asked by telephone by a research assistant to participate. All subjects were offered $20 to participate. Approximately 600 eligible patients were referred; of these, 60 agreed to participate. The major reason for refusal to partici-
250 pate was the patient's or their family's perception that the patient was too ill to comply with the study protocol. In fact, the target group for the study was a very frail group with repeated hospitalizations. Randomization occurred using a table of random numbers after the
255 elderly individuals agreed to participate and finished an in-person baseline data-collection interview. Subsequent to randomization, four patients died, two sets of caps were lost, and four people withdrew before completing the study. These 10 subjects were excluded
260 from the analysis.

*Data Collection Procedures*

After consent was obtained, a research assistant went to the subjects' homes to complete the mental status screen (Folstein et al., 1975) and collect the baseline battery data, which included the SF-36 (Ware & Sherbourne, 1992) and the MLHF (Rector et al., 1987).

The MMSE was selected for its clinical brevity and widespread use in the field. It is a 30-item inventory divided into two sections which gives a gross measure of cognition (Folstein et al., 1975). A score of 20 or less greatly increases the chance of cognitive impairment; therefore, the authors selected a cut score of 20 to exclude individuals who may be very impaired, and yet enroll the maximum number of subjects into the study (Siu, Reuben, & Moore, 1994). The SF-36 contains eight scales that measure both physical and mental dimensions of health status: physical functioning, role limitations secondary to physical functioning, bodily pain, general health perception, vitality, social functioning, role limitations because of emotional problems, and mental health. Each scale is scored separately, resulting in a profile of eight scores for each respondent. Items are answered in a Likert-response format. This measure was selected to obtain a baseline of physical and mental function to compare the groups. Similarly, the MLHF questionnaire (Rector et al., 1987), a 21-item survey based on a range of ranking from 0 to 5, was administered at baseline and at the end of the study to determine the degree of symptom management difficulty across groups. All of the aforementioned instruments have extensive psychometric testing (Folstein et al., 1975; Rector et al., 1987; Ware & Sherbourne, 1992). After the questionnaires were completed, MEMS caps were placed on a maximum of four medication bottles for each enrolled elderly patient. The number four was selected to provide an average across medications and control for variance. The cost of the caps precluded capping all pill bottles. Medications selected for capping were: ACE inhibitors, calcium channel blockers, beta-blockers, and thereafter, cardiac-related medications such as digoxin, diuretics, and vasodilators. Some elderly patients were taking fewer than four medications and, therefore, had fewer caps. The protocol included a 2-week period of baseline compliance monitoring, a 6-week intervention phase with daily telephone or videotelephone calls, and a 2-week postintervention compliance monitoring period. Caps were picked up by the research assistant at the end of the 2-week postintervention period. At that time, a postinterview was conducted, consisting of the SF-36, MLHF, and a set of questions regarding the patient's experience with the study.

*The Intervention*

After the 2-week baseline compliance monitoring period had ended, patients were randomized to one of the three study arms. The research assistant went to the home of those in the videotelephone group, installed the videotelephone apparatus, and taught the patients how to use it. At that point, the research assistant also determined a convenient time for the patient to receive daily medication reminder calls. Patients in the standard telephone group provided this information via the telephone. Thereafter, during the 6-week intervention period, a telephone or a videotelephone call was made daily (Monday through Friday) during the time window agreed on by the patient and the research assistant. Whether by telephone or videotelephone, the research assistant's reminder call consisted of a brief greeting, and the patients then were asked whether they had taken their medications the previous day. No effort was made to conduct directly observed therapy, and this was not a goal of the study. Calls usually lasted from 3 to 5 minutes, with longer calls occurring when the patient had questions. If there was no answer, the call was placed at regular intervals for the remainder of the day until contact was made. When no contact was made, a notation was made on the study protocol records, and calls were resumed the next day. The only difference between the videotelephone and regular telephone reminder was that the videotelephone group could see the image of the research assistant on the videotelephone screen and vice versa. The videotelephone images are limited by a 2-second frame delay, which can make motion choppy for the individual on the other end of the phone but allows the two individuals to see each other as they speak.

*Data Analysis*

Using the Statistical Package for the Social Sciences-Personal Computer (SPSS-PC) and MANOVA, the three groups were compared to determine any differences in medication compliance as recorded by the MEMS caps. The cap printouts were reviewed, and a percent compliance rate was calculated for each of three time periods: T1 (average of 2-week baseline percent compliance), T2 (average of 6-week intervention compliance), and T3 (average of 2-week postintervention compliance). Compliance was calculated using the approach described by Kruse et al. (1992), and expanded by Rohay et al. (1998). Using the daily events adherence method of calculation, which is based on the number of events that occur each day and then averaged over the interval, the method is stated to be comparable to the average of daily pill counts. An average compliance measure was calculated for each of the three time periods using repeated measures ANOVA. The compliance rates were compared in a three-by-three design (i.e., control, telephone, and videotelephone at T1, T2, and T3). Preintervention and postintervention scores were calculated for the MLHF and SF-36.

## Results

*Baseline Equivalence*

Table 1 reports selected demographic data for the

370 study sample. The mean age was 74.2 (SD = 6.8), with a median age of 72. The mean number of years of education was 9.3 (SD = 4.9; median, 10.5). More than 70% of subjects were either widowed or divorced. Only two individuals were working for pay outside of

375 the home on a part-time basis. The group was 14% White, 30% Black, 54% other, and 2% "missing," reflecting the diversity of New York and the limitations of racial labels. Half of the interviews were conducted in Spanish to accommodate the language of preference.

380 There were no statistically significant demographic differences between the experimental and control groups.

Table 1
*Selected Demographics\**

| Variable number | Control 18 | Telephone 15 | Video-telephone 17 |
|---|---|---|---|
| Race | | | |
| White | 0 | 3 | 4 |
| Black | 6 | 5 | 4 |
| Other | 11 | 7 | 9 |
| Marital status | | | |
| Married | 1 | 4 | 3 |
| Widowed | 7 | 6 | 8 |
| Divorced or separated | 8 | 2 | 5 |
| Never married | 0 | 3 | 1 |
| Years of education | mean = 7.8 (SD = 5.7) | mean = 11.5 (SD = 3.8) | mean = 9 (SD = 4.7) |
| Age | mean = 73.7 (SD = 5.3) | mean = 76.2 (SD = 8.8) | mean = 73.1 (SD = 6.5) |

\* Not significant across groups.

### Intervention Effects

During the 2-week baseline compliance monitoring period, there were no statistically significant differ-

385 ences in the compliance rates of the intervention and control groups. The average compliance rates across the three groups were: 81% for the controls, 76% for the telephone group, and 82% for the videotelephone group. During the subsequent two time periods (6

390 weeks intervention and 2 weeks postintervention), the compliance rate of the control group dropped significantly (from 81% at T1 to 57% at T3, $p < .04$), while the compliance rates of the two intervention groups remained steady (Figure 1, Table 2). Thus, there was a

395 statistically significant time effect during the course of the study from baseline to postintervention ($F[2, 34] = 4.08, p < .05$). Over time, the elderly patients who were called either by telephone or videotelephone showed enhanced medication compliance relative to the control

400 group, demonstrating an effect from the calling interventions. However, there was no significant difference in compliance rates between the two intervention groups. The enhanced technology offered by the video-

telephone images apparently did not offer a relative

405 advantage over regular telephone reminders regarding the elderly patients' compliance behavior. Multiple regression analysis did not yield any demographic predictors for better compliance.

Both the SF-36 scores and the MLHF scores im-

410 proved from baseline to postintervention for all groups. There was no significant change in the SF-36 scores for the sample, but there was improvement in the MLHF scores ($p < .001$), indicating improved self-reported clinical status. Group membership did not make a dif-

415 ference for either score (Table 3).

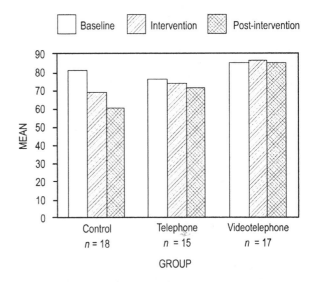

*Figure 1.* The effects of telephone call intervention in medication compliance for three experimental groups of community-dwelling elderly individuals during 2-week baseline, 6-week intervention, and 2-week postintervention.

Table 2
*Intervention Effects on Medication Compliance of Community-Dwelling Elderly Individuals*

| Time | Control | Telephone | Videotele-phone |
|---|---|---|---|
| Time 1 | 81% | 76% | 82% |
| Time 3 | 57% | 74% | 84% |

*Note.* The Time 1 to Time 3 difference for the control group was significant at $p < .04$.

### Discussion and Nursing Implications

The most striking finding of this study is the significant falloff in the control group's medication compliance rate over time, compared to the rates of the two intervention groups. Between T1 and T3, compliance

420 in the control group fell 24 percentage points, while compliance in the two reminder groups fluctuated by no more than 2 percentage points. By the end of the 10-week period during which compliance rates were measured, the control group was taking on average

425 only 57% of prescribed medication doses, while the

Table 3
*Intervention Effects*

| | Measure | | | | | | | |
| | SF-36 scores | | | | MLHF scores | | | |
| | Preintervention | | Postintervention | | Preintervention | | Postintervention | |
| Group | Mean | *SD* | Mean | *SD* | Mean | *SD* | Mean | *SD* |
| Control (*n* = 14) | 87.3 | 24.3 | 91.7 | 22.7 | 46.6 | 27.7 | 32.9 | 22.9 |
| Telephone (*n* = 13) | 81.0 | 15.2 | 90.1 | 20.6 | 54.4 | 21.1 | 32.9 | 25.2 |
| Videotelephone (*n* = 15) | 86.1 | 17.0 | 85.9 | 18.9 | 43.1 | 20.8 | 36.7 | 19.9 |

other two groups—exposed to daily medication reminders—were taking between 74% to 84%. With the advent of managed care and cuts in home care reimbursement, the ability to enhance medication compli-
430 ance by such simple means as a telephone call is important. The usual practice of prepouring medications for the week, often performed by home care nurses at the cost of a visit, may be replaced by telephone calls by the home care nurse, saving travel time, increasing
435 the number of contacts, and obtaining better compliance. In large part, these are patients who are quite ill, and the daily reminder to take medications could have a positive effect on overall symptom management and well-being, which should be investigated in the future.
440 One may ask why the baseline compliance rates across the three groups were so high, ranging from 76% to 82%, and why the pattern of compliance observed in the study involved differential falloff from a relatively high percentage of doses completed rather
445 than a differential improvement from a relatively low level of initial compliance. One plausible explanation is that the compliance rates observed during the 2-week baseline monitoring period may have been an artifact of the study's measurement technology. One could
450 argue that the action of placing MEMS caps on patients' pill bottles—an action necessary for measuring compliance throughout the study—was itself an intervention and could have produced a Hawthorne effect that raised compliance beyond its natural level in the
455 study population. Because the protocol of placing caps on bottles was identical across the three groups, this effect was observed more or less uniformly across the control and intervention groups at baseline. As the presence of the electronic bottle caps became routine,
460 its effect could be expected to wear off, leaving compliance rates to fall to what was presumably their prior level. In the absence of any other intervention, this is apparently what happened in the control group. In contrast, the introduction of the telephone and videotele-
465 phone reminders in the two intervention groups evidently worked to sustain the relatively high levels of compliance that were observed at baseline. Why these levels were sustained during the 2 weeks postintervention (after daily reminders were no longer received)
470 and for how long the apparent benefit associated with

the reminders will endure are questions for future study.
The second substantive finding of this study is the absence of a significant difference between the two
475 intervention groups. The opportunity afforded by the videotelephone for the patient and the individual providing the medication reminder to see each other was presumed to establish greater rapport through visual contact and was expected to yield a stronger compli-
480 ance effect relative to regular telephone communication. However, no significant advantage could be detected, although the trend for a greater effect was there. This may be partly because of the small sample participating in the study because the trend toward a stronger
485 effect with the videotelephone is evident. It may also be partly because of perceived limitations of the videotelephone technology. The videotelephones are somewhat more awkward to use than regular phones and the images are neither vivid nor in real time. In any case,
490 the small magnitude of the discernable difference between the two types of reminders suggests that either technology could be used to positive effect. Since this study, technology has improved and the "CU-SeeMe" (Cornell University, Ithaca, NY) systems along with
495 Internet television hold promise as creative venues for personal contact. Finally, the change in the MLHF scores cannot be interpreted meaningfully in this study because of sample size but warrant further consideration in a larger trial. Further, in a next phase, the inves-
500 tigators hope to explore the question of "dose." That is, how frequently must calls be made to get the desired enhanced compliance effect.
This study has at least two important limitations. First is the extremely low participation rate (approxi-
505 mately 10%), which reflects national trends in heart failure studies (Goodyer, Miskelly, & Milligan, 1996). The refusal-to-participate rate is a concern. Focus groups using potential subjects to help understand their hesitation to participate would be of value. Selecting
510 younger, healthier subjects is always an option but would result in a different study. Given the large numbers of very frail community-dwelling elderly individuals in the United States, it makes more sense to focus on their participation. The modest stipend for
515 enrollees ($20) did not provide a strong incentive for

90

participation, although elderly individuals were not asked specifically if more money would change their minds. Furthermore, the severity of illness of the patients referred to the study was clearly a deterrent to 520 participation. Sicker individuals were more likely to decline to participate, and sensory impairments such as hearing and vision deficits further reduced participation.

The second limitation of the study was the exclu-525 sion of individuals who routinely relied on prepoured medications, such as daily or weekly pillboxes and dosing dispensers. Because the MEMS compliance measurement methodology requires that computerized medication caps be placed on the patients' medication 530 bottles, individuals who did not routinely take their pills from the bottle, but rather from a special pillbox, could not be included. It should be stressed that this exclusion was a requirement of the research measurement methodology and not the reminder strategy per 535 se. There is inherently no obvious reason why such individuals could not benefit from daily medication reminders. However, any research study designed to include this group would have to rely on some other method of measuring compliance.

540 Given the mixed results of patient education interventions designed to increase medication compliance among frail elderly individuals, increasing attention has focused on stimulant strategies designed to augment medication information and to prompt pill-taking be-545 havior. Despite its small sample, this study demonstrated that daily telephone calls or electronic home visits could improve medication compliance significantly in a sample of elderly individuals with CHF who took, on average, 3 to 15 doses of medication every 550 day. In addition, monitoring with computerized medication caps provided an accurate and consistent method of electronic observation. Patients who have been hospitalized for CHF have a high rate of rehospitalization, which may be attributable in part to poor medication 555 compliance and to resultant illness. This pilot study demonstrated a simple, inexpensive approach with promising results. These results suggest the importance of conducting the intervention on a larger scale.

### References

Cargill, J. M. (1992). Medication compliance in elderly people: Influencing variables and interventions. *Journal of Advanced Nursing, 17*, 422–426.

Cramer, J. A., Mattson, R. H., Prevey, M. L., Scheyer, R. D., & Ouellette, V. L. (1989). How often is medication taken as prescribed? A novel assessment technique. *Journal of the American Medical Association, 261*, 3273–3277.

DeGeest, S., Dunbar-Jacob, J., & Vanhaeckel, J. (1998). *Diagnostic value of structured interviews in assessing non-compliance with immunosuppressive therapy in heart transplant patients.* Manuscript submitted for publication.

Fineman, B., & DeFelice, C. (1992). A study of medication compliance. *Home Healthcare Nurse, 10*(5), 26–29.

Fitten, L. J., Coleman, L., Siembieda, D. W., Yu, M., & Ganzell, S. (1995). Assessment of capacity to comply with medication regimens in older patients. *Journal of the American Geriatrics Society, 43*, 361–367.

Folstein, M. F., Folstein, S. E., & McHugh, P. R. (1975). Mini-Mental State: A practical guide for grading the cognitive state of patients for the clinician. *Journal of Psychiatric Research, 12*, 189–198.

Goodyer, L. I., Miskelly, F., & Milligan, P. (1996). Does encouraging good compliance improve patients' clinical condition in heart failure? *British Journal of Clinical Pharmacology, 49*, 173–176.

Isaac, L. M., & Tamblyn, R. M. (1993). Compliance and cognitive function: A methodological approach to measuring unintentional errors in medication compliance in the elderly. *The Gerontologist, 33*, 772–781.

Klein, L. E., German, P. S., McPhee, S. J., Smith, C. R., & Levine, D. M. (1982). Aging and its relationship to health knowledge and medication compliance. *The Gerontologist, 22*, 384–387.

Kruse, W., Koch-Gwinner, P., Nikolaus, T., Oster, P., Schlierf, G., & Weber, E. (1992). Measurement of drug compliance by continuous electronic monitoring: A pilot study in elderly patients discharged from hospital. *Journal of the American Geriatrics Society, 40*, 1151–1155.

Kruse, W., & Weber, E. (1990). Dynamics of drug regimen compliance—Its assessment by microprocessor-based monitoring. *European Journal of Clinical Pharmacology, 38*, 561–565.

Lee, J. Y., Kusek, J. W., Greene, P. G., Bernhard, S., Norris, K., Smith, D., Wilkening, B., & Wright, J. T. (1996). Assessing medication adherence by pill count and electronic monitoring in the African American Study of Kidney Disease (AASK) pilot study. *The American Journal of Hypertension, 9*, 719–725.

Matsuyama, J. R., Mason, B. J., & Jue, S. G. (1993). Pharmacists' interventions using an electronic medication-event monitoring device's adherence data versus pill counts. *Annals of Pharmacotherapy, 27*, 851–855.

McKinney, J. M., Munroe, W. P., & Wright, J. T. (1992). Impact of an electronic medication compliance aid on long-term blood pressure control. *Journal of Clinical Pharmacology, 32*, 277–283.

Murray, M. D., Birt, J. A., Manatunga, A. K., & Darnell, J. C. (1993). Medication compliance in elderly outpatients using twice-daily dosing and unit-of-use packaging. *Annals of Pharmacotherapy, 27*, 616–621.

Raynor, D. K., Booth, T. G., & Blenkinsopp, A. (1993). Effects of computer generated reminder charts on patients' compliance with drug regimens. *British Medical Journal, 306*, 1158–1161.

Rector, T. S., Kubo, S. H., & Cohn, J. N. (1987). Patients' self-assessment of their congestive heart failure: Part 2: Content, reliability and validity of a new measure, the Minnesota Living with Heart Failure Questionnaire. *Heart Failure, 124*, 198–209.

Rohay, J. M., Dunbar-Jacob, J., Sereika, S., Kwoh, K., & Burke, L. E. (1998). *The impact of method of calculation of electronically monitored adherence data controlled clinical trials.* Manuscript submitted for publication.

Salzman, C. (1995). Medication compliance in the elderly. *Journal of Clinical Psychiatry, 56*(Suppl. 1), 18–22.

Siu, A. L., Reuben, D. B., & Moore, A. A. (1994). Comprehensive geriatric assessment. In W. R. Hazzard, E. L. Bierman, J. P. Blass, W. H. Ettinger, & J. B. Halter (Eds.), *Principles of geriatric medicine and gerontology* (pp. 203–211). New York: McGraw-Hill.

Spiers, M. V., & Kutzik, D. M. (1995). Self-reported memory of medication use by the elderly. *American Journal of Health-System Pharmacy, 52*, 985–990.

Ware, J. E., & Sherbourne, C. D. (1992). The MOS 36-item short-form health survey (SF-36), I: Conceptual framework and item selection. *Medical Care, 30*, 473–483.

Wolfe, S. C., & Schirm, V. (1992). Medication counseling for the elderly: Effects on knowledge and compliance after hospital discharge. *Geriatric Nursing, 13*(3), 134–138.

**Note**: This project was funded by The Merck Company Foundation, Merck-Medco Managed Care LLC, West Point, Pennsylvania, and the Frederick and Amelia Schimper Foundation, New York, New York.

**Address correspondence to**: Terry T. Fulmer, PhD, RN, FAAN, Professor, New York University, Division of Nursing, 429 Shimkin Hall, 50 West 4th Street, New York, NY 10012.

# Exercise for Article 13

## Factual Questions

1. Which one of the three types of strategies for enhancing compliance is intended to *prompt* pill taking?

2. Participants were referred from what two sources?

3. How many of the original subjects in this study withdrew before completing it?

4. What precluded capping all pill bottles?

5. Which one of the three groups had the highest average years of education?

6. Was the drop in the control group's compliance rate from Time 1 to Time 3 statistically significant?

7. According to the researchers, what is the "second substantive finding" of the study?

## Questions for Discussion

8. Speculate on what the researchers mean by "Likert-response format." (See lines 283–284.)

9. The footnote to Table 1 indicates that the differences in demographics across groups were not significant. Is this important information? Explain.

10. In the paragraph beginning on line 440, the researchers speculate on why the initial (baseline) compliance rates were so high. Does their speculation make sense? Why? Why not?

11. In the paragraph beginning on line 503, the researchers identify the low participation rate as an "important limitation." Do you agree that it is important? Explain.

12. If you were to conduct another study on the same topic, what changes in the research methodology, if any, would you make?

## Quality Ratings

Directions: Indicate your level of agreement with each of the following statements by circling a number from 5 for strongly agree (SA) to 1 for strongly disagree (SD). If you believe an item is not applicable to this research article, leave it blank. Be prepared to explain your ratings. When responding to criteria A and B, keep in mind that brief titles and abstracts are conventional in published research.

A. The title of the article is appropriate.

   SA   5   4   3   2   1   SD

B. The abstract provides an effective overview of the research article.

   SA   5   4   3   2   1   SD

C. The introduction establishes the importance of the study.

   SA   5   4   3   2   1   SD

D. The literature review establishes the context for the study.

   SA   5   4   3   2   1   SD

E. The research purpose, question, or hypothesis is clearly stated.

   SA   5   4   3   2   1   SD

F. The method of sampling is sound.

   SA   5   4   3   2   1   SD

G. Relevant demographics (for example, age, gender, and ethnicity) are described.

   SA   5   4   3   2   1   SD

H. Measurement procedures are adequate.

   SA   5   4   3   2   1   SD

I. All procedures have been described in sufficient detail to permit a replication of the study.

   SA   5   4   3   2   1   SD

J. The participants have been adequately protected from potential harm.

   SA   5   4   3   2   1   SD

K. The results are clearly described.

   SA   5   4   3   2   1   SD

L. The discussion/conclusion is appropriate.

   SA   5   4   3   2   1   SD

M. Despite any flaws, the report is worthy of publication.

   SA   5   4   3   2   1   SD

# Article 14

*Independent*
*- cause*
*← dependent*

# Effectiveness of Nursing Counseling
# On Coping and Depression in Women
# Undergoing In Vitro Fertilization

**Nermin Gürhan, Aygül Akyüz, Fahriye Oflaz, Derya Atici, GulsenVural**[*]

ABSTRACT. The purpose of the present study was to evaluate the effectiveness of counseling provided by nurses on depression and coping strategies of infertile women undergoing *in vitro* fertilization ($N = 67$). Of the 84 women who were interviewed, 30 were accepted as a comparison group, and 37 were included in the study group. The study group women were given counseling in addition to routine nursing care services, including group education and individual interviews about treatment and coping strategies. The nurses also provided support by accompanying the women during the invasive procedures. The Beck Depression Inventory and Jalowiec's Coping Strategies Form were used for measurements. All the women were using emotional coping and had moderate depression prior to the study. There was no statistically significant difference between the comparison and study groups before or after the counseling with respect to depression and coping strategies. Parameters to evaluate the efficacy of counseling are discussed.

From *Psychological Reports*, 100, 365–374. Copyright © 2007 by Psychological Reports. Reprinted with permission.

Infertility can be a major health problem for some couples. In the last few decades, through the development of assisted reproduction technologies, new treatment techniques such as *in vitro* fertilization (IVF)
5 have given infertile couples the opportunity to have a baby. Many studies indicate that infertility itself can be a major problem, particularly for women, and can have negative effects on their emotional well being and social interactions (Akyüz, İnanç, & Pabuçcu, 1999; Lee,
10 2003; Olshansky, 2003; Sherrod, 2004). Since the distress has effects before and after the babies are born, counseling is recommended for these couples (Anderheim, Holter, Bergh, & Moller, 2005; Fisher, Hammarberg, & Baker, 2005).
15 In Turkey, similar to some other societies and communities, having a baby is an important aspect of being a "real family." Within this perspective, the purpose of marriage is seen as coming together to have

and raise a child. In some communities, childlessness
20 can be perceived as a disability of women more than a health problem of couples. Not having a child can be seen as a major failure in the role of being a wife and can also decrease the social status of a woman in her own community (Peterson, Newton, & Rosen, 2003;
25 Saydam, 2003).
As a result of these complicated issues, it is more likely that infertile women will have marital problems, experience distress and difficulties in interpersonal relationships, avoid social interactions, and have emo-
30 tional problems such as anxiety, depression, hopelessness, helplessness, and hostility (Bush, 2001; Lee, 2003; Olshansky, 2003; Sherrod, 2004). Studies indicate that infertile women particularly show subclinically raised scores for depression and anxiety (Pook,
35 Röhrle, Tuschen-Caffier, & Krause, 2001). IVF treatment is a last resort to raise the probability of pregnancy for infertile couples, and requires time- and money-consuming procedures for diagnosis and treatment. In addition, the treatment process can be tiring
40 and stressful for the women given repeated invasive interventions (Bush, 2001; Lee, 2003; Olshansky, 2003; Peterson et al., 2003; Venkatesan, 2005). Anderheim et al. (2005) stated that everyone who undergoes IVF treatment and other infertility procedures is
45 stressed.
Lee (2003) emphasized that women undergoing IVF treatment use different coping strategies in different stages of the treatment. The coping strategies of infertile women are generally categorized into two
50 subgroups: emotional coping and problem-solving strategies. Emotional coping strategies, such as avoidance, crying, or denial, include responses to maintain emotional balance and to have control over emotions related to the stressors. Problem-solving strategies
55 (thinking of the event directly) include efforts to deal with or to change the sources of stress (Demyttenaere, Bonte, Gheldof, Vervaeke, Meuleman, Vanderschuerem, & D'Hooghe, 1998; Eugster & Vinger-

---

[*]*Address correspondence to*: Dr. A. Akyüz, Obstetric and Gynecological Nursing Department, Gulhane Military Medical Academy, School of Nursing, Etlik-Ankara, Turkey 06018. E-mail: aygulakyuz@yahoo.com

hoests, 1999). Research has shown that individuals who avoid stress in general are poorly adjusted, whereas those individuals using more active, constructive coping methods experience better psychological adjustment and engage in healthier behavior (Roesch, Weiner, & Vaughn, 2002). These psychological issues and stress management strategies of women have an effect on well being, quality of daily life, and marital relationships. In many infertile women, regardless of the exact cause and effect, depression and stress require attention. When stress starts to disrupt a woman's daily life, it is recommended that she get counseling (Pook et al., 2001; Olshansky, 2003; Anderheim et al., 2005).

As Pook et al. (2001) stated, given the general distress, it is important for infertile couples to get counseling, and couples with marital problems can be reached better if psychological help is not described as "therapy." That is why nurses can be beneficial to infertile women in the process of IVF treatment by taking a counselor role besides other nursing roles. Nurses have important roles and responsibilities in every stage of IVF treatment. Therefore, they are in a very advantageous position by being with the patients during all the processes. Nurses trained in counseling for this specific group can help women cope with medical procedures and psychosocial distresses by using their communication and counseling skills and teaching roles. However, there are very few studies conducted with nurses demonstrating the effects of their interventions both on psychosocial difficulties of women and on the results of IVF. Therefore, in the present study, infertile women who participated in counseling by nurses were compared to infertile women who did not participate in these counseling services.

The aim of the research was to determine the effectiveness of a nursing counseling protocol in improving the coping strategies and alleviating the depression of infertile women undergoing IVF. The hypotheses of the study were that counseling can improve coping strategies and decrease the depression of infertile women.

**Method**

This study has a quasi-experimental design. The study was conducted between October 2001 and April 2002 at the Gazi University IVF Center in Ankara. Five obstetrics and gynecology specialists (M.D.), one consultant urologist (M.D.), three embryologists (M.D.), and two nurses work at this center. Approximately 15 IVF-ICSI (intracytoplasmic sperm injection) treatment cycles are carried out per month at the center.

*Participants*

A total of 84 infertile women who were about to begin IVF treatment were interviewed and informed about the study by the investigators, and verbal consent was provided by each of the women to participate in the study. Since it did not seem appropriate to randomize the women, the investigators divided the study duration (six months) into two parts. The women who applied to the center within the first 3-mo. period were defined as the comparison group, and the women who applied to the center in the next 3 mo. formed the study group. The first 42 women to volunteer were assigned to the comparison group, and the next 42 women were the study group. All of the women applying to the center during the study period volunteered to participate in the study. The exclusion criteria were not progressing to the embryo transfer stage, having a diagnosed psychiatric disorder, or being under psychiatric treatment. None of the women who were interviewed had a diagnosed current psychiatric disorder. During the study, 17 women who could not progress to the embryo transfer stage for lack of sperm, not developing adequate oocytes, or no fertilization were excluded from study. At the end of the study, the comparison group included 30 women and the study group included 37 women.

*Procedure*

The pretests and the study questionnaire were distributed to both the comparison and the study groups on their first day, just before treatment was started (the day on which controlled ovarian hyperstimulation was started), after information about the study was provided by the investigators and verbal consent was given by participants. The institution does not require written consent or ethical committee permission for studies that do not have invasive interventions or any medical treatments. Posttests were performed before the embryo transfer, and the duration between the pre- and posttest was approximately 12 days for each measurement. The women in the study group were given counseling by two nurses in addition to receiving the routine nursing care services at the center. Routine nursing care at this center includes describing the doses and names of the medicines the women will take, administering the medicines, drawing blood samples, and preparing the women for ultrasound and collecting oocytes. The women in the comparison group did not participate in the additional counseling service.

The counseling service did not require any additional fee from the couples. The counselor nurses were the investigators, who work as faculty (assistant professors) in the Psychiatric and Gynecological and Obstetric Nursing Departments at the School of Nursing. They had courses on counseling in their doctorate program and were experienced in working with infertile couples.

After being given the pretests and study questionnaire, the women in the study group participated in structured counseling. This counseling program included (a) a group education session given by the obstetric and gynecologic nursing faculty, where information about the treatment and procedures was given and discussed (approximately 60 min.); (b) individual interviews carried out by psychiatric nursing faculty, where each person was interviewed twice to evaluate and to

*— operational definition* [handwritten]

*categorical* [handwritten]

170 meet the needs of coping. Each session lasted approximately 20 min. Within these interviews, the participants were encouraged to talk about their feelings, concerns, psychosocial distress, and coping strategies. Relaxation techniques were taught. When the support of
175 the husband was needed, he was invited to participate in these sessions. In general, husbands were not included in the counseling process; they were invited to the individual interviews when their wives needed them or when the counselors asked them to come to-
180 gether; (c) support was provided by staying with the participants during the invasive procedures and the participants were encouraged to use the relaxation techniques taught in the first education session.

*Measures*

*CATEGORICAL or OrdinaL*

The study questionnaire developed by the investi-
185 gators included demographics and the infertility history of the women. Depression was measured by the Beck Depression Inventory (BDI) (Savaşir & Şahin, 1997). The reliability and validity of the Turkish version of the scale was checked by Savaşir and Şahin (1997),
190 and the Cronbach alpha of the scale was .74. This 4-point Likert-type rating scale is used for measuring depression in individuals. The patients are asked to mark the statement that shows their feelings during the last week, including the day the scale was filled out.
195 Scores range between 0–63, with higher scores meaning higher depression. The Cronbach alpha of this scale was .77 in the present study.

Coping strategies were measured with the Jalowiec's Coping Strategies Form. This form was de-
200 veloped in 1984, and the reliability and validity of the Turkish version were tested by Gürhan in 1995, and the Cronbach alpha was .82. The Jalowiec's Coping Strategies Form measures emotional coping strategies and problem-solving abilities of the subjects when facing
205 stress. It is composed of 40 questions on coping strategies rated on a 5-point scale. Twenty items measure emotional coping, and the other 20 items measure problem solving. Higher scores show higher utilization of those coping strategies on the scale. The Cronbach
210 alpha value in the present study was .73.

*Data Analysis*

All of the statistical analyses were performed using the SPSS 11.0 software. Descriptive findings were given either as means or frequencies. Relations between groups and the categorical variables were analyzed by
215 the chi-square test. Pre- and posttest values of the scales were compared by the paired samples $t$ test. Differences between the groups were analyzed by using the independent samples $t$ test. A $p$ value of .05 or less was considered statistically significant.

**Results**

220 As shown in Table 1, the women in both groups were mostly in the 30- to 39-yr. age group. The average age of the participants was 33.3 yr. ($SD$ = 5.40). Length of marriage was 10.3 yr. ($SD$ = 6.0) in both groups. Most of the women in the study sample had
225 completed higher education. There was no significant difference between the study group and the comparison group in age, length of marriage, education, and duration of infertility. Additionally, 55.2% of the women were coming from different cities to receive treatment.

Table 1
*Women's Demographic Characteristics By Group*

| Characteristic | Comparison group ($n$ = 30) | | Study group ($n$ = 37) | | Total ($N$ = 67) | | $\chi^2$ |
|---|---|---|---|---|---|---|---|
| | $n$ | % | $n$ | % | $n$ | % | |
| Age, yr. | | | | | | | 1.82 |
| 29 and younger | 5 | 16.7 | 10 | 27.0 | 15 | 22.4 | |
| 30–39 | 20 | 66.7 | 24 | 64.9 | 44 | 65.7 | |
| 40 and older | 5 | 16.7 | 3 | 8.1 | 8 | 11.9 | |
| Length of marriage, yr. | | | | | | | 2.94 |
| 1–8 | 14 | 46.7 | 15 | 40.5 | 29 | 43.3 | |
| 9–16 | 14 | 46.7 | 14 | 37.8 | 28 | 41.8 | |
| 17 and greater | 2 | 6.6 | 8 | 21.6 | 10 | 14.9 | |
| Education | | | | | | | 5.63 |
| Primary school | 6 | 20.0 | 16 | 43.2 | 22 | 32.8 | |
| Secondary | 1 | 3.3 | 3 | 8.1 | 4 | 6.0 | |
| High school | 9 | 30.0 | 6 | 16.2 | 15 | 22.4 | |
| University | 14 | 46.7 | 12 | 32.4 | 26 | 38.8 | |
| Duration of infertility, yr. | | | | | | | 7.11 |
| 1–3 | 11 | 36.7 | 6 | 16.2 | 17 | 25.4 | |
| 4–6 | 4 | 13.3 | 13 | 35.1 | 17 | 25.4 | |
| 7–10 | 7 | 23.3 | 5 | 13.5 | 12 | 17.9 | |
| 11 and higher | 8 | 26.7 | 13 | 35.1 | 21 | 31.3 | |

*$p$ > .05.

95

Table 2
*Concerns of Women About Being Infertile*

| Concern | Comparison group ($n = 30$) | | Study group ($n = 37$) | | Total ($N = 67$) | | $\chi^2$ |
|---|---|---|---|---|---|---|---|
| | $n$ | % | $n$ | % | $n$ | % | |
| When is being infertile most disturbing? | | | | | | | 0.16 |
| When I see couples with a child | 11 | 36.7 | 12 | 32.4 | 23 | 34.3 | |
| When I am questioned about the reason for my infertility | 17 | 56.7 | 22 | 59.5 | 39 | 58.2 | |
| When my husband expresses his wishes to have a child | 2 | 6.7 | 3 | 8.1 | 5 | 7.5 | |
| Who applies the pressure? | | | | | | | 2.12 |
| Husband | 0 | 0.0 | 2 | 10.0 | 2 | 6.1 | |
| Family of husband | 4 | 30.8 | 5 | 25.0 | 9 | 27.3 | |
| Relatives | 9 | 69.2 | 13 | 65.0 | 22 | 66.7 | |
| What is she doing to cope? | | | | | | | 0.18 |
| Talking with others | 2 | 15.4 | 5 | 25.0 | 7 | 21.2 | |
| Avoiding talking | 6 | 46.2 | 12 | 60.0 | 18 | 54.5 | |
| Ignoring the problem | 5 | 38.5 | 3 | 15.0 | 8 | 24.2 | |

*$p > .05$.

230 During the first interview, the participants were questioned about their concerns and distress regarding being infertile. Most of the participants expressed feeling distressed mostly when they were questioned about the reason for being infertile in a social interpersonal 235 situation. In addition, they also stated that relatives and acquaintances were more likely to ask these kinds of questions and that they usually preferred to avoid answering these kinds of questions (Table 2).

At the initial stage of the study, there were no sta-240 tistical differences between the participants in the comparison group and the study group for depression ($p > .05$). Depression was moderate in both groups (Table 3). The evaluation of effectiveness of counseling service on depression and coping strategies is re-245 ported in Tables 3 and 4. Following counseling, there was no statistically significant difference between the comparison and study groups for depression. Depression did not change within the groups either.

As demonstrated in Table 4, the participants used 250 emotional coping strategies when faced with stress. Following counseling, there was no statistically significant difference between the comparison group and study group in use of coping strategies.

### Discussion

Based on the results of this study, there was no sta-255 tistically significant difference in demographic characteristics, depression, and coping strategies of participants between the groups at the initial stage. These findings demonstrate that the women had similar characteristics in the two groups, and this makes the com-260 parisons reliable.

In different studies, researchers have found that infertile women experienced mild to moderate depression (Demyttenaere et al., 1998; Pook et al., 2001; Emery,

Beran, Darwiche, Oppizzi, Joris, Capel, Guex, & Ger-265 mond, 2003). The present findings are consistent with the results of these studies. As Olshansky (2003) stated, infertility causes psychosocially adverse effects as a life stress, and its treatment also causes additional distress because of invasive interventions and affects 270 the adjustment of the women. However, at the beginning of the IVF treatment, there are also some positive effects, such as the hope of having a child and possibly reducing particular stresses in the environment by changing the city they live in. Having the IVF treat-275 ment facilitates meeting other people experiencing similar problems, which could reduce stress (Lee, 2003). These positive effects of treatment may help the couples feel less stress during the procedures (Eugster & Vingerhoests, 1999). Similarly, during the interviews 280 in this study, women stated that beginning to receive the treatment, changing their environment, and sharing emotions and concerns with others reduced their distress. However, despite their positive thoughts about the treatment, many still had significant depression. 285 The presence of depression in infertile women warrants attention. The psychological symptoms are important, not only for the adjustment to the procedures and pregnancy, but also regarding the risk for developing emotional problems related to parenting (Pook et al., 2001; 290 Anderheim et al., 2005; Fisher et al., 2005). In addition, it is likely that these women could have severe depression in case of IVF failure.

Evaluating the coping strategies, it was found that the participants most frequently used emotional coping 295 strategies. This finding is supported by the expressions of the women participants about avoidance of relationships (Table 2). Similarly, Lee (2003) has suggested that infertile women avoid talking about the issue of childlessness and are often isolated from

Table 3

*Depression By Group Before and After Counseling*

*Continuous*

| Group | Before counseling | | After counseling | | t |
|---|---|---|---|---|---|
| | M | SD | M | SD | |
| Comparison group (n = 30) | 11.10 | 4.93 | 11.27 | 7.25 | 0.88 |
| Study group (n = 37) | 11.35 | 7.04 | 12.24 | 6.41 | 0.84 |
| t | 0.17 | | 0.57 | | |

\* p > .05.

Table 4

*Coping Strategies of Women By Group Before and After Counseling*

| Strategies | Comparison group (n = 30) | | Study group (n = 37) | | t |
|---|---|---|---|---|---|
| | M | SD | M | SD | |
| Emotional coping | | | | | |
| Before counseling | 88.86 | 8.75 | 91.86 | 11.01 | −1.20 |
| After counseling | 86.20 | 13.37 | 89.40 | 14.93 | −0.90 |
| t | 1.17 | | 1.39 | | |
| Problem solving | | | | | |
| Before counseling | 70.03 | 14.18 | 69.35 | 12.27 | −0.45 |
| After counseling | 67.72 | 14.31 | 69.13 | 10.81 | 0.21 |
| t | 0.41 | | 0.15 | | |

\* p > .05.

friends and relatives. It is considered that emotional coping can contribute to depression. Supporting this concern, Demyttenaere et al. (1998) found that women using more emotional coping had higher depression scores and that it affected the results of pregnancy negatively. However, Anderheim et al. (2005) claimed that stress does not have any effect on the chances of becoming pregnant.

Both groups mostly used emotional coping strategies. However, the women could have ceased thinking about the issue when they started the treatment, and this could appear as emotional coping on the scale. In addition, it is notable that the participants stated that the emotional coping strategies reduced distress in their interpersonal relationships.

On the other hand, despite the higher emotional coping scores, deciding to receive and receiving IVF treatment, which is very expensive and requires painful invasive procedures, can be considered a direct problem-solving strategy for the couples. As stated in Lee (2003) and Eugster and Vingerhoest's (1999) article, the couples who receive the treatment are the couples who cope better and take actions to change their situation. This may mean that they are not avoiding solving the problem directly but are avoiding talking about it in their social life. Also, accepting the presented counseling service can be seen as a determined attitude towards solving the problem. Individuals differ in their interpretation of what is stressful and their construal of a stressful event as being a threat (a negative perception) or a challenge (a positive perception). These initial cognitive interpretations can be observed both directly and indirectly via various coping strate-

gies (Roesch et al., 2002). The infertility itself can be seen as a threat, but the IVF treatment can be seen as a challenge for the infertile individuals. Thus, the IVF treatment is more likely to have a positive influence on the individuals.

It was remarkable that the counseling service did not change either depression scores or coping strategies of the participants. Similarly, in the studies of Lee (2003) and Emery et al. (2003), although the participants stated that they were satisfied with the counseling service, their scores on depression or coping strategies [did] not change. Only a few studies indicate that infertility patients might benefit from counseling[1] (Anderheim et al., 2005; Fisher et al., 2005). Although it is recommended that emotional support before and after their babies are born is both therapeutic and preventive, it still remains unclear what specific programs or components could be beneficial for this population.

It is likely that the time period of the counseling was not sufficient to change the perspectives and attitudes of the women. The amount of decrease in depression and the improvement of coping skills might not be observable in the scores. In light of the results of the present study and the literature, it is difficult to evaluate the universal effect of intervention since women received treatment during various time spans with various content for individual sessions according to their needs. Well-structured programs including longer time

[1] Bartlik, B., Greene, K., Graf, M., Sharma, G., & Melnick, H. (1999). Examining PTSD as a complication of infertility. *Medscape General Medicine, 1*(2). [Formerly published in *Medscape Women's Health eJournal, 2*(3). 1997]. Available at http://www.medscape.com/viewarticle/408851

periods are needed to see the effects of these kinds of interventions. In addition, it is recommended that different measurements or different study methods like qualitative methods be used in future research to be able to show the effectiveness of such interventions.

365

### References

Akyüz, A., İnanç, N., & Pabuçcu, R. (1999). IVF ünitesinde eşlere yönelik hemşirelik faaliyetlerinin planlanmasında temel almacak deneyim ve gereksinimlerin belirlenmesi. *Gülhane Tip Dergisi, 1*(41), 37–45. [in Turkish]

Anderheim, L., Holter, H., Bergh, J., & Moller, A. (2005). Does psychological stress affect the outcome of *in vitro* fertilization? *Human Reproduction, 20,* 2969–2975.

Bush, S. (2001). Chasing a miracle: Why infertile women continue to stay in treatment. *ABNF (The Association of Black Nursing Faculty) Journal, 12,* 116–120.

Demyttenaere, K., Bonte, L., Gheldof, M., Vervaeke, M., Meuleman, C., Vanderschuerem, D., & D'Hooghe, T. (1998). Coping style and depression level influence outcome in *in vitro* fertilization. *Fertility and Sterility, 69,* 1026–1033.

Emery, M., Beran, M. D., Darwiche, J., Oppizzi, L., Joris, V., Capel, R., Guex, P., & Germond, M. (2003). Results from a prospective, randomized, controlled study: Evaluating the acceptability and effects of routine pre-IVF counseling. *Human Reproduction, 18,* 2647–2653.

Eugster, A. V, & Vingerhoests, A. J. J. M. (1999). Psychological aspects of *in vitro* fertilization: A review. *Social Science & Medicine, 48,* 575–578.

Fisher, J. R., Hammarberg, K. & Baker, H. W. (2005). Assisted conception is a risk factor for postnatal mood disturbance and early parenting difficulties. *Fertility and Sterility, 84,* 426–430.

Gürhan, N. (1995). Şizofren hastalarin sosyal destek, hastalik ve stresle baş etmelerinin değerlendirilmesi, Hacettepe Üniversitesi Sağlik Bilimleri Enstitüsü Hemşirelik Programi Doktora Tezi. [Dissertation in Turkish]

Lee, S. H. (2003). Effects of using a nursing crisis intervention program on psychosocial responses and coping strategies of infertile women during *in vitro* fertilization. *Journal of Nursing Research, 11,* 197–207.

Olshansky, E. (2003). A theoretical explanation for previously infertile mothers' vulnerability to depression. *Journal of Nursing Scholarship, 35,* 263–268.

Peterson, B. D., Newton, C. R., & Rosen, K. H. (2003). Examining congruence between partners' perceived infertility-related stress and its relationship to marital adjustment and depression in infertile couples. *Family Process, 42,* 59–70.

Pook, M., Röhrle, B., Tuschen-Caffier, B., & Krause, W. (2001). Why do infertile males use psychological couple counseling? *Patient Education and Counseling, 42,* 239–245.

Roesch, S. C., Weiner, B., & Vaughn, A. A. (2002). Cognitive approaches to stress and coping. *Current Opinion in Psychiatry, 15,* 627–632.

Savaşir, I., & Şahin, N. H. (1997). Bilişsel terapilerde değerlendirme: Sik kullanilan ölçekler, "Beck Depresyon Envanteri." *Türk Psikologlar Derneği Yayinlari,* Ankara, 23–28. [in Turkish]

Saydam, B. K. (2003). Türk toplumunda kisir kadinin statüsü. *Sağlik ve Toplum, 13*(1), 30–34. [in Turkish]

Sherrod, R. A. (2004). Understanding the emotional aspects of infertility: Implications for nursing. *Journal of Psychosocial Nursing & Mental Health Services, 42,* 40–47.

Venkatesan, L. (2005). Self-concept in infertile women. *Nursing Journal of India, 96,* 55–56.

# Exercise for Article 14

## Factual Questions

1. Is this study an example of a "true experiment" *or* a "quasi-experiment"?

2. What are the explicitly stated hypotheses for this study?

3. Of the 42 women initially assigned to the comparison group, how many remained at the end of the study?

4. What is the name of the measure used to measure depression?

5. What is the name of the inferential test reported in Table 3?

6. Which table reports on changes in coping strategies?

## Questions for Discussion

7. Do you believe verbal consent is adequate for a study of this type? Would you recommend using written consent? Explain. (See lines 108–112 and 136–141.)

8. Is it important to know the researchers did not assign the women to the two groups at random? Why? Why not? (See lines 112–120.)

9. In your opinion, is the structured counseling provided to the study group described in sufficient detail? Explain. (See lines 162–183.)

10. If you had planned this study, would you have expected to find significant differences between the two groups? Explain. (See Tables 2 and 3.)

11. Do you agree that the time period might not have been sufficient? Explain. (See lines 351–353.)

12. Do you agree that it might be useful to conduct a qualitative study on this topic in the future? Explain. (See lines 362–365.)

## Quality Ratings

Directions: Indicate your level of agreement with each of the following statements by circling a number from 5 for strongly agree (SA) to 1 for strongly disagree (SD). If you believe an item is not applicable to this research article, leave it blank. Be prepared to explain your ratings. When responding to criteria A and B, keep in mind that brief titles and abstracts are conventional in published research.

A. The title of the article is appropriate.

SA   5   4   3   2   1   SD

B. The abstract provides an effective overview of the research article.

SA   5   4   3   2   1   SD

C. The introduction establishes the importance of the study.

SA   5   4   3   2   1   SD

D.  The literature review establishes the context for the study.

       SA   5   4   3   2   1   SD

E.  The research purpose, question, or hypothesis is clearly stated.

       SA   5   4   3   2   1   SD

F.  The method of sampling is sound.

       SA   5   4   3   2   1   SD

G.  Relevant demographics (for example, age, gender, and ethnicity) are described.

       SA   5   4   3   2   1   SD

H.  Measurement procedures are adequate.

       SA   5   4   3   2   1   SD

I.  All procedures have been described in sufficient detail to permit a replication of the study.

       SA   5   4   3   2   1   SD

J.  The participants have been adequately protected from potential harm.

       SA   5   4   3   2   1   SD

K.  The results are clearly described.

       SA   5   4   3   2   1   SD

L.  The discussion/conclusion is appropriate.

       SA   5   4   3   2   1   SD

M.  Despite any flaws, the report is worthy of publication.

       SA   5   4   3   2   1   SD

# Article 15

*Independent*

# Effects of Two Educational Methods on the Knowledge, Attitude, and Practice *—dependent* of Women High School Teachers in Prevention of Cervical Cancer

**Mahin Baradaran Rezaei**, MSc, **Simin Seydi**, MSc, **Sakineh Mohammad Alizadeh**, MSc[*]

ABSTRACT. Because of the increased emphasis on prevention and early detection of cervical cancer, we studied the effects of 2 educational methods on the knowledge, attitude, and practice, regarding prevention of cervical cancer, of women high school teachers in Tabriz. This study was a semiexperimental research. Samples were 129 female teachers divided into 3 groups: experimental 1 (educated by pamphlets), experimental 2 (educated by a lecture and flash cards), and control group (not manipulated). After doing pretest in the 3 groups, investigators used 2 educational methods for experimental groups. Data regarding the knowledge and attitude of 3 groups were gathered after 14 days and data regarding practice were gathered after 2 months. Chi-square and 1-way ANOVA were used for data analysis. Before education, knowledge, attitude, and practice of the 3 groups were the same, but after education there were significant differences in mean scores of knowledge and attitude of 2 experimental groups as compared with the control group and also between the 2 experimental groups ($p < .001$). Education by lecture and flash cards was more effective than by pamphlets. In regard to Pap smear practice, there was a significant difference between the 2 experimental groups as compared with the control group ($p = .001$), but there was no significant difference between the 2 experimental groups. Therefore, educational methods were effective on knowledge, attitude, and practice of teachers regarding prevention of cervical cancer, and education by lecture and flash cards was more effective than by pamphlets in increasing knowledge and inducing a positive attitude, but the 2 educational methods had the same effect on practice of teachers.

From *Cancer Nursing*, 27, 364–369. Copyright © 2004 by Lippincott Williams & Wilkins. Reprinted with permission.

The report of the WHO (World Health Organization) in 1998 categorized cervical cancer as the fourth widespread cancer among women.[1] Seventy percent of the cases of genital cancer among women are of cervi-

5  cal cancer.[2] The report of the cytology unit of the Ira-

nian Ministry of Health, Treatment, and Medical Education in 1999 indicated that 0.2% of the microscopic slides received from women between the ages of 20 and 45, who had been referred to the health centers,

10  contained some degree of dysplasia and cervical cancer. This rate in the East Azerbaijan Province was 0.2%. (It should be noted that women experiencing menopause and other women at risk were not included in the statistics.)[3]

15  Pap smear is an effective test for cervical cancer screening, and women can get 3 Pap smears done in 1 year; if the test is repeated once in 3 years, up to 90% mortality from cancer can be prevented.[4,5] Although the efficiency of regular cytology tests such as Pap smear

20  has already proved to reduce the rate of mortality from cervical cancer, its application in the developing countries is less than that in the developed countries. This is because of the low knowledge of this important factor among women.[2]

25  The lack of knowledge concerning cervical cancer, the possibility of its diagnosis, the possibility of its full treatment in case of an early detection, and the lack of awareness of the existence of Pap smear as a means of diagnosis are all obstacles for Pap smear. Several stud-

30  ies indicate that the practice of getting Pap smears done in women is dependent on the degree of their sensitivity to the disease, their attitudes toward cancer, their beliefs, and also their awareness of the advantages of early detection.[6] To achieve a permanent change in

35  behavior and to bring about changes in personal practices, one finds that it is necessary to give people proper knowledge and to establish logical attitudes through health education programs.[7] One of the effective policies concerning the best use of cervical cancer

40  screening by women is the accessibility of cervical cancer screening programs for the community and instructing people about cervical cancer, and a change in the attitude of the community toward this cancer.[8]

[*]*Mahin Baradaran Rezaei is an instructor of basic sciences, Nursing & Midwifery, Tabriz University of Medical Sciences, Tabriz, Iran. Sakineh Mohammad Alizadeh is the deputy dean of Research, Nursing & Midwifery, Tabriz University of Medical Sciences, Tabriz, Iran.*

Table 1
*Teachers' Demographics*

| Characteristics | % | | |
| --- | --- | --- | --- |
| | Experimental group 1 | Experimental group 2 | Control group |
| Age | | | |
| ≤ 34 | 39.6 | 39.6 | 37.2 |
| 35–39 | 34.9 | 32.6 | 18.6 |
| 40–44 | 14.0 | 7.0 | 27.9 |
| ≥ 45 | 11.6 | 21.0 | 16.3 |
| First marriage, age | | | |
| < 20 | 14.0 | 9.3 | 4.7 |
| 20–24 | 44.0 | 39.5 | 46.5 |
| 25–29 | 34.9 | 34.9 | 25.6 |
| ≥ 30 | 7.0 | 16.3 | 23.3 |
| Number of pregnancies | | | |
| None | 2.3 | 11.6 | 7.0 |
| 1–2 | 81.4 | 11.6 | 81.4 |
| ≥ 3 | 16.3 | 20.9 | 11.6 |
| Main source for information | | | |
| Intermedia | 55.8 | 46.5 | 65.1 |
| Health workers | 14.0 | 9.3 | 27.9 |
| Friends | 23.3 | 9.3 | 0.0 |
| Others | 11.6 | 16.3 | 20.9 |

Groups: Experimental group 1 was educated by pamphlets, experimental group 2 was educated by a lecture and flash cards, and the control group was not manipulated (number of participants in each group was 43).

Through the application of these programs, the use of Pap smear has increased 3 times in the developed countries.[2]

In the developing countries where people are not sufficiently informed of the screening tests, especially Pap smear, the basic role of public health education and awareness of community should be emphasized.[9]

The variety of the methods of education is not only very effective in the process of teaching and learning, but it is also necessary to produce an interest and attract the cooperation of the addressee.[10,11]

Several studies that determined the knowledge, attitude, and practice of women regarding the prevention of cervical cancer were not appropriate.[12] The urgency of the problem caused the present researchers to study the effects of 2 educational methods on the knowledge, attitude, and practice of women high school teachers in Tabriz in prevention of cervical cancer.

Teachers are believed to be a group of women who play a fundamental role in the education of young girls in this region of the country and they should necessarily be conscious of the ways to prevent cervical cancer[13] so that they can teach the ways of its prevention to the members of their own society.

Researchers hope that the findings of this study will lead the authorities of the Education Department, and those in charge of education in the Departments of Health, Treatment, and Medical Education, to include effective cervical cancer screening programs in their schedules. It is also hoped that the minds will be oriented to the methods of prevention in order to lengthen, as much as possible, the lives of human beings, the invaluable treasures walking on Earth.

**Literature Review**

Researchers had frequently realized that women's knowledge, attitude, and practice in terms of the prevention of cervical cancer and undergoing Pap smear are not satisfactory.

Findings of Kottke et al., titled "Cancer screening behaviors and attitudes of women in southeastern Minnesota," showed that in women aged 18 years and older, 60% reported having had a Pap smear within the preceding year. More than 90% of the respondents expressed a willingness to have this test if their physicians were to advise them that the tests were needed.[14]

Another study was performed in China, titled "The knowledge and attitude of cancer prevention among junior high school teachers," by National Yang-Ming Medical College. The results showed that the cognizance rate of cervical cancer as the leading cancer (by that time) and the most curable for women in Taiwan was 69.3% and 37.5%, respectively. Pap smear was known to 96.8% of the teachers.[15]

Seyami and her colleagues studied the "knowledge and behavior (Pap smear) of women who referred to Tehran Health Centers." Findings showed that the knowledge of the majority of the participants (75.7%) was low and the knowledge of 18.29% of the participants was moderate.[16]

The study done by Baradaran and Alizadeh in Tabriz, Iran, on the topic "Nurses' and teachers' knowledge, attitude, and practice regarding prevention

Table 2

*Teachers' Knowledge by Groups\* at Preeducation and Posteducation*

*continuous→ordinal*

| Knowledge | Preeducation[†] | | | Posteducation[‡] | | |
|---|---|---|---|---|---|---|
| | Experimental group 1 | Experimental group 2 | Control group | Experimental group 1 | Experimental group 2 | Control group |
| Knowledge level, % | | | | | | |
| Low (0–8) | 32.6 | 23.3 | 37.2 | 0.0 | 0.0 | 49.5 |
| Moderate (9–16) | 65.1 | 72.1 | 62.8 | 27.9 | 9.3 | 60.5 |
| High (17–24) | 2.3 | 4.7 | 0.0 | 72.1 | 90.7 | 0.0 |
| Knowledge score | | | | | | |
| Mean | 10.49 | 10.19 | 8.65 | 18.76 | 19.93 | 9.28 |
| SD | 4.27 | 4.51 | 5.0 | 2.83 | 1.91 | 4.38 |

\*Groups: Experimental group 1 was educated by pamphlets, experimental group 2 was educated by a lecture and flash cards, and the control group was not manipulated (number of participants in each group was 43).
[†]Difference between groups is statistically not significant ($p > .05$).
[‡]Difference between groups is statistically significant ($p = .0001$).

105 of cervical cancer" enhances the subject in this respect. They indicated that 73.9% of nurses and 33.3% of teachers had appropriate knowledge and 17.4% of nurses and 20% of teachers had a positive attitude in this regard. Regarding regular performing of Pap
110 smear, 95.6% of nurses and 90% of teachers had poor practice.[12]

Dignan et al. performed a survey on the topic "Effectiveness of health education to increase screening for cervical cancer among Eastern-band Cherokee In-
115 dian women in North Carolina." The results showed that women who received the educational programs exhibited a greater knowledge about cervical cancer prevention and were more likely to have reported having had a Pap smear within the past year than did
120 women who did not receive the educational programs.[17]

Mcavoy and her colleagues showed that health education interventions increased the uptake of cervical cytology among Asian women in Leicester who had
125 never been tested. Personal visits were most effective, irrespective of the health education materials used, but there was some evidence that home videos may be particularly effective in one of the most hard to reach groups.[18]

## Method

130 This study is a quasi-experimental research. To do this, 129 teachers were chosen as the sample, all from among women high school teachers teaching in Tabriz.

The sample was randomly divided into 3 groups, each group comprising 43 teachers. Thus, 43 teachers
135 were included in the control group, 43 teachers in experimental group 1, being educated by pamphlets, and 43 teachers in experimental group 2, being educated by a lecture and flash cards.

Cluster sampling was used for data gathering.
140 Three high schools from each of the 5 education districts in Tabriz were chosen and overall 15 high schools were randomly selected. From the 3 high schools in each district, randomly one was assumed as control group, the second as experimental group 1, and

145 the third as experimental group 2. Regarding the number of teachers in each district, the samples were chosen via stratification sampling from each high school.

The self-structured questionnaire was evaluated by 10 experts in nursing and midwifery science, and on-
150 cology practitioners and its format were also considered by a statistics expert. Another factor that contributed to content validity was the theoretical concepts that were operationalized on the basis of previous studies. Reliability was measured by test-retest. The Pear-
155 son correlation coefficient for knowledge items was $r = 0.87$ and for attitude items was $r = 0.85$.

The questionnaire contained 4 parts: there were 7 questions on demographic characteristics, 24 relating to knowledge, 16 on attitude, and 11 questions on prac-
160 tice. The questionnaires were completed by the teachers. After reviewing them, the researchers identified the educational requirements of the teachers. Based on the information collected and following the opinions of experts, books, and various articles, pamphlets and the
165 texts of lectures together with 10 flash cards that included basic points related to Pap smear were provided. Pamphlets were then distributed among the teachers in group 1, and the teachers in group 2 were educated, in a session of 30 minutes, through a lecture and flash
170 cards. The control group did not receive any education. The part of the questionnaire related to knowledge and attitude was again completed after 2 weeks and the part related to practice was completed after 2 months for the 3 groups.

175 Only married teachers (who have sexual activity) were included in the study as Iranian culture and religious norms permit women to have sexual activity only after marriage.

To analyze the data, descriptive statistics such as
180 mean and standard deviation and analytical statistics such as test and 1-way ANOVA were used.

*Operational - definition*

*Categorical - definition*

Table 3
*Teachers' Attitude by Groups\* at Preeducation and Posteducation*

| Attitude | Preeducation[†] | | | Posteducation[‡] | | |
|---|---|---|---|---|---|---|
| | Experimental group 1 | Experimental group 2 | Control group | Experimental group 1 | Experimental group 2 | Control group |
| Attitude, % | | | | | | |
| Negative (16–48) | 34.9 | 39.5 | 44.2 | 20.9 | 0.0 | 39.5 |
| Positive (49–80) | 65.1 | 60.5 | 55.8 | 79.1 | 100 | 60.5 |
| Attitude score | | | | | | |
| Mean | 51.16 | 49.84 | 49.35 | 54.19 | 58.21 | 50.28 |
| SD | 5.17 | 5.81 | 5.87 | 5.02 | 5.84 | 7.25 |

\*Groups: Experimental group 1 was educated by pamphlets, experimental group 2 was educated by a lecture and flash cards, and the control group was not manipulated (number of participants in each group was 43).
[†]Difference between groups is statistically not significant ($p > .05$).
[‡]Difference between groups is statistically significant ($p = .0001$).

## Results

The average age of the teachers in group 1 was 36.28 years, 36.17 in group 2, and 37.74 in the control group. The average age at the first marriage was 23.93 in group 1, 24.79 in group 2, and 25.16 in the control group. The average number of pregnancies was 1.84 in group 1, 1.81 in group 2, and 1.79 in the control group.

No significant difference was observed among the groups in age, the age at the first marriage, and the numbers of pregnancies through a 1-way variance analysis. All the teachers had bachelor's degrees and all had married only once (Table 1).

Before education, the majority of the teachers had a moderate knowledge related to cervical cancer; very few had high knowledge. There was not a significant difference among the groups in the mean of knowledge scores. No person in groups 1 and 2 had a low knowledge after education; however, 49.5% of the control group had low knowledge. A significant difference was observed between the control and the experimental groups in knowledge ($p = .0001$). In a one-to-one comparison, there was a significant difference between groups 1 and 2 and the control group ($p < .0001$) and between group 1 and group 2 ($p < .05$) (Table 2).

Concerning the attitude toward the prevention of cervical cancer, approximately one-third of the samples had negative attitudes. There was no significant difference between the groups in terms of the degree of their attitudes before education; however, there was a significant difference between the groups after education ($p = .0001$). In a one-to-one comparison, a meaningful difference was observed between groups 1 and 2 and the control group ($p < .0001$) and between group 1 and group 2 ($p < 0.05$) (Table 3).

In terms of the practice of Pap smear, approximately 46% of the teachers had no practical experience of Pap smear, and there seemed to be no significant difference among the groups. However, 74.4% of the experimental groups 1 and 2 had gotten Pap smear done after education, while only 46.5% of the control group had gotten Pap smear done only once. There was a significant difference between the groups ($p = .0001$); and in a one-to-one comparison, there was a significant difference between experimental groups 1 and 2 and the control group ($p = .0001$). There was no significant difference between group 1 and group 2 (Table 4).

## Discussion

Regarding the results of the research, both methods managed to increase the knowledge of the teachers about the prevention of cervical cancer. Nevertheless, education through flash cards and giving lectures had been more effective than using the pamphlets.

The study done by Gremiel and colleagues in England is indicative of the positive effect of 4 different education methods on the degree of women's knowledge in this respect; however, the degree of knowledge of women educated through lectures and educational figures was more than that of women educated through other methods. In terms of the degree of effectiveness, education through lectures alone was the second best, and education through the use of video films was the third, over education through written materials.[19] Gremiel et al.'s research enhances the results gained in the present research concerning the priority of education through lectures and flash cards over education through giving written texts. Because of the face-to-face encounter between the educator and the receiver of education in the process of education through lectures and flash cards, the communication is reciprocal and the flash cards impart more objectivity to the issue under consideration, letting the samples use both sight and hearing senses. The result is an increase in learning.

The research proved that both of the educational methods managed to induce positive attitudes toward the prevention of cervical cancer, education through lectures and flash cards being more effective than education through the use of pamphlets.

The study of Heydarnia and his colleagues showed that education with a synthetic method (including face-to-face meeting, the use of posters and pamphlets) had caused a positive change in the attitudes of the participants.[20]

Table 4
*Teachers' Practice in Relation to Doing Pap Smear by Groups\* at Preeducation and Posteducation*

| Behavior (Pap smear) | Preeducation[†] | | | Posteducation[‡] | | |
|---|---|---|---|---|---|---|
| | Experimental group 1 | Experimental group 2 | Control group | Experimental group 1 | Experimental group 2 | Control group |
| Yes | 62.1 | 51.2 | 46.5 | 74.4 | 74.4 | 46.5 |
| No | 34.9 | 48.8 | 53.5 | 7.0 | 2.3 | 44.2 |
| Intended to get a Pap smear during the next time[§] | — | — | — | 18.6 | 23.3 | 9.3 |

\*Groups: Experimental group 1 was educated by pamphlets, experimental group 2 was educated by a lecture and flash cards, and the control group was not manipulated (number of participants in each group was 43).
[†]Difference between groups is statistically not significant ($p > .05$).
[‡]Difference between groups is statistically significant ($p = .0001$).
[§]This has not been considered in preeducation practice.

It would seem that the effectiveness of the education through lectures and flash cards on attitude is because of the face-to-face encounter of the educator and the receiver of education, the lecturer's emphasis on the significance of early diagnosis and treatment of the disease, and the confidence gained by the teachers in believing that the treatments are not aggressive in case of early diagnosis and that this cancer can be completely cured. The lectures highlight the texts and the flash cards prove and substantiate what is taught, although these issues are written in the pamphlets. The present study showed that both methods had equal impact on the practice of Pap smear. A study by Mcavoy and colleagues indicated that 47% of the women educated through video films together with face-to-face meetings and 37% of women educated by flash cards and face-to-face meetings underwent Pap smear. The rate of getting Pap smear done in the group that had received pamphlets was only 11%, while only 5% of the control group had gotten Pap smear done.[21] The lack of difference between the effects of the 2 methods in the present study may be due to the insufficiency of a 2-month period for practice (because of the limit on the time of the research) and also of the insufficiency of the number of samples.

Considering the results of this research, the health personnel should employ appropriate methods for every occasion and encourage people to receive the Pap smear. The lecture and flash cards method may be very appropriate for illiterate people (especially in rural communities), because it is very objective. The use of pamphlets can be useful in urban areas with educated people, because the pamphlets are cheap, the education is done very fast, and it covers a vast group of people.

The value and importance of screening are not well known in the developing countries. The people often do not visit the doctor unless they are ill.[18] Therefore, to encourage women to do Pap smear regularly, the authorities should pay due attention to the practice of Pap smear in their educational programs. The belief should be internalized in the women that they should primarily visit a doctor to prevent the disease by getting a Pap smear done. This will be very effective in the prevention of cancer, and it will also decrease the mortality rate.

## Suggestions

Regarding the unpleasant physical and mental outcomes in people suffering from malignant diseases, educating people through various effective methods to visit the doctors for early detection of the probable cancer can be one of the basic attempts to increase the public knowledge, attitude, and practice, and it can solve a fatal problem.

To achieve the objectives of the WHO and to conduct practically the motto "Health for All" up to 2000, teachers should receive proper health education, because they are impressive persons in the society and they encounter a large group of prospective mothers and women. Thus, a suitable and effective education for teachers can lead to the promotion of screening programs and their success.

It is hoped that the Department of Education and those in charge of the school textbooks will consider the teaching of this aspect of health to the very important half of the population.

Moreover, the managers and the authorities of the local health centers should provide necessary pamphlets and flash cards with high quality and distribute them among women.

They should also prepare suitable booklets and pamphlets for the health personnel in order to use them to increase the information of the women.

## References

1. *The World Health Organization (WHO) Report.* 1998.
2. Baheiraei Azam. *Methods of Cervical Cancer Prevention.* 1st ed. Tehran: Boshra Co; 1996:6–24.
3. Iranian Ministry of Health Cytology Unit. *Treatment and Medical Education: Family Health Word.* Iranian Ministry of Health Cytology Unit; 2000.
4. Ryan KJ, Robert W. *Kistner's Gynecology and Women's Health.* 7th ed. St Louis, Mo: Mosby; 1999:93–118.
5. Recommendations of frequency of Pap test screening. *Int J Gynecol Obstet.* March 1995;152:210–211.
6. Lobeal M, Bay C. Barriers to cancer screening in Mexican American women. *Mayo Clin Proc.* 1998;73(4):307–308.
7. Darmalingum T, Ramachandran L. *Health Education.* Fourogh S, trans. Tehran: Tehran University Press; 1992:20–23.
8. Miller AB. Cervical cancer screening, International Agency for Research on Cancer, Lyon, France. In: XV Asia Pacific Cancer Conference; December 12–15, 1999; Madras, India.

9.  Mehdeezadeh KH, Mohammadalizadeh S, Forudnia F. Effect of education of girls' primary school teachers on their knowledge about the importance and practice of Pap smear test. *J Kerman Univ Med Sci.* 1996; 3(1):28–34.

10. Helmserresht P, Delpishe E. *Health Education and Healthy Preferences for Education.* Tehran: Chahr Co; 1996:119–162.

11. Ewles L, Simnet I. *Health Education: A Practical Guide for Health Professionals.* Shidfar MA, trans. Tehran: Cyaroosh Co; 1993:28–50.

12. Baradaran M, Mohammad Alizadeh S. Study of knowledge, attitude, and practice regarding prevention of cervical cancer in female nurses and teachers. In: Seminar on Cancer: From Prevention to Rehabilitation. 1997; Tabriz.

13. Julaei S, Amin M. Effect of education on knowledge and practice regarding breast self-examination and Pap smear test in teachers. *J Hyat.* 1998;5(9):19–27.

14. Kottke TE, Trapp MA, Fores MM, et al. Cancer screening behaviors and attitudes of women in Southeastern Minnesota. *JAMA.* 1995;273(74):1099–1105.

15. Cheng Ch, Choupp G. The knowledge and attitude of cancer prevention among junior high school teachers. *Chung Hua I Hsueh Isa Chin Taipie.* 1994;53(6, suppl):1–8 (abstract for Med).

16. Seyami SH, Shafiey F. The knowledge & behavior (Pap smear) of women about cervical cancer who referred to Tehran health centers. *Med J Shahid Beheshty Univ.* 12:25–32.

17. Dignan M, Michelutee R, Bliason K. Effectiveness of health education to increase screening for cervical cancer among Eastern-band Cherokee Indian women in North Carolina. *J Natl Cancer Inst.* 1996;88(22):70–73.

18. Mcavoy BR, Raza R. Can health education increase uprate of cervical smear testing among Asian women? *BMJ.* 1991;302(6):833–836.

19. Gremiel ER, Gappmayer-Locker E, Girardi FL, et al. Increasing women's knowledge and satisfaction with cervical cancer screening. *J Psychosom Obstet Gynecol.* 1997;18(4):273–279.

20. Heydarnia A, Faghih-Zadeh S, Asgari H. The investigation about health education effectiveness on knowledge, attitude and practices of mothers who have children under age of five in rural areas of Central Province. *J Shahed Univ.* 1998;5(20):9–12.

21. Kelly AW, Wollan PC, Trapp MA. A program to increase breast and cervical cancer screening for Cambodian women in a Midwestern community. *Mayo Clin Proc.* 1996;72:437–444.

**Acknowledgments**: It is a desirable duty to thank the high school officials in Tabriz and also to thank all the teachers who took part in this research.

# Exercise for Article 15

## Factual Questions

1. How many questions on the questionnaire related to knowledge?

2. How was experimental group 2 educated?

3. What was the mean knowledge score for experimental group 1 on the pretest (i.e., preeducation) and on the posttest (i.e., posteducation)?

4. Did the mean attitude score for experimental group 2 go up from pretest (i.e., preeducation) to posttest (i.e., posteducation)? Explain.

5. At the preeducation stage of this study, the majority of which group had not had a Pap smear test?

6. Was a significant difference observed between the control and the experimental groups in knowledge? If yes, at what probability level was it significant?

## Questions for Discussion

7. The researchers refer to this study as "quasi-experimental." What is your understanding of the meaning of this term? (See line 130.)

8. In your opinion, is the design of the study clearly described in lines 130–147?

9. The researchers discuss the content validity of the questionnaire in lines 148–154. In your opinion, is this discussed in sufficient detail?

10. The researchers state that reliability was measured by the test-retest method and that the Pearson correlation coefficient for knowledge items was $r = 0.87$ and for attitude items was $r = 0.85$. Based on what you know about reliability, are the coefficients at an acceptable level? (See lines 154–156.)

11. Do you believe that this study has important practical implications? Explain.

12. If you were conducting a study on the same topic, what changes, if any, would you make in the research methodology?

## Quality Ratings

Directions: Indicate your level of agreement with each of the following statements by circling a number from 5 for strongly agree (SA) to 1 for strongly disagree (SD). If you believe an item is not applicable to this research article, leave it blank. Be prepared to explain your ratings. When responding to criteria A and B, keep in mind that brief titles and abstracts are conventional in published research.

A. The title of the article is appropriate.

   SA   5   4   3   2   1   SD

B. The abstract provides an effective overview of the research article.

   SA   5   4   3   2   1   SD

C. The introduction establishes the importance of the study.

   SA   5   4   3   2   1   SD

D. The literature review establishes the context for the study.

   SA   5   4   3   2   1   SD

E. The research purpose, question, or hypothesis is clearly stated.

   SA   5   4   3   2   1   SD

F. The method of sampling is sound.

   SA   5   4   3   2   1   SD

G.  Relevant demographics (for example, age, gender, and ethnicity) are described.

SA    5    4    3    2    1    SD

H.  Measurement procedures are adequate.

SA    5    4    3    2    1    SD

I.  All procedures have been described in sufficient detail to permit a replication of the study.

SA    5    4    3    2    1    SD

J.  The participants have been adequately protected from potential harm.

SA    5    4    3    2    1    SD

K.  The results are clearly described.

SA    5    4    3    2    1    SD

L.  The discussion/conclusion is appropriate.

SA    5    4    3    2    1    SD

M.  Despite any flaws, the report is worthy of publication.

SA    5    4    3    2    1    SD

Article 15  Effects of Two Educational Methods on the Knowledge, Attitude, and Practice of Women High School Teachers
in Prevention of Cervical Cancer

106

# Article 16

# Physical Restraint Reduction in the Acute Rehabilitation Setting: A Quality Improvement Study

**Shelly Amato**, MSN, RN, CNS, CRRN, **Judy P. Salter**, MSN, RN, CNS, CRRN,
**Lorraine C. Mion**, PhD, RN, FAAN[*]

ABSTRACT. A prospective, continuous quality improvement study was implemented at a hospital on two rehabilitation units: stroke and brain injury. The purpose of the study was to decrease restraint use by 25% and to maintain fall rates no greater than 10% over baseline. A multicomponent restraint reduction program was implemented that focused on administrative support, education, consultation, and feedback. Monthly restraint rates and fall rates were monitored and compared to the previous year's rates. Both units reduced restraint use. Importantly, this reduction was accomplished at the same time as a decline in fall rates.

From *Rehabilitation Nursing*, *31*, 235–241. Copyright © 2006 by the Association of Rehabilitation Nurses. Reprinted with permission.

Nurses have utilized physical restraints as part of patient care for many years in a variety of settings. For example, acute care nurses use physical restraints to prevent delirious or agitated patients from prematurely
5 disrupting therapy devices (Minnick, Mion, Leipzig, Lamb, & Palmer, 1998). Nurses in acute rehabilitation settings physically restrain patients to prevent falls, to manage agitation, and to manage impulsive behavior (Mion, Frengley, Jakovcic, & Marino, 1989; Schleen-
10 baker, McDowell, Moore, Costich, & Prater, 1994). Many patients in acute rehabilitation suffer from neurological conditions, such as brain injury or stroke, that increase their risk for falls and agitated behavior.

Although they are considered beneficial, physical
15 restraints do not necessarily prevent patient falls. Indeed, up to 34% of rehabilitation patients who fall do so while in physical restraint (Arbesman & Wright, 1999; Mion et al., 1989; Schleenbaker et al., 1994). In addition, physical restraints can have adverse effects
20 and may even cause death (Bromberg & Vogel, 1996; Miles & Irvine, 1992). Given the questionable risk-benefit ratio of physical restraints, federal regulation and accreditation standards have restricted the use of

physical restraint in all patient settings (Health Care
25 Financing Administration [HCFA], 1999; Joint Commission on Accreditation of Healthcare Organizations [JCAHO], 2005). As a result, many healthcare organizations have actively pursued reducing their use of physical restraints.

30 Studies have shown that restraint reduction programs in both acute care and long-term care settings have been effective in reducing restraint use while maintaining patient safety (Evans et al., 1997; Mion et al., 2001; Neufeld, Libow, Foley, & White, 1995). A
35 review of the literature yielded a descriptive report (Weeks, 1997) but found that no studies have systematically examined physical restraint reduction in the rehabilitation setting.

To establish the feasibility and effectiveness of
40 nonrestraint strategies in an acute rehabilitation setting, a continuous quality improvement (CQI) study was implemented on two acute rehabilitation units: brain injury and stroke. The study's purpose was to determine whether a multicomponent intervention strategy,
45 adapted from strategies used in long-term care and acute care settings, could safely reduce the use of physical restraints in acute rehabilitation units.

## Methods

### Setting

The Restraint Reduction Program (RRP) was implemented from March 2004 through March 2005 on
50 two acute rehabilitation units at a 732-bed county teaching hospital in the Midwest. The two units involved were the stroke rehabilitation unit (a 16-bed unit) and the brain injury rehabilitation unit (an 18-bed unit.)

### Restraint Reduction Program (RRP)

55 Interventions in the RRP were adapted from programs successfully implemented in acute and long-term care settings (Evans et al., 1997; Mion et al., 2001). The planning committee for the program con-

---

[*]*Shelly Amato* is a clinical nurse specialist for the Brain Injury and Stroke Rehabilitation Units at MetroHealth Medical Center. *Judy P. Salter* is a clinical instructor, Lorain County Community College. *Lorraine C. Mion* is director of research at MetroHealth Medical Center.

sisted of clinical nurse specialists, unit nurse managers,
60  nurse-patient care coordinators, physical therapists,
occupational therapists, and staff nurses.

The program consisted of four components: administration, education, consultation, and feedback.
The administrative component involved gaining the
65  active support of the director of nursing, nurse managers, patient care coordinators, physician leaders, and
therapists prior to implementation of the program. The
clinical nurse specialists met with the leadership group
to discuss the high use of restraints on both rehabilita-
70  tion units, the significance of the restraint use issue,
and the proposed Restraint Reduction Program. Updates given during regularly scheduled meetings included progress reports on the program, barriers to
implementation, and suggestions for facilitating staff
75  adoption of the program.

The education component consisted of both formal
and informal information sessions for all levels of nursing staff. These sessions focused on the restraint and
seclusion policy as well as the hospital's philosophy
80  regarding restraint use. A local vendor demonstrated
restraint alternatives available for purchase. Staff
members chose the devices that they felt would be
most effective for their patient population, then tested
the devices on a trial basis for effectiveness, after
85  which the selected devices were purchased for the program. The staff received training on proper use of the
devices. Staff also received formal education on falls:
risk factors, universal precautions, and targeted interventions using the selected physical restraint alterna-
90  tives. Content for those sessions was drawn from best
evidence and practice guidelines (American Geriatrics
Society, 2001; Leipzig, Cumming, & Tinetti, 1999a;
Leipzig, Cumming & Tinetti, 1999b) and from the
hospital's own Fall Prevention Protocol.

95  For the consultation component of the program, the
clinical nurse specialists went on rounds with staff
nurses, initially biweekly and then weekly after the
RRP was firmly established. Rounds focused on patients who were restrained, patients who had fallen, or
100  patients judged to be at risk for falling. For example,
the clinical nurse specialist and the nurse caring for a
restrained patient might discuss issues for that particular patient such as impulsivity, steadiness of gait, and
cognition. When a nurse identified that a patient was
105  starting to use the call light appropriately, or if a patient's gait was improving, a wheelchair and/or bed
alarm, respectively, would be recommended. The nurse
caring for the patient would then make the final decision to remove the restraint based on the nurse's as-
110  sessment of the patient. During the next consultation
session, the clinical nurse specialist would evaluate
whether recommendations had been carried out. For
any patient who had experienced a fall, the clinical
nurse specialist would explore circumstances leading to
115  the fall and discuss any interventions nurses may have
put in place following the fall. Fall-prevention strate-

gies found to be most effective in reducing restraint use
included using alarms (for the bed or wheelchair), increased surveillance techniques (such as 15-minute
120  checks or moving patients closer to the nurses' station),
and changing patient routines to facilitate surveillance
and staff contact.

The feedback component was twofold. First, the
nurses' adherence to the plan of care was monitored
125  and reviewed during the ongoing consultation rounds,
at which time individual nurse-to-nurse feedback was
provided. Second, the quality management department
provided aggregate data in the form of monthly run
charts for fall rates and physical restraint use on each
130  unit (see Figure 1).

The institutional review board (IRB) approved the
study in late 2003. The administrative and education
components began on both units in early 2004, with the
consultation component starting in March 2004 and the
135  feedback component in April of that year.

### Outcome Variables

The outcome variables for this study were the rates
of physical restraint use and patient falls. Physical restraint was defined as "any device, material, or equipment attached or adjacent to the patient's body that the
140  patient cannot remove easily, that restricts freedom of
movement, and that is not intended as part of the standard practice of care" (HCFA, 1999). Restraints included mitt(s), wrist restraints, waist restraints, pelvic
restraints, and full side rails. Monthly restraint rates
145  were calculated as the total number of restraint hours
per 100 patient days. Patient falls were defined as any
witnessed or unwitnessed event in which the patient
was found on the ground secondary to an unplanned
event. Fall rates were calculated as the number of pa-
150  tient falls per 1,000 patient days.

### Data Collection Procedures

Physical restraint data were collected from nursing
documentation. Unit secretaries input the information
into a computer database. At this hospital, quality management department personnel conduct ongoing audits
155  to ensure data collection consistency; any noted deviations are addressed at the time of the audit. Falls data
were collected using the incident reports that nurses
completed following any patient fall.

### Analysis

Monthly prevalence rates for both restraint use and
160  falls were calculated for the year prior to implementation of the study (baseline: March 2003 through February 2004) and compared with the rates observed during
the RRP (post: March 2004 through February 2005).
Physical restraint benchmarks were established for
165  both units using a 25% reduction rate from baseline.
Relative reduction rates were calculated using the mean
yearly rates with the following equation: [(baseline-
post)/baseline] × 100. An upper safety limit for fall
rates was established as a 10% relative increase over

---

**What Is Quality Improvement (QI)?**

- Also called performance improvement (PI), quality management (QM) and continuous quality improvement (CQI), QI is a disciplined approach to continuously improve outcomes using management techniques, existing improvement efforts, and technical tools.

**QI in Nursing**

- Florence Nightingale was the first healthcare professional that used and encouraged systematic inquiry into practices that might explain variation in outcomes.
- National organizations, such as the Joint Commission on Accreditation of Healthcare Organizations and the American Nurses Credentialing Center for Magnet Hospital designation, determine whether QI processes are a part of the nursing department's activities.

**• What Outcomes Are Important to Nursing?**

- A number of patient outcomes have been shown to be affected by either nursing structure and resources or by nursing practices. These nurse-sensitive outcomes include patient falls, physical restraints, nosocomial infections, pressure ulcers, and medication errors.

**• How Does One Determine Whether Outcomes Need to Be Improved or if Processes Have Improved Chosen Outcomes?**

- Many outcomes have national benchmarks established by which to compare your organization's rates to those considered to be "best practice." Most outcomes are reported as a prevalence rate per patient-days (either per 100 patient-days or 1,000 patient-days) rather than as an incidence rate (percentage of patients developing an outcome). This is done in order to maintain an "apple-to-apple" comparison since hospitals and units vary in size and characteristics. Outcomes can be expressed as a duration (e.g., number of hours/patient-days), or as an event (e.g., number of falls/patient-days).
- If an organization's outcome is worse than the national benchmark (the baseline value), then a team is assembled and possible sources or reasons for the problem are identified.
- The team brainstorms on possible solutions for improving the outcome and implements these actions.
- Outcome results are monitored continuously, typically in monthly reports.
  Run or Trend Charts (see figures in this article) display the data points over time. A target or benchmark value can be added to the chart as a horizontal line. Healthcare providers monitor whether their practices or processes bring the outcome rates close to or better than the targeted benchmark value. If outcome rates continue to be worse than benchmark for more than a predetermined amount of time (e.g., three months, five months, etc.), then the process improvement activities are reevaluated and modified.

  Statistical control charts also display the points over time. Month-to-month fluctuations in the outcome rate are normal. To determine if there are times when the fluctuation is greater or lesser than expected, two additional horizontal lines are added. These horizontal lines are typically three standard deviations above and below the mean, and are referred to as upper and lower control limits. If a monthly outcome rate occurs that is abnormally high or low (greater than three standard deviations), then the team immediately examines potential causes to explain the excessive variation (root cause analysis) and institutes changes in processes as needed.

---

From Claflin, N., DaMert, L., Hughes, J.D., Spath, P., Stephan, M., & Guthmann, I. (1998). NAHQ Guide to Quality Management, 8th Edition. Glenview, IL: National Association for Healthcare Quality; Langley, G.J., Nolan, K., Nolan, T.W., Norman, C.L., & Provost, L. P. (1996). The Improvement Guide: A Practical Approach to Enhancing Organizational Performance. San Francisco, CA: Jossey-Bass.

---

*Figure 1.* Understanding and utilizing quality improvement techniques.

---

170 baseline. The quality management office aggregated the data and reported it to the units.

## Results

Both the stroke rehabilitation unit and the brain injury rehabilitation unit reduced their overall restraint rates (Figures 2 and 3). The stroke rehabilitation unit 175 reduced restraint use from 216.6 hours per 100 patient days to 153.3 hours per 100 patient days, representing a 29.2% relative reduction in overall restraint use. The brain injury unit reduced restraint use from 1054.3 hours per 100 patient days to 883.3 hours per 100 pa-180 tient days—a 16.2% relative reduction.

Fall rates also decreased on both units (Figures 4 and 5). Stroke rehabilitation patients' fall rates declined from 11.4 to 6.1 falls per 1,000 patient days, a 45.5% relative reduction. Fall rates on the brain injury reha-185 bilitation unit declined from 9.1 to 3.3 falls per 1,000 patient days, a 64.2% relative reduction.

## Discussion

Federal regulations mandate the restriction of physical restraints in all patient settings, including rehabilitation (HCFA, 1999). Thus, rehabilitation nurses 190 must examine other ways to prevent falls among these high-risk patients. A restraint reduction program, fo-cusing on fall risk and impulsive or agitated behavior in stroke and brain injury rehabilitation patients, proved safe as well as effective. Our aim was to reduce 195 restraints while maintaining fall rates within 10% of baseline. Our achievement of both objectives demonstrates the feasibility and effectiveness of this systematic approach.

We found that the RRP program was more success-200 ful on the stroke unit than on the brain injury unit. Several factors may account for this. First, the units are shaped differently. The stroke unit is circular, while the brain injury unit is a rectangular space with only a few beds visible from the nurses' station. Indeed, the two 205 most common strategies on the brain injury unit involved surveillance: moving a patient to a room closer to the nurses' station and/or instituting 15-minute surveillance checks. Another published report of a restraint reduction program also emphasized surveillance 210 strategies (Weeks, 1997). The nature of patients' medical conditions may also explain the differences in reduction rates. Although stroke patients may have cognitive deficits, such as poor judgment or lack of insight, brain injury patients tend to have greater impulsivity 215 and agitation.

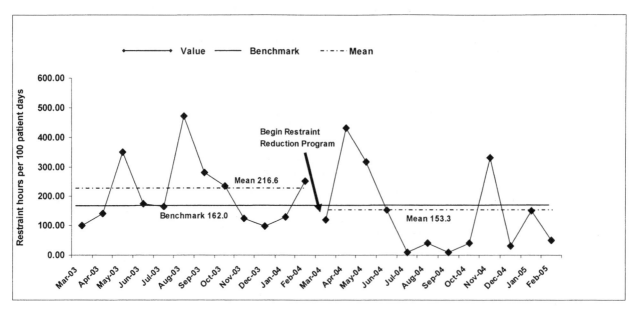

*Figure 2.* Changes in physical restraint rates—stroke rehabilitation unit.

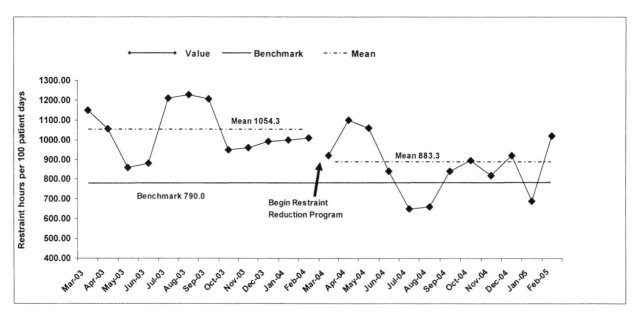

*Figure 3.* Changes in physical restraint rates—brain injury unit.

Of note, both units had spikes in restraint use upon the initiation of the RRP as well as at later points in the program. These occasional increases were not associated with falls, and the rates were within the upper control limits of the mean (see Figure 1 for explanation). The initial spikes may reflect staff resistance toward implementing a new program, but the initial and later occasional spikes may simply reflect normal variations in restraint use over time. Given the successful results in restraint reduction, future plans for the stroke unit are to continue monitoring restraint use and fall rates and to ensure that restraint reduction strategies continue to be implemented in a safe manner.

Although restraint reduction was also successful on the brain injury unit, the outcome difference was not as great as that seen on the stroke unit. The brain injury unit staff will implement a unit-based restraint committee, which will be led by the clinical nurse specialist and will meet monthly. Membership will include all nursing staff as well as the nurse manager. The committee will focus on restraint reduction, examination of the causes of falls, and restraint documentation. In response to the challenge of reducing restraints while maintaining safety in the high-risk brain injury population, a "day room" has been designated and is under current remodeling on the brain injury unit. The room,

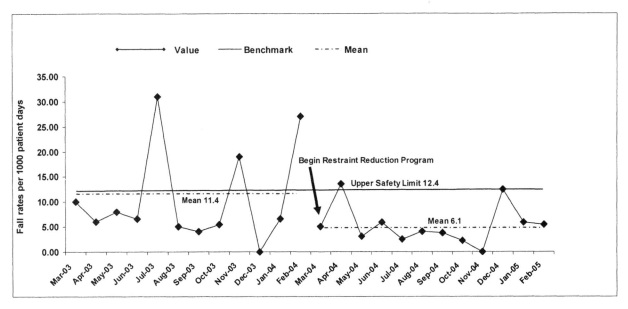

*Figure 4.* Changes in fall rates—stroke rehabilitation unit.

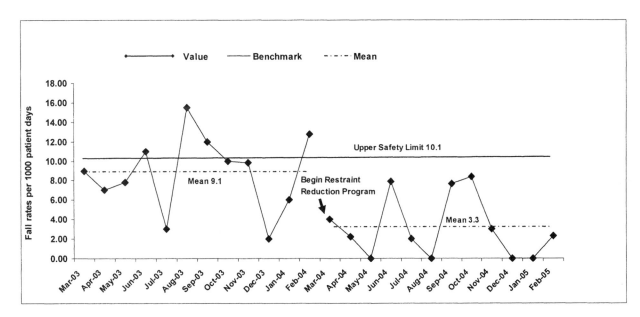

*Figure 5.* Changes in fall rates—brain injury rehabilitation unit.

which is to be staffed by a patient care provider, will provide a place where high-risk patients can be monitored closely during the daytime hours that they are not 245 in therapy.

In summary, in an acute rehabilitation setting, a restraint reduction program that emphasizes restraint alternatives can provide safe care that is effective in preventing falls while preserving patients' rights and 250 dignity.

### References

American Geriatrics Society, British Geriatrics Society, and American Academy of Orthopaedic Surgeons Panel on Falls Prevention. (2001). Guideline for the prevention of falls in older persons. *Journal of the American Geriatrics Society, 49*, 664–672.

Arbesman, M. C., & Wright, C. (1999). Mechanical restraints, rehabilitation therapies, and staffing adequacy as risk factors for falls in an elderly hospitalized population. *Rehabilitation Nursing, 24*, 122–128.

Bromberg, M. B., & Vogel, C. M. (1996). Vest restraint palsy. *Archives of Physical Medicine and Rehabilitation, 77*, 1316–1319.

Evans, L. K., Strumpf, N. E., Allen-Taylor, S. L., Capezuti, E., Maislin, G., & Jacobsen, B. (1997). A clinical trial to reduce restraints in nursing homes. *Journal of the American Geriatrics Society, 45*, 675–681.

Health Care Financing Administration. (1999). *Medicare and Medicaid Programs. Hospital Conditions of Participation: Patients' Rights; Interim Final Rule.* 42 CFR Part 482. *Federal Register* (64:127).

Joint Commission on Accreditation of Healthcare Organizations. (2005). *2006 Comprehensive Accreditation Manual for Hospitals: The Official Handbook.* Oakbrook Terrace, IL: Author.

Leipzig, R. M., Cumming, R. G., & Tinetti, M. E. (1999a). Drugs and falls in older people: A systematic review and meta-analysis: I. Psychotropic Drugs. *Journal of the American Geriatrics Society, 47,* 30–39.

Leipzig, R. M., Cumming, R. G., & Tinetti, M. E. (1999b). Drugs and falls in older people: A systematic review and meta-analysis: II. Cardiac and analgesic drugs. *Journal of the American Geriatrics Society, 47,* 40–50.

Miles, S. H., & Irvine, P. (1992). Deaths caused by physical restraints. *Gerontologist, 32,* 762–766.

Minnick, A. F., Mion, L. C., Leipzig, R., Lamb, K., & Palmer, R. M. (1998). Prevalence and patterns of physical restraint use in the acute care setting. *Journal of Nursing Administration, 28,* 19–24.

Mion, L. C., Fogel, J., Sandhu, S., Palmer, R. M., Minnick, A. F., & Cranston, T. (2001). Outcomes following physical restraint reduction programs in two acute care hospitals. *The Joint Commission Journal on Quality Improvement, 27,* 605–618.

Mion, L. C., Frengley, J. D., Jakovcic, C. A., & Marino, J. A. (1989). A further exploration of the use of physical restraints in hospitalized patients. *Journal of the American Geriatrics Society, 37,* 949–956.

Mion, L. C., Gregor, S., Buettner, M., Chwirchak, D., Lee, O., & Paras, W. (1989). Falls in the rehabilitation setting: Incidence and characteristics. *Rehabilitation Nursing, 14,* 17–22.

Neufeld, R. R., Libow, L. S., Foley, W. J., & White, H. (1995). Can physically restrained nursing-home residents be untied safely? Intervention and evaluation design. *Journal of the American Geriatrics Society, 43,* 1264–1268.

Schleenbaker, R. E., McDowell, S. M., Moore, R. W., Costich, J. F., & Prater, G. (1994). Restraint use in inpatient rehabilitation: Incidence, predictors, and implications. *Archives of Physical Medicine and Rehabilitation, 75,* 427–30.

Weeks, S. K. (1997). RAP: A Restraint Alternative Protocol that works. *Rehabilitation Nursing, 22,* 154–156.

**Acknowledgments**: The authors wish to acknowledge the staff nurses on the stroke and brain injury rehabilitation units for implementing the Restraint Reduction Program, Kathleen McCarthy for the data analysis portion of this study, and the MetroHealth Foundation (grant no. 57-2003) for the funding to purchase restraint alternatives for this study.

**Address correspondence to**: Shelly Amato, MetroHealth Medical Center, 2500 MetroHealth Drive, Cleveland, OH 44109. E-mail: samato@metrohealth.org

# Exercise for Article 16

## Factual Questions

1. The brain injury rehabilitation unit had how many beds?

2. How was "patient falls" defined?

3. How long did the baseline last?

4. As a percentage, what was the relative reduction in overall restraint use?

5. Fall rates on the brain injury rehabilitation unit had what percentage relative reduction?

## Questions for Discussion

6. Is the intervention described in sufficient detail? (See lines 55–135.)

7. How important was Figure 1 in helping you understand the background for this study? Would the report be as effective without the figure? Explain.

8. How important were Figures 2 through 5 in helping you understand the results of this study? Would the report be as effective without the figures? Explain.

9. To what extent has this study convinced you of the effectiveness of the intervention? Explain.

10. If you were planning a follow-up study on this topic, would you include a control group? Explain.

## Quality Ratings

Directions: Indicate your level of agreement with each of the following statements by circling a number from 5 for strongly agree (SA) to 1 for strongly disagree (SD). If you believe an item is not applicable to this research article, leave it blank. Be prepared to explain your ratings. When responding to criteria A and B, keep in mind that brief titles and abstracts are conventional in published research.

A. The title of the article is appropriate.

 SA   5   4   3   2   1   SD

B. The abstract provides an effective overview of the research article.

 SA   5   4   3   2   1   SD

C. The introduction establishes the importance of the study.

 SA   5   4   3   2   1   SD

D. The literature review establishes the context for the study.

 SA   5   4   3   2   1   SD

E. The research purpose, question, or hypothesis is clearly stated.

 SA   5   4   3   2   1   SD

F. The method of sampling is sound.

 SA   5   4   3   2   1   SD

G. Relevant demographics (for example, age, gender, and ethnicity) are described.

 SA   5   4   3   2   1   SD

H. Measurement procedures are adequate.

 SA   5   4   3   2   1   SD

I. All procedures have been described in sufficient detail to permit a replication of the study.

 SA   5   4   3   2   1   SD

J. The participants have been adequately protected from potential harm.

 SA   5   4   3   2   1   SD

K. The results are clearly described.

 SA   5   4   3   2   1   SD

L.   The discussion/conclusion is appropriate.

    SA   5   4   3   2   1   SD

M.  Despite any flaws, the report is worthy of publication.

    SA   5   4   3   2   1   SD

# Article 17

## Sleep Disturbances in Women With HIV or AIDS: Efficacy of a Tailored Sleep Promotion Intervention

**Angela L. Hudson**, PhD, FNP-C, **Carmen J. Portillo**, PhD, RN, FAAN,
**Kathryn A. Lee**, PhD, RN, FAAN.[*]

### ABSTRACT

*Background*: Poor sleep is a frequent complaint of persons with HIV infection.

*Objectives*: To pilot test a tailored sleep promotion intervention protocol based on principles of sleep hygiene in a convenience sample of 30 HIV seropositive women.

*Methods*: At baseline and 1 week after implementing the intervention, sleep was assessed by self-report measures and wrist actigraphy. Objective sleep measures include total sleep time, number of awakenings, and sleep efficiency, as well as level of daytime activity, 24-hr activity rhythm, and amount of sleep during the day.

*Results*: Prior to the intervention, women averaged 6.4 hr (*SD* = 1.99) of sleep, and 67% (*n* = 20) of the sample napped more than 30 min per day. After allowing 1 week to implement sleep hygiene principles to promote healthy sleep behaviors, there was a significant improvement in their perception of sleep and a significant change in their 24-hr activity rhythm. This involved more activity and less napping during the day.

*Discussion*: Although there was minimal change in objective measures of nighttime sleep for the group as a whole, those with initiation insomnia and maintenance insomnia benefited most from the intervention. These findings support the utility of a tailored sleep promotion intervention for women who are HIV positive to address their unique form of sleep disturbance.

From *Nursing Research*, 57, 360–366. Copyright © 2008 by Lippincott Williams & Wilkins. Reprinted with permission.

Sleep disturbance is a common complaint among persons living with HIV infection and occurs in all stages of HIV-related illnesses (Reid & Dwyer, 2005). Sleep disturbance affects quality of life and daytime functioning (Nokes & Kendrew, 2001), and it has been reported that the proportion of persons with HIV and AIDS who experience problems with sleep is higher than that of the general population (Lee, Portillo, & Miramontes, 2001; Nokes, Chidekel, & Kendrew, 1999; Rubinstein & Selwyn, 1998).

Sleep disturbance, often categorized as *insomnia*, includes difficulty falling asleep (initiation insomnia) and nighttime awakenings (maintenance insomnia) that result in poor sleep efficiency. Early morning awakening or feeling sleepy and poorly rested after a night's sleep can also be related to poor sleep and is included in some definitions of insomnia (Lee, 2006). In HIV infection, poor sleep has been associated with disease progression, highly active antiretroviral therapy, lack of employment, and fatigue (Koppel & Bharel, 2005; Nokes & Kendrew, 2001; Nunes et al., 2001; Phillips et al., 2004; Wheatley & Smith, 1994). Other associated problems include anxiety, depressive symptoms, nonadherence to antiretroviral medications, and decreased immune function (Irwin, Clark, Kennedy, Christian Gillin, & Ziegler, 2003; Nokes & Kendrew, 2001; Perkins et al., 1995).

Reports of insomnia among individuals who are HIV positive range from 29% to 74% (Reid & Dwyer, 2005; Rubinstein & Selwyn, 1998; Vogl et al., 1999). One of the first studies of HIV infected women found moderate sleep efficiency when assessed objectively with wrist actigraphy in the home environment (Lee et al., 2001). Sleep disturbance is not only prevalent but also one of the more debilitating symptoms in intensity and severity (Hudson, Kirksey, & Holzemer, 2004; Wheatley & Smith, 1994).

Despite many observational studies on sleep disturbance in this population, little is known about nonpharmacologic interventions for sleep complaints. Phillips and Skelton (2001) found that sleep quality significantly improved in a sample of 21 HIV positive men and women after receiving a 5-week course of acupuncture. A group of 44 persons, HIV positive adults who decreased their caffeine intake by 90%, significantly improved their sleep quality and well-

---

[*] *Angela L. Hudson* is an assistant professor, Los Angeles School of Nursing, University of California. *Carmen J. Portillo* is a professor, Department of Community Health Systems. *Kathryn A. Lee* is a professor, Department of Family Health Care Nursing, San Francisco School of Nursing, University of California.

being compared with 44 controls (Dreher, 2003). More research, however, is needed on nonpharmacologic interventions to manage insomnia and improve sleep quality among persons who are HIV positive experiencing sleep disturbance.

### Sleep Promotion Behavioral Education

Sleep promotion, also known as sleep hygiene, is a set of behavioral principles delivered as an educational intervention to promote healthy sleep habits. In addition to a healthy diet and reduced caffeine intake, sleep promotion includes attention to environmental factors such as light and noise reduction, temperature control, and mattress comfort (McCall, 2005). Exercise is encouraged but should be avoided within 3 to 4 hr before bedtime. Establishing a regular schedule for going to bed and getting up is important, and avoiding daytime naps is emphasized, particularly if the client is complaining of difficulty falling asleep at night (Eddy & Walbroehl, 1999; Hauri, 1997).

Several studies include sleep hygiene interventions for older persons with sleep disturbance and caregivers of persons with chronic illness. Behaviors such as structured physical exercise and nighttime incontinence care produced significant improvements in sleep quality among elderly nursing home residents (Alessi, Yoon, Schnelle, Al-Samarrai, & Cruise, 1999). After receiving sleep promotion behaviors, elderly residents living in a continuous-care retirement facility had significant improvements in memory-oriented tasks (Naylor et al., 2000). Sleep hygiene also is effective in decreasing insomnia and depressive symptoms in family caregivers of persons with advanced cancer (Carter, 2006), and sleep hygiene significantly reduced nocturnal wake time and improved pain and mood in a sample of adults with fibromyalgia (Edinger, Wohlgemuth, Krystal, & Rice, 2005).

### Actigraphy

A wrist actigraph is a device used in sleep research studies to measure body movements during sleep and is an appropriate method for documenting sleep disturbance, especially among individuals who are unable to participate in gold standard polysomnography (Coffield & Tryon, 2004). The actigraph monitors movement or activity to estimate various sleep variables, such as sleep efficiency, total sleep time (TST), latent sleep onset, and time awake after sleep onset (Edinger et al., 2005). Actigraphy as an objective measure of sleep has been validated with polysomnography (Edinger et al., 2005; Landis et al., 2003), and wrist actigraphy is a feasible way to estimate sleep in the home environment (Bauldoff, Ryan-Wenger, & Diaz, 2007).

The purpose of this pilot study, therefore, was to test the efficacy of a tailored sleep promotion intervention protocol based on principles of sleep hygiene (Hauri, 1997). In the intervention, subjective and objective measures were incorporated to assess sleep quality.

## Methods

### Sample

The last 32 women participating in a cross-sectional descriptive sleep study of 100 women with HIV or AIDS were included in this pilot study after obtaining the descriptive baseline data. To increase the validity of the findings, women were excluded if there was a confirmed AIDS dementia diagnosis—as they would be unable to reliably complete the diary and questionnaires—and excluded if they had moderate (Grade II) neuropathy because the intervention would not address sleep problems due to neuropathy. They also were excluded if they currently used illicit substances or were hospitalized within the past week, so that measures of mood and sleep would not be affected by these confounding issues. Because they were part of the initial larger descriptive study of 100 women, they were not screened for sleep problems or excluded from participation on the basis of sleep complaints. Baseline data on the entire sample are published elsewhere (Lee et al., 2001). One of the 32 women had actigraphy equipment failure during the postintervention study, and another participant was excluded from analysis based on questionable gender; therefore, the final sample is composed of 30 women.

The sample included 18 African American, 6 Mexican American, and 6 Caucasian women between 31 and 54 years ($M = 40.4 \pm 6.3$ years) with CD4 cell counts between 40 and 930 mm$^3$. The mean CD4 cell count was $373 \pm 220.3$ mm$^3$, and 26% had CD4 cell counts below 200 mm$^3$. The sample did not differ significantly from the first 70 women who participated in the descriptive phase of the study (Lee et al., 2001).

### Procedures

Approval for the study was obtained from the institutional review board of the University of California, San Francisco. Participants receiving ambulatory care in clinic settings throughout the San Francisco Bay Area were accessed through their healthcare provider and presented with the details of the study. After expressing interest in participating, they subsequently were given explanation of the study purpose by the principal investigator or research assistant. After giving informed consent, they were instructed in wearing a wrist motion sensor to monitor sleep and activity continuously for the next 48 hr, and the most recent CD4 cell count was obtained from their clinic record. The participants in this pilot study signed an additional consent form for the intervention pilot study; no one refused to participate in the pilot intervention study.

Data were collected between January and June 1997. Standardized instruments were administered by a member of the research team in a private area within the clinic setting or at a mutually agreed-upon location. Instruments took approximately 30 min to complete. At the end of 48 hr, the wrist actigraph was collected, the participant was paid $25.00 for her participation, and the participant contracted with the researcher to try two of the potential six sleep hygiene behaviors for 1 week. At the end of the week, participants returned for a follow-up assessment using the same standardized instruments and an additional 48 hr of sleep monitoring on the same two nights of the week to control for variability in social week wake-sleep patterns. Upon return of the equipment after the second 48-hr assessment, each participant was paid an additional $25.00.

*Measures*

*Sleep and Activity.* Continuous noninvasive monitoring of activity was accomplished with a wrist motion sensor (Mini Motionlogger Actigraph, AAM-32 Ambulatory Monitoring, Inc., Ardsley, NY). This wrist actigraphy has been validated with electroencephalograph measures of sleep and awakenings on men and women and on healthy and disturbed sleepers (Hauri & Wisbey, 1992; Walsh et al., 1991). It provides continuous motion data using a battery-operated wristwatch-size microprocessor that senses motion with a piezo-electric beam and detects movement and acceleration in all three axes.

Moderate to high correlations are documented between polysomnographic laboratory measures (gold standard for measuring sleep-wake patterns) and wrist actigraphy measures in various groups of research participants (Cole, Kripke, Gruen, Mullaney, & Gillin, 1992; Sadeh, Hauri, Kripke, & Lavie, 1995). Actigraphy is a valid measure of sleep on four out of five sleep parameters (Lichstein et al., 2006). The ability to detect sleep disturbance (specificity) was 90% in nursing home patients with dementia (Ancoli-Israel, Clopton, Klauber, Fell, & Mason, 1997). One-minute intervals were used to calculate TST (minutes), number of awakenings, and percentage of wake time during the night on both nights using an automatic sleep scoring program (Action4 Software Program, Ambulatory Monitoring Inc., Ardsley, NY). The average of the two nights was used for analysis. A sleep diary also was completed each evening, which included a brief description of activity, meals, beverages consumed, stressors, and symptoms experienced during the day. In the morning, the diary asked for bedtimes and wake times as well as perception of the night's sleep. This diary was used to confirm bedtimes and final wake times for the actigraphy sleep analyses as well as assess any discrepancies in behaviors or medications between the two time points.

To estimate activity patterns, the mean level of activity (mesor or 24-hr adjusted mean level) and amplitude of the rhythm pattern for the 48 hr of activity data were calculated using cosinor analysis, with an expected 24-hr period length. Daytime sleep was assessed for a 12-hr period during the day (typically the 720 min between 09:00 and 21:00 hours) between Night 1 and Night 2 and expressed as a percentage of the 720 min possible. Those who spent more than 4% of the day

asleep were considered nappers. Rhythm strength, which indicates the consistency of the participant's sleep and activity pattern, was estimated by autocorrelated data points with the data point 24 hr later. On the basis of the 2,880 data points obtained in 48 hr of continuous activity monitoring, these estimates result in an autocorrelation coefficient for a 24-hr rhythm that can range from 0 (*no strength*) to .99 (*highly regular and consistent*). An autocorrelation coefficient of 0 to .25 is considered generally a weak 24-hr rhythm, with no consistent pattern from one night or day to the next. A coefficient of .26 to .5 is considered moderate, whereas a coefficient greater than .5 is considered to be a strong and consistent rhythm.

To estimate women's general perception of sleep problems, two self-report measures were utilized. The Pittsburgh Sleep Quality Index (PSQI) was used to describe their sleep history (Buysee, Reynolds, Monk, Berman, & Kupfer, 1989). The items in this instrument ask respondents to think about how often, on a 4-point scale from 0 (*not during the past month*) to 3 (*three or more times a week*), they experienced sleep problems, such as trouble falling asleep within 30 min or trouble staying awake while driving, eating, or socializing, and how much of a problem it is to keep up enough enthusiasm to get things done, from 0 (*no problem at all*) to 3 (*a very big problem*). The PSQI has been validated with laboratory polysomnography and found to have adequate validity and reliability. A cutoff score of 5 was sensitive (84.4%) and specific (86.5%) for distinguishing controls from patients with disorders of initiation and maintenance of sleep. Scores can range from 0 to 21, and scores greater than 5 indicate substantial sleep disturbance (Buysee et al., 1989). Because participants are asked to think about the past month, however, it was not a sensitive or valid assessment for change after only 1 week of sleep hygiene and was used as a descriptor for their baseline sleep characteristics. Cronbach's alpha coefficient for the seven subscales was .844 for this sample at baseline.

To obtain a more sensitive estimate of changes in sleep, the investigators asked the participants to complete the 21-item General Sleep Disturbance Scale (GSDS; Lee, 1992), which was administered preintervention and postintervention. The GSDS asks participants to indicate frequency of various sleep-related behaviors during the past week from 0 (*not at all*) to 7 (*every day*). Items refer to the multidimensional aspects of falling asleep and maintaining sleep and aspects of daytime functioning, such as feeling tired or sleepy during the day. Items are summed to obtain a total mean score that can range from 0 (*no sleep disturbance*) to 7 (*frequent sleep disturbance*). The scale was validated originally with women shift workers (Lee, 1992) and was internally consistent in this sample (Cronbach's α coefficient = .82). It also was correlated highly with the PSQI at the preintervention measure

($r = .77$, $p < .001$), indicating adequate validity for this subjective measure of sleep disturbance.

*Intervention*

The intervention was an educational and behavioral set of sleep-promoting behaviors based on principles of sleep hygiene. The intervention consisted of a 30- to 45-min session in which six primary principles of sleep hygiene were reviewed with each individual participant. The educational session was adapted from various versions of sleep hygiene, in which there are from 11 to 22 principles (Espie, Inglis, Tessier, & Harvey, 2001; Hauri, 1997), and framed within the context of *Sleep B.E.T.T.E.R.* (Table 1). Each principle is followed by a detailed 1-page discussion, with space for an individualized contract. For example, under E for eating and drinking, one woman reported drinking a 6-pack of Dr Pepper each day. When educated about caffeine's effect on sleep, she responded that she drank Diet Dr Pepper, indicating that she needed to understand that diet Dr Pepper also has caffeine. After correcting her confusion about calories and caffeine, she agreed to try Diet Sprite for the next week, and it was written as her contract in the space provided.

*Data Analyses*

Measures of central tendency were used to describe sample characteristics. The actigraphy data were analyzed for each participant using Action4 software. This software allows for automatic sleep scoring, cosinor analysis, and autocorrelation, as described earlier. These data were then entered into SPSS, Version 14.0 software, for group analyses. Using paired $t$ tests with significance set at $p < .05$, results were analyzed for significant differences in sleep variables between baseline and postintervention. Results were analyzed by intention to treat, which assumes that all participants tried the intervention during the next 7 days.

## Results

*Sample Characteristics*

Of the 30 women in this pilot study, 25 (81%) had a history of poor sleep, as indicated by PSQI scores greater than 5 at baseline. Sleep variables for the sample of 30 women with HIV or AIDS before and after the intervention are shown in Table 2. Although 10 of the 30 women did not experience sleep disturbance at baseline, they were included in the analysis to demonstrate that the pilot intervention would not worsen an already adequate sleep experience. Others may or may not have initiated their contracted intervention during the week but were also included in all analyses by intention to treat.

Table 1

*Principles of Sleep Hygiene: How to Sleep B.E.T.T.E.R.*

**Sleeping B.E.T.T.E.R.** uses the letters in the word *b e t t e r* to help you remember the six basic rules of sleep hygiene.

| | |
|---|---|
| **B**edroom. | The noise, light, and temperature in the room where you sleep needs to be considered. |
| **E**xercise. | Having some type of daily activity is important for a good night's sleep. |
| **T**ension. | Reducing your tension with relaxing activities in the evening will help you fall asleep faster and sleep better. |
| **T**ime to sleep. | Not everyone needs 8 hours of sleep. |
| | Spending time trying to fall asleep, or trying to go back to sleep when you wake up too early, is not relaxing. Your time is better spent getting up and reading or doing another quiet activity. |
| **E**ating, drinking, and drugs. | Sleep is affected by what you eat or drink, and medications you take. |
| **R**hythm. | Keep a consistent day and night schedule. Avoid light at night, but get light during the day. |

*Clinical nurse asks:*      *What are you already doing to get better sleep?*
                               *Which of these are you willing to work on during the next week?*

CONTRACT:

     1. *B E T T E R*    No caffeine after 6 PM
     2. *B E T T E* **R**    Up every morning by 7 AM

Table 2

*Changes in Sleep Quality Variables After Sleep Hygiene Intervention (n = 30)*

| Sleep and activity | Preintervention $M \pm SD$ | Postintervention $M \pm SD$ | Significance |
|---|---|---|---|
| Perception of sleep onset (diary minutes) | $33.0 \pm 25.8$ | $33.5 \pm 30.2$ | |
| General Sleep Disturbance (GSDS) | $3.11 \pm 1.08$ | $2.50 \pm 0.78$ | $t = 4.10, p < .001$ |
| Sleep onset (actigraph minutes) | $22.8 \pm 29.9$ | $20.5 \pm 20.0$ | |
| Total sleep time at night (hours) | $6.4 \pm 1.99$ | $5.9 \pm 1.93$ | $t = 1.40$, not significant |
| Sleep efficiency (% of total sleep time) | $72.7 \pm 18.7$ | $71.9 \pm 15.7$ | |
| Number of awakenings | $20.6 \pm 9.7$ | $19.1 \pm 8.8$ | |
| Wake after sleep onset (% of total sleep) | $23.3 \pm 17.6$ | $25.2 \pm 16.8$ | |
| Daytime sleep (% time) | $10.0 \pm 11.5$ | $8.1 \pm 9.9$ | |
| Circadian rhythm parameters | | | |
|      Mesor (Hz) | $67.3 \pm 10.1$ | $73.1 \pm 12.9$ | $t = 2.58, p = .015$ |
|      Amplitude (Hz) | $49.2 \pm 10.7$ | $48.9 \pm 9.6$ | |
|      Autocorrelation ($r$) | $0.37 \pm 0.18$ | $0.45 \pm 0.13$ | $t = 2.12, p = .043$ |

*Effect of the Intervention on Initiation Insomnia*

315    Sleep onset was highly variable, and there was no significant change in perception of sleep onset or objectively measured time to fall asleep with wrist actigraphy (Table 2) when the total sample was analyzed. When the sample was dichotomized by those who took 320 30 min or longer to fall asleep, 6 women (20%) had initiation insomnia by wrist actigraphy measures prior to the intervention. As seen in Figure 1, repeated-measures analysis of variance revealed a significant, $F(1, 29) = 9.9$, $p = .004$, improvement in sleep onset 325 latency for the 6 women with initiation insomnia (from 72 ± 38.4 to 35 ± 37.7 min) compared with the 24 without initiation insomnia (from 11 ± 7.04 to 17 ± 11.9 min) when assessed by wrist actigraphy. The woman who switched from Dr Pepper to Sprite, for 330 example, reduced her sleep onset time from an average of 35 min on the two preintervention nights to 12 min on the two postintervention nights.

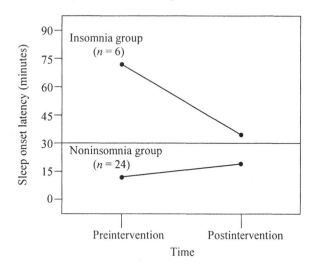

*Figure 1.* Change in sleep onset latency (minutes after turning out the lights) assessed by wrist actigraphy. The 6 women 335 who took more than 30 min to fall asleep are compared with the 24 women who fell asleep in less than 30 min on average for the two nights of monitoring during the preintervention assessment. The reference line at 30 min on the *y* axis indicates the cut point for designating the two groups at the initial 340 preintervention assessment.

*Effect of the Intervention on Maintenance Insomnia and TST*

There was no significant change in number of awakenings or duration of awakenings, and no change in the TST because of the intervention when assessed by objective sleep monitoring for the entire group of 30 345 women (Table 2). When the group was categorized on the basis of good (less than 10% wake time), fair (between 11% and 30% wake time), and poor (>30% wake time) sleep, the intervention had a significant effect. As seen in Figure 2, those with the poorest sleep 350 maintenance (*n* = 7) had significant improvement

compared with the other two groups, $F(2, 26) = 6.2$, $p = .006$, particularly the good sleepers ($p < .001$) and, to a lesser extent, also the fair sleepers ($p = .075$) based on post hoc Scheffé analysis.

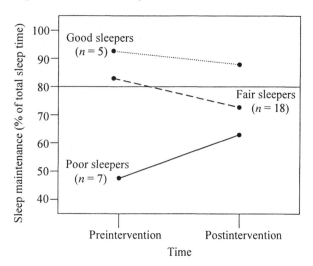

355    *Figure 2.* Change in sleep maintenance (percentage of total sleep time) assessed by wrist actigraphy. The 5 good sleepers who averaged more than 90% sleep and the 18 fair sleepers who averaged 70%–90% sleep during the night are compared with the 7 poor sleepers who averaged less than 70% sleep 360 during the night. The reference line at 80% on the *y* axis indicates the cut point for good sleep maintenance in a population with chronic illness with this type of actigraphy methodology.

*Effect of the Intervention on Daytime Activity*

Prior to the intervention, 67% (*n* = 20) napped. Af-365 ter the sleep hygiene intervention was introduced, there was a significant decrease ($\chi^2 = 6.0$, $p = .02$) in the percentage who napped (42%), likely in response to education about *R* or rhythm and the importance of being active during the day to improve sleep at night. There 370 was a significant increase in the average level of activity (mesor) and improvement in rhythm strength as ascertained by the autocorrelation for a 24-hr rhythm, but there was no change in activity amplitude (Table 2). As seen in Figure 3, the poor sleepers initially slept 375 more during the day, $F(1, 24) = 15.2$, $p = .001$, and, although all three groups decreased their daytime sleep in response to the education about napping, there was no significant difference between preintervention and postintervention daytime sleep.

380    In addition to objective indicators of improved rest-activity rhythm, there was a significant improvement in participants' perception of their sleep after 1 week of a tailored sleep hygiene intervention. As indicated in Table 2, there was a significant improvement in their 385 self-reported sleep (GSDS) compared with the prior week's baseline measure.

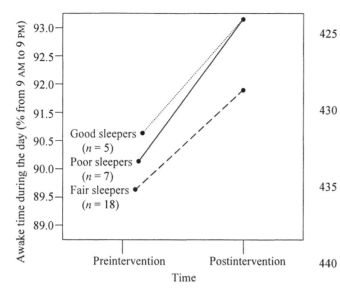

*Figure 3.* Change in time spent awake during the day (percentage of time in 12 hr from 09:00 to 21:00 hours) assessed by wrist actigraphy. All three groups of sleepers increased the
390   amount of time spent awake during the day from preintervention to 1 week later at postintervention.

## Discussion

This study utilized a cross-sectional convenience sample of women with HIV or AIDS to pilot test an educational and behavioral intervention to improve
395   sleep in a sample of women with chronic illness. Their sleep was very poor (6.4 hr and 73% sleep efficiency), considering the minimal monitoring equipment used in their own home. After the intervention, they averaged approximately 30 min less total sleep, as recorded by
400   wrist actigraphy. Although this reduction was not statistically significant, it was less recorded sleep time rather than more. This decrease may, in part, reflect the actigraph's overestimation of time spent asleep in inactive adults (the preintervention condition). Because one
405   of the principles of sleep hygiene, $T$ for time in bed, emphasizes only being in bed to sleep, this overestimation would be eliminated in the postintervention assessment because they were instructed to increase their activity and spend less time in bed while awake.
410   Naps were more frequent, even after the intervention, in comparison with that reported for a community sample of healthy women in which 31% reported naps (Lee, Lentz, Taylor, Mitchell, & Woods, 1994), but similar to a sample of men with AIDS (Darko,
415   McCutchan, Kripke, Gillin, and Golshan, 1992), in which 50% reported napping. Rather than only 7 hr of sleep at night, however, those men reported an average of 9 hr of sleep at night.

It was the group with the poorest nighttime sleep
420   who slept the most during the day prior to initiating the intervention. If napping does not interfere with sleep at night, a nap should not be discouraged. However, rather than a nap during the day, exercise and daytime

activity may be better for healthy circadian rhythms
425   and deeper stages of sleep at night. Results from this pilot study would indicate that foregoing naps may have a beneficial effect on the next night's sleep maintenance and serve to reduce maintenance insomnia.

Like one of the participants in the pilot study, pa-
430   tients may confuse calories with caffeine or be unaware of the caffeine in chocolate, tea, dark colas such as Pepsi or light colas such as Mountain Dew, some analgesics, and even some herbal teas and decaffeinated coffees. There are also bottled waters that contain caf-
435   feine. The high use of caffeine is likely to manifest as jittery and anxious feelings resulting in delayed sleep onset. Yet, the patient who experiences difficulty falling asleep at 11 PM may not relate it to the caffeine taken at 6 or 7 PM.
440   Further research is needed to ascertain why women with HIV infection experience a high frequency of awakenings during the night. Interventions that can be targeted toward reducing the number of awakenings, as well as the length of time spent awake, are needed. The
445   high amounts of fluid intake may result in urinary frequency during the night, and medications used in the treatment of HIV often produce adverse side effects such as nausea, vomiting, and diarrhea. These side effects can also exacerbate a patient's problem with sleep
450   maintenance.

### Limitations

Although the data were collected in 1997, there is no indication from the literature that sleep disturbance has become a primary focus for HIV practitioners in the care of women with HIV. Moreover, little is docu-
455   mented in the literature regarding interventions for sleep disturbance in persons living with HIV or AIDS since the time this study was conducted. Currently known are the various symptoms that women with HIV experience, which typically include sleep disturbance.
460   Hence, the results from this study are relevant and meaningful. Findings from this small convenience sample of women should not be generalized to the larger population of all women with HIV or AIDS, particularly when there was no placebo attention control
465   group in this pilot study. Although changes during a 1-week period do not predict long-term positive effects on sleep, the significant changes for the poorest of sleepers and the significant changes in perception of sleep and distressful symptoms are encouraging. Be-
470   cause some of these women had a history of substance abuse, they welcomed the opportunity for a nonpharmacologic intervention for self-care management of their insomnia. Nonetheless, tailoring the information and strategies to their specific needs may have pro-
475   duced a Hawthorne effect or provided them with better coping and control over their symptom experience.

Sleep promotion interventions are more effective than placebo and hypnotics in persons with insomnia, but those with chronic illnesses often are excluded

480  from intervention trials (Edinger, Wohlgemuth, Radtke, Marsh, & Quillian, 2001; Morin et al., 1999; Murtagh & Greenwood, 1995). Results from this study of women living with chronic health problems associated with HIV or AIDS demonstrate that sleep hygiene
485  has high potential benefit for subjective sleep and objective sleep when poor sleepers are targeted specifically for a tailored educational and behavioral intervention.

## References

Alessi, C. A., Yoon, E. J., Schnelle, J. F., Al-Samarrai, N. R., & Cruise, P. A. (1999). A randomized trial of a combined physical activity and environmental intervention in nursing home residents: Do sleep and agitation improve? *Journal of the American Geriatrics Society, 47*(7), 784–791.

Ancoli-Israel, S., Clopton, P., Klauber, M. R., Fell, R., & Mason, W. (1997). Use of wrist activity for monitoring sleep/wake in demented nursing-home patients. *Sleep, 20*(1), 24–27.

Bauldoff, G. S., Ryan-Wenger, N. A., & Diaz, P. T. (2007). Wrist actigraphy validation of exercise movement in COPD. *Western Journal of Nursing Research, 29*(7), 789–802.

Buysee, D. J., Reynolds, C. F., Monk, T. H., Berman, S. R., Kupfer, D. J. (1989). The Pittsburgh Sleep Quality Index: A new instrument for psychiatric practice and research. *Psychiatric Research, 28*, 193–213.

Carter, P. A. (2006). A brief behavioral sleep intervention for family caregivers of persons with cancer. *Cancer Nursing, 29*(2), 95–103.

Coffield, T. G., & Tryon, W. W. (2004). Construct validation of actigraphic sleep measures in hospitalized depressed patients. *Behavioral Sleep Medicine, 2*(1), 24–40.

Cole, R. J., Kripke, D. F., Gruen, W., Mullaney, D. J., & Gillin, J. C. (1992). Automatic sleep/wake identification from wrist activity. *Sleep, 15*(5), 461–469.

Darko, D. F., McCutchan, J. A., Kripke, D. F., Gillin, J. C., & Golshan, S. (1992). Fatigue, sleep disturbance, disability, and indices of progression of HIV infection. *American Journal of Psychiatry, 149*(4), 514–520.

Dreher, H. M. (2003). The effect of caffeine reduction on sleep quality and well-being in persons with HIV. *Journal of Psychosomatic Research, 54*(3), 191–198.

Eddy, M., & Walbroehl, G. S. (1999). Insomnia. *American Family Physician, 59*(7), 1911–1918.

Edinger, J. D., Wohlgemuth, W. K., Krystal, A. D., & Rice, J. R. (2005). Behavioral insomnia therapy for fibromyalgia patients. *Archives of Internal Medicine, 165*(21), 2527–2535.

Edinger, J. D., Wohlgemuth, W. K., Radtke, R. A., Marsh, G. R., & Quillian, R. E. (2001). Cognitive behavioral therapy for treatment of chronic primary insomnia: A randomized controlled trial. *JAMA, 285*(14), 1856–1864.

Espie, C. A., Inglis, S. J., Tessier, S., & Harvey, A. (2001). The clinical effectiveness of cognitive behaviour therapy for chronic insomnia: Implementation and evaluation of a sleep clinic in general medical practice. *Behaviour Research and Therapy, 39*(1), 45–60.

Hauri, P. J. (1997). Can we mix behavior therapy with hypnotics when treating insomniacs? *Sleep, 20*(12), 1111–1118.

Hauri, P. J., & Wisbey, J. (1992). Wrist actigraphy in insomnia. *Sleep, 15*(4), 293–301.

Hudson, A., Kirksey, K., & Holzemer, W. (2004). The influence of symptoms on quality of life among HIV-infected women. *Western Journal of Nursing Research, 26*(1), 9–23.

Irwin, M., Clark, C., Kennedy, B., Christian Gillin, J., & Ziegler, M. (2003). Nocturnal catecholamines and immune function in insomniacs, depressed patients, and control subjects. *Brain, Behavior, and Immunity, 17*(5), 365–372.

Koppel, B. S., & Bharel, C. (2005). Use of amitryptyline to offset sleep disturbances caused by efavirenz. *AIDS Patient Care and STDs, 19*(7), 419–420.

Landis, C. A., Frey, C. A., Lent, M. J., Rothermel, J., Buchwald, D., & Shaver, J. L. (2003). Self-reported sleep quality and fatigue correlates with actigraphy in midlife women with fibromyalgia. *Nursing Research, 52*(3), 140–147.

Lee, K. A. (1992). Self-reported sleep disturbances in employed women. *Sleep, 15*(6), 493–498.

Lee, K. A. (2006). Sleep dysfunction in women and its management. *Current Treatment Options in Neurology, 8*(5), 376–386.

Lee, K. A., Lentz, M. J., Taylor, D. L., Mitchell, E. S., & Woods, N. F. (1994). Fatigue as a response to environmental demands in women's lives. *Image: The Journal of Nursing Scholarship, 26*(2), 149–154.

Lee, K. A., Portillo, C. J., & Miramontes, H. (2001). Influence of sleep and activity patterns on fatigue in women with HIV/AIDS. *Journal of the Association of Nurses in AIDS Care, 12*(Suppl.), 19–27.

Lichstein, K. L., Stone, K. C., Donaldson, J., Nau, S. D., Soeffing, J. P., Murray, D., et al. (2006). Actigraphy validation with insomnia. *Sleep, 29*(2), 232–239.

McCall, W. V. (2005). Diagnosis and management of insomnia in older people. *Journal of the American Geriatrics Society, 53*(Suppl. 7), S272–S277.

Morin, C. M., Hauri, P. J., Espie, C. A., Spielman, A. J., Buysee, D. J., & Bootzin, R. R. (1999). Nonpharmacologic treatment of chronic insomnia: An American Academy of Sleep Medicine review. *Sleep, 22*(8), 1134–1156.

Murtagh, D. R., & Greenwood, K. M. (1995). Identifying effective psychological treatments for insomnia: A meta-analysis. *Journal of Consulting and Clinical Psychology, 63*(1), 79–89.

Naylor, E., Penev, P. D., Orbeta, L., Janssen, I., Ortiz, R., Colecchia, E. F., et al. (2000). Daily social and physical activity increases slow-wave sleep and daytime neuropsychological performance in the elderly. *Sleep, 23*(1), 87–95.

Nokes, K. M., Chidekel, J. H., & Kendrew, J. (1999). Exploring the complexity of sleep disturbances in persons with HIV/AIDS. *Journal of the Association of Nurses in AIDS Care, 10*(3), 22–29.

Nokes, K. M., & Kendrew, J. (2001). Correlates of sleep quality in persons with HIV disease. *Journal of the Association of Nurses in AIDS Care, 12*(1), 17–22.

Nunes, M., de Requena, D. G., Gallego, L., Jimenez-Nacher, I., Gonzalez-Lahoz, J., & Soriano, V. (2001). Higher efavirenz plasma levels correlate with development of insomnia. *Journal of Acquired Immune Deficiency Syndromes, 28*(4), 399–400.

Perkins, D. O., Leserman, J., Stern, R. A., Baum, S. F., Liao, D., Golden, R. N., et al. (1995). Somatic symptoms and HIV infection: Relationship to depressive symptoms and indicators of HIV disease. *American Journal of Psychiatry, 152*(12), 1776–1781.

Phillips, K. D., & Skelton, W. D. (2001). Effects of individualized acupuncture on sleep quality in HIV disease. *Journal of the Association of Nurses in AIDS Care, 12*(1), 27–39.

Phillips, K. D., Sowell, R. L., Rojas, M., Tavakoli, A., Fulk, L. J., & Hand, G. A. (2004). Physiological and psychological correlates of fatigue in HIV disease. *Biological Research for Nursing, 6*(1), 59–74.

Reid, S., & Dwyer, J. (2005). Insomnia in HIV infection: A systematic review of prevalence, correlates, and management. *Psychosomatic Medicine, 67*(2), 260–269.

Rubinstein, M. L., & Selwyn, P. A. (1998). High prevalence of insomnia in an outpatient population with HIV infection. *Journal of Acquired Immune Deficiency Syndromes and Human Retrovirology, 19*(3), 260–265.

Sadeh, A., Hauri, P. J., Kripke, D. F., & Lavie, P. (1995). The role of actigraphy in the evaluation of sleep disorders. *Sleep, 18*(4), 288–302.

Vogl, D., Rosenfeld, B., Breitbart, W., Thaler, H., Passik, S., McDonald, M., et al. (1999). Symptom prevalence, characteristics, and distress in AIDS outpatients. *Journal of Pain and Symptom Management, 18*(4), 253–262.

Walsh, J. K., Schweitzer, P. K., Anch, A. M., Muehlbach, M. J., Jenkins, N. A., & Dickins, Q. S. (1991). Sleepiness/alertness on a simulated night shift following sleep at home with triazolam. *Sleep, 14*(2), 140–146.

Wheatley, D., & Smith, K. (1994). Clinical sleep patterns in human immune virus infection. *Psychopharmacology, 9*, 111–115.

**Acknowledgments:** This research was supported by the National Institute of Nursing Research Grant R01 NR03969. Thank you to Helen Miramontes, Lili Tom, and Mary Ellen Zaffke.

**Address correspondence to**: Kathryn A. Lee, PhD, RN, FAAN, Department of Family Health Care Nursing, University of California, 2 Koret Way, #N-411, San Francisco, CA 94143-0606. E-mail: kathy.lee@nursing.ucsf.edu

# Exercise for Article 17

## *Factual Questions*

1. Why were women with confirmed AIDS dementia diagnosis excluded?

2. Of the 30 women sampled, how many were Caucasians?

3. Continuous noninvasive monitoring of sleep activity was accomplished with what type of device?

4. How many self-report measures were utilized to estimate the women's general perception of sleep problems?

5. Was the difference from preintervention to postintervention on the GSDS statistically significant? If so, at what probability level?

6. Was the decrease in the percentage of those who napped statistically significant after the intervention? If yes, at what probability level?

## Questions for Discussion

7. Do you think that paying the participants might have affected the results of the study? Explain. (See lines 154–164.)

8. Was having a sleep diary an important feature of the study? Explain. (See lines 193–202.)

9. In your opinion, was the intervention described in sufficient detail? (See lines 271–290.)

10. How helpful are Figures 1, 2, and 3 in helping you understand the results? Explain. (See Figures 1, 2, and 3.)

11. Was the study successful in determining if the intervention can improve sleep in women with chronic illness? Explain. (See lines 392–409.)

12. Do you agree that further research is needed to ascertain why women with HIV infection experience a high frequency of awakening during the night? Explain. (See lines 440–450.)

## Quality Ratings

Directions: Indicate your level of agreement with each of the following statements by circling a number from 5 for strongly agree (SA) to 1 for strongly disagree (SD). If you believe an item is not applicable to this research article, leave it blank. Be prepared to explain your ratings. When responding to criteria A and B, keep in mind that brief titles and abstracts are conventional in published research.

A. The title of the article is appropriate.

    SA  5  4  3  2  1  SD

B. The abstract provides an effective overview of the research article.

    SA  5  4  3  2  1  SD

C. The introduction establishes the importance of the study.

    SA  5  4  3  2  1  SD

D. The literature review establishes the context for the study.

    SA  5  4  3  2  1  SD

E. The research purpose, question, or hypothesis is clearly stated.

    SA  5  4  3  2  1  SD

F. The method of sampling is sound.

    SA  5  4  3  2  1  SD

G. Relevant demographics (for example, age, gender, and ethnicity) are described.

    SA  5  4  3  2  1  SD

H. Measurement procedures are adequate.

    SA  5  4  3  2  1  SD

I. All procedures have been described in sufficient detail to permit a replication of the study.

    SA  5  4  3  2  1  SD

J. The participants have been adequately protected from potential harm.

    SA  5  4  3  2  1  SD

K. The results are clearly described.

    SA  5  4  3  2  1  SD

L. The discussion/conclusion is appropriate.

    SA  5  4  3  2  1  SD

M. Despite any flaws, the report is worthy of publication.

    SA  5  4  3  2  1  SD

# Article 18

# An Intervention to Enhance Nursing Staff Teamwork and Engagement

**Beatrice J. Kalisch**, PhD, RN, FAAN, **Millie Curley**, MS, RN, **Susan Stefanov**, BSN, RN[*]

ABSTRACT. Numerous studies have concluded that work group teamwork leads to higher staff job satisfaction, increased patient safety, improved quality of care, and greater patient satisfaction. Although there have been studies on the impact of multidisciplinary teamwork in healthcare, the teamwork among nursing staff on a patient care unit has received very little attention from researchers. In this study, an intervention to enhance teamwork and staff engagement was tested on a medical unit in an acute care hospital. The results showed that the intervention resulted in a significantly lower patient fall rate, staff ratings of improved teamwork on the unit, and lower staff turnover and vacancy rates. Patient satisfaction ratings approached, but did not reach, statistical significance.

From *The Journal of Nursing Administration*, 37, 77–84. Copyright © 2007 by Lippincott Williams & Wilkins. Reprinted with permission.

The importance of quality teamwork in healthcare has been the subject of a number of studies in healthcare. Teamwork has been associated with a higher level of job staff satisfaction,[1–6] a higher quality of care,[4,7–13]
5  an increase in patient safety,[5,14–19] greater patient satisfaction with their care,[11,20] more productivity,[21] and a decreased stress level.[22,23] Highly functioning teams have also been shown to offer a wider range of support to inexperienced staff.[22]
10  Outside healthcare, there have been a plethora of studies highlighting the value of teamwork. For example, one investigation of flight crews demonstrated the link between teamwork and safety. These researchers evaluated the impact of fatigue on error rate and found
15  that staff who had flown together for several days made fewer errors than teams who were rested and had not worked together for very long. The fatigued team actually made more errors, but because the team had worked together, they were able to compensate and
20  catch one another's near misses. This is due to less stress, knowledge of the vulnerabilities and strengths of other team members, and the practice of monitoring performance and giving feedback to one another.[22]

Many studies have tested interventions to improve
25  teamwork. Approaches which have been found to enhance teamwork include cross training,[24,25] teamwork skills training,[26] Crew Resource Training,[14,27–31] role playing,[32] simulation,[33,34] automation,[35] posttraining feedback,[36] team-building activities,[37,38] and a combi-
30  nation of training and action groups.[39]

Specifically within healthcare, there has been a growing awareness of the need to improve teamwork. The Joint Commission on Accreditation of Healthcare Organizations (JCAHO) in July 2004 released a Senti-
35  nel Event Alert on the prevention of infant deaths. Its database showed that nearly three-quarters of hospitals cited communication breakdown and teamwork problems as a major reason for these deaths. The JCAHO recommended that hospitals conduct formal team train-
40  ing to the obstetrical/perinatal team.[40] In a study conducted by Dynamics Research Corporation, weaknesses and error patterns in emergency department teamwork were assessed, and a prospective evaluation of a formal teamwork training intervention was con-
45  ducted. Improvements were obtained in five key teamwork measures, and most important, clinical errors were significantly reduced.[41] Hope et al.[42] found that a team-building initiative for health profession students resulted in an improved interdisciplinary understand-
50  ing, team atmosphere, and teamwork skills. In another study, teamwork training of emergency department physicians and nurses significantly increased the quality of team behaviors, attitudes toward teamwork, and decreased clinical errors.[16]
55  Only a few studies have tested methods of increasing nursing teamwork. Amos et al.[43] found that the introduction of team-building activities resulted in greater staff communication, stronger interpersonal relationships, and greater job satisfaction. Britton[44]
60  reported that a team development program conducted for hospital nurse managers led to greater understanding and clarity of work roles and improved cohesion and teamwork at the management level. In another study, a team-building intervention showed an im-

[*]*Beatrice J. Kalisch* is director, Nursing Business and Health Systems and Titus distinguished professor of nursing, School of Nursing, University of Michigan, Ann Arbor, MI. *Millie Curley* is vice president nursing, and *Susan Stefanov* is nursing project manager, Parrish Medical Center, Titusville, FL.

65 provement in group cohesion, nurse satisfaction, and turnover rates.[45]

This article reports the results of a study that will add to the body of knowledge about nursing teamwork. It evaluates the impact of an intervention designed to 70 enhance teamwork and promote staff engagement. The staff engagement component was considered an essential element of the intervention in that teamwork could not be achieved without the involvement and commitment of the staff. The aim of this project was to deter- 75 mine the impact of an intervention designed to enhance teamwork and staff engagement on the rate of patient falls, patient satisfaction, the staff's assessment of level of teamwork on their unit, and vacancy and turnover rates.

**Project Method**

*Study Subjects*

80 The study was conducted on a 41-bed medical–oncology unit in a community hospital in 2004/2005. There were 55 staff members on the unit—32 registered nurses (RNs), 2 licensed practical nurses, 15 certified nurse assistants (CNAs), and 6 unit secretaries.

*Measures*

85 Measures for this project were patient fall rates, patient satisfaction scores, staff assessment of level of teamwork, staff vacancy, and turnover rates.

*Patient falls* per 1,000 patient days were collected before (January 2000–August 2004) and after (Sep- 90 tember 2004–June 2005) the teamwork and engagement intervention.

*Patient satisfaction* was measured with the Professional Research Consultants Patient Satisfaction Survey Tool, which has been utilized in hospitals through- 95 out the United States for 20 years.[46] Scoring is based on a point scale with weighting factors: Excellent (100), Very Good (80), Good (60), Fair (40), and Poor (20). In terms of validity of the instrument, Professional Research Consultants reports that they have per- 100 formed various tests of internal validity. The Cronbach $\alpha$ was .936 ($n = 824$) for the data from the medical unit utilized in this investigation. Professional Research Consultants also reports that they have conducted "side-by-side studies to compare various methodolo- 105 gies" and that by "utilizing norm data, they have demonstrated stability and consistency across various groups."[46]

*Staff ratings of level of teamwork* were completed 6 months after the intervention implementation. Confi- 110 dential interviews were conducted with 48 of 55 of the unit's staff by an external data collector who had no previous contact with the organization. The interviews were a combination of structured questions (e.g., "Has teamwork improved, stayed the same, or gotten 115 worse?") and semistructured, open-ended questions (e.g., "How do you assess the RN and CNA relationships at this time compared to before the project? Give specific examples").

*Staff turnover*, exclusive of relocation, return to 120 school, retirement, or death, was calculated by dividing the preventable turnover FTEs by the budgeted FTEs for full-time and part-time RNs, licensed practical nurses, and CNA employees minus the open positions for the period before (March–August 2004) and after 125 the intervention (March–August 2005). Staff *vacancy rates* were calculated by determining the average of the vacant positions each pay period divided by the budgeted positions. This was collected for the 6 months before and 6 months after the teamwork and engage- 130 ment project.

**Description of the Intervention**

The teamwork and engagement enhancement intervention tested in this study was based on principles of teamwork,[11,14,16,19,30] change in management,[47] train- 135 ing,[32–34,36,39,42] and staff engagement.[47] The steps in the intervention can be seen in Figure 1.

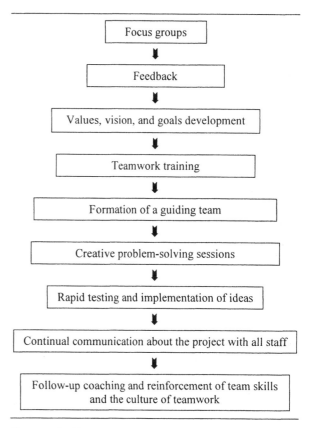

*Figure 1.* Staff teamwork and engagement enhancement intervention.

In the first step, 11 focus groups were conducted with RNs (5 groups), licensed practical nurses (1 group), CNAs (4 groups), and unit secretaries (2 groups) to determine their perceptions of the level of 140 teamwork on the unit and issues that inhibit and enhance teamwork. A total of 56 staff were interviewed, a participation rate of 97% of the unit staff. The purpose of the focus groups was to assess the level and nature of teamwork on the unit as well as the staff educational needs in the area of teamwork. Focus groups and interviews were also conducted with key stakeholders. Two focus groups with former unit patients were selected randomly from a list of discharged patients from the unit for a month prior to the implementation of the intervention. In addition, individual interviews were conducted with the 6 physicians who admitted the most patients to the unit. All of the focus groups and interviews were transcribed and analyzed using the N-Vivo qualitative research software. Major themes were identified.

### Feedback

These focus group data were compiled into a report which was presented in several feedback sessions, making it possible for each staff member on the unit to attend. The purpose of this second step in the process was not only to give the staff a report of the results of the focus groups they participated in but also to create a need for change. According to Kotter,[47] the first step in any change process is to create a sense of urgency. He notes that "we underestimate the enormity of the task [of change], especially the first step, establishing a sense of urgency."[47(p35)] It is not uncommon for teams to deny that they have problems working together effectively even when they are obvious. Kotter[47(p36)] points out: "People will find a thousand ingenious ways to withhold cooperation from a process" they do not buy into. Focus group data using quotations from staff members themselves, their patients, and the physicians they work with were designed to be compelling and mitigate tendencies of staff to discount reality. These data were referred to repeatedly during the project.

After each presentation, staff members were asked if they were interested in working on a project to improve teamwork. As noted above, it is crucial in a change process to overcome complacency in order to gain the cooperation of those involved. Each group of staff indicated that they were committed to improving teamwork and supporting a project designed to improve it.

### Values, Vision, and Goals

The next step was to conduct values, vision, and goals sessions, involving all unit staff in the process. Values (enduring beliefs which determine behavior) and vision (a compelling, inspirational, achievable, and comprehensible picture of the unit at some point in the future) gave direction to the unit staff and allowed the team to share in the development of a common unified direction.[48] Once the values and vision were finalized, the entire staff engaged in a gap analysis. They looked at where they were now and compared it to their vision statement or where they wanted to be. They then identified the goals for the project or the first priorities they felt they should work on to achieve their vision.

### Training

Each staff member then attended a day-long team training program. As mentioned above, the focus groups served as the needs analysis for the teamwork-training requirements of the staff and also as a source of scenarios used in the role-playing aspects of the training program. This information was used to specify the objectives, content, and posttraining evaluation of the program. Major deficiencies in teamwork knowledge, skills, and abilities—namely, feedback, conflict management, listening, and understanding of team information processing styles—were evident and formed the focus for the teamwork training.

### Guiding Teams

Two guiding teams (which were soon combined into one due to confusion over overlapping efforts) were created to address the specified project goals of improving staff relationships (with an emphasis on the relationship between nurses and CNAs) and redesigning the work to facilitate teamwork and improve quality of care. Following Kotter's guidelines, guiding team membership included managers (with position power), representatives from the different job categories so that all viewpoints would be represented, credible staff with good reputations on the unit so that their ideas would be taken seriously by other employees, and staff with leadership capabilities.[47(p57)] In addition, staff with different information processing styles were selected to balance the talents of the group.[49]

The guiding team initiated their work with several intense day and half-day meetings, which focused on creative idea generation and the classification of ideas into a 4-cell diagram in which "easy- to hard-to-implement" was on one axis and "high and low cost" on the other axis.[50] The idea was to assist the staff in selecting the easy-to-implement, low-cost ideas first so that early successes, or what Kotter refers to as "short term wins," could be achieved.[47] A major change like this one takes a considerable amount of time. Yet unit staff members look for convincing evidence that the work of the guiding team is paying off. By addressing the easy/low-cost items first, the guiding team met the needs of the staff, thus making it easier for the guiding team to take the time necessary to work on the more complex issues.

### Rapid Testing and Implementation

Rapid testing of ideas was the next step. For example, ideas, such as redesign of the patient change-of-shift report, were tested on one of 3 of the unit's wings before being adapted unit-wide. A similar approach was used when the team decided to move all staff to 12-hour shifts from a mix of 8- and 12-hour shifts to decrease the number of handoffs between staff members and the number of different people they worked with.[51] Implementation of permanent changes occurred when the testing of ideas proved successful. Maintenance of the changes was monitored on an ongoing basis by the guiding team.

*Communication*

Communication was a vital component of the project. The guiding teams adopted the assumption that they needed to communicate their messages in at least 4 ways before they could expect that staff members actually would hear and understand the messages. Kotter[47(p94)] notes that "effective information transferral almost always relies on repetition." Each guiding team member was assigned to five to six of the unit staff members (constituents) who were not on the team, and was responsible for keeping these staff members informed of the work of the team and gaining feedback from them. At the end of each meeting, a decision was made about what would be reported to the constituent staff members about the meeting, as well as what areas of feedback from the staff were needed for the next meeting. This communication occurred within 24 hours of the end of each guiding team meeting. A second method of communication involved the development of a special bulletin board in the staff lounge devoted to keeping everyone informed about the work of the project. The third method was an e-mail sent by the nurse manager to all staff members at the end of each meeting, and the fourth communication tool was a report about the project in each monthly unit staff meeting.

*Coaching*

The ninth element of the project involved a systematic reinforcement by managers and guiding team members on the knowledge, skills, and attitude taught in the training programs. This step was considered essential because training is a learning process and not a one-time event. Like any skill, teamwork competencies will decay without periodic reinforcement and practice. Thus, the awareness training (which focused on knowledge and attitudes) was followed by skills practice and recurrent skills maintenance.[26]

**Project Results**

*Patient Falls*

As can be seen in Figure 2, the 2-sample $t$ test showed that the patient fall rates dropped significantly from a mean of 7.73 per 1,000 patient days before the team intervention to 2.99 after the intervention ($t = 3.98$, $p < .001$).

*Patient Satisfaction*

Comparisons of the "excellent" scores on the Professional Research Consultants Patient Satisfaction Survey Tool for the study unit for quarters before and after the intervention approached but did not reach statistical significance. Patients' perceptions of nurses' promptness in responding to calls increased from 32.0% to 49.0%; nurses' communication with patients and family increased from 36.7% to 48.0%; and overall quality of nursing care increased from 46.0% to 52.0%.

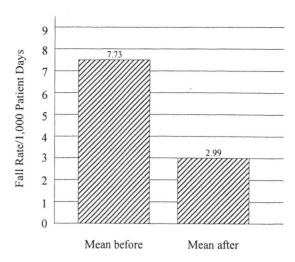

*Figure 2.* Mean fall rates before and after intervention. $t = 3.98$, $df = 64$, $p = .00$.

*Staff Ratings of Level of Teamwork*

The staff ratings of level of teamwork were completed in July 2005, and showed that staff felt that teamwork had improved ($\chi^2 = 36.065$, $p = .000$). Figure 3 contains a graphic distribution of the responses to the question "Has teamwork improved, stayed the same, or gotten worse since the teamwork intervention?" When analyzed by shift, 84% of the nurses and 80% of the CNAs on days and 35% of the nurses and 60% of the CNAs on nights reported that teamwork had improved on the unit. The discrepancy between shifts was reported to be due to the fact that the night shift felt that their level of teamwork was higher than the day shift before the project was initiated. Figure 4 shows more changes that staff felt had helped to improve teamwork.

*Staff Turnover and Vacancy Rates*

As can be seen in Figure 5, 2-sample $t$ test showed that there was a significant drop in staff turnover rates after the intervention from 13.14 to 8.05 ($t = 2.18$, $p = .033$). Similarly, the vacancy rates declined significantly from before to after the teamwork enhancement project from 6.14 to 5.23 ($t = 4.55$, $p = .0000$).

**Limitations**

The major limitation of this study centered on the measurement of patient satisfaction. Not only was the number of patients surveyed small but the tool is proprietary and the data were collected by the company rather than by the researchers. In future studies, patient satisfaction should be measured directly by the researchers to ensure accuracy in data collection and analysis. This study needs to be replicated with other nursing teams and in other settings. Exploration of additional measures of teamwork and patient outcomes needs to be developed.

**Discussion**

This study tests a specific intervention for improving nursing staff teamwork and engagement on a hospi-

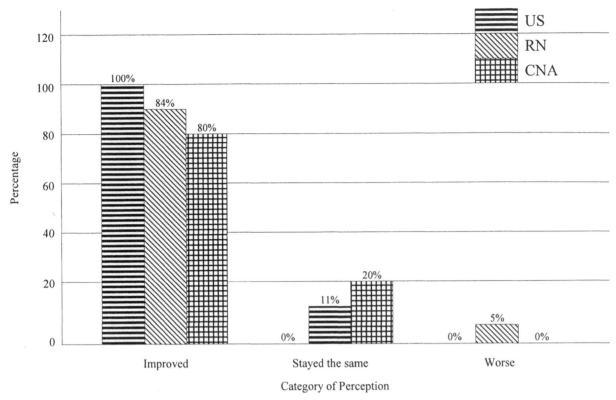

*Figure 3.* Staff perception of changes in teamwork after the intervention. $\chi^2 = 36.065$, $df = 2$, $p = .000$.

---

**Moving to an all 12-hour shift as opposed to the mix of 8- and 12-hour shifts** (RN: The 12-hour shifts have helped significantly. There are only one CNA and RN working together. You can follow up easier. It helps with continuity of care and patient satisfaction increases.)

**Greater team awareness of one another and more back-up behaviors** (RN: We are working really well with each other. It is a mentality of "our patients" not just "my patients"; RN: We are more aware of each of their problems and issues, more open to helping each other than before; CNA: People are finding out more about each other. RN: The CNA/RN relationship is better; CNA: Nurses are helping out more with patient care. Nurses will help with things I cannot do on my own, like turning a patient or doing a bath. They didn't used to.)

**Eliminating the different call light colors for the nurse and CNA** (RN: Everyone is answering all of the call lights.)

**Redistribution of certain tasks across both shifts and the development of a belief that the patients are "all of ours, no matter what shift we work"** (CNA: The night shifts are doing the baths, and it takes some of the workload off the day shift.)

**Clarification of roles of team members** (RN: I feel like everyone is much clearer about our roles. There is much less of this feeling that the CNAs think we are goofing off when we are at the computer documenting.)

**Improved ability to give feedback and deal with conflict** (RN: We are much more likely to tell each other when there is a problem. We used to pass it to the manager.)

---

*Figure 4.* Staff perception of changes that improved teamwork. RN indicates registered nurse, CNA, certified nursing assistant.

tal medical unit. The intervention was based on established principles of change, training, teamwork, and empowerment. It involved extensive upfront efforts to establish a sense of urgency among a large proportion of the unit staff undergoing the change. The intervention included involvement of the entire unit staff in the development of values, vision, and goals to guide the project; a teamwork training needs assessment; training in teamwork knowledge, skills, and attitudes customized to the unit; the appointment of a guiding team made up of unit staff and managers who engaged in creative idea generation, testing, and implementation of ideas for change; a comprehensive communication strategy to keep the entire unit staff informed and involved in the project; and follow-up after training by managers and guiding team members to reinforce the new behaviors and ultimately change the culture of the unit to one that supports and expects teamwork.

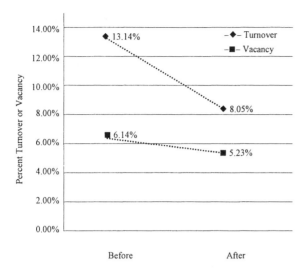

*Figure 5.* Turnover and vacancy rate before and after intervention. Turnover $t = 2.18$, $df = 63$, $p = .033$; vacancy $t = 4.55$, $df = 58$, $p = .0000$.

The team enhancement and engagement intervention followed a specific protocol developed before the initiation of the project but still allowed for flexibility 355 within it to meet the specific needs of the participants. For example, unit staff made the decisions as to what specific changes they wished to make on their unit to foster teamwork.

The outcomes of this study are promising in that 360 there was a significantly lower patient fall rate, lower turnover and vacancy rates, as well as staff self-reports of improved teamwork. Patient satisfaction improved but did not reach statistical significance, perhaps because the number surveyed was small.

365 Although this intervention was relatively extensive in scope, the potential to increase the quality of nursing care, avoid errors, decrease staff turnover, lower staff vacancy rates, and increase productivity makes the time and effort expended in this intervention worthy of 370 the effort. Potential cost savings, although not measured in this study, would appear to be substantial (e.g., decreased staff turnover, fewer errors, decreased length of stay, etc.).

The results of the staff interviews, as well as ongo-375 ing observations of work behavior, demonstrate a continual need to work with staff in the areas of listening, feedback, and conflict management. The team is currently working on dividing themselves into smaller units in an effort to reduce the number of different in-380 dividuals they are working with so that they can develop the culture necessary to function as a high-performing team and to be able to monitor one another's performance, give feedback, conduct closed loop communication, put the team above the individ-385 ual, and provide the team leadership needed.

## References

1. Rafferty AM, Ball J, Aiken LH. Are teamwork and professional autonomy compatible, and do they result in improved hospital care? *Qual Saf Health Care.* 2001;10(II): 32–37.
2. Gifford BD, Zammuto RF, Goodman EA. The relationship between hospital unit culture and nurses' quality of work life. *Health Care Manag.* 2002;47:13–26.
3. Collette JE. Retention of staff—a team-based approach. *Aust Health Rev.* 2004;28(3):349–356.
4. Horak BJ, Guarino JH, Knight CC, Kweder SL. Building a team on a medical floor. *Health Care Manage Rev.* 1991;16(2):65–71.
5. Leppa CJ. Nurse relationships and work group disruption. *J Nurs Adm.* 1996;26(10):23–27.
6. Cox KB. The effects of unit morale and interpersonal relations on conflict in the nursing unit. *J Adv Nurs.* 2001;35(1):17–25.
7. Knaus WA, Draper EA, Wagner DP, Zimmerman JE. An evaluation of outcomes from intensive care in major medical centers. *Ann Intern Med.* 1986;104(3):410–419.
8. Shortell SM, O'Brien JL, Carman JM. Assessing the impact of continuous quality improvement/total quality management: Concept versus implementation. *Health Serv Res.* 1995;30(2):377–401.
9. Shortell SM, Zimmerman JE, Rousseau DM, Gillies RR. The performance of intensive care units: Does good management make a difference? *Med Care.* 1994;32(5):508–525.
10. Young GJ, Charns MP, Desai KR, et al. Patterns of coordination and clinical outcomes: A study of surgical services. *Health Serv Res.* 1998;33(5):1211–1236.
11. Mickan S, Rodger S. Characteristics of effective teams: A literature review. *Aust Health Rev.* 2000;23(3):201–208.
12. Grumbach K, Bodenheimer T. Can health care teams improve primary care practice? *JAMA.* 2004;291(10):1246–1251.
13. Wheelan SA, Burchill CN, Tilin F. The link between teamwork and patients' outcomes in intensive care units. *Am J Crit Care.* 2003;12(6):527–534.
14. Baker DP, Gustafson S, Beaubien JM, Salas E, Barach P. Medical team training programs in healthcare. In: Henriksen K, Battles JB, Marks ES, Lewin DI, eds. *Advances in Patient Safety: From Research to Implementation. Volume 4: Programs, Tools and Products.* Rockville, MD: Agency for Healthcare Research and Quality; 2005:253–267.
15. Firth-Couzens J. Cultures for improving patient safety through learning: The role of teamwork. *Qual Health Care.* 2001;10(2):26–31.
16. Morey JC, Simon R, Jay GD, et al. Error reduction and performance improvement in the emergency department through formal teamwork training: Evaluation results of the MedTeams Project. *Health Serv Res.* 2002;37(6):1553–1581.
17. Silen-Lipponen M, Tossavainen K, Hannele T, Smith A. Potential errors and their prevention in operating room teamwork as experienced by Finnish, British and American nurses. *Int J Nurs Pract.* 2005;11(1):21–32.
18. Gristwood J. Seeing the benefits of teamwork on falls prevention programmes. *Nurs Times.* 2004;100(26):39.
19. Kaissi A, Johnson R, Kirschbaum MS. Measuring teamwork and patient safety attitudes of high-risk areas. *Nurs Econ.* 2003;21(5):211–219.
20. Meterko M, Mohr DC, Young GJ. Teamwork culture and patient satisfaction in hospitals. *Med Care.* 2004;42(5):492–498.
21. Rondeau KV, Wagar TH. Hospital chief executive officer perceptions of organizational culture and performance. *Hosp Top.* 1998;76:14–21.
22. Carter AJ, West MA. Sharing the burden: Teamwork in the healthcare setting. In: Firth-Cozens J, Payne RL, eds. *Stress in Health Professionals.* Chichester: Wiley; 1999:191–201.
23. Sonnetag S. Work group factors and individual well-being. In: West MA, ed. *Handbook of Work Group Psychology.* Chichester: Wiley; 1996.
24. Volpe CE, Cannon-Bowles JA, Salas E. The impact of cross training on team functioning: An empirical investigation. *Hum Factors.* 1996;38(1):87.
25. Cannon-Bowers JA, Salas E, Blickensderfer E, Bowers CA. The impact of cross-training and workload on team functioning: A replication and extension of initial findings. *Hum Factors.* 1998;40(1):92–101.
26. Beaubien JM, Baker DP. The use of simulation for training teamwork skills in healthcare: How low can you go? *Qual Saf Health Care.* 2004;13:51–56.
27. Salas E, Fowlkes JE, Stout RJ, Milanovich DM, Prince C. Does CRM training improve teamwork skills in the cockpit? Two evaluation studies. *Hum Factors.* 1999;41(2):326–343.
28. Salas E, Rhodenizer L, Bowers CA. The design and delivery of crew resource management training: Exploiting available resources. *Hum Factors.* 2000;42(3):490–511.
29. Salas E, Burke CS, Bowers CA, Wilson KA. Team training in the sky: Does crew resources management training work? *Hum Factors.* 2001;43:641–674.
30. Grogan EL, Stiles RA. The impact of aviation-based teamwork training on the attitudes of health-care professionals. *J Am Coll Surg.* 2004;199(6):843–848.

31. Blum RH, Raemer DB, Carroll JS, Sunder N, Feinstein DM, Copper JB. Crisis resource management training for an anesthesia faculty: A new approach to continuing education. *Med Educ.* 2004;38:45–55.

32. Beard RI, Salas E, Prince C. Enhancing transfer of training: Using role plays to foster teamwork in the cockpit. *Int J Aviat Psychol.* 1995;5(2):131–143.

33. Swezey RW, Owens JM, Bergondy ML, Salas E. Task and training requirements analysis methodology (TTRAM): An analytic methodology for identifying potential training uses of simulator networks in teamwork-intensive task environments. *Ergonomics.* 1998;41:1678–1697.

34. Shapiro MJ, Morey JC, Small SD, et al. Simulation-based teamwork training for emergency department staff: Does it improve clinical team performance when added to an existing didactic teamwork curriculum? *Qual Saf Health Care.* 2004;13:417–421.

35. Wright MC, Kaber DB. Effects of automation of information-processing functions on teamwork. *Hum Factors.* 2005;47(1):20–66.

36. Beaubien JM, Baker DP. Post-training feedback: The relative effectiveness of team- versus instructor-led debriefs. *Proceedings of the 47th Annual Meeting of the Human Factors and Ergonomic Society.* Santa Monica, CA: Human Factors and Ergonomics Society; 2003:2033–2036.

37. Stoller JK, Dolgan C, Hoogwerf BJ, Rose M, Lee R. Teambuilding and leadership training in an internal medicine residency training program. *J Gen Intern Med.* 2004;19(6):692–697.

38. Horak BJ, Kerns J, Pauig J, Keidan B. Patient safety: A case study in team building and interdisciplinary collaboration. *J Healthc Qual.* 2004;26(2):6–12.

39. Ellis APJ, Bell BS, Ployhart RE, Hollenbeck DR. An evaluation of generic teamwork skills training with action teams: Effects on cognitive and skill-based outcomes. *Pers Psychol.* 2005;58(3):641–672.

40. Joint Commission on Accreditation of Healthcare Organizations. Available at: http://www.jcaho.org/SentinelEvents. Accessed July 2004.

41. Barrett J, Gifford C, Morey J, Risser D, Salisbury M. Enhancing patient safety through teamwork training. *J Healthc Risk Manag.* 2001;21(4):57–65.

42. Hope JM, Lugassy D, Meyer R, et al. Bringing interdisciplinary and multicultural team building to health care education: The downstate team-building initiative. *Acad Med.* 2005;80(1):74–83.

43. Amos MA, Hu J, Herrick CA. The impact of team building on communication and job satisfaction of nursing staff. *J Nurses Staff Dev.* 2005;21(1):10–16.

44. Britton L. Use of behavioral science concepts and processes to facilitate change: A team building program for nursing supervisors. *Aust Health Rev.* 1984;7(3):162–179.

45. DiMeglio K, Padula C, Korber S, et al. Group cohesion and nurse satisfaction: Examination of a team-building approach. *JONA.* 2005;35(3):110–120.

46. Inguanzo JM. Professional Research Consulting. Reliability and validity of the patient satisfaction tool. Unpublished document; 2005.

47. Kotter J. *Leading Change.* Boston: Harvard Business School Press; 1996.

48. Ingersoll GI, Witzel PA, Smith TC. Using organizational mission, vision, and values to guide professional practice model development and measurement of nurse performance. *JONA.* 2005;35(2):86–93.

49. Kalisch B, Begeny S. The informational processing styles of nurses and nurse managers: Impact on change and innovation. Unpublished document; 2006.

50. Institute for Health Care Improvement. Transforming care at the bedside: Sparking innovation and excitement on the hospital unit. Available at: http://www.IHI.org. Accessed July 2006.

51. Kalisch B, Begeny S. Improving nursing unit team work. *JONA.* 2005;35(12):550–556.

**Acknowledgments**: The authors acknowledge the contributions of the study unit staff and managers and Suzanne Begeny, MS, RN, for conducting and analyzing the staff interviews.

**Address correspondence to**: Beatrice J. Kalisch, Nursing Business and Health Systems, School of Nursing, University of Michigan, 400 N. Ingalls Street, Ann Arbor, MI 48109. E-Mail: bkalisch@umich.edu

# Exercise for Article 18

## Factual Questions

1. How many of the participants were certified nurse assistants?

2. Was the difference in fall rates statistically significant? If yes, at what probability level?

3. Was the difference in turnover rates statistically significant? If yes, at what probability level?

4. According to the researchers, a major limitation centered on what?

5. Do the researchers call for replication of this study?

## Questions for Discussion

6. In your opinion, is the Patient Satisfaction Survey Tool described in sufficient detail? Explain. (See lines 92–107.)

7. Do you think it was a good idea to have the interviews conducted by an external data collector who had no previous contact with the organization? Explain. (See lines 109–112.)

8. In your opinion, is the intervention described in sufficient detail? Explain. (See lines 131–286.)

9. This research is classified as "Pre-Experimental Research" in the Contents of this book. Do you agree with the classification? Explain.

10. Do you think that "potential cost savings" is an important issue to examine in future studies? Explain. (See lines 370–373.)

11. If you were to conduct a follow-up study on the same topic, what changes, if any, would you make in the research methodology?

## Quality Ratings

Directions: Indicate your level of agreement with each of the following statements by circling a number from 5 for strongly agree (SA) to 1 for strongly disagree (SD). If you believe an item is not applicable to this research article, leave it blank. Be prepared to explain your ratings. When responding to criteria A and B, keep in mind that brief titles and abstracts are conventional in published research.

A. The title of the article is appropriate.

SA   5   4   3   2   1   SD

B. The abstract provides an effective overview of the research article.

SA   5   4   3   2   1   SD

C. The introduction establishes the importance of the study.

SA   5   4   3   2   1   SD

D. The literature review establishes the context for the study.

SA   5   4   3   2   1   SD

E. The research purpose, question, or hypothesis is clearly stated.

SA   5   4   3   2   1   SD

F. The method of sampling is sound.

SA   5   4   3   2   1   SD

G. Relevant demographics (for example, age, gender, and ethnicity) are described.

SA   5   4   3   2   1   SD

H. Measurement procedures are adequate.

SA   5   4   3   2   1   SD

I. All procedures have been described in sufficient detail to permit a replication of the study.

SA   5   4   3   2   1   SD

J. The participants have been adequately protected from potential harm.

SA   5   4   3   2   1   SD

K. The results are clearly described.

SA   5   4   3   2   1   SD

L. The discussion/conclusion is appropriate.

SA   5   4   3   2   1   SD

M. Despite any flaws, the report is worthy of publication.

SA   5   4   3   2   1   SD

# Article 19

# Vaccine Risk/Benefit Communication: Effect of an Educational Package for Public Health Nurses

**Terry C. Davis**, PhD, **Doren D. Fredrickson**, MD, PhD, FAAP, FACPM,
**Estela M. Kennen**, MA, **Sharon G. Humiston**, MD, MPH, **Connie L. Arnold**, PhD,
**Mackey S. Quinlin**, BS, **Joseph A. Bocchini Jr.**, MD[*]

ABSTRACT. The purpose of this study was to determine whether an in-service for public health nurses (PHNs) and accompanying educational materials could improve vaccine risk/benefit communication. The content and timing of vaccine communication were recorded during 246 pre- and 217 postintervention visits in two public health immunization clinics. Pre-/postintervention comparisons showed PHN communication of severe side effects (13% vs. 44%, $p < .0001$) and their management (29% vs. 60%, $p < .0001$) increased. There was no significant change in discussion of vaccine benefits (48% vs. 51%) or common side effects (91% vs. 92%), screening for contraindications (71% vs. 77%), or distribution of written information (89% vs. 92%). More parents initiated vaccine questions postintervention (27% vs. 39%, $p < .01$) and were more satisfied with vaccine-risk communication (8.1 vs. 8.9 on a 10-point scale, $p < .01$). Average vaccine communication time increased from 16 to 22 seconds ($p < .01$).

From *Health Education & Behavior, 33*, 787–801. Copyright © 2006 by SOPHE. Reprinted with permission.

Risk communication is receiving increased attention in public health and clinical medicine (Leask, 2002; National Vaccine Advisory Committee, 2003). Clear risk/benefit communication may be particularly important for childhood immunization. As the number of childhood immunizations increases and the incidence of vaccine-preventable diseases decreases, parental concern about vaccine risks is increasing (Gellin, Maibach, & Marcuse, 2000; Marshall & Gellin, 2001). Risk/benefit issues may be heightened because both health care professionals and parents have a diminishing level of experience with the diseases that vaccines prevent, and vaccine information widely available to parents may be inaccurate and/or misleading (National Vaccine Advisory Committee, 2003). A national telephone survey found that although 87% of parents believed that immunizations were extremely important, almost one-fourth had misconceptions about vaccines (Gellin et al., 2000).

Limited or inaccurate information could undermine parent confidence in vaccine safety and affect parents' immunization decision making. A recent survey of pediatricians and family physicians found that more than two-thirds reported a substantial increase in parental concern about vaccine safety in the past year (Freed, Clark, Hibbs, & Santoli, 2004). The National Childhood Vaccine Injury Act (U.S. Government, 1986) mandates that all immunization providers give parents the applicable Vaccine Information Statements (VIS) developed by the Centers for Disease Control and Prevention (CDC) with each vaccine dose and provide appropriate verbal explanation (American Academy of Pediatrics, 2000; Evans, 2000; Freed et al., 2004; Simpson, Suarez, & Smith, 1997). Printed VISs are written at a 10th-grade level in English and are available in 30 languages through the Immunization Action Coalition (http://www.immunize.org/vis/).

Vaccine risk/benefit information needs to be communicated as simply as possible. The Institute of Medicine (2004) reported that most health information is unnecessarily complex and that 90 million Americans have trouble understanding and using health information. The report recommended that both written and spoken information be given to patients in everyday language. Clear vaccine communication is important in all childhood immunization settings, but recent findings indicate that parents at public health clinics (PHCs) in particular may need plain language information about vaccine risks and benefits. A notable proportion of U.S. children are immunized in the public sector. Gellin et al. (2000) found that parents who were Black, were Hispanic, or had less than a high school

[*]*Terry C. Davis*, Louisiana State University Health Sciences Center, Shreveport. *Doren D. Fredrickson*, University of Kansas School of Medicine, Wichita. *Estela M. Kennen*, Louisiana State University Health Sciences Center, Shreveport. *Sharon G. Humiston*, University of Rochester School of Medicine and Dentistry, New York. *Connie L. Arnold, Mackey S. Quinlin*, and *Joseph A. Bocchini Jr.*, Louisiana State University Health Sciences Center, Shreveport.

education—those more likely to attend PHCs—were more likely to be concerned about vaccine side effects. In a separate study, parents in Texas attending PHCs had more concerns about vaccine safety than those attending private offices (Simpson et al., 1997).

Much of the background of the present study has been previously reported research by this team. The sequence of those studies included the following.

- Focus groups: We elicited feedback on written and spoken vaccine risk/benefit communication from health care providers and demographically diverse groups of parents in six U.S. cities (T. C. Davis et al., 2001; Fredrickson, Davis, & Bocchini, 2001; Page, Eason, Humiston, & Baker, 2000). Parents noted that VISs often "disintegrated in the diaper bag" and remained unread. Parents wanted a sturdy, to-the-point reference booklet before the child's first immunization visit as well as verbal information. They were particularly interested in practical information such as which shots their child would receive, common side effects, and the vaccine schedule, but they also wanted brief information on severe side effects. As noted in other studies (Ball, Evans, & Bostrom, 1998; Gellin & Schaffner, 2001), we found that parents wanted concise vaccine risk/benefit information from their own trusted provider. In provider focus groups (T. C. Davis et al., 2001), physicians and nurses stated that they rarely discussed severe vaccine side effects. Physicians felt such discussions would "open a can of worms," which in turn would cause them to be "in the exam room all day," whereas nurses felt that they lacked sufficient knowledge to address severe side effects.

- National survey: We mailed questionnaires that we developed based on focus group findings to a random national sample of immunizing private practice physicians (pediatricians and family physicians) and their nurses and to a geographically stratified, random national sample of public health nurses (PHNs) (T. C. Davis et al., 2001). Results showed that although the majority of providers reported discussing common side effects, severe side effects, and vaccine benefits, PHNs reported higher rates of communication than did private providers. Although most pediatricians (54%) reported lacking time to discuss risks and benefits, only 37% of PHNs reported time constraints. Almost half of PHNs (48%) reported having no barrier to risk/benefit communication. Health care providers of all types expressed the need for practical materials to help improve vaccine communication.

- Private physician office-based intervention: An immunization education package was developed based on the aforementioned studies and a review of the literature on improving provider adherence to health guidelines (Cabana et al., 1999; Dugan & Cohen, 1998; D. A. Davis, Thomson, Oxman, & Haynes, 1995; D. A. Davis et al., 1999). The package included a clinic-based in-service that reviewed current vaccine guidelines, provided feedback on the clinics' current vaccine communication performance, and introduced educational materials. The educational materials included a poster titled "7 Questions Parents Need to Ask About Baby Shots" aimed at both providers and parents, an accompanying answer sheet for providers, and a contraindication screening sheet for providers. We assessed the efficacy of this educational package among pediatricians and their nurses in two private pediatric offices. The pediatric office-based package significantly increased six aspects of vaccine communication (discussion of contraindications, common side effects, treatment of common side effects, severe side effects, management of severe side effects, and schedule of the next vaccination), with less than a minute increase in visit time (T. C. Davis, Fredrickson, et al., 2002).

The purpose of the present study was to determine whether an intervention similar to the private office-based intervention, but tailored to PHNs and with the addition of an immunization booklet designed for parents, could improve vaccine risk/benefit communication in a timely manner among PHNs.

## Method

### The Intervention

We designed an intervention that included five components: a clinic-based in-service tailored for PHNs and four educational materials (a poster for the clinic, a vaccine information handout for PHNs, a contraindication screening sheet for PHNs, and a baby shot booklet for parents). Each of the materials was reviewed and supported by a national advisory board representing 14 agencies.[1] Materials were available for use only after the in-service session.

*Poster.* The poster was developed using patient education and health literacy principles (Doak, Doak, & Root, 1996; McGee, 1999; Rudd & Comings, 1994). It contained a brief list of what parents and providers indicated needed to be included in vaccine communication (T. C. Davis et al., 2001; Fredrickson et al., 2001). Designed to trigger provider/parent vaccine communication, it was formatted as seven simple questions. The colorful poster included age-specific photographs of vaccine-eligible children. It used a conversational tone including specific wording suggested by parents and providers in the demographically diverse focus groups in six U.S. cities (T. C. Davis, Frederickson, et al., 2002). For example, the poster used the term "severe side effects" rather than "risks" and "baby shots" rather than "immunizations" because more parents understood those terms. The poster was written at a fourth-grade reading level and was scored 100 (*very easy*) on

the Flesch Reading Ease Scale (0-100; Flesch, 1949).
165 Based on health literacy guidelines (Doak et al., 1996; Institute of Medicine, 2004; McGee, 1999; Rudd & Comings, 1994), the poster was extensively pilot tested for clarity, comprehension, cultural appropriateness, and appeal.

170 *Vaccine information handout.* A vaccine information handout titled "Answers to the Seven Questions" was designed specifically for providers to help them answer the questions on the poster. The handout included a brief discussion of the information on the VIS.

175 *Contraindication screening sheet.* We modified a self-administered contraindication screening sheet originally developed by the Immunization Action Coalition (http:// www.immunize.org/catg.d/p4060scr.pdf) and tailored it to be easily administered by PHNs and
180 to be included in the clinic record.

*Educational session.* The clinic in-service was based on adult learning principles and effective continuing education strategies (D. A. Davis et al., 1995; Dugan & Cohen, 1998). The interactive academic
185 in-service was taught by a local opinion leader (an infectious-disease physician who was head of the local medical school Department of Pediatrics [Louisiana] or the medical director of the Public Health Clinic [Kansas]). The leader reviewed the requirements of the Na-
190 tional Childhood Vaccine Injury Act, the national data concerning compliance with the mandates, and the local clinic results from the preintervention observation of vaccine communication.

The leaders then introduced each of the educational
195 materials. PHNs were encouraged to tailor the vaccine communication to fit their practice style and time demands as well as the knowledge, previous childhood immunization experience, and communication needs of each parent. In-service leaders encouraged PHNs to
200 elicit parent concerns and discuss poster questions. They recommended providing the simplest layer of information first and modifying communication based on parent questions or concerns.

The leader elicited questions and concerns through-
205 out the in-service. For example, although PHNs felt very comfortable mentioning common side effects, they felt unskilled in discussing severe risks. PHNs were encouraged to provide simple, general information about risks, such as, "There's a very small possi-
210 bility that the vaccine could cause seizures or death."

*Baby Shot Booklet.* The parent-centered booklet was also developed using patient education and health literacy principles (Doak et al., 1996; Institute of Medicine, 2004; McGee, 1999; Rudd & Comings,
215 1994). The focus groups revealed that parents wanted a single, colorful, and durable easy-to-read source for all childhood vaccine information, organized sequentially by the child's age (T. C. Davis et al., 2001; Fredrickson et al., 2001; Page et al., 2000). They also requested
220 immunization information that would not disintegrate in the diaper bag. The *Baby Shot Booklet* was designed

as such. Written at a fourth-grade level, it simplified and reformatted age-specific information from the VISs, including shots for that visit, possible side ef-
225 fects, instructions for follow-up care, and how to reach both the National Vaccine Injury Compensation Program and the Vaccine Adverse Event Reporting System. Photos were used to illustrate ages at which each vaccine should be administered. The booklet was ex-
230 tensively pilot tested for clarity, comprehension, organization, and appeal.

*Study Design and Setting*

The study was a pre-post trial in two immunization-only clinics in urban PHCs, one in Louisiana and one in Kansas. The sites were chosen because they served
235 racially mixed populations of working poor families typical of PHCs and were in two distinct geographic areas. The Louisiana public health unit employed 1 clerk and 12 PHNs, all registered nurses (RNs), who rotated through the immunization clinic. Depending on
240 clinic volume, 1 to 3 RNs were assigned to the immunization clinic each day. The Kansas unit employed 1 administrative aide, 9 clerks, and 3 immunization nurses, all RNs. These nurses did not rotate through other sections of the PHC. In Louisiana, 3 of the 12
245 PHNs missed the training and were separately in-serviced by the head nurse. In Kansas, all 3 immunization nurses attended the training.

The Louisiana clinic's immunization practices were determined by a state Public Health Immunization Pol-
250 icy, which requires that the appropriate VIS be distributed with each dose of vaccine and that PHNs tell parents which vaccines are to be administered that visit, their contraindications, and side effects; review recommended comfort measures; and give the date of the
255 next visit. The Kansas clinic immunization practices were determined locally; nurses had been given CDC guidelines to follow.

From June 2000 through August 2001, research assistants (RAs) shadowed a convenience sample of 463
260 immunization visits of children younger than 5 years of age. RAs shadowed 246 preintervention and 217 postintervention visits. Clinic staff members were aware of the observer's presence and the general topic of the study (i.e., childhood immunizations) but not of
265 the specific communication variables recorded.

After clinic check-in, RAs asked parents for consent to participate in a study about how nurses communicate with parents. Parents were asked whether they would be willing to answer a few questions and allow
270 the RA to shadow the visit. Fewer than 5% of parents refused to participate. The most common reasons given were being too busy with the children and not wanting to complete the literacy assessment. Consenting parents signed a consent form before the RA collected demo-
275 graphic information and measured literacy. The RA then became a silent observer during the clinic visit. After the visit, RAs assessed the parent's satisfaction.

The Institutional Review Board at Louisiana State University Health Sciences Center–Shreveport (LSUHSC-S) and the Committees on the Rights of Human Subjects at University of Kansas School of Medicine–Wichita (UKSM–W) both approved the study design and instruments.

*Outcome Variables and Data Collection Instruments*

Variables were recorded using a 41-item checklist, which included parent demographics, immunizations given, information about VIS distribution, what risk/benefit communication took place, who initiated it, and how long it lasted. We chose specific aspects of vaccine risk/benefit communication to study based on previous studies (T. C. Davis et al., 2001; Page et al., 2000). The items included mention of rare severe risks, what to do if they occurred, common side effects, how to treat them, benefits, contraindication screening, the next immunization visit, and the long-term vaccination schedule. We used the term "side effect" to refer to common side effects of childhood vaccinations, such as fever of less than 105°, soreness, swelling, and fussiness. Rare severe side effects, such as seizures, fever higher than 105°, and brain damage were referred to as "severe risks." Visit length and vaccine communication were timed using silent stopwatches

Parent literacy was assessed using the Rapid Estimate of Adult Literacy in Medicine (REALM), a commonly used health word recognition test (T. C. Davis, Long, & Jackson, 1993; T. C. Davis, Michielutte, Askov, Williams, & Weiss, 1998). The REALM is highly correlated with other standardized reading tests and the Test of Functional Health Literacy (T. C. Davis et al., 1993; Parker, Baker, & Williams, 1995).

Parent satisfaction with three specific aspects of vaccine communication (benefits, common side effects, and severe risks), their confidence in handling possible side effects and risks, and their trust in the PHN were assessed with 10-point, Likert-type scales. Pilot testing had revealed that very specific questions were required for parents to discriminate their degree of satisfaction regarding vaccine communication. During the postintervention period, parent satisfaction with, and perceived helpfulness of, the poster and *Baby Shot Booklet* were assessed with open-ended questions and 10-point, Likert-type scales. The checklist and survey questions were pilot tested in the LSUHSC-S Pediatric Resident Continuity Clinic.

*Procedures for Quality Assurance*

RAs were trained and supervised by an author at each site. Conference calls between sites were conducted to ensure standardized data collection procedures.

*Data Management and Analysis*

Data recording and analysis were completed using Statistical Analysis Software SAS 9.1 (2002). Visit records were grouped as pre- or postintervention. Cate-gorical variables were compared across the intervention groups using chi-square. Normally distributed continuous variables were compared using unpaired *t* tests. Child and family demographics and immunizations given were compared across the two study sites and among the pre- and postintervention groups to determine whether potential selection bias was present.

Response to the intervention by the special subgroup of parents bringing their first child for first immunization were compared with those of more experienced parents without such characteristics using stratified analysis. Demographic independent variables were compared with outcome measures using chi-square for categorical and student *t* test for continuous variables to determine whether any association was present which might indicate potential confounding.

*Poststudy PHN Site Visit*

One year after the intervention, we revisited the sites and conducted interviews with the PHNs at each clinic. Scripted probes were used to discover PHNs' satisfaction with each of the intervention materials, whether parents asked more questions (particularly those on the poster), influence on vaccine communication and time demands, and suggestions for improvement.

## Results

Parent demographic characteristics are shown in Table 1. The only significant difference between pre- and postintervention groups was that more parents were in the self-pay category during the postintervention period. On average, parents in both groups had completed 12.4 years of school, but approximately one-quarter of parents tested were reading below a ninth-grade level.

As expected, the study population demographics were somewhat different at the two study sites. Compared to Kansas, the Louisiana study participants were more likely to be Black and pay with Medicaid, whereas Kansas participants were more likely to be White and pay with cash. No differences in child age, number of vaccines, or other variables were detected. The demographics at each site remained stable between pre- and postintervention periods, so study data from the two sites were merged and described as one study population for outcomes evaluation.

Vaccines administered by PHNs during the study included diphtheria/tetanus/acellular pertussis (DTaP), hepatitis B (HBV), *Haemophilus influenzae* type b (Hib), measles/mumps/rubella (MMR), inactivated polio (IPV), and varicella. A mean of 3.5 vaccine doses were given per visit in both pre- and postintervention time periods. No vaccines were refused during the study.

133

*(handwritten margin notes: "many topic", "Extraneous Factors", "variable pre & post", "mean", "paired T-test", "chi square", "chi square test")*

Table 1

*Parent Demographic Characteristics: Comparison of Parents in the Pre- and Postintervention Groups*

| | Pre-intervention (n = 246) | Post-intervention (n = 217) | Significance of difference |
|---|---|---|---|
| Parent present | | | |
|   Mother | 86% | 87% | ns |
|   Father | 17% | 16% | ns |
| Parent race | | | |
|   White | 41% | 46% | ns |
|   Black | 56% | 50% | ns |
|   Other | 3% | 3% | ns |
| Parent literacy | | | |
|   Ninth grade and higher | 70% | 78% | ns |
|   Seventh to eighth grade | 22% | 16% | ns |
|   Sixth grade and lower | 8% | 6% | ns |
| Payment method | | | |
|   Medicaid | 53% | 50% | ns |
|   Self-pay | 30% | 42% | p < .01 |
|   Free | 13% | 6% | ns |
|   Private insurance | 4% | 1% | ns |
| Parent's first baby | 33% | 33% | ns |
| Baby's first visit | 13% | 9% | ns |
| | M (SD) | M (SD) | |
| Parent age in years | 26.8 (7.8) | 27.5 (8.6) | ns |
| Parent education | 12.4 (2.0) | 12.4 (1.9) | ns |
| No. of children in family | 2.3 (1.3) | 2.5 (1.6) | ns |

*Note.* ns = not significant.

During both pre- and postintervention periods, the VIS distribution (89% vs. 92%) as well as communication about side effects (91% vs. 92%) and treatment of
385  side effects (91% vs. 93%) occurred frequently. Providers significantly improved discussion of severe side effects (13% vs. 44%, p < .001) and their management (29% vs. 60%, p < .001). The proportion of visits in which specific side effects and severe side effects were
390  addressed is shown in Table 2. Mention of the Vaccine Injury Compensation Program (VICP) increased to 11% from a baseline of 0% (p < .0001).

Discussion of the schedule of the next visit dropped significantly (93% vs. 81%, p < .001), although it was
395  commonly addressed in both periods. Screening for contraindications was moderately high throughout and did not change significantly (71% vs. 77%). In Louisiana, an electronic immunization registry was introduced during the study and, although the Louisiana
400  nurses referred to the contraindication sheet, they did not incorporate the results into the electronic record. Communication about vaccine benefits occurred in about half of visits pre- and postintervention (48% vs. 51%); the most commonly mentioned benefit was pro-
405  tection against disease.

The amount of time spent discussing vaccines ranged from 0 to 120 seconds preintervention and from 0 to 240 seconds postintervention; mean vaccine communication time increased by 6 seconds from a mean
410  of 16 seconds to 22 seconds (p < .001), median time

increased from 11 seconds to 15 seconds. This included time spent referring to the contraindication sheet in Louisiana and using it as a checklist in Kansas. In the 19 visits in which communication lasted more than 60
415  seconds (8 pre and 11 post), mothers tended to be younger (24 years vs. 29, p < .05). There was no difference by race, parent's education, or child's age.

Comparison of demographic variables (e.g., first or subsequent visit, first child, presence of father, mater-
420  nal age, race, high vs. low maternal education, number of vaccines given, and child insurance status) with outcome variables showed no statistically significant confounders present.

Table 2

*Proportion of All Visits in Which Specific Side Effects Were Discussed Pre- and Postintervention*

| | Pre-intervention (n = 246) | Post-intervention (n = 217) | Significance of difference |
|---|---|---|---|
| Common side effects discussed: | | | |
|   Fever | 70% | 73% | ns |
|   Soreness | 70% | 65% | ns |
|   Fussiness | 36% | 33% | ns |
|   Mean number discussed | 2.00 | 2.41 | ns |
| Severe side effects discussed: | | | |
|   Fever of 105 degrees or higher | 10% | 34% | p < .0001 |
|   Seizures/severe brain reactions | 7% | 25% | p < .0001 |
|   Severe allergic reaction | 2% | 10% | p < .0001 |
|   Permanent brain damage | 0% | 4% | p < .01 |
|   Pneumonia | 0% | 1% | ns |
|   Other | 6% | 21% | p < .0001 |
|   No rare/severe side effect discussed | 87% | 56% | p < .0001 |
|   Mean number discussed | 0.24 | 0.97 | p < .0001 |

*Note.* ns = not significant.

### Parent Questions and Parent Satisfaction

A higher proportion of parents asked questions
425  postintervention (27% pre versus 39% post, p < .005). When stratified by literacy level, this increase was seen only in parents reading above the sixth-grade level (28% pre versus 41% post, p < .01). Forty percent of parents who asked a question wanted to know about the
430  schedule, making it the most frequently asked type of question.

Table 3 shows the mean scores (highest score = 10) for parents' satisfaction, confidence, and trust. The only significant change was in the parents' satisfaction
435  with discussion of rare severe side effects, in which the percentage of dissatisfied parents (those who rated their

134

satisfaction level below 6) dropped significantly from 17% to 9% ($p < .05$).

Table 3

*Mean Scores for Parent Satisfaction, Confidence, and Trust Pre- and Postintervention*

|  | Pre-intervention ($n = 246$) | Post-intervention ($n = 217$) | Significance of difference |
|---|---|---|---|
| Parent satisfaction with discussion of: |  |  |  |
| Severe side effects | 8.1 | 8.9 | *p* < .01 |
| Common mild side effects | 9.1 | 9.4 | *ns* |
| Vaccine benefits | 9.0 | 8.9 | *ns* |
| Parent level of confidence with their own ability to handle: |  |  |  |
| Mild side effects | 9.6 | 9.6 | *ns* |
| Severe side effects | 9.3 | 9.4 | *ns* |
| Parent level of trust in the PHN | 9.4 | 9.3 | ns |

*Note.* PHN = public health nurse. For mean scores, low = 0, high = 10; *ns* = not significant.

At the conclusion of the immunization visit, parents were asked for their responses to the material. Seventy-four percent recalled seeing the poster. Of parents receiving both the *Baby Shot Booklet* and the VIS prior to the visit with the nurse administering the immunization, 36% were observed reading the VISs and 42% reading the *Baby Shot Booklet*. Parents who reported looking at the materials rated them highly. On a 10-point scale, mean usefulness scores were 8.9 for the poster, 9.3 for the VIS, and 9.4 for the *Baby Shot Booklet*.

In response to an open-ended question on the poster, parents reported liking the photographs and finding the poster helped them know both what questions to ask and when their child should return. Some parents felt that the poster had too many words or admitted not having read all the poster questions. In response to an open-ended question about the booklet, parents reported that they liked the size, color, and sturdiness of the book. Many mothers suggested that the *Baby Shot Booklet* should be given before the visit, ideally at birth, so they could read it more thoroughly and/or show it to their husband or mother.

Provider discussion of vaccine benefits; the number of questions parents asked; parent satisfaction with the providers' discussion of benefits, common side effects, and rare side effects; and parent confidence in their ability to manage common or severe side effects did not increase after the intervention among the 20 parents with a first baby with first immunization. Time spent discussing all topics increased from 16 seconds to 21 seconds (*ns*) among these parents and from 16 to 22 seconds ($p < .01$) among all other parents.

*Postintervention Site Visits*

A year after the study ended, the posters were still hanging in the waiting room and exam rooms in both PHCs. In individual interviews, PHNs noted that parents and children were attracted to the poster photographs. PHNs felt that the poster was particularly helpful in structuring the discussions of vaccines. The nurses indicated that the poster and in-service helped them fine-tune their vaccine discussion and include mention of severe risks. In addition, although the nurses reported an increase in the number of parent questions, they did not perceive this to slow them down or add to visit time. They said that they felt more prepared to answer the questions and believed that the content of the questions needed to be discussed.

The PHNs felt that all parents should receive the booklet (ideally when their child was born) and found both the content and physical aspects of the booklet practical and inviting. PHNs at both sites gave booklets to parents as long as supplies lasted and then requested more booklets. Nurses also reported that parents continued to bring booklets to future visits and that new parents requested the booklets after having seen other parents use them. PHNs appreciated the contraindication screening sheets and found them quick and easy to use. PHNs said that they shifted from dreading the process to feeling confident that they knew specific contraindication questions to ask. They felt they were doing a more thorough screening.

**Discussion**

Providers and public health policymakers agree that parents need clear language explanations of vaccine risks and benefits. Our study found that vaccine communication materials developed with input from parents and providers could easily be introduced into PHCs and would be well received by PHNs and parents. As a tool to improve specific aspects of vaccine communication, the intervention package was effective in some ways, ineffective in some, and had no impact in others.

There were several positive effects of this intervention, the main one being a threefold increase in PHNs' discussion of severe side effects and how to manage them and parents' corresponding increase in satisfaction with the discussion of severe side effects. In this study of preschool visits to public health immunization clinics, the increase in provider communication of severe side effects did not lead to vaccine refusals. The frequency with which PHNs discussed the VICP also increased significantly but was still minimal (11%) postintervention. Another positive finding was that the poster may have served as both a reminder and encouragement for parents to ask questions; the proportion of parents who read above a sixth-grade level asking questions increased from 27% to 40%.

525　　Provider discussion of the vaccine schedule decreased postintervention. This may have occurred because the PHNs focused on improving the risk/benefit message. The most common parent questions pre- and postintervention involved the vaccine schedule, which
530　validates parent desire for practical information. Because information about the next visit and long-term schedule are important aspects of vaccine communication to parents, they need to be clearly emphasized during the in-services.

535　　In our present study, PHNs discussed side effects and gave the VIS in approximately 9 of 10 immunization visits, both pre- and postintervention, and screened for contraindications 75% of the time. This observational study corroborated our previous finding that
540　PHNs self-reported that they consistently distributed VISs and discussed common side effects and that screening for contraindications was also frequent (T. C. Davis et al., 2001).

　　This study was conducted in public health immuni-
545　zation-only clinics. No parents refused a vaccine in the pre- or postintervention periods. This is consistent with results of a national survey of public health clinics showing that the median refusal rate at these clinics was 0.4 refusals per 1,000 children immunized a year
550　(Fredrickson et al., 2004).

*Comparisons with Previous Studies*

　　In a previous study, a very similar intervention was tested in two private pediatric offices (T. C. Davis, Fredrickson, Bocchini, et al., 2002) and was found to dramatically increase the overall content of provider
555　vaccine communication. The size of the gains, with relatively little extra time required, indicate that little additional staff time is needed for this to-the-point communication.

　　It is important to note that although the educational
560　in-services for the private pediatric practices and PHCs contained similar content, each was tailored according to clinic characteristics (time demands and the needs of their patients) and provider-initiated communication.

　　Findings from this and other studies indicate that
565　vaccine communication concerning rare severe side effects and vaccine benefits is not common (T. C. Davis et al., 2001; T. C. Davis, Fredrickson, Bocchini, et al., 2002; Gellin et al., 2000). Potential severe risks are included in the VISs and so, from a legal stand-
570　point, should be discussed. From a parent's standpoint, this discussion is also important as a way for providers to express respect and build trust (T. C. Davis et al., 2001; Fredrickson et al., 2001). Health care providers may also overlook the discussion of vaccine benefits,
575　believing that the serious morbidity and mortality of vaccine-preventable diseases is common knowledge (T. C. Davis et al., 2001; T. C. Davis, Fredrickson, Bocchini, et al., 2002). This may not be the case; most parents today have limited experience with vaccine-
580　preventable diseases. They may be more motivated to immunize their child because of school and day care admission rules, rather than disease prevention (Gellin et al., 2000). A simple, affirming message about vaccine benefits needs to be a standard aspect of every
585　immunization visit to help parents understand why routine immunizations are recommended for all children.

　　Previous research has found that parents— especially those with limited literacy—tend to want
590　information that is relevant to them, that emphasizes what they need to do, and that explains why this action would benefit them or their child (Doak et al., 1996). Abstract facts and statistics are usually not useful to parents with limited health literacy. Concrete, practical
595　information is preferred (T. C. Davis, Williams, Marin, Parker, & Glass, 2002; Doak et al., 1996). These principles were corroborated in our study.

*The Seven Question Poster*

　　Previous research has indicated that individuals' ability to independently comprehend material is usually
600　two or three grade levels lower than their reading recognition level, which is measured by tests such as the REALM. Individuals with low literacy tend to ask fewer questions, often because they feel that they do not have the right words (Doak et al., 1996). Based on
605　this information, the poster was designed with three things in mind. First, it invited parents to ask common vaccine questions. Second, it was envisioned as a potentially effective, low-cost method of triggering and structuring vaccine communication for nurses and phy-
610　sicians. Third, because the poster offered general questions appropriate to all vaccines, it would not need to be replaced despite continuing changes in the vaccine schedule. The poster could become outdated, however, if immunizations are recommended for ages not indi-
615　cated by the pictures on the poster.

　　Even though the poster used in this study was brief (100 words) and was written on a fourth-grade level according to the Flesch Kincaid scale, parents in public health clinics indicated that it had too many words (in-
620　cluding the title) and it looked too busy. In response to this feedback, we have modified the poster: We decreased it to 60 words and increased the amount of white space to increase readability. The new poster has a second-grade reading level and a perfect score (100)
625　on the Flesch Reading Ease scale. Ideally, these modifications would be tested in future trials. In addition, it would be of interest to test the poster and provider information sheet without the in-service and other materials to see whether similar results could be obtained at
630　a lower cost.

*Limitations*

　　The generalizability of our findings is limited by the fact that the study was conducted in only two PHCs, both urban and both conducted only in English. Translation of materials and testing in a wider variety
635　of public health clinics are needed. General limitations

of this simple, low-cost study design were typical of observational pre-post comparison studies that do not control for temporal trends.

The PHNs' vaccine communication and time allotted may have been influenced by the presence of the observer in the immunization visit. However, PHNs were not aware of the objective of the study or that certain aspects of the visit would be timed. Because observers were present both before and after the in-service, parent satisfaction ratings may have been inflated in both time periods, potentially blunting the demonstrated efficacy of the intervention.

The time spent on discussion of predetermined vaccination topics was measured by trained RAs using silent stopwatches, but the beginning and ending of these conversations were subjective. More accurate measurements using audio- or videotapes were beyond the scope of this project. Interrater reliability between sites was not tested. There was, however, no difference in the mean time increase reported at our two sites. In a future study, the interactions may be audiotaped to allow more comprehensive coding and to minimize observer bias.

Because the intervention included a set of five components (the education session and four materials), we could not separate the effects of each component, which in future studies could be tested separately.

The small number of parents (6% to 8%) reading below a sixth-grade level may have limited our ability to detect changes in this group's asking questions. However, patient education literature indicates that patients with limited literacy tend to ask fewer questions (Doak et al., 1996).

*Implications for Practitioners*

One of the health objectives for the nation in Healthy People 2010 is improving health communication and health literacy (U.S. Department of Health and Human Services, 2000). Improved vaccine risk/benefit communication and subsequent parent understanding may be important components of immunization delivery and overlooked aspects of building parent confidence in vaccine safety. In the United States today, approximately 45% of young children receive at least one vaccine in a public health clinic (National Immunization Program, 2001). Parents at these clinics are more likely to have limited literacy skills and may require repeated, plain-language, oral vaccine risk and benefit information in addition to the VISs. Simple, appealing patient education materials developed with input from providers and parents and organized from a parent's perspective might augment provider vaccine communication and subsequent parent understanding by encouraging parents to ask questions.

Vaccine risk/benefit communication has been mandated since 1986, but content based on what parents and providers request and how it is most effectively delivered has not been adequately addressed (Page et

al., 2000; Simpson et al., 1997). The National Vaccine Advisory Committee (2003) Standards for Child and Adolescent Immunization indicate that health care professionals should allow sufficient time to discuss the vaccines, the diseases they prevent, known risks, the immunization schedule, the need to receive vaccines at the recommended ages, and the importance of bringing the child's vaccine record to each health care visit. Our research suggests that an efficient and systematic approach to discussion of risks and benefits can be done by busy PHNs in public health settings at every visit in a short amount of time.

In this study, we found that PHNs were doing a good job of distributing the VIS and discussing common mild side effects, as mandated by their clinics' guidelines, but needed improvement in communication of vaccine risks and benefits. Our intervention, which used an academic outreach visit that included feedback on baseline performance and provided PHNs with easy-to-use educational materials and prompts, significantly increased communication of severe side effects and increased parent vaccine questions and parent satisfaction with little expenditure of additional time.

The implications of this study have broader applications. As the number of licensed vaccines expands to include those for more common illnesses (e.g., rotavirus diarrhea), sexually transmitted infections (e.g., human papilloma virus), and frightening potential illnesses (e.g., pandemic influenza), communication with patients and their parents will require even greater skill and more carefully tailored and tested messages. The effective continuing education strategies used in this study and the educational materials, which were designed to be provider- and patient-centered, can be used with a wide array of health professionals. One of the important aspects of this study is that it explored creative approaches to making continuing education more provider-centered and health communication more parent-centered. This study shows that it is possible to engage parents and providers in health communication without increasing the time burden or responsibility of either party.

## Note

[1]The 14 agencies are as follows: American Academy of Pediatrics, Ambulatory Pediatric Association, American Academy of Family Physicians, Society of Teachers of Family Medicine, American College of Obstetricians and Gynecologists, American Nurses Association, National Association of Pediatric Nurses and Practitioners, Association of Faculties of Pediatric Nurse Practitioner/Associate Programs, National Association of Community Health Centers Inc., Association of Teachers of Preventive Medicine, Health Resources and Service Administration, Centers for Disease Control and Prevention, Food and Drug Administration, and McKesson Bioservice Corporation.

## References

American Academy of Pediatrics. (2000). Informing patients and parents. In L. K. Pickering (Ed.), *Red book: Report of the Committee on Infectious Diseases* (25th ed., pp. 4–6). Elk Grove Village, IL: Author.

Ball, L., Evans, G., & Bostrom, A. (1998). Risky business: Challenges in vaccine risk benefit communication. *Pediatrics, 101,* 453–458.

Cabana, M. D., Rand, C. S., Powe, N. R., Wu, A. W., Wilson, M. H., Abboud, P. A. C., et al. (1999). Why don't physicians follow clinical practice guidelines? A framework for improvement. *Journal of the American Medical Association, 282,* 1458–1465.

Davis, D. A., O'Brien, M. A. T., Freemantle, N., Wolf, F. M., Mazmanian, P., & Taylor-Vaisey, A. (1999). Impact of formal continuing medical education: Do conferences, workshops, rounds, and other traditional continuing education activities change physician behavior or health care outcomes? *Journal of the American Medical Association, 282,* 867–874.

Davis, D. A., Thomson, M. A., Oxman, A. D., & Haynes, R. B. (1995). Changing physician performance: A systematic review of the effect of continuing medical education strategies. *Journal of the American Medical Association, 274,* 700–705.

Davis, T. C., Fredrickson, D. D., Arnold, C. L., Cross, J. T., Humiston, S. G., Green, K., et al. (2001). Childhood vaccine risk/benefit communication in private practice office settings: A national survey. *Pediatrics, 107,* E17.

Davis, T. C., Fredrickson, D. D., Bocchini, C., Arnold, C. L., Green, K., Humiston, S., et al. (2002). Improving vaccine risk/benefit communication with an immunization education package: A pilot study. *Ambulatory Pediatrics, 2,* 193–200.

Davis, T. C., Long, S., & Jackson, R. (1993). Rapid estimate of adult literacy in medicine: A shortened screening instrument. *Family Medicine, 25,* 391–395.

Davis, T. C., Michielutte, R., Askov, E. N., Williams, M. V., & Weiss, B. (1998). Practical assessment of adult literacy in health care. *Health Education & Behavior, 25,* 613–624.

Davis, T. C., Williams, M., Marin, E., Parker, R. M., & Glass, J. (2002). Health literacy and cancer communication. *CA: A Cancer Journal for Clinicians, 52,* 134–149.

Doak, C. C., Doak, L. G., & Root, J. H. (1996). *Teaching patients with low-literacy skills* (2nd ed.). Philadelphia: J. B. Lippincott.

Dugan, E., & Cohen, S. J. (1998). Improving physicians' implementation of clinical practice guidelines: Enhancing primary care practice. In S. A. Shumaker, J. K. Ockene, & W. L. McBee (Eds.), *The handbook of health behavior change* (2nd ed., pp. 238–304). New York: Springer.

Evans, G. (2000). Pediatricians must use official Vaccine Information Statements. *American Academy of Pediatrics News, 16,* 14.

Flesch, R. (1949). *The art of readable writing.* New York: Harper & Row.

Fredrickson, D. D., Davis, T. C., Arnold, C. L., Kennen, E., Humiston, S. G., Cross, J. T., et al. (2004). Childhood immunization refusal: Provider and parent perceptions. *Family Medicine, 36,* 431–439.

Fredrickson, D. D., Davis, T. C., & Bocchini, J. A. (2001). Explaining the risks and benefits of vaccines to parents. *Pediatric Annals, 30,* 400–406.

Freed, G. L., Clark, S. J., Hibbs, B. F., & Santoli, J. M. (2004). Parental vaccine safety concerns: The experiences of pediatricians and family physicians. *American Journal of Preventive Medicine, 26,* 11–14.

Gellin, B. G., Maibach, E. W., & Marcuse, E. K. (2000). Do parents understand immunizations? A national telephone survey. *Pediatrics, 106,* 1097–1102.

Gellin, B. G., & Schaffner, W. (2001). The risk of vaccination: The importance of "negative" studies. *New England Journal of Medicine, 344,* 372–373.

Institute of Medicine. (2004). *Health literacy: A prescription to end confusion* (L. Nielson-Bohlman, A. Panzer, & D. A. Kindig, Eds.). Washington, DC: National Academies Press.

Leask, J. L. (2002). Vaccination and risk communication: Summary of a workshop, Arlington, Virginia, USA, 5–6 October 2000. *Journal of Paediatrics and Child Health, 38,* 124–128.

Marshall, G. S., & Gellin, B. G. (2001). Challenges to vaccine safety. *Primary Care, 28,* 853–868.

McGee, J. (1999). *Writing and designing print materials for beneficiaries: A guide for state Medicaid agencies* (HFCA Publication No. 10145). Baltimore: U.S. Department of Health and Human Services, Health Care Financing Administration, Center for Medicaid and State Operations.

National Immunization Program. (2001). *National Immunization Survey, Q3/2000–Q2/2001.* Atlanta, GA: Centers for Disease Control.

National Vaccine Advisory Committee. (2003). Standards for child and adolescent immunization practices. *Pediatrics, 112,* 978–981.

Page, D., Eason, P., Humiston, S., & Barker, W. (2000). Notes from the Association of Teachers of Preventive Medicine: Vaccine risk/benefit communication project. *American Journal of Preventive Medicine, 18,* 176–177.

Parker, R. M., Baker, D., & Williams, M. V. (1995). The Test of Functional Health Literacy in Adults (TOFHLA): A new instrument for measuring patients' literacy skills. *Journal of General Internal Medicine, 10,* 537–545.

Rudd, R. E., & Comings, J. P. (1994, Fall). Learner developed materials: An empowering product. *Health Education Quarterly, 21,* 313–327.

Simpson, D. M., Suarez, L., & Smith, D. R. (1997). Immunization rates among young children in the public and private health care sectors. *American Journal of Preventive Medicine, 13,* 84–88.

Statistical Analysis Software. 9.1 ed. (2002). Cary, NC: SAS Institute.

U.S. Department of Health and Human Services. (2000). Health communication. In *Healthy People 2010: Understanding and Improving Health* (2nd ed.). Washington, DC: Government Printing Office.

U.S. Government. (1986). National Childhood Vaccine Injury Act of 1986 (Publication No. 99-660), *42,* USC Sect 300aa-26.

**Acknowledgments**: The authors wish to acknowledge the nurses, clinic staff, and patients who participated in this study. They also would like to thank their research assistants Vicky Specian, Catherine Davis, Amanda McConnell, Cathy Lott, Terri Jones, Cameron Fahrenholtz, and Kim Hooten for their hard work and colleague Linda Martin for her careful reading of the article. This project was partially funded by the Health Resources and Services Administration (HRSA) through Cooperative Agreement 6U76 AH 00001 to the Association of Teachers of Preventive Medicine (ATPM).

**Address correspondence to**: Terry C. Davis, Louisiana State University Health Sciences Center–Shreveport, Departments of Pediatrics and Internal Medicine, 1501 Kings Hwy., Shreveport, LA 71130. E-mail: tdavis1@lsuhsc.edu

# Exercise for Article 19

## Factual Questions

1. The Kansas unit had how many immunization nurses?

2. What percentage of the parents refused to participate?

3. What percentage of the postintervention parents had Medicaid?

4. Was the pre-to-post difference in discussing severe allergic reactions statistically significant? If yes, at what probability level?

5. At the conclusion of the immunization visits, what percentage of the parents recalled seeing the poster?

6. How was time spent on discussion of predetermined vaccination topics measured?

## Questions for Discussion

7. Are the educational sessions described in sufficient detail? Explain. (See lines 181–210.)

8. Could the fact that the staff members were aware of the observer's presence have affected the results of this study? Explain. (See lines 262–265.)

9. Is the fact that the research was approved by a board and committee important? Explain. (See lines 278–283.)

10. Is it important to know that the pre- and postintervention groups were similar in demographic characteristics? Explain. (See lines 355–362 and Table 1.)

11. Do you think it would be worthwhile to conduct a future study on each of the five components separately? Explain. (See lines 659–662.)

12. Do you think it would be worthwhile to include a control group in a future study on this topic? Why? Why not?

## Quality Ratings

Directions: Indicate your level of agreement with each of the following statements by circling a number from 5 for strongly agree (SA) to 1 for strongly disagree (SD). If you believe an item is not applicable to this research article, leave it blank. Be prepared to explain your ratings. When responding to criteria A and B, keep in mind that brief titles and abstracts are conventional in published research.

A. The title of the article is appropriate.

   SA   5   4   3   2   1   SD

B. The abstract provides an effective overview of the research article.

   SA   5   4   3   2   1   SD

C. The introduction establishes the importance of the study.

   SA   5   4   3   2   1   SD

D. The literature review establishes the context for the study.

   SA   5   4   3   2   1   SD

E. The research purpose, question, or hypothesis is clearly stated.

   SA   5   4   3   2   1   SD

F. The method of sampling is sound.

   SA   5   4   3   2   1   SD

G. Relevant demographics (for example, age, gender, and ethnicity) are described.

   SA   5   4   3   2   1   SD

H. Measurement procedures are adequate.

   SA   5   4   3   2   1   SD

I. All procedures have been described in sufficient detail to permit a replication of the study.

   SA   5   4   3   2   1   SD

J. The participants have been adequately protected from potential harm.

   SA   5   4   3   2   1   SD

K. The results are clearly described.

   SA   5   4   3   2   1   SD

L. The discussion/conclusion is appropriate.

   SA   5   4   3   2   1   SD

M. Despite any flaws, the report is worthy of publication.

   SA   5   4   3   2   1   SD

# Article 20

# A Comparison Pilot Study of Public Health Field Nursing Home Visitation Program Interventions for Pregnant Hispanic Adolescents

**Jody Duong Nguyen**, RN, MSN/MPH, **Michael L. Carson**, MS, **Kathleen M. Parris**, RN, MSN, **Patricia Place**, BSN, BCRN, PHN[*]

## ABSTRACT

*Objective*: Improve pregnancy outcomes in first-time Hispanic adolescent mothers and their infants.

*Setting*: Urban communities in Orange County, California.

*Design and Methods*: A comparison of the Nurse–Family Partnership pilot study home visitation program with traditional Public Health Field Nursing (PHFN) home visitation.

*Participants*: Two hundred twenty-five Hispanic adolescent mothers and their infants.

*Interventions*: Participants in the control group received the traditional PHFN services; the intervention group received interventions from advanced trained public health nurses. The control group received a minimum of three home visits: one initial client assessment and family profile, one antepartum visit, and one postpartum visit including newborn assessment. Participants in the intervention group received weekly home visits for the first 4 weeks, followed by visits every other week until delivery, weekly visits for the next 6 weeks, visits every other week until the child was 20 months, and monthly visits until the child was 24 months of age.

*Results*: Preliminary results indicate that home visitation by public health nurses (PHNs) positively affected the health of adolescent mothers and their infants. The incidence of premature births to adolescent mothers in the intervention group was lower than that found in the California population of adolescent mothers.

*Conclusion*: Preliminary results from this program showed that PHN home visitation (control and intervention groups) positively affects the birth outcomes of adolescent mothers and their infants.

From *Public Health Nursing*, 20, 412–418. Copyright © 2003 by Blackwell Publishing, Inc. Reprinted with permission.

Reduction of adolescent pregnancies has been identified as a public health priority. In 2000, President Clinton released a statement saying that he was encouraged by the new birth data released by the Centers for Disease Control and Prevention. The data showed that teen birth rates in the United States were at their lowest level since record keeping began 60 years before. Nevertheless, the president encouraged every sector of society to continue its efforts in reducing adolescent pregnancy. He called on Congress to enact his budget initiative to provide $25 million to support living arrangements for teen parents, help reduce repeat pregnancies, and improve the health of mothers and their children (U.S. Department of Health and Human Services [USDHHS], 2000). In addition, one of the Healthy People 2010 goals is to improve pregnancy planning, increase spacing between pregnancies, and prevent unintended pregnancy occurring within 24 months of a previous birth (USDHHS, 2000).

The primary focus of this article is not on prevention of adolescent pregnancy but rather on developing an intervention program that focuses on the health and well-being of pregnant adolescents and their children. This includes assisting teen mothers in preparing to deliver a healthy full-term baby, promoting healthy growth and development of the child, and identifying and accomplishing the mother's life goals. The federal government estimates that approximately $40 billion per year is spent on helping families that begin with a teenage birth. Studies show that providing early-intervention programs serving low-income mothers and their children can reduce federal government spending on adolescent pregnancy. The Nurse Home Visitation Program in Elmira, New York, based on the David Olds Home Visitation Model, shows a taxpayer savings of more than $18,000 per low-income first-time mother (Karoly, Greenwood, Everingham, Hoube, Kilburn, Rydell, Sanders, & Cheisa, 1998). Studies have demonstrated the effectiveness of the Olds Home Visitation Model in reducing the number of repeat pregnancies;

[*]*Jody Duong Nguyen* is supervising public health nurse, Orange County Health Care Agency, Santa Ana, CA. *Michael L. Carson* is senior epidemiologist, Orange County Health Care Agency, Santa Ana, CA. *Kathleen M. Parris* is public health nursing manager, Orange County Health Care Agency, Santa Ana, CA. *Patricia Place* is supervising public health nurse, Orange County Health Care Agency, Santa Ana, CA.

child abuse; and maternal behavioral problems due to use of alcohol and drugs, sexual partners, cigarettes smoked, and alcohol consumption in 15-year-old girls (Karoly et al., 1998). This article presents an overview
45 of the Nurse-Family Partnership (NFP) Pilot Study in Orange County, California, and reviews early results of the pilot study. NFP is based on the Olds Home Visitation Model and is designed to improve adolescent pregnancy outcomes and early childhood health and
50 development. NFP is a comprehensive program in which specially trained public health nurses visit women and families in their homes and link them with services they need during pregnancy and the first 2 years of their child's life.

## Significance of the Problem

55      Despite the recent decline in the teen birth rate, adolescent pregnancy remains a significant problem in the United States. The U.S. teen birth rate is nearly double Great Britain's, at least four times that of France and Germany, and more than 10 times that of
60 Japan (Singh & Darroch, 2000). Most teen pregnancies are unintended. Statistics show that four in 10 American teenage girls become pregnant at least once before they reach age 20, leading to almost 1 million pregnancies a year (National Campaign to Prevent Teen Preg-
65 nancy, 1997). Their babies are often low birthweight and have disproportionately high mortality rates. Approximately 80% of adolescent mothers who drop out of high school are likely to be poor. In contrast, just 8% of children born to married high school graduates aged
70 20 or older live in poverty (Maynard, 1997). Even though teen pregnancy is a problem affecting all populations, there are some subgroups that are more profoundly affected than others. Nationally, Hispanic adolescents now have the highest teen birth rates and are
75 more likely to drop out of school and become pregnant than their non-Hispanic white and African American counterparts (Manlove, 1998).

Repeat births account for 22% of adolescent pregnancies. The percentage of repeat births of all teen
80 births within specific racial groups was 20% for whites, 28% for blacks, 22% for American Indians, and 21% for Asians. Of births to Hispanic adolescents of all races, 25% were repeat births (USDHHS, 2000). Teen multiparas have short pregnancy intervals, which could
85 affect maternal and infant health. A study of 3,400 first-time teenage mothers who received public assistance in Chicago showed that 64% had at least one pregnancy during the follow-up period of approximately 29 months, and 21% had two or more pregnan-
90 cies (Maynard & Rangarajan, 1994). Of the adolescent mothers who became pregnant again, 35% did so within one year of the birth of their first child, and 75% became pregnant again within 2 years. Three-quarters of the repeat pregnancies resulted in a live birth. In a
95 study of almost 10,000 adolescents who had repeat live births between 1980 and 1988, 36% had pregnancy intervals shorter than 7 months, and 26% were pregnant again between 7 and 12 months after the first birth (Hellerstedt & Perie, 1994). Adolescent mothers with
100 the lowest education, skills, and economic circumstances are likely to have more repeat pregnancies during their adolescent years. Furthermore, studies have shown that adolescent mothers do not use an effective contraceptive method, which puts them at risk for rapid
105 repeat pregnancies (Maynard & Rangarajan, 1994).

### Consequences of Early Childbearing for Mothers

Adolescent mothers experience more pregnancy and delivery problems and have less healthy babies than adult mothers. These risks are associated with poverty and the environmental and social circum-
110 stances of young mothers. Adolescents experience a maternal death rate 2.5 times greater than that of mothers aged 20 to 24 years (Brown & Eisenberg, 1995). They may be disproportionately exposed to violence and have high rates of physical and sexual abuse histo-
115 ries (Bayatpour, Wells, & Holford, 1992). They are also at a higher risk for sexually transmitted diseases (STDs). At least 60% of all cases of STDs in the United States are in individuals who are 25 years old or younger. Furthermore, they are at a higher risk for sub-
120 stance abuse, stress, and depression (USDHHS, 2000). Common prenatal and obstetrical problems in adolescent mothers include inadequate prenatal care, poor weight gain and nutrition, hypertension, and anemia. Alternatively, excessive prenatal weight gain predis-
125 poses young mothers to adult obesity. Lactation may also adversely affect bone density in still-growing adolescents (National Campaign to Prevent Teen Pregnancy, 1997).

### Consequences of Adolescent Childbearing for the Child

Children born to adolescent mothers have greater
130 health and medical risks than children of adult mothers. They suffer from higher rates of low birthweight, intrauterine growth retardation, and preterm birth (Ventura, Martin, Curtin, & Mathews, 2001). Low birthweight increases the risk of infant mortality, blindness,
135 deafness, chronic respiratory problems, mental retardation, mental illness, and cerebral palsy. Children of adolescent mothers receive less well-baby and preventive care and more medical treatment than children of adult mothers (Maynard, 1997). Furthermore, they are
140 at risk of poor parenting skills, are often victims of abuse and neglect, and may suffer from poor school performance (National Campaign to Prevent Teen Pregnancy, 1997).

## Target Population

As previously mentioned, adolescent pregnancy
145 rates have decreased in the United States, but there are some racial/ethnic populations in which adolescent pregnancy rates remain the same and have not decreased when compared with other racial/ethnic

groups. In the United States, three out of five Hispanic
150 adolescent girls become pregnant at least once as a
teen. Currently, California has more than 33 million
residents, and the Hispanic population is the fastest-
growing racial/ethnic group. Hispanic adolescents have
the highest birth rates in California (Manlove, 1998). In
155 Orange County, Hispanic teens (15 to 19 years old)
have the highest birth rate compared with other ra-
cial/ethnic groups. In 1999, the Orange County Hispanic teen birth rate was 105.9 per 1,000 live births,
followed by African American (36.6), American Indian
160 (28.0), white (14.3), and Asian/Pacific Islander (11.3).
The overall county birth rate for 15- to 19-year-olds in
1999 was 44.40 per 1,000 live births (Orange County
Health Care Agency, 2001).

## Setting

The setting is predominantly urban Orange County,
165 California. The 2000 U.S. Census report showed the
population to be more than 2.8 million, 24.4% of the
population is aged 18 and under, and 30% is of Hispanic or Latino origin (U.S. Census Bureau, 2001). The
Hispanic population is considered to be the largest ra-
170 cial/ethnic population in Orange County. In Santa Ana
city, for example, Hispanics account for 71% of the
overall population, compared with 17.1% non-Hispanic
whites (Center for Demographic Research, 2000). In
the next 20 years, the Hispanic adolescent population
175 will grow much faster than the overall adolescent
population in the United States. The projected 13- to
19-year-old Hispanic adolescent population growth in
the United States for 2000–2020 is 60%, compared
with 8% growth for all adolescents (Day, 1996).

## Theoretical Framework

180 To affect the target population and to achieve program goals and objectives, the program must have a
well-developed theoretical base to provide the foundation and context for program design, implementation,
and evaluation. The theoretical framework for this pro-
185 gram is based on the self-efficacy theory introduced by
Albert Bandura (1977). The theory is grounded in his
early work on social cognitive theory. The self-efficacy
theory provides a useful framework for improving and
promoting the adolescent's health behavior during
190 pregnancy and childcare and her own personal growth
and development.

Self-efficacy is defined as the individual's judgments of his or her capabilities to organize and execute
courses of action required to successfully attain desig-
195 nated types of performances or behavior. Self-efficacy
is the most influential authority in human nature and
plays a powerful role in determining the choices people
make, the effort they expend, how long they persist
when confronted with obstacles, and the degree of
200 anxiety or confidence they will bring to the task at
hand. Self-efficacy helps explain why people's behavior differs widely even when they have similar knowledge and skills. What people do and how they behave

is better predicted by their beliefs. Bandura (1977)
205 identifies and distinguishes efficacy expectation from
outcome expectations. A belief in one's own competence to execute a task is required to produce a desired
outcome expectation. Self-efficacy expectations are
derived from several sources of information: previous
210 performance accomplishments, modeling, verbal persuasion, and emotional arousal (Bandura, 1977).

Successful accomplishment increases expectations
of mastery, and repeated failures decrease it. Teenagers
may recognize the outcome expectation that a subse-
215 quent pregnancy during the 12 months postpartum is
damaging to their health. Modeling by a variety of personally significant individuals in adverse situations will
encourage behavior changes.

The success of this program will depend on the
220 public health nurses' reinforcement of the adolescents'
behaviors that are consistent with the program's goal.
Public health nurses hope to build the self-confidence
of the adolescents and reinforce the positive behaviors
and accomplishments. Verbal persuasion is employed
225 to educate the adolescents about healthy practices,
available health care services, and support resources.
Public health nurses also serve as role models for adolescent mothers and provide reinforcement of previous
accomplishments to increase the mothers' self-efficacy.

## Design and Methods

230 Providers that serve pregnant adolescents in the
community refer pregnant adolescents to the NFP. Providers include physicians, community clinics, schools,
social services agencies, probation departments, pregnancy testing clinics, juvenile health services, and the
235 supplemental food program for women, infants, and
children (WIC). Participants for this pilot study were
randomly assigned to the control or intervention group
by the drawing of colored blocks. To participate in the
study, participants needed to be on or eligible for
240 Medi-Cal, at less than 28 weeks' gestation, younger
than 20 years old, and pregnant with their first child.
Participants assigned to the control group received the
traditional Public Health Field Nursing (PHFN) services, while the intervention group received services
245 from advanced trained public health nurses (ATPHNs).
Informed consent was obtained from all participants.

PHFN nurses are Bachelor of Science in Nursing
(BSN)-prepared with maternal and child health experience and receive general field nursing orientation. In
250 addition to general field orientation, ATPHNs receive 1
week of extensive training in Denver and two follow-
up trainings; the follow-up trainings include a 3-day
training on Partners in Parenting Education and a 2-day
training on toddler protocols. The ATPHNs also re-
255 ceive training in home visitation protocols, clinical
record keeping, the information management system,
and the theoretical framework upon which the NFP is
based.

Participants in the control group received a minimum of three PHFN home visits: one for initial assessment of the client and family profile, one antepartum visit (during which the PHN provides physical assessment, education, referral, and encourages compliance with prenatal care), and one postpartum and newborn visit. Participants in the intervention group received weekly ATPHN home visits for the first 4 weeks, followed by visits every other week until delivery, weekly for the next 6 weeks, every other week until the child was 21 months old, and monthly until the child was 24 months old. ATPHNs promote the self-efficacy of adolescents during the structured home visits by encouraging the adolescents to set personal goals. Adaptive behavior changes are encouraged to promote healthy outcomes of pregnancy, develop positive parenting skills, and optimize the developmental potential of the infant. The ATPHNs assist the adolescents in identifying and developing informal support systems of family and friends. In addition, they serve as a link for adolescents to community services for health care and welfare. Home visits usually last from 60 to 90 minutes and focus on personal health, environmental health, maternal role development, maternal life course development, child and family functioning, and knowledge and use of health and human service agencies.

## Results

Preliminary results of the study from pregnancy through postpartum are discussed here. A total sample of 225 Hispanic adolescents was enrolled in the study: 121 in the control group and 104 in the intervention group. Initial demographic data for both groups are presented in Table 1. Significantly more control group adolescents than intervention group adolescents (74/121 vs. 45/103) were born outside the United States ($p = 0.007$). All 74 control group adolescents and 43 of the 45 (95.6%) intervention group adolescents born outside the United States were born in Mexico; the remaining two intervention group adolescents born outside the United States were born in Central/South America. Adolescents in both groups were more likely to be single, never married, enrolled in school, and planning to continue education postpartum. Median number of years of education completed was the same for adolescents in both groups: 10 years (range 2–14 years). Only 32 of 225 (14.2%) adolescents in the study were employed part-time or full-time at initial interview. Adolescents in both groups reported being "somewhat likely" or "very likely" to return to or find work within 6 months after giving birth. Sixty-eight percent and 69.3% of adolescents in the study reported receiving Medi-Cal and WIC, respectively. Only 5.3% of participants reported receiving food stamps. When asked to select their total household income from a predefined list, many participants declined or refused to answer. For the 97 control

(80.2%) and 81 intervention (77.9%) group adolescents answering the question, the median total household income range was $12,001 to $15,000.

Table 1
*Initial Demographics*

| Variable | Control group | Intervention group | p value[*] |
|---|---|---|---|
| Place of birth (*n* = 224) | | | |
| United States | 47 | 58 | 0.007 |
| Other | 74 | 45 | |
| Marital status (*n* = 225) | | | |
| Single, never married | 112 | 92 | NS |
| Married | 9 | 12 | |
| Education (*n* = 225) | | | |
| Enrolled in school | 61 | 63 | NS |
| Not enrolled in school | 60 | 41 | |
| Educational plan (*n* = 223) | | | |
| Continue education | 103 | 92 | NS |
| No further education | 17 | 11 | |
| Employment (*n* = 225) | | | |
| Full- or part-time work | 20 | 12 | NS |
| Not working | 101 | 92 | |
| Likelihood of returning to or finding work within 6 months postpartum (*n* = 224) | | | |
| Not/not very likely | 53 | 40 | NS |
| Somewhat/very likely | 68 | 63 | |
| Receive Medi-Cal (*n* = 225) | | | |
| Yes | 78 | 74 | NS |
| No | 43 | 30 | |
| Receive aid from Women, Infants, and Children (*n* = 225) | | | |
| Yes | 83 | 73 | NS |
| No | 38 | 31 | |
| Receive food stamps (*n* = 225) | | | |
| Yes | 8 | 4 | NS |
| No | 113 | 100 | |

[*]*p* values are based on chi-square tests of significance.
NS = not significant.

Of the 225 Hispanic adolescents enrolled in the study, information on infant birth outcome was available for 152 (67.6%): 82 (67.8%) in the control group and 70 (67.3%) in the intervention group. Twenty-seven of the mothers were still pregnant at the time of data analysis. Four mothers (3 in the control group and 1 in the intervention group) gave birth to twins; therefore, birth outcome information was available on 156 infants.

Of the 225 Hispanic adolescents, 49 were lost to follow-up. The most prevalent reasons for dropping out of the study during pregnancy included declined further participation, moved out of state/program area, and excessive missed appointments.

Adolescents in the control and intervention groups gave birth to more girls (55%) than boys. As shown in Table 2, adolescents in both groups had similar mean weight gain during pregnancy (40 pounds) and infant gestational age at birth (39 weeks), but a larger percentage of adolescents in the control group (8.2%) gave

Table 2
*Birth Outcome Data*

| Outcome | *n* Mean (range) *SD* | |
| --- | --- | --- |
| | Control group | Intervention group |
| Maternal weight gain during pregnancy, pounds (*n* = 137) | 69<br>40.35 (0–156)<br>73.89 | 68<br>39.87 (13–275)<br>35.00 |
| Gestational age, weeks (*n* = 154) | 85<br>38.92 (21–42)<br>2.70 | 69<br>38.88 (27–41)<br>2.23 |
| Birth weight, grams (*n* = 156) | 85<br>3130.06 (652.05–4422.60)<br>570.78 | 71<br>3294.32 (1077.30–5159.70)<br>567.56 |

birth to premature infants (< 37 weeks gestation) than did adolescents in the intervention group (Table 3). Overall, the percentage of premature births in the study was 6.5%, which is a considerably smaller proportion than the 13.7% of California teens giving birth to premature infants (California Maternal and Child Health Branch, 1997).

Table 2 also shows that infants born to adolescents in the intervention group had a higher mean birthweight than infants born to adolescents in the control group (3294 g vs. 3130 g). As shown in Table 4, a larger percentage of infants born to mothers in the intervention group had a birthweight of 3500 g or greater; two infants in each group weighed more than 4000 g, and one infant in the intervention group weighed more than 5000 g. A larger percentage of infants born to mothers in the control group had low birth weight (< 2500 g) (10.6% vs. 5.6%). Overall, the percentage of low birth weight infants in the study was 8.3%, which is higher than the 7.7% of California teens giving birth to infants weighing less than 2500 g (California Maternal and Child Health Branch, 1997).

Table 3
*Gestational Age Group by Study Group*

| Gestational age group | *n* (%) | | Total |
| --- | --- | --- | --- |
| | Control group | Intervention group | |
| < 37 weeks | 7 (8.2) | 3 (4.3) | 10 |
| 37 weeks | 78 (91.8) | 66 (95.7) | 144 |
| Total | 85 | 69 | 154 |

Table 4
*Birthweight Group by Study Group*

| Birthweight group | *n* (%) | | Total |
| --- | --- | --- | --- |
| | Control group | Intervention group | |
| < 2500 grams | 9 (10.6) | 4 (5.6) | 13 |
| 2500–3499 grams | 58 (68.2) | 41 (57.8) | 99 |
| ≥ 3500 grams | 18 (21.2) | 26 (36.6) | 44 |
| Total | 85 | 71 | 156 |

Apgar scores were available for 24 control group infants and 44 experimental group infants. Mean 1-minute and 5-minute Apgar scores were similar for both groups (8.00 and 8.30 and 8.56 and 9.07, respectively); the range of 1-minute and 5-minute Apgar scores was 2 to 10. No birth defects were reported in infants born to adolescents in either group, but birthing complications were reported in 19 (22.4%) control group deliveries and 16 (22.5%) intervention group deliveries. Birth complications identified included cesarean section (due to failure to progress; slow heart rate or respiratory distress; or breech, transverse, or face-up position), abruptio placenta, sepsis, cord around the neck, 3+ meconium aspiration, pregnancy-induced hypertension, and maternal fever.

**Implications**

Previously published studies support the notion that home visitation by PHNs improves the health and well-being of adolescents and their infants and families (Olds, Henderson, Kitzman, Eckenrode, Cole, & Tatelbaum, 1999; Kitzman, Olds, Henderson, 1997; Kitzman, Olds, Sidora, Henderson, Hanks, Cole, Luckey, Bondy, Cole, & Glazner, 2000). Preliminary results from this program indicate that home visitation by PHNs positively affects the health of Hispanic adolescents and their infants. The prevalence of premature birth is lower than in the general California teen population. Furthermore, both groups' results showed significant improved perinatal outcomes (e.g., initial birthweight, gestational age).

Public health nurses in the intervention group encountered many challenges during their home visits. Maintaining the schedule of home visits is sometimes difficult, especially the time of the visit. Before delivery, the clients are generally quite available; most attend school, and the home visit is planned around the school schedule. Some of the adolescents work, which complicates the home visit dates and times. Many clients forget their scheduled visits. Program attrition of clients during pregnancy and during infancy is a concern and needs to be strengthened. The reasons mothers dropped out during perinatal services were excessive

405 missed appointments, unable to locate client, and declined to participate. There are many reasons for the high rate of attrition. The main reason was that Orange County has a mobile population. Another reason was that it is difficult to determine and control adolescent behavior.

A significant challenge was that some clients had not yet revealed their pregnancies to family members. Some wanted the PHN to tell the family for them. The

410 program also received more referrals than the available trained staff could accommodate. The PHNs reported it was sometimes difficult to explain to clients during the initial home visit that to participate in the program they would be randomly selected for the intervention or

415 control group and that the same nurse who visited them at the initial intake might not be their follow-up nurse. With this knowledge, many clients declined to participate.

Results from this program are preliminary. Addi-

420 tional study is needed to measure the effect of interventions at 12, 18, and 24 months postpartum. We hope to show statistically significant effects between the two groups at 12 months', 18 months', and 24 months' follow-up. Two well-known studies on prenatal and

425 infancy home visitation by nurses conducted in Elmira, New York, and Memphis, Tennessee, showed effects at program termination as well as 3 to 4 and 15 years after (Olds, Henderson, Kitzman, Eckenrode, Cole, & Tatelbaum, 1999; Olds, Eckenrode, Henderson, Kitzman,

430 Powers, Cole, Sidora, Morris, Pettitt, & Luckey, 1997; Kitzman et al., 1997, 2000).

In conclusion, preliminary results from this program showed that PHN home visitation (both control and intervention groups) can positively affect the birth

435 outcomes of Hispanic adolescent mothers. Generalizability of these findings is limited to first-time pregnant adolescents in Orange County, California.

## References

Bandura, A. (1977). *Social Learning Theory.* Englewood Cliffs, NJ: Prentice Hall.

Bayatpour, M., Wells, R. D., & Holford, S. (1992). Physical and sexual abuse as predictors of substance use and suicide among pregnant teenagers. *Journal of Adolescent Health, 13,* 128–132.

Brown, S., & Eisenberg, L. (Eds.). (1995). *The Best Intentions. Unintended Pregnancy and the Well-Being of Children and Families.* Washington, DC: National Academy Press.

California Maternal and Child Health Branch. (1997). The adolescent's family life program: Reporting of selected outcomes for clients active in AFLP as of November 30, 1997. Available online: http://www.dhs.ca.gov/pcfh/mchb/pdfs/AFLP_Report.pdf Accessed April 23, 2001.

Center for Demographic Research. (2000). *Orange County Progress Report.* California State University, Fullerton. Available on-line: http://www.fullerton.edu/cdr/ Accessed April 23, 2001.

Day, J. C. (1996). Population projections of the United States by Age, Sex, Race, and Hispanic Origin, 1995–2050. *Current Population Reports: P25-1130.*

Hellerstedt, W. L., & Perie, P. L. (1994). *The Association of Pregnancy Intervals and Infant Growth Among Infants Born to Adolescents.* American Public Health Association (annual meeting). Washington, DC, October 30–November 3, 1994.

Karoly, L. A., Greenwood, P. W., Everingham, S. S., Hoube, J., Kilburn, M. R., Rydell, C. P., Sanders, M., & Cheisa, J. (1998). *Investing in our children: What we know and don't know about the costs and benefits of early childhood interventions.* Washington, DC: RAND.

Kitzman, H., Olds, D. L., Henderson, C. R. Jr., Hanks, C., Cole, R., Tatebaum, R., McConnochie, K. M., Sidora, K., Luckey, D. W., Shaver, D., Engelhardt, K., James, D., Barnard, K. (1997). Effect of prenatal and infancy home visitation by nurses on pregnancy outcomes, childhood injuries, and repeated childbearing: A randomized controlled trial. *Journal of the American Medical Association, 278,* 644–652.

Kitzman, H., Olds, D., Sidora, K., Henderson, C., Hanks, C., Cole, R., Luckey, D., Bondy, J., Cole, K., & Glazner, J. (2000). Enduring effects of nurse home visitation on maternal life course. *Journal of the American Medical Association, 283,* 1983–1989.

Manlove, J. (1998). The influence of high school dropout and school disengagement on the risk of school age pregnancy. *Journal of Research on Adolescence, 8,* 187–220.

Maynard, R. (Ed.). (1997). *Kids Having Kids: A Robin Hood Foundation Special Report on the Costs of Adolescent Childbearing.* New York: Robin Hood Foundation.

Maynard, R., & Rangarajan, A. (1994). Contraceptive use and repeat pregnancies among welfare-dependent teenage mothers. *Family Planning Perspectives, 26,* 198–205.

National Campaign to Prevent Teen Pregnancy. (1997). *Whatever happened to childhood? The problem of teen pregnancy in the United States.* Washington, DC: National Campaign to Prevent Teen Pregnancy.

Olds, D. L., Eckenrode, J., Henderson, C. R. Jr., Kitzman, H., Powers, J., Cole, R., Sidora, K., Morris, P., Pettitt, L. M., & Luckey, D. (1997). Long-term effects of home visitation on maternal life course and child abuse and neglect: 15-year follow-up of a randomized trial. *Journal of the American Medical Association, 278,* 637–643.

Olds, D. L., Henderson, C. R. Jr., Kitzman, H., Eckenrode, J., Cole, R., & Tatelbaum, R. (1999). Prenatal and infancy home visitation by nurses: Recent findings. *Future of Children, 9,* 44–65.

Orange County Health Care Agency. (2001). Orange County, California, birth outcomes, 1999. Orange County Health Care Agency, Santa Ana, CA.

Singh, S., & Darroch, J. E. (2000). Adolescent pregnancy and childbearing: Levels and trends in developed countries. *Family Planning Perspectives, 32,* 14–23.

U.S. Census Bureau. (2001). *Population by sex, age, Hispanic origin, and race.* Washington, DC: Author. Available online: http://www.census.gov/population/socdemo/hispanic/p20-535/tab01-3.txt Accessed May 23, 2001.

U.S. Department of Health and Human Services. (2000). *Healthy People 2010: Understanding and Improving Health,* 2nd Ed. Washington, DC: U.S. Government Printing Office, Available online: http://www.health.gov/healthypeople Accessed May 23, 2001.

U.S. Department of Health and Human Services. (2000). *HHS fact sheet: Preventing teenage pregnancy.* Available online: http://www.hhs.gov/topics/teenpreg.html Accessed May 23, 2001.

Ventura, S. J., Martin, J. A., Curtin, S. C., & Mathews. T. J. (2001). Births: Final data for 1997. *National Vital Statistics Reports, 47(18).*

**Address correspondence to**: Jody Duong Nguyen, County of Orange Health Care Agency, 1725 W. 17th Street, Santa Ana, CA 92706. E-mail: jnguyen@hca.co.orange.ca.us

# Exercise for Article 20

## Factual Questions

1. According to the literature, which of the following experience more pregnancy and delivery problems and have less healthy babies than the other?
   A. Adolescent mothers
   B. Adult mothers

2. According to Bandura (1977), self-efficacy expectations are derived from what four sources of information?

3. How many participated in the control group, and how many participated in the intervention group?

4. Did the infants born to adolescents in the intervention group *or* the infants born to adolescents in the control group have a higher mean birthweight?

5. Of the 225 Hispanic adolescents, how many were unavailable for follow-up?

6. The researchers state that the generalizability of these findings is limited to what group?

## Questions for Discussion

7. In your opinion, how important is the theoretical framework presented in lines 180–229 as a background for understanding this program evaluation?

8. An important characteristic of a report on a program evaluation is a clear explanation of the program components and how they work. In your opinion, are they sufficiently clear in this program evaluation? Consider the entire article when answering this question, especially lines 230–285.

9. In your opinion, was the random assignment to groups an important part of the research methodology in this evaluation? Explain. (See lines 236–238.)

10. Table 1 shows the initial demographics on nine variables. The two groups were significantly different on only one of them. Is it important to know that, to a large extent, the two groups were initially similar? Explain.

11. The researchers report that they asked participants to select their total household income from a predefined list; however, many declined or refused to answer? Does this surprise you? Explain. (See lines 312–314.)

12. The researchers state that the results from this program are preliminary, and additional study is needed. Do you agree? Explain. (See lines 419–424.)

## Quality Ratings

Directions: Indicate your level of agreement with each of the following statements by circling a number from 5 for strongly agree (SA) to 1 for strongly disagree (SD). If you believe an item is not applicable to this research article, leave it blank. Be prepared to explain your ratings. When responding to criteria A and B, keep in mind that brief titles and abstracts are conventional in published research.

A. The title of the article is appropriate.

SA   5   4   3   2   1   SD

B. The abstract provides an effective overview of the research article.

SA   5   4   3   2   1   SD

C. The introduction establishes the importance of the study.

SA   5   4   3   2   1   SD

D. The literature review establishes the context for the study.

SA   5   4   3   2   1   SD

E. The research purpose, question, or hypothesis is clearly stated.

SA   5   4   3   2   1   SD

F. The method of sampling is sound.

SA   5   4   3   2   1   SD

G. Relevant demographics (for example, age, gender, and ethnicity) are described.

SA   5   4   3   2   1   SD

H. Measurement procedures are adequate.

SA   5   4   3   2   1   SD

I. All procedures have been described in sufficient detail to permit a replication of the study.

SA   5   4   3   2   1   SD

J. The participants have been adequately protected from potential harm.

SA   5   4   3   2   1   SD

K. The results are clearly described.

SA   5   4   3   2   1   SD

L. The discussion/conclusion is appropriate.

SA   5   4   3   2   1   SD

M. Despite any flaws, the report is worthy of publication.

SA   5   4   3   2   1   SD

# Article 21

# Culturally Tailored Diabetes Education Program for Chinese Americans: A Pilot Study

**Chen-Yen Wang**, PhD, APRN, CDE, **Siu Ming Alain Chan**, RN, MSN[*]

### ABSTRACT

*Background*: The prevalence of type 2 diabetes among Chinese Americans is rising, and cultural and socioeconomic factors prevent this population from achieving optimal diabetes management.

*Objective*: To assess the feasibility and acceptability of a culturally appropriate diabetes management program tailored to Chinese Americans with type 2 diabetes and the preliminary outcomes of the intervention.

*Method*: Forty eligible subjects were recruited from the community to participate in this 10-session program developed by integrating Chinese cultural values into an established Western diabetes management program. Feasibility and acceptability of the program were evaluated by the percentage of participants meeting the course objectives and satisfaction with the program. Outcome measurements included the Diabetes Quality-of-Life (DQOL) survey, body weight, blood pressure, and HbA1c levels measured before, after, and 3 months after the intervention.

*Results*: Thirty-three participants completed all 10 sessions and the outcome measurements. Attrition rate was 17.5%. The majority of the participants understood the course content (75%) and identified and demonstrated various diabetes management skills (70% and 82.5%, respectively). All participants who completed the program were "very satisfied" with the program. With regard to the outcome variables, 43.6% of the participants lost more than 5 pounds and most had a reduction in blood pressure at 3 months after completion of the program. Mean HbA1c decreased from 7.11 to 6.12 postintervention. Significant improvements on the DQOL also were reported.

*Discussion*: Culturally tailored diabetes management may be effective in Chinese Americans with type 2 diabetes. Further study, with a larger sample size and a control group, is recommended.

From *Nursing Research*, *54*, 347–353. Copyright © 2005 by Lippincott Williams & Wilkins. Reprinted with permission.

Type 2 diabetes among Chinese Americans is rising. Statistics have shown that diabetes prevalence rates in the Asia-Pacific region already exceed 8% in 12 countries and areas within the region (Cockram, 2000). A study of progression to diabetes in 657 Chinese showed that the crude annual rate of progression to diabetes in participants with impaired fasting glucose was 8.38% per year (Ko, Chan, & Cockram, 2001), whereas the conversion rate in most Western countries was 1.5–13.8% per year. The prevalence of diabetes in Chinese people in Hawaii in 1993 was four times higher than in 1989 (Centers for Disease Control and Prevention, 1993; Shim, 1995).

The literature regarding obstacles to achieving optimal diabetes management in Chinese Americans indicates that traditional American diabetes management strategies remain difficult for Chinese Americans to access, largely due to language barriers, difficulty in lifestyle transitions (Fujimoto, 1996), financial constraints (Cockram, 2000), and incomplete acculturation (Jang, Lee, & Woo, 1998).

Culturally tailored interventions have been successful for diabetes management in African American and Latino adults. In a study of 23 adult African Americans, culturally competent dietary education significantly improved fat intake, HbA1c and fasting blood glucose levels, and frequency of acute care visits (Anderson-Loftin, Barnett, Sullivan, Bunn, & Tavakoli, 2002). In a prospective study (Brown, Garcia, Kouzekanani, & Hanis, 2002) of 256 Mexican Americans, culturally tailored diet, social emphasis, family participation, and cultural health beliefs were incorporated into the intervention. The intervention consisted of 52 contact hours over 12 months provided by bilingual Mexican American nurses, dietitians, and community workers. At 6 months, participants in the experimental group had significantly lower levels of HbA1c and fasting blood glucose levels (1.4% below the control group mean).

The preferred learning style of Chinese American adults is similar to other American adults, who prefer to learn by attaching meaning to their experience (Cranton, 1994) and practice (Wlodkowski, 1985). Group classes (Jiang et al., 1999) are culturally appropriate for educating Chinese adults. Various studies

---

[*]*Chen-Yen Wang* is an associate professor, and *Siu Ming Alain Chan* is a graduate student, School of Nursing and Dental Hygiene, University of Hawaii at Manoa, Honolulu.

(Arseneau, Mason, Bennett-Wood, Schwab, & Green, 1994; Gagliardino & Etchegoyen, 2001) using adult Latin Americans with type 2 diabetes have shown that participants in group classes had a significantly greater reduction in HbA1c levels than the control group who received individual consultations.

However, the literature regarding diabetes mellitus management in Chinese Americans in the United States is limited. A study of diabetes knowledge and compliance among 52 Chinese with type 2 diabetes (Chan & Molassiotis, 1999) showed no association between diabetes knowledge and compliance with treatment regimen. There was a gap between what the patients were taught and what they were doing. Strategies are needed to close this "knowledge-action gap" in this population. Therefore, the purpose of this pilot study was to assess the feasibility and acceptability of a culturally appropriate diabetes management program tailored to Chinese Americans with type 2 diabetes and to evaluate the preliminary efficacy of the interventions.

## Methods

### Theoretical Framework

The *empowerment model* guided the development of this study. The empowerment model was used to help a patient explore and develop his or her inherent ability to manage his or her life and disease (Funnell, Nwankwo, Gillard, Anderson, & Tang, 2005). The empowerment model was used in this study to provide culturally tailored diabetes management information to equip patients with the knowledge to make informed decisions regarding lifestyle choices, diabetes control, and consequences. Therefore, patients became responsible to manage diabetes in a way that best fit their lives (Funnell et al., 2005).

### Design

A single group pretest and posttest quasiexperimental design was used to meet the objectives of this study. Course content was adapted from the American Diabetes Association's Standards of Medical Care of Diabetes guidelines (American Diabetes Association, 2004).

### Setting and Sample

Forty participants were recruited from Chinese American social clubs, religious organizations, clinics, referrals from private physician offices, and newspaper advertisements. The participants had not received any organized diabetes education prior to this program. All of the participants were (a) previously diagnosed with type 2 diabetes and managing the diabetes with diet, oral hypoglycemic agents or insulin, or both, (b) 44–87 years of age, (c) residents of Hawaii, and (d) speakers of Mandarin, Cantonese, or Taiwanese. Exclusion criteria included persons who had self-reported cardiac conditions or cancer.

During the 10 weeks of the program, four sessions were offered on different days of the week to accommodate participants' schedules. The investigator and a registered nurse delivered the group sessions. A maximum of 10 persons was allowed for each session to enhance the interaction between the program leader and the participants. Information presented in each session strictly adhered to a predetermined agenda and was delivered in a standardized manner to minimize variations between different sessions.

### Feasibility and Acceptability Measures

Feasibility of this program was determined by the ability to recruit and retain participants, the ability to deliver the materials in 10 weeks, and the ability of participants to meet the in-class objectives. Ability to meet in-class objectives was assessed at the end of each lesson by skills demonstration and questions and answers; each participant used the same set of evaluation criteria. An investigator-developed tool utilizing Chinese languages was used to measure acceptability. At the 3-month follow-up interview, participants were asked to respond to three questions that served as single-item measures of their satisfaction with the culturally tailored intervention. Responding on a 5-point scale (1 = Very satisfied to 5 = Very dissatisfied), participants were asked the following questions: "In general, how satisfied were you with the culturally tailored intervention?" and "How satisfied were you with the integration of Chinese medicine, exercise, and diet into your diabetes management?" Participants were asked to offer a yes or no answer for the following question: "If you had the opportunity, would you recommend this intervention to a friend or relative?" These questions were used previously to assess patients' satisfaction with automated telephone disease management (Piette, 2000). The satisfaction scales had a Cronbach's alpha of .82.

### Outcome Measures

The Diabetes Quality of Life (DQOL) survey was administered before and immediately after the intervention program. The DQOL was originally created for the Diabetes Control and Complications Trial, but it was culturally adapted (Cheng, Tsui, Hanley, & Zinman, 1999) for an elderly Chinese population. The Chinese version of DQOL is a 42-item, multiple-choice tool with three primary scales including satisfaction, impact, and diabetes-related worry. Test-retest reliabilities of three subscales ranged from .94 to .99 (Cheng et al., 1999). Content validity (Cronbach's alpha = .76–.92) was performed with an expert panel (Cheng et al., 1999). Questions on the DQOL survey are related to diabetes management and how it affects an individual's life. A low score on the DQOL survey is indicative of high quality of life.

Glycosylated hemoglobin levels (HbA1c) were analyzed before and 3 months after the group sessions using the Metrika A1cNow test kits. Due to budget limitations, participants' HbA1c levels were not evaluated at the 10-week course completion time. The Metrika A1cNow test kit was certified by the National

Glycohemoglobin Standardization Program as a viable method in testing a client's HbA1c value (Metrika, 2003; National Glycohemoglobin Standardization Program, 2003).

Body weight was measured before, immediately after, and 3 months after the program using an upright scale in light indoor clothing to the nearest 10th of a pound. In accordance with the American Heart Association recommendations (Pickering et al., 2004), blood pressure was taken twice after sitting in a quiet room for 5 min. If the difference between two readings was larger than 2 mmHg, a third blood pressure reading was taken. Palpable obliterated pressure plus 30 mmHg was used to measure systolic blood pressure and the pressure at first heard muffling sound was used as the diastolic pressure.

*Procedures*

Human subject approval was received from the Internal Review Board of the university. Written permission of participation was obtained from each participant at the first session. Baseline data (e.g., questionnaires, HbA1c, weight, and blood pressure) were collected at the first session. Participants then participated in 10 educational sessions (once a week). Questionnaires (except demographics) and outcome measures were collected again at the end of the program and at 3 months after the program. A certified diabetes educator taught the group sessions in Mandarin, Cantonese, or Taiwanese as required by the participants. Each group session lasted for 60 min and was held at the primary investigator's clinic in Chinatown, Hawaii. The group session agenda is shown in Table 1. A monetary incentive was given to the participants at the third month follow-up visit. Handouts of lecture notes in Chinese were given to all participants. Cultural values in dietary practice, exercise, medication, and diabetes-related self-care behavior were integrated into handouts.

To facilitate effective communications for clients with low literacy skills, the investigators included hands-on activities and presented information using videos and Microsoft PowerPoint slides. Participants with low literacy were encouraged to ask questions as needed during class; however, no additional time was offered to this group, to maintain treatment integrity across all of the participants. In addition, participants were encouraged to involve their family in the learning process outside of the classroom setting. Peer-to-peer assistance was an unexpected phenomenon during the course, as participants enthusiastically helped each other to understand the course content. This type of mutual support was another way to overcome the literacy barriers.

*Dietary Education*

During the first session, the investigators introduced participants to the food guide pyramid and then explained the nature of carbohydrates and their impact on blood glucose levels. A comprehensive list of carbohydrate and nutrition content of common Chinese foods was provided for the participants; this list was intended to assist them in making appropriate food selection. In addition, a placemat printed with common Chinese food nutritional values written in Chinese, a handy nutrition guide during meal times, was offered to clients. Other Chinese-oriented tools such as rice bowls, soup bowls, and Chinese-style dining utensils were used to illustrate serving sizes. Measuring cups and spoons were given to participants to assist them with food serving measurements. A knowledge empowerment and self-determination approach was used to facilitate participants' dietary changes. Throughout the program, participants engaged in hands-on activities such as packing their own lunch boxes and measuring food serving sizes.

*Exercise*

The second component of the program was to encourage participants to develop a regular exercise routine. The energy expenditure of various types of exercise, including Taichi and Chi-gong, was discussed with the participants, which empowered them with the knowledge to select types of exercise suitable for individual conditions and interests. Tudor-Locke, Bell, Myers, Harris, Lauzon, and Rodger (2002) demonstrated that the pedometer is a valid tool in quantifying the levels of physical activities for adults with type 2 diabetes. An activity log and pedometer were provided for each participant to record their exercise quantity.

*Medication*

Medication compliance was the third focus of this program, as many participants expressed concern about medication cost, efficacy, side effects, and compatibility with other Chinese medicines. Medication cost prohibited medication compliance for some participants, as many of them were retired and lived on a limited income. To lessen participants' financial burden, they were assisted in applying to medication assistance programs from various drug manufacturers or provided drug samples if it was deemed appropriate by the program's advanced practice registered nurse. However, no changes were made to participants' medication regimens until 3 months after the classes, in order to minimize variations in data. A detailed discussion on various types of insulin and oral agents was held to assist participants in understanding the purpose, actions, and potential side effects of these medications, and ways to deal with hypoglycemia induced by medications.

*Self-care*

Chinese values were incorporated into the diabetes self-care education program. The program offered information on how to manage diabetes during sickness; the yin and yang concept was used to illustrate types of food to consume in the event of illness. Because many participants traveled to their native countries fre-

Table 1
*Objectives and Content for the Culturally Tailored Diabetes Intervention Program*

| Objectives | Content |
| --- | --- |
| 1. Verbalize understanding of this program | a) Introduce the Chinese recipe books, exercise books, and some Chinese pamphlets regarding diabetes |
| | b) Give handout in Chinese about this program |
| 2. Verbalize understanding of research findings | a) Translate the research findings into Chinese |
| | b) Application of research findings within Chinese Culture |
| | c) Ask participants to bring their favorite recipes to the next session |
| 3. Demonstrate healthy food choice | a) Explain Chinese dietary patterns with detailed analysis on the starch food group in terms of rice, noodle, yam, and dumpling |
| | b) Analyze 5 recipes brought by the participants |
| 4. Demonstrate self-monitoring blood glucose (SMBG) with accurate skills | a) Recognize the uneasiness doing self-monitoring in the Chinese |
| | b) Describe the relationship between SMBG and changes in serum glucose levels |
| | c) Ask participants to bring in information about their preferred exercise in the next session |
| 5. Verbalize benefits of exercise | a) Analyze pros and cons of 5 common Chinese exercises |
| | b) Explain the calorie utilization of each listed exercise and their relationships with blood glucose control |
| | c) Ask participants to bring in medicine taken in the next session |
| 6. Verbalize understanding of oral agents | a) Analyze pros and cons of the Chinese medicine and the Western medicine used by participants |
| | b) Ask participants to bring in a list of symptoms and complications they experienced in the next session |
| 7. Develop plans for preventing/treating diabetic complications | a) Compile symptoms and complications brought by the participants on the clipboard |
| | b) Explain the possible methods of prevention |
| | c) Help participants to develop individualized plans |
| 8. Develop plans for sick days/traveling | a) Compile the treatment plans used by the participants |
| | b) Explain the principle of handling sick days and traveling |
| 9. Verbalize plans of foot and skin care | a) Show a video on the foot/skin care and its importance |
| | b) Ask participants to bring in preferred stress management methods in the next session |
| 10. Demonstrate skills of stress management | a) Group sharing about the benefits of stress management |
| | b) Summarize the benefits of stress management |

quently, information was offered on synchronizing medications or an insulin regimen for a different time zone, managing blood glucose during flight, and converting different measurement units for blood glucose.
265  Participants were also helped to explore methods of stress management; various types of Chinese-specific activities were suggested to the participants, such as meditation, Taichi, and Chi-gong. Foot and skin care activities were demonstrated to the participants.

*Data Analysis*
270  Descriptive statistics were used to describe and summarize central tendency and variability of demographic variables. Feasibility of this culturally tailored diabetes management program was evaluated by percentages of (a) educational sessions having more than
275  85% of participants attending, (b) participants who attended all 10 educational sessions, and (c) participants who met at least 9 of the 10 class objectives. The acceptability of the culturally tailored diabetes program was determined by program satisfaction. Percentiles
280  were used to measure the variability of satisfaction and

participation rate, and mode and median were used to describe central tendency.

The DQOL was measured on an ordinal scale. Difference in total score between pretest and posttest was
285  computed with a student's $t$ test. Differences in means between pretest and posttest for each item were computed with a $t$ test of paired sample statistics with SPSS software. Study outcome measures were determined by the percentage of persons showing a decrease of
290  Hb1Ac levels, degree of weight loss in 3 months (if appropriate), and blood pressure reduction.

**Results**

The native language of most participants was Cantonese (57.6%) (Table 2). Most participants were married with a living partner (66.7%), retired (75.8%), had
295  less than $1,001 combined monthly household income (81.8%), and had an education level of high school graduate and beyond (57.6%).

Thirty-three out of the 40 recruits completed the 10-session program. The attrition rate was 17.5%. The
300  seven participants who departed cited that traveling plans were the primary reason for their inability to

complete the program. However, it was interesting to note that the seven participants who did not complete the program had all returned for the 3-month post-program evaluation appointments.

Table 2
*Frequency Distribution of Demographic Data (n = 33)*

| Demographic data | Frequency |
|---|---|
| Gender | |
| Male | 48.5% |
| Female | 51.5% |
| Length of time (years) in the United States (*n* = 33), *M (SD)* | 16.5 (9.3) |
| 1–5 years | 5.0% |
| 6–10 years | 25.0% |
| 11–20 years | 40.0% |
| 21–30 years | 22.5% |
| 31–35 years | 7.5% |
| Native language | |
| Cantonese | 57.6% |
| Mandarin | 36.4% |
| Taiwanese | 6.1% |
| Preferred medical treatment | |
| Western medicine only | 66.7% |
| Chinese medicine only | 9.1% |
| Western medicine plus Chinese medicine | 7.5% |
| Home remedies and self-treatment | 3.0% |
| Travel to home country for care | 3.5% |
| Duration of DM (years), *M (SD)* [range] | 9.03 (8.74) [1–40] |
| Age (years), *M (SD)* [range] | 68.8 (10.1) [44–87] |

*Note.* DM = diabetes management.

Upon the completion of this program, the 33 remaining participants were able to meet 4 to 10 (*M* = 8.22, *SD* = 2.18) course objectives. Most of the group members were able to demonstrate healthy food choices (82.5%), tell the benefits of frequent exercise (90%), identify ways to prevent or treat diabetes complications (82.5%), demonstrate stress management skills (70%), verbalize plans for foot and skin care (90%), and verbalize plans for diabetes self-management on sick days or during travel (70%). On the other hand, only 57.5% of the participants were able to demonstrate accurate self-monitoring of blood glucose levels, and only 55% of the group were able to verbalize understanding of oral hypoglycemic agents. According to the course evaluation, 100% of the participants were "very satisfied" with this culturally tailored diabetes program and would recommend this program to friends and family who have type 2 diabetes. Ninety-two percent of the group were "very satisfied" or "somewhat satisfied" with the Chinese-oriented course content and 8% remained neutral on this item.

Table 3 shows the participants' averages of HbA1c level, systolic blood pressure, diastolic blood pressure, and body weight at the start of the program, immediately after the intervention, and at 3 months after the program. Comparison of participants' weight revealed that 20.5% of the participants were able to lose 5 pounds or more during the course of the program, and

this increased to 43.6% 3 months after the completion of the program. About two-thirds of the participants weighed over 128 pounds at baseline, and 53.6% of them were able to lose 5 pounds or more 3 months after the program. The weight loss was greater among those in the upper-third weight class (weight >148 pounds); 71% of the participants who weighed more than 148 pounds at baseline were able to lose 5 pounds or more in 3 months. In contrast, only 12.6% of the participants reported weight gain during the program, of which only one participant was in the upper-third weight class at baseline. Body mass index (BMI) of the participants ranged 18.4–37.9 with a mean of 26.4 prior to the start of the program. At baseline, 18% of participants had a BMI less than 23 and 37% of participants had BMI more than 27. Forty-two percent of the participants had a reduction in BMI with the program; 24% of the participants achieved a BMI equal to or less than 23 at 3 months postintervention. The mean BMI reduced to 25.8 *(n* = 33; *SD* = 4.16) 3 months after the class. The mean HbA1c level decreased from 7.11 *(SD* = 1.1) to 6.12 *(SD* = 2.4) at 3 months after the completion of the program.

Table 3
*Physiological Variables of Participants (n = 33) at Baseline, at the End of Classes, and at 3 Months Following the Intervention*

| | *M (SD)* | Range |
|---|---|---|
| Weight at baseline (lbs) | 139.3 (26.7) | 77–210 |
| Weight after classes (lbs) | 122.8 (48.9) | 80–207 |
| Weight at the third month (lbs) | 121.8 (48.6) | 80–202 |
| HbA1c at baseline (%) | 7.11 (1.1) | 5.4–11.0 |
| HbA1c at the third month (%) | 6.12 (2.4) | 5.4–8.4 |
| Systolic BP at baseline (mmHg) | 131.5 (13.6) | 100–162 |
| Systolic BP after classes (mmHg) | 118.9 (42.1) | 100–160 |
| Systolic BP at 3rd month (mmHg) | 113.7 (46.2) | 100–190 |
| Diastolic BP at baseline (mmHg) | 69.4 (10.9) | 48–90 |
| Diastolic BP after classes (mmHg) | 63.4 (23.4) | 50–88 |
| Diastolic BP at 3rd month (mmHg) | 63.2 (25.9) | 50–92 |

*Note.* HbA1c was not assessed at the end of class due to study design.

## Discussion

This culturally tailored diabetes program was developed to address obstacles that prevent Chinese Americans from receiving optimal diabetes management. The results from this program confirmed that by approaching diabetes management from a culturally specific perspective, diabetes self-care can be effectively enhanced. It was hypothesized that by integrating Chinese cultural values into the diabetes regimen, there would be an improvement in compliance of Chinese Americans' self-care practices related to diabetes management. Findings of this culturally tailored diabetes management program were congruent with the outcomes of a structured group education mode, called Programa de Educación de Diabéticos No Insulinodependientes en América Latina (PEDNID-LA), used in several Latin American countries (Gagliardino & Etchegoyen, 2001). Similarities between our diabetes management program and PEDNID-LA include: (a) the interactive group method was used; (b) general concepts about type 2 diabetes and physiological changes were introduced; (c) educational materials were provided in the native language; and (d) photographs of cultural foods were used.

An important feature of this program was the language of instruction. The classes were conducted in Cantonese, Mandarin, or Taiwanese. The use of participants' native languages helped facilitate communication and the learning process. Due to the mixture of participants, some of the classes were conducted with a combination of the above languages. By coincidence, all of the Taiwanese-speaking participants were able to speak and understand Mandarin fluently, so the use of Taiwanese during class instruction was minimal. However, it was interesting to note that many participants were more open to discussions and interactions when the class consisted of only Cantonese speakers or Mandarin speakers. It appeared that a language divide existed among the participants. Some participants attended different group sessions because of a change in working hours. They still communicated openly with participants in the new group when all participants spoke the same dialect. Therefore, if resources permit, it would be optimal to set up classes based on participants' dialectical preference rather than grouping participants on their cultural background alone. Also such criteria may apply to other cultures; for example, it may be feasible to group Filipino clients based on their dialectical preference (e.g., Ilocano, Tagalog, or Visayan).

Appropriate diet selection is one of the keys to successful diabetes management. However, it is also one of the major obstacles for Chinese Americans. As mentioned previously, most of the diabetes education materials were developed for the Western cultures and the Chinese dietary habits varied greatly from their Western counterparts. Because the Chinese translation for diabetes is "sugar urine disease," many participants took the term literally and thought that they had to avoid only sweet-tasting foods. Many participants reported that their physicians instructed them to consume less rice; subsequently, some participants avoided rice but consumed other carbohydrates (e.g., noodles or buns). Hence, the dietary education component of the program emphasized the concept of carbohydrates.

In this program, participants were empowered by providing information about the nutrition content of common Chinese foods and appropriate serving sizes. The pedometer was a useful tool in encouraging participants to exercise, as evidenced by participants' enthusiasm in comparing the number of steps shown on the pedometer with their peers. This type of mutual comparison created a motivation to exercise. Findings supported previous studies in which understanding the determinants of exercise led to behavioral change (Plotnikoff, Brez, & Hotz, 2000).

Concurrent use of Western medicine and Chinese medicine to treat elevated serum blood glucose levels may affect patients' adherence in Western medicine treatments. The percentage of participants (7.5%) using Chinese medicine was slightly lower than the 9% in the study by Wai, Lan, and Donnan (1995). In 1999, percentages of Chinese Americans living in Houston and Los Angeles who used traditional Chinese clinics, used Western clinics in the United States, and traveled to the origin country for care were 25.3%, 21.3%, and 32%, respectively (Ma, 1999).

Literacy was a limitation of the study. Although informative, the handouts provided for the participants were word-intensive, which may have created a problem for those with limited literacy skills. Some of the participants hesitated in revealing their limitations in reading comprehension skills. Various studies have shown that individuals with low health literacy incur as much as four times the healthcare cost over the individuals with adequate literacy skills (AMA-MSS Community Service Committee, 2004). Hence, it was imperative for this group of participants to be able to comprehend the course content.

Another obstacle that can affect health literacy is the use of different writing systems. In general, Mainland Chinese use simplified Chinese characters, whereas clients from Taiwan and Hong Kong use traditional Chinese characters. Because most of the participants originated from Taiwan or Hong Kong, the course handouts comprised traditional Chinese characters. Fortunately, most of the participants from Mainland China were able to comprehend the course materials, as they were an older generation educated prior to the era of simplified Chinese characters. However, as Mainland China becomes the major source of Chinese immigration to the United States, it will be necessary to have simplified Chinese educational materials available.

The timing of the education sessions was another potential limitation to the study. The classes were held during a holiday season, and the seven participants who did not complete the classes left because of their travel plans. Therefore, it would be optimal to hold classes during a period with minimal holidays. In the case of the Chinese population, program coordinators should avoid holding classes during the Chinese New Year, because it is a period of frequent travel and festivities for many Chinese, which may affect the overall attendance rate and blood glucose control.

Language barriers, difficulty in lifestyle transitions (Fujimoto, 1996), financial constraints (Cockram, 2000), and incomplete acculturation (Jang, Lee, & Woo, 1998) were some of the obstacles preventing Chinese Americans from accessing optimal diabetes care. This culturally tailored diabetes education program was developed to address these concerns by integrating Eastern values into Western diabetes management strategies. Results indicated that most of the par-

ticipants were able to decrease their body weight, blood pressure, and HbA1c values. Course materials were delivered in participants' native languages. Most of the participants were able to gain knowledge about diabe-
495   tes, medications, prevention strategies, and self-care skills. Participants also formed a support network with some of their peers through this program. Results indicated that this culturally tailored diabetes management pilot study could be an effective tool in reducing the
500   health disparities in the Chinese American population.

## References

Aiken, L. H., Clarke, S. P., Cheung, R. B., Sloane, D. M., & Silber, J. H. (2003). Educational levels of hospital nurses and surgical patient mortality. *Journal of the American Medical Association, 290*, 1617–1623.

AMA-MSS Community Service Committee. (2004). *The abc's of health literacy. A proposal for the AMA-MSS 2004–2006 national service project.* Retrieved August 14, 2005, from http://www.ama-assn.org/ama1/pub/upload/mm/15/health_literacy.doc

American Diabetes Association. (2004). Standards of medical care of diabetes. *Diabetes Care, 27,* 15S–35S.

Anderson-Loftin, W., Barnett, S., Sullivan, P., Bunn, P. S., & Tavakoli, A. (2002). Culturally competent dietary education for southern rural African Americans with diabetes. *Diabetes Educator, 28*, 245–257.

Arseneau, D. L., Mason, A. C., Bennett-Wood, O., Schwab, E., & Green, D. (1994). A comparison of learning activity packages and classroom instruction for diet management of patients with NIDDM. *Diabetes Educator, 20,* 509–514.

Brown, S. A., Garcia, A. A., Kouzekanani, K., & Hanis, C. L. (2002). Culturally competent diabetes self-management education for Mexican Americans: The Starr County border health initiative. *Diabetes Care, 25,* 259–268.

Centers for Disease Control and Prevention. (1993). *Diabetes surveillance, 1991.* Washington, DC: US Government Printing Office.

Chan, Y. M., & Molassiotis, A. (1999). The relationship between diabetes knowledge and compliance among Chinese with non-insulin dependent diabetes mellitus in Hong Kong. *Journal of Advanced Nursing, 30*, 431–438.

Cheng, A. Y., Tsui, E. Y., Hanley, A. J., & Zinman, B. (1999). Cultural adaptation of the diabetes quality-of-life measure for Chinese patients. *Diabetes Care, 22*, 1216–1217.

Cockram, C. S. (2000). Diabetes mellitus: Perspective from the Asia-Pacific region. *Diabetes Research and Clinical Practice, 50* (Suppl. 2), S3–S7.

Cranton, P. (1994). *Transformative learning: A guide for educators of adults.* San Francisco, CA: Jossey-Bass.

Fujimoto, W. Y. (1996). Overview of non-insulin-dependent diabetes mellitus (NIDDM) in different population groups. *Diabetes Medicine, 13* (9 Suppl. 6), S7–S10.

Funnell, M. M., Nwankwo, R., Gillard, M. L., Anderson, R. M., & Tang, T. S. (2005). Implementing an empowerment-based diabetes self-management education program. *Diabetes Educator, 31*, 53, 55–56, 61.

Gagliardino, J. J., & Etchegoyen, G. (2001). A model educational program for people with type 2 diabetes: A cooperative Latin American implementation study (PEDNID-LA). *Diabetes Care, 24,* 1001–1007.

Jang, M., Lee, E., & Woo, K. (1998). Income, language, and citizenship status: Factors affecting the health care access and utilization of Chinese Americans. *Health & Social Work, 23*, 136–145.

Jiang, Y. D., Chuang, L. M., Wu, H. P., Shiau, S. J., Wang, C. H., Lee, Y. J., Juang, J. H., Lin, B. J., & Tai, T. Y. (1999). Assessment of the function and effect of diabetes education programs in Taiwan. *Diabetes Research and Clinical Practice, 46*, 177–182.

Ko, G. T., Chan, J. C., & Cockram, C. S. (2001). Change of glycaemic status in Chinese subjects with impaired fasting glycaemia. *Diabetic Medicine, 18,* 745–748.

Ma, G. X. (1999). Between two worlds: The use of traditional and Western health services by Chinese immigrants. *Journal of Community Health, 24,* 421–437.

Metrika, Inc. (2003). *Clinical accuracy.* Retrieved July 20, 2003, from http://www.metrika.com/3medical/accuracy.html

National Glycohemoglobin Standardization Program. (2003). *List of NGSP certified methods.* Retrieved July 22, 2003, from http://web.missouri.edu/-diabetesingsp/index.html

Pickering, T. G., Hall, J. E., Appel, L. J., Falkner, B. E., Graves, J., Hill, M. N., Jones, D. W., Kurtz, T., Sheps, S. G., Roccela, E. J. (2004). *Recommendations for blood pressure measurement in humans and experimental animals. Part 1: Blood pressure measurement in humans: A statement for professionals from the Subcommittee of Professional and Public Education of the American Heart Association Council on High Blood Pressure Research.* Retrieved February 28, 2005, from http://hyper.ahajournals.org/cgi/content/full/45/1/142

Piette, J. D. (2000). Satisfaction with automated telephone disease management calls and its relationship to their use. *Diabetes Educator, 26*, 1003–1010.

Plotnikoff, R. C., Brez, S., & Hotz, S. B. (2000). Exercise behavior in a community sample with diabetes: Understanding the determinants of exercise behavior change. *Diabetes Educator, 26*, 450–459.

Shim, M. J. (1995). *Self-reported diabetes in Hawaii* (pp. 1988–1993). Manoa, HI: University of Hawaii at Manoa.

Tudor-Locke, C. E., Bell, R. C., Myers, A. M., Harris, S. B., Lauzon, N., & Rodger, N. W. (2002). Pedometer-determined ambulatory activity in individuals with type 2 diabetes. *Diabetes Research and Clinical Practice, 55,* 191–199.

Wai, W. T., Lan, W. S., & Donnan, S. P. (1995). Prevalence and determinants of the use of traditional Chinese medicine in Hong Kong. *Asian Pacific Journal of Public Health, 8,* 167–170.

Wlodkowski, R. J. (1985). *Enhancing adult motivation to learn: A guide to improving instruction and increasing learner achievement.* San Francisco, CA: Jossey-Bass.

**Acknowledgments**: This project was funded by the University of Washington, Center for Women's Health Research (NR04001). Authors would like to give appreciation to Margaret Heitkemper, PhD, RN, FAAN, Chairperson and Professor of University of Washington, Department of Biobehavioral Nursing and Health Systems, for mentoring and finalizing this manuscript.

**Address correspondence to**: Chen-Yen Wang, PhD, APRN, CDE, 1702 Kewalo Street, Apt. 1103, Honolulu, HI 96822. E-mail: chen-wang@ hawaii.edu.

# Exercise for Article 21

## Factual Questions

1. In addition to social clubs, religious organizations, clinics, and referrals from physicians, how else were participants recruited?

2. How many questions were asked to determine participants' satisfaction with the intervention?

3. Why were the participants' HbA1c levels not evaluated at the 10-week course completion time?

4. What was the attrition rate?

5. What was the mean age of the participants?

6. Upon completion of the program, what percentage of the participants were able to demonstrate accurate self-monitoring of blood glucose skills?

7. According to the researchers, was timing of the education sessions a potential limitation of the study?

## Questions for Discussion

8. The researchers characterize their research as a "pilot study." Do you agree with this characterization? Explain. (See line 61.)

9. Potential participants who had self-reported cardiac conditions or cancer were excluded. Do you think this was appropriate? Explain. (See lines 92–94.)

10. Test-retest reliabilities for the DQOL ranged from .94 to .99. What is your understanding of the meaning of test-retest reliability? Are .94 and .99 high *or* low values? (See lines 139–141.)

11. In your opinion, is the program described in sufficient detail? (See lines 169–269.)

12. Do you agree that literacy is a limitation of this study? (See lines 444–455.)

13. If you were to conduct a follow-up evaluation of this program, would you include a control group? Why? Why not?

## Quality Ratings

Directions: Indicate your level of agreement with each of the following statements by circling a number from 5 for strongly agree (SA) to 1 for strongly disagree (SD). If you believe an item is not applicable to this research article, leave it blank. Be prepared to explain your ratings. When responding to criteria A and B, keep in mind that brief titles and abstracts are conventional in published research.

A. The title of the article is appropriate.

   SA   5   4   3   2   1   SD

B. The abstract provides an effective overview of the research article.

   SA   5   4   3   2   1   SD

C. The introduction establishes the importance of the study.

   SA   5   4   3   2   1   SD

D. The literature review establishes the context for the study.

   SA   5   4   3   2   1   SD

E. The research purpose, question, or hypothesis is clearly stated.

   SA   5   4   3   2   1   SD

F. The method of sampling is sound.

   SA   5   4   3   2   1   SD

G. Relevant demographics (for example, age, gender, and ethnicity) are described.

   SA   5   4   3   2   1   SD

H. Measurement procedures are adequate.

   SA   5   4   3   2   1   SD

I. All procedures have been described in sufficient detail to permit a replication of the study.

   SA   5   4   3   2   1   SD

J. The participants have been adequately protected from potential harm.

   SA   5   4   3   2   1   SD

K. The results are clearly described.

   SA   5   4   3   2   1   SD

L. The discussion/conclusion is appropriate.

   SA   5   4   3   2   1   SD

M. Despite any flaws, the report is worthy of publication.

   SA   5   4   3   2   1   SD

# Article 22

# Effect of a Medical-Surgical Practice and Certification Review Course on Clinical Nursing Practice

**Cindy Sayre**, MN, ARNP, **Sheri Wyant**, MSN, RN, OCN,
**Colleen Karvonen**, MN, RN, CMSRN, CWON[*]

ABSTRACT. The purpose of this study was to describe the effects of participation in a medical-surgical certification and practice review course on the participants' clinical nursing practice. A descriptive survey was mailed to 119 nurses 4 months after the completion of the 2005 course. The majority responding agreed that participation in the course had a positive effect on their self-confidence, competence, leadership, and initiative. The written clinical examples demonstrated the efficacy of the course in the domains of knowledge acquisition and validation, enhancement of confidence, and the ability to contribute to collegial discussions. These results demonstrate successful achievement of the ultimate goal of staff education: to see nurses translate newly acquired knowledge into practice.

From *Journal for Nurses in Staff Development*, 26, 11–16. Copyright © 2010 by Lippincott Williams & Wilkins. Reprinted with permission.

*Certification* has been defined as "the formal recognition of specialized knowledge, skills, and experience demonstrated by the achievement of standards identified by a nursing specialty to promote optimal
5 health outcomes" (American Board of Nursing Specialties, 2005). Nursing certification has been shown to be important for protecting the public (Cary, 2001) and distinguishing nursing practice. Certification is a means by which nurses show their commitment to patients
10 and to lifelong learning. Certification benefits the individual, the profession, and the public through promotion of quality patient care, expanded career opportunities, and increased self-esteem and satisfaction. Medical-surgical nursing certification is available
15 through the American Nurses Credentialing Center (ANCC) and the Academy of Medical Surgical Nurses.

Cary (2001) studied more than 19,000 certified nurses from across the United States and Canada. The study was the first to elucidate the perceived benefits of

20 certification as reported by nurses who were certified. Some of the benefits that were cited include "feeling more confident in my ability to detect early signs and symptoms of complications in my patients" and being able to "initiate early and prompt interventions for pa-
25 tients experiencing complications." An interesting finding was that the nurses who were most recently certified reported the greatest changes to their practice. Cary stated that these findings "provide initial evidence that certification may give nurses the means or oppor-
30 tunity to practice in a manner likely to improve outcomes."

Nurse educators and clinical nurse specialists at an academic medical center were interested in enhancing nursing practice for medical-surgical nurses and poten-
35 tially improving patient outcomes. A 14-week medical-surgical certification and practice review course has been offered at the medical center since 2002. The course consists of 14 sessions, each lasting 3 hours. The classes include content from the core curriculum
40 provided by the certifying bodies (see Table 1). The classes are didactic in format, with a 2- to 3-hour lecture and a facilitated test-taking session. Supplemental online content is available for participants, including steps on applying for certification, nursing process,
45 test-taking tips, research and quality improvement, discharge planning, and domestic violence. Participants are encouraged to share a written summary of a clinical example(s) that demonstrates the application of content from the class to a clinical event(s). The examples
50 might include an event where the nurse believes that the intervention(s) really made a difference in a patient's outcome, an "aha!" experience, or the application of critical thinking to a complex case. Some clinical examples are shared each week with all the partici-
55 pating sites.

---
[*]*Cindy Sayre*, MN, ARNP, is medical-surgical clinical nurse specialist, Patient Care Services, University of Washington Medical Center, Seattle, Washington and currently director of Professional Practice and Patient and Family Centered Care, University of Washington Medical Center. *Sheri Wyant*, MSN, RN, OCN, is pain management clinical nurse specialist, Patient Care Services, University of Washington Medical Center, Seattle, Washington. *Colleen Karvonen*, MN, RN, CMSRN, CWON, is wound ostomy clinical nurse specialist, Patient Care Services, University of Washington Medical Center, Seattle, Washington.

Table 1
*Content of the 14-Week Medical-Surgical Certification and Practice Review Course*

| Week | Content |
|------|---------|
| 1 | Fluid/electrolytes/acid/base |
| 2 | Wound care |
| 3 | Nursing process, ethical/legal issues/cultural competency |
| 4 | Cardiovascular impairment |
| 5 | Renal system |
| 6 | Hematology |
| 7 | Neurological impairment |
| 8 | Gastrointestinal disorders |
| 9 | Caring for older adults research/QA/QI |
| 10 | Endocrine disorders |
| 11 | Respiratory impairment |
| 12 | Arthritis/immobility |
| 13 | Pain/HIV |
| 14 | Psychosocial nursing |

*Note.* QA = quality assurance; QI = quality improvement.

Further details about the course development are described in a previous article (Karvonen, Sayre, & Wyant, 2004). In 2005, in collaboration with the continuing nursing education department of the University of Washington School of Nursing, the course was expanded to include six sites from Washington and Alaska via videoconferencing. A total of 146 participants from all the sites were enrolled in the course. One hundred nineteen (82%) successfully completed the course. Participating sites were facilitated by an agency coordinator. Agency coordinators are educators and certified nurses who received additional training from the course planners. The agency coordinators meet for a full-day training session annually. One of the topics discussed is mentoring or coaching. For the purposes of this program, mentoring is understood to be a time-limited relationship wherein the coordinator assists the participant to identify potential barriers to success and collaborates with the participant in making a plan to address the barriers. Both the agency coordinator workshop and the medical-surgical certification and practice review course were supported in part by funds from a training grant from the Division of Nursing, Bureau of Health Professions, Health Resources and Services Administration, Department of Health and Human Services.

The national certification examination pass rate for participants from the 2005 medical-surgical certification and practice review course was 86%. Statistics provided by the ANCC demonstrate a national pass rate of 71.7% for all baccalaureate-level and higher-level specialty examinations combined and 64.6% for all diploma- and associate-degree-level specialty examinations combined. Statistics were not available from the Academy of Medical Surgical Nurses. Anonymous demographic data were collected from the course participants on the first day of class. The collected demographic data are summarized in Table 2.

In previous years, participants described unanticipated benefits from the course, such as enhanced self-confidence, competence, and initiative. Course facilitators also noted enhanced leadership qualities in those who participated. For the purposes of this study, participants were asked to reflect on the impact of the course on their self-confidence, competence, leadership, and initiative.

Table 2
*Demographic Data of Course Registrants*

| Demographics | n |
|--------------|---|
| Practice setting | |
| Urban | 109 |
| Rural | 5 |
| Type of setting | |
| Hospital | 108 |
| Clinic | 13 |
| Other | 11 |
| Gender | |
| Male | 10 |
| Female | 114 |
| Years in clinical practice | |
| Less than 1 | 1 |
| 1–5 | 41 |
| 6–10 | 22 |
| 11–20 | 28 |
| More than 20 | 29 |
| Primary position | |
| Staff nurse | 104 |
| Nurse educator | 4 |
| Administrator/manager | 1 |
| Clinical nurse specialist | 8 |
| Other | 7 |
| Highest degree | |
| Associate | 38 |
| Diploma | 12 |
| Baccalaureate | 65 |
| Master's | 7 |
| Doctorate | 1 |
| Heritage | |
| American Indian or Alaska Native | 11 |
| Black or African American | 9 |
| Hispanic/Latino | 5 |
| Asian | 17 |
| Native Hawaiian or Pacific Islander | 2 |
| White | 88 |

## Review of the Literature

Nursing certification has been shown to have many potential benefits, including personal and professional growth, professional recognition, and increased opportunity for career advancement (Cary, 2001; Prowant et al., 2007). The four benefits selected for this study included the qualities of self-confidence, competence, leadership, and initiative. A review of the literature to identify standardized definitions for each of the qualities was completed.

*Self-confidence* is defined for the purpose of this study as the belief in yourself that you know what to do to provide nursing care. A literature review did not reveal any standardized definitions of self-confidence in nursing. Many articles interchange the terms *self-confidence* and *self-efficacy*. Bandura (1986) defined *perceived self-efficacy* as a belief in one's capabilities to organize and execute the course of action required to

attain a goal. The underlying premise of self-efficacy is
120 self-regulation of behavior by cognitive, affective, and
motivational processes. Bandura's *self-efficacy* construct includes a broader scope of behavior than that of
the term *self-confidence*. Several self-confidence scales
are reported in the literature, but none is specific to the
125 content of interest for this study.

*Competence* is defined in the dictionary (http://
dictionary.reference.com/browse/competence) as pos-
session of required skill, knowledge, qualification, or
capacity to perform a certain task. It can encompass
130 one's knowledge, skills, and behaviors. *Nursing competence* was defined for this study as being "effective,
capable and skilled to provide nursing care." This definition is consistent with del Bueno's (2001) definition
of *competence*: the "ability to meet job expectations
135 and subsequent continuous effective care for assigned
patients."

*Leadership* is defined as the ability to positively influence others in the provision of patient care. This
definition is consistent with Cook's (1999) definition
140 of a *leader* as "an expert clinician, involved in providing direct clinical care, who influences others to continuously improve the care they provide."

*Initiative* is defined as the power to begin a process
to improve patient care. Initiative allows an individual
145 to identify problems and implement solutions. A literature review did not reveal any standardized definitions
of initiative. Anecdotal examples from students in the
review course include the following: A nurse in the
2004 class decided to learn dialysis after taking the
150 course; prior to the class, she did not think she could do
it. In the 2005 class, a nurse helped change a standardized order set after learning about the indications for
the various IV fluids.

## Methodology

### Survey

A research proposal was submitted and approved
155 by the institutional review board. A descriptive survey
was developed and reviewed by expert medical-
surgical nurses for face validity.

The survey tool included two sections: a 5-point
Likert scale and an open-ended question. Participants
160 were asked to read the definitions for each domain provided (see Table 3) and to rate the degree to which the
course affected their medical-surgical nursing practice
using the definitions for *self-confidence, competence,
leadership,* and *initiative.*

165 The second section of the survey was structured to
elicit a written example of the impact of the course on
nurses' medical-surgical nursing practice. The survey
included this question: "Provide a brief example of
how your participation in the medical-surgical cer-
170 tification review has affected your medical-surgical
nursing practice." Space was provided for the participants to write their responses, including the back of the
survey page.

### Sample

The sample was composed of registered nurses
175 ($n = 119$) who completed $\geq 80\%$ of the review course
offered in 2005. These nurses were employed in the
states of Washington and Alaska.

### Method

An anonymous survey including an introduction
cover letter was mailed 4 months after the conclusion
180 of the course to all course participants who completed
80% or more of the course. A follow-up reminder letter
was sent 2 weeks later. The surveys were mailed back
to a central nursing office, where an administrative
staff member not associated with the study opened
185 them. The surveys were placed in a blank envelope for
the researchers.

Table 3
*2005 Medical-Surgical Review Course Questionnaire*

Read the definitions for each of the following concepts.

**Self-confidence**: the belief in yourself that you know what to do to provide nursing care.

**Competence**: being effective, capable, and skilled to provide nursing care.

**Leadership**: the ability to positively influence others in the provision of patient care.

**Initiative**: the power to begin a process to improve patient care.

Using the definitions above, circle the number that best represents your response to the following statement:
"Participation in the medical-surgical certification review course had a positive effect on my **medical-surgical nursing practice** in the following areas":

| Concept | Strongly disagree | Disagree | Neutral: no effect | Agree | Strongly agree |
|---|---|---|---|---|---|
| Self-confidence | 1 | 2 | 3 | 4 | 5 |
| Competence | 1 | 2 | 3 | 4 | 5 |
| Leadership | 1 | 2 | 3 | 4 | 5 |
| Initiative | 1 | 2 | 3 | 4 | 5 |

*Data Analysis*

The Likert-scale data were summarized using percentage of response for each concept. The written examples were analyzed using content analysis. Downe-Wamboldt (1992) described the content analysis research method as generally encompassing the following with the goal of external validity: selecting the unit of analysis, creating and defining categories, pretesting the category definitions/rules, assessing reliability and validity, revising the coding rules as needed, pretesting the revised categories, coding the data, and reassessing reliability and validity. All of the written examples were reviewed by the researchers to identify mutually exclusive themes (entire ideas or thoughts). A set of rules for classification of the themes into categories was developed and tested on a sample of written responses by the researchers and revised. The researchers then used the revised rules to independently code the data. In addition, another nurse researcher, skilled in qualitative research methodologies and content analysis, was asked to participate in the coding process. Comparison of results demonstrated strong agreement (100%) between the coders with both the second and third rating rounds.

## Results

Surveys were returned by 39 of the 119 nurses sampled, representing a 33% return rate. Thirty-eight nurses responded to the Likert scale question, "Participation in the medical-surgical certification review course had a positive effect on my medical-surgical nursing practice in the following areas: self-confidence, competence, leadership, and initiative."

Survey results demonstrated a positive effect on the nurses' self-confidence (87%), competence (82%), leadership (60%), and initiative (82%). Seventy-six percent of participants agreed that the course positively affected all four qualities. Five of the participants (13%) *strongly agreed* that they experienced a positive effect on their medical-surgical practice for all four concepts.

Three participants responded that the course had *no effect* on the four domains tested. One participant *disagreed* that participation in the course had a positive effect on competence and leadership. This same respondent *agreed* that the course had a positive effect on initiative.

Using content analysis as described by Downe-Wamboldt (1992), the written exemplars were rank ordered into seven theme categories (see Table 4).

The exemplars demonstrated the efficacy of the course in the domains of knowledge acquisition and validation, enhancement of confidence, and the ability to contribute to collegial discussions. Nurses became a resource for their peers and were inspired to strive for more. Some, however, remained unconvinced about the benefits of certification.

Table 4
*Rank-Ordered Themes and Percentages of Responses*

| Rank-ordered themes | % | Quotes from written examples |
|---|---|---|
| Boosted my confidence | 25 | "I feel that I got reinforcement of and deeper knowledge in all areas of nursing. This has improved critical thinking for me, increasing self-confidence." |
| I learned something new | 20 | "After class, nurses and I would discuss new stuff we learned and I could see us applying the new 'pearls of wisdom.'" |
| I became a resource, a nurse among nurses | 16 | "...this habit of articulating rationales has caused me to become an informal resource among coworkers." |
| I knew more than I thought I did | 11 | "I had validation of my prior skills through the course in addition to new knowledge." |
| I am better able to contribute to collegial conversations | 10 | "I had a patient who had a dramatic change in respiratory status and vital signs. Came to my mind right away that this could be a P.E. Collaborated with team surgery. Tests were done (CT scan) and patient was transferred to ICU." |
| Inspired me to strive for more | 9 | "I feel this course was very effective in increasing my initiative to improve patient care." |
| I am still not convinced about the need for certification | 9 | "I do not agree strongly if you'll mandate certification." |
| | | "Licensure and the daily nursing experience and my patients' satisfaction with my care make me whole. Every day is a learning experience." |

## Discussion

Survey results are consistent with the previous findings of Cary and Prowant et al. The study found that nurses who prepared for certification reported both increased confidence and increased competence in their
245 role as nurses. This led to enhanced collaboration, which has been found to improve patient outcomes (Baggs, 1992). Survey comments such as, "The course broadened my knowledge base, I am more willing to participate in troubleshooting with doctors and fellow
250 co-workers" and "The med–surg course improved my competence and in turn helped me be a better nurse and give better care to my patients," speak clearly of the impact of the course. A clinical example shared during the course exemplifying this is the following:

255 Following the neurology session, I had a patient post stroke with elevated blood pressure. The nurse I got [the] report from did not understand why the parameters for giving hydralazine were so high. I was able to use the information from this class to explain why they wanted her
260 blood pressure to be higher than normal and to have a much better understanding of her care issues.

### Limitations

It could be argued that the nurses in the study were a motivated group based on their commitment to taking on and completing at least 80% of a 14-week certifica-
265 tion review course. Therefore, these participants may have grown personally and professionally even with a different review model. In addition, the mentoring and coaching that participants received as individuals and as a group may have contributed to their success. The
270 effect of mentoring and coaching was not studied. As the course progressed, so did the sense of community within the group. This may have affected the participants but was not studied. Some of the participants were mandated by employers to complete the course,
275 which may have affected their overall level of satisfaction with the course. Finally, content analysis methodology is limited to only the written communication provided, and there are limited types of statistical analysis that may be applied to the data.

### Conclusion

280 Participation in the medical-surgical certification review course had a positive effect on medical-surgical nursing practice for the concepts of self-confidence, competence, leadership, and initiative for most participants responding to the survey. These results demon-
285 strate successful achievement of the ultimate goal of staff education to see nurses translate newly acquired knowledge into practice, thus enhancing the quality of patient care.

### References

American Board of Nursing Specialties. (2005). *Position statement on the value of specialty nursing certification.* Retrieved June 9, 2008, from http://www.nursingcertification.org/position_statements.htm

Baggs, J. G. (1992). The association between interdisciplinary collaboration and patient outcomes in a medical intensive care unit. *Heart & Lung, 21*(1), 18–24.

Bandura, A. (1986). *Social foundations of thought and action: A social cognitive theory.* Englewood Cliffs, NJ: Prentice-Hall.

Cary, A. H. (2001). Certified registered nurses: Results of the study of the certified workforce. *American Journal of Nursing, 101*(1), 44–52.

Cook, M. J. (1999). Improving care requires leadership in nursing. *Nurse Education Today, 19*(4), 306–312.

del Bueno, D. J. (2001). Buyer beware: The cost of competence. *Nursing Economic$, 19*(6), 250–257.

*Dictionary.com Unabridged. (v 1.1).* Retrieved November 02, 2004, from Dictionary.com Web site: http://dictionary.reference.com/browse/competence

Downe-Wamboldt, B. (1992). Content analysis: Method, applications, and issues. *Health Care for Women International, 13*(3), 313–321.

Karvonen, C., Sayre, C., Wyant, S. (2004). Building a medical surgical certification review course: A blueprint for success. *Journal for Nurses in Staff Development, 20*(5), 213–218.

Prowant, B. F., Niebuhr, B., & Biel, M. (2007). Perceived value of nursing certification—summary of a national survey. *Nephrology Nursing Journal, 34*(4), 399–402.

**Acknowledgments:** The authors wish to thank to Kristen Swanson, PhD, RN, FAAN, and Elizabeth Bridges, PhD, RN, CCNS, for their assistance with data analysis. This research was made possible by Grant D11HP03123-01-00, "Expanded Practice in Medical-Surgical Nursing," Division of Nursing, Bureau of Health Professions, Health Resources and Services Administration, Department of Health and Human Services.

**Address correspondence to:** Cindy Sayre, MN, ARNP, Patient Care Services, University of Washington Medical Center, 1959 NE Pacific Ave, Seattle, WA 98195. E-mail: casayre@u.washington.edu

# Exercise for Article 22

## Factual Questions

1. How many of the course registrants were Asian?

2. The second section of the survey questionnaire was structured to elicit what?

3. The survey was mailed to participants who completed at least what percentage of the course?

4. When was a follow-up reminder letter sent?

5. What was the return rate?

6. What percentage of participants endorsed the theme of boosting confidence?

## Questions for Discussion

7. In your opinion, is the review course described in sufficient detail? Explain. (See lines 37–55 and Table 1.)

8. What is your understanding of the meaning of the term "face validity"? (See lines 155–157.)

9. Do you think it was a good idea to use an anonymous survey? Explain. (See lines 178–186.)

10. Do you think the method of data analysis is described in sufficient detail? Explain. (See lines 187–209.)

11. To what extent does Table 4 help you understand the results of this study?

12. In future studies of this type, would you recommend including a control group? Explain.

## Quality Ratings

Directions: Indicate your level of agreement with each of the following statements by circling a number from 5 for strongly agree (SA) to 1 for strongly disagree (SD). If you believe an item is not applicable to this research article, leave it blank. Be prepared to explain your ratings. When responding to criteria A and B, keep in mind that brief titles and abstracts are conventional in published research.

A.  The title of the article is appropriate.

    SA   5   4   3   2   1   SD

B.  The abstract provides an effective overview of the research article.

    SA   5   4   3   2   1   SD

C.  The introduction establishes the importance of the study.

    SA   5   4   3   2   1   SD

D.  The literature review establishes the context for the study.

    SA   5   4   3   2   1   SD

E.  The research purpose, question, or hypothesis is clearly stated.

    SA   5   4   3   2   1   SD

F.  The method of sampling is sound.

    SA   5   4   3   2   1   SD

G.  Relevant demographics (for example, age, gender, and ethnicity) are described.

    SA   5   4   3   2   1   SD

H.  Measurement procedures are adequate.

    SA   5   4   3   2   1   SD

I.  All procedures have been described in sufficient detail to permit a replication of the study.

    SA   5   4   3   2   1   SD

J.  The participants have been adequately protected from potential harm.

    SA   5   4   3   2   1   SD

K.  The results are clearly described.

    SA   5   4   3   2   1   SD

L.  The discussion/conclusion is appropriate.

    SA   5   4   3   2   1   SD

M.  Despite any flaws, the report is worthy of publication.

    SA   5   4   3   2   1   SD

# Article 23

# HIV Medication Adherence Programs: The Importance of Social Support

**Jean M. Breny Bontempi**, PhD, MPH, **Laura Burleson**, MPH, **Melissa Hofilena Lopez**, MPH[*]

ABSTRACT. Since the advent of medical treatments for HIV, the promotion of adherence to these difficult treatment regimens has proven critical to disease management. Three Connecticut state-funded HIV medication adherence programs were evaluated. The purpose of this process evaluation was to explore and compare the goals and modality of each adherence program, assess client and staff satisfaction, and provide recommendations for the improvement of these programs.

Focus group interviews with clients and individual interviews with staff were conducted at each of the programs. Interviews were transcribed, coded, and analyzed with a code-and-retrieve method of theme identification. Focus group themes included the importance of social support on medication adherence and the "lifesaving" effect the program has had. The staff expressed that although complete adherence should be the long-term objective, more intermediate objectives should be considered (e.g., behavioral changes to increase clients' ability, self-esteem, and self-efficacy to take medications).

Along with success of prolonging life with new combination therapies for HIV comes the worry of adherence and the maintenance of a high quality of life while these medications are taken (Chesney, Morin, & Sherr, 2000). This aspiration is something that challenges health care professionals, patients, and persons involved with patients who are infected with HIV. Because HIV can now be managed as a long-term and chronic disease due to advances in pharmacotherapy, it is important to evaluate the effectiveness of public health interventions geared toward the control of the disease in infected persons (Chesney, 2003).

HIV therapy is complex. There are different characteristics of the treatment regimen to consider that may affect medication adherence; these include the number of medications, the frequency of dosing, the complexity of the schedule, the duration of the therapy, and side effects (Chesney, 2003; Friedland & Williams, 1999). It is not uncommon for a lifelong treatment regimen to include four to five different drugs at any one time (Frank & Miramontes, 1999). Scheduling complex regimens into daily activities is a problem that persons infected with HIV have discussed in relation to antiretroviral adherence (Golin, Isasi, Breny Bontempi, & Eng, 2002). Because of this, it is understandable that medication adherence programs are constantly reinventing themselves to strive for interventions that will result in 100% adherence among their clients.

The evaluation of adherence programs allows planners to identify areas that need improvement to increase adherence behaviors. The types of evaluation that are used in HIV medication adherence programs are varied. Reports on the progress of the programs include participation rates; biological markers, such as viral load and measurements of healthy white blood cells (or CD4 counts); patient reports; and patient satisfaction measures. Strategies for obtaining evaluation information include pill counts, patient interviews and focus groups, and, in the case of some hospital interventions, chart review and the number of clinic appointments kept (Chesney et al., 2000).

These strategies are in line with impact and outcome program evaluation, which shows the success (or failure) of a program by the examination of intermediate (impact) or long-term (outcome) measures of adherence. Although these evaluation procedures provide important information, why a given program has such outcomes is not clear. A process evaluation can answer the question of why program outcomes were (or were not) realized and is recognized as a critical part of program design and evaluation (Steckler & Linnan, 2002).

This article presents the results of a process evaluation conducted of three state-funded HIV medication adherence programs in Connecticut. The evaluation took place over the course of 1 year, between February 2001 and January 2002. The methods, results, and recommendations for the adherence programs are presented here.

[*]*Jean M. Breny Bontempi*, Department of Public Health, Southern Connecticut State University. *Laura Burleson*, Department of Community Health, Brown University. *Melissa Hofilena Lopez*, Connecticut Department of Public Health.

Table 1
*Summary of Determinants of and Challenges to Program Success*

| Programs | Determinants | Challenges |
|---|---|---|
| Atlas | • Conducts individual assessments on all clients.<br>• Located in a medical setting. | • Staff turnover in past year. |
| Crossroads | • Uses behavior change framework as an approach to increase adherence.<br>• Conducts individual assessments on all clients.<br>• Located in a medical setting. | • Overburdened staff because of a large number of clients. |
| La Familia | • Conducts individual assessments on all clients.<br>• Covers large geographic area and serves large Hispanic population.<br>• Community-based setting. | • Difficulty accessing medical data.<br>• Overburdened staff because of a large number of clients spread across a large geographic area. |

## Description of Program Strategies

Three HIV medication adherence programs were
60  evaluated for this article; they are referred to here as
Atlas, Crossroads, and La Familia. To protect anonymity, the real names of programs, staff, and locations
were changed. All three programs were located in metropolitan areas of Connecticut, and because they were
65  state funded, they were each required to follow a protocol developed by the Connecticut Department of
Public Health (DPH). Although the overall goal identified by each program was identical (i.e., to improve
HIV medication adherence), the methods used to
70  achieve this goal were diverse and, hence, too varied to
compare across programs. Each program staff developed its intervention methods on the basis of what it
thought could best achieve adherence among its own
group of clients. The unique aspects of the program
75  methods are described here. Although this evaluation
was not for the purpose of measuring the outcomes of
these programs, we briefly highlight the diversity
across the programs with regard to their stated outcomes, intervention methods, and processes of collect-
80  ing data to measure program success. A summary table
of the determinants of and challenges to the programs'
success is provided (see Table 1).

*Atlas*

The Atlas medication adherence program used a
home care approach to facilitate medication adherence.
85  Strategies used included an in-depth assessment of
each client, the prefilling of pill boxes for clients, and
comprehensive education with regard to the HIV disease process and medications. The program visiting
nurse used HIV viral load and CD4 counts to evaluate
90  the success of the program.

*Crossroads*

Crossroads was a hospital-based program situated
within an infectious disease clinic where medications
were also distributed. Unlike the other programs evaluated, the clients had the ability to meet and schedule
95  appointments with their infectious disease provider at

the same site. Staff for this adherence program included an adherence counselor (a Registered Nurse)
and a treatment advocate (an Advanced Practice Registered Nurse). The Crossroads medication adherence
100  program used a behavior change model (with a focus
on information, motivation, skill building, and behavioral change) as a framework for the program. This
program had as its goal a decrease in viral load because
of medication adherence. Strategies used within the
105  framework to foster medication adherence included
education, motivational techniques, and skill building.
Specific goals relative to these strategies were identified individually for each client.

*La Familia*

The La Familia program was an HIV treatment ad-
110  vocacy program serving Hispanic clients in the community. The program had three goals for its adherence
program:

  • To foster independence in each client.
  • To have each client realize the importance of
115  medication adherence.
  • To keep clients healthy and avoid hospitalization.

The staff included a monolingual nurse and a bilingual
treatment advocate. An individualized approach was
120  used with each client, and a visit plan was set up after
the initial visit. The strategies used were home visits,
medication prepours, education and teaching about the
importance of medication adherence, and referrals to
appropriate social service agencies. Evaluation meth-
125  ods included the presence of improved viral load and
CD4 counts and the checking of medicine boxes or
necessary refills on individual medications.

## Method

The three aims of this process evaluation were to
(a) explore and compare the goals and modalities of
130  each program, (b) assess client and staff satisfaction,
and (c) provide recommendations for the improvement
of current programs. Through a competitive bid process, our evaluation team was hired to conduct this pro-

Table 2
*Data Collection Overview*

| Data collection method | Data source |
| --- | --- |
| Focus groups | • Sample of clients from two state-funded programs. |
| Interviews | • Two staff persons of state-funded programs.<br>• Department of Public Health staff for overall goals of programs. |
| Secondary data | • Client data collected at all three state-funded programs.<br>• Quarterly reports from all three programs.<br>• Independent evaluation of one state-funded program. |

gram evaluation and met quarterly with an HIV Medi-
135  cation Advisory Committee at the Connecticut State
DPH for guidance and clarification of the evaluation
focus.

To explore and compare program modalities, data
were collected from the DPH and medication adher-
140  ence program staff with regard to the goals, methods,
and reporting mechanisms of each program. The ex-
trapolation of medical data on individual clients was
also completed through the review of medical charts.
Client and staff satisfaction were assessed through in-
145  depth qualitative research methods. Table 2 shows an
overview of the collected data.

Qualitative process evaluation methods were used
to explore the goals and modalities of each adherence
program, to assess client and staff satisfaction, and to
150  provide recommendations for improving programs.
Focus group interviews were conducted with the clients, and individual interviews were conducted with
the staff from each of these programs.

*Focus Groups*

The evaluation team conducted focus groups with
155  clients from two of the adherence programs. The results from an independent focus group with the third
program were used in this evaluation. The recruitment
of focus groups was done by the program staff, who
invited all their clients to attend the focus groups, in-
160  forming them of the length of time of the group, the
topics that would be covered, and that each participant
would be paid $25.00 for their participation.

Semistructured focus group guides were developed.
These guides provided a logical sequence of question-
165  ing and open-ended questions, making it possible to
obtain deeper and richer information. Focus groups
were staffed by both a moderator and a note taker. The
role of the moderator was to facilitate the discussion
around the questions of the focus group guide. The
170  note taker's role was to assist the moderator with follow-up questions and to take notes for the transcription
of the focus group tape. The identities of the focus
group participants were kept anonymous. Focus groups
lasted approximately 2 hr.

*Staff Interviews*

175  Staff interviews were conducted with the primary
medication adherence staff person from each program.

Interviews were tape-recorded. Staff were asked about
their satisfaction with the program, their program's
goals, and what improvements they felt could be made
180  to their program.

*Data Analysis*

Each focus group and interview tape was transcribed verbatim. The transcribed data were entered
into the qualitative analysis software package QSR
NVivo for an analysis of the themes. Three coders (the
185  principal investigator and two research assistants) conducted a content analysis of the transcripts with the
open-coding technique to examine conceptual patterns,
or themes, in the text. To ensure accuracy in the content analysis, the transcripts were read and coded sepa-
190  rately by the three coders, who then compared and revised the coding scheme. Specifically, concepts that
were salient and repeated in the text were identified
and used as codes to organize the text into categories.
QSR NVivo was used to organize, code, and translate
195  the data into the results for this evaluation.

*Human Participants' Approval*

Before data collection, all of the consent forms and
focus group and interview questions were included in
an application submitted to the Institutional Review
Board for Human Subject Research at Southern Con-
200  necticut State University. Data collection began on
approval from the Institutional Review Board.

All the focus group participants were asked to read
and sign a consent form before the start of data collection. Any member of the focus groups needing assis-
205  tance with reading the consent form had it read to
them. Each participant received a copy of the consent
form.

**Results**

*Focus Groups*

A total of 14 participants participated in the two focus groups we conducted, and 15 participants took part
210  in the independent focus group with the third program
(More, 2002). These numbers represented approximately 20% of program clients at the time of the focus
groups. Across all three of the focus groups, participants included 9 women and 20 men; 22 were His-
215  panic, 6 were African American, and 1 was White. All

the focus groups were conducted at the program's primary site.

Four themes emerged from the focus groups with regard to program satisfaction and needed improvements. They were (a) the provision of emotional and social support, (b) the provision of education on medication, (c) the need for staff to liaise between clients and medical providers, and (d) additional needs not currently being met. There was much discussion in the focus groups about adherence issues related to side effects of the medications; however, this was beyond the scope of this article.

Clients stated several ways in which their participation in the program had been helpful to them both personally and in taking their medications. Across all focus groups, clients spoke specifically about the adherence program nurses when talking about the program. There was not one comment made with regard to the program that was not specifically about the nurse. Comments about the program staff were always positive.

There was an overwhelmingly positive response to the adherence programs and staff. Clients stated that participation in the program had increased their knowledge about their HIV medications; provided them assistance with reminders to take medications; increased their social support, self-esteem, and self-confidence; and provided hope and encouragement that they would continue living. Nonadherence to medication, doctor referral, financial status, and need for support were all stated as reasons for being in the programs. Discussion around reasons for being in the adherence program initiated further dialogue on medication barriers, including side effects and forgetting to take medications.

Additionally, the La Familia evaluation included a survey with two foci: to determine the efficacy of the medication adherence program implementation and to examine variables that correlated with effective adherence to antiretroviral medication (More, 2002). With regard to client satisfaction, respondents were asked to rate the importance they gave to the kinds of support they received. Five respondents rated the medication adherence counselor to be "extremely important" to their adherence, whereas other supports included providers, family, and other professionals. "Primary care" and "respect" were noted by clients as the most critical issues influencing medication adherence (More, 2002).

*Provision of social support and trust.* The ways in which the adherence program nurses had been helpful to clients were many and included the provision of social support, instilling of trust, and provision of positive reinforcement. Focus group participants emphasized that the nurses were always available to them and that their contact with the nurses was among the most beneficial aspects of their participation in the program. Participants stressed that they had come to rely on the nurses' visits and phone calls and needed their continued support in living with HIV.

One participant stated, "They [the nurses] take care of me. I love the people; they go to your home, like they're my friends. Every time they say, how are you doing? Do you need anything?" Another said, "I felt so alone. It's nice to know that somebody does understand what it is all about and you can depend on that person."

Participants in the focus groups expressed many competing life issues that had previously acted as barriers in their medication adherence. These life issues included drug and alcohol abuse, insufficient housing, unhealthy interpersonal relationships, unemployment, financial constraints, poor nutrition, and the experience of stigma because of their HIV status. Either through direct support or referring support, program staff assisted clients in taking their medications by targeting each of these life issues. This attention to these other competing life issues was a significant benefit of the adherence programs according to focus group participants.

Further highlighting the importance and appreciation of social support, we asked the focus group members about their attendance in the focus group. Sentiment among focus group participants was that talking in groups about their medication adherence experiences was very helpful. Some participants were active members of support groups, whereas others were looking for groups to join.

*Provision of education on medication.* Education about the benefits and side effects of the medications, the provision of clear instruction and tools to assist with adherence, clarification of confusing drug regimens, and the reduction of information overload from medical providers were key elements of the adherence programs. With regard to the clarification of the adherence regimen, one client stated, "[Name of nurse] really walked me through it. Today I stand a little stronger. And I'm grateful because many things were shot to me all at once and [Name of nurse] has helped me to digest it little by little and has helped me understand."

Others expressed that the nurses keep them honest by being persistent in asking about missed doses. "[Name of nurse] snagged me one time I stopped taking the meds and I took the blood test and she goes, 'Have you been taking your meds?' and I said 'Yes.' She said, 'You sure you've been taking it? Because we got the blood back and there is no trace of it.'" This participant went on to explain that her adherence improved because of this.

*Staff as liaison.* The adherence nurse serving as "a close tie to the doctor" was important to patients and helped them adhere to their medications. Adherence program nurses assisted clients by either talking to providers for them or encouraging them to ask questions of their doctors. This tie to the medical providers allowed patients to feel more empowered about their medication regimen and gave them a sense of control over their destiny.

*Additional needs.* Clients stressed the importance of the role of adherence program nurses to their adherence success. They expressed concern about burnout among the staff and suggested that more staff be hired to continue to provide the program services. Other improvements suggested by focus group participants included increasing staff visits to more than weekly, having programs provide more referral information, increasing the availability of protection for sexually active clients, and improving access to food and housing. Additional needs mentioned by clients included increasing access to reminder devices, such as beepers and pill boxes.

*Staff Interviews*

Across the two interviews, three common themes emerged. They were (a) program aspects of success, (b) the provision of social and emotional support, and (c) nurses acting as a liaison for their clients.

*Program aspects of success.* The staff interviewed stated that the overall program goal was total adherence to medication. This included reducing viral load, increasing CD4 counts, and decreasing missed doses and appointments. Additional patient-specific goals were described, including increasing patient knowledge about HIV medications, increasing self-empowerment to take medications, and changing individual client behavior to increase adherence. In one staff interview, the adherence program nurse stated, "The goal for me of course would be total adherence. The reality is that I don't think that's going to happen. But I would say even to achieve between 80 and 90% adherence and education, that's a large goal of this program and self-empowerment, too." Both of the program adherence nurses stated that although total medication adherence should be the long-term objective, more immediate objectives should be measured, including individual behavioral changes that would increase clients' ability, self-esteem, and self-efficacy to take their medications.

The adherence nurses stated that they felt their programs were meeting the goals, so stated by one interviewee, "If one patient has benefited, then the program is meeting its goal." Although there was not 100% adherence among all clients, other aspects of improvement showed that goals were being met.

Both of the staffs interviewed expressed feelings of satisfaction and success with their respective medication adherence programs. Quarterly adherence meetings with the state and continuing education, which was necessary for their work, were highlighted as extremely helpful ways to provide social support to program staff. Desired improvements centered on ways to better help clients adhere to their medications. Both interviewees stated that they continuously sought out ways to improve education and understanding of the importance of taking medications, found ways to help patients remember to take their medications, and provided support in other ways to make taking medications easier.

*Providing social and emotional support.* Time spent developing trust was a key component of the job of the medication adherence nurses. The program nurses stressed the importance of gaining client trust because of clients' competing life issues and the fact that many clients had been mistreated by the medical community. As stated by one staff member, "My place is to build relationships with [my clients]. So to me, that's the first step in compliance, trust and being able to trust what I say, being able to listen to me."

*Acting as a liaison.* Stated as a benefit of the adherence program by clients, the staffs also expressed the importance of staying abreast of clients' needs with their providers. As one interviewee stated,

> So, I do keep in contact with all practitioners if I see any other issues, a psychological issue or I refer clients to home care if I think they need it. And I discuss everything with a social worker. I keep in touch with providers at the clinic. I mean, it's a collaborative thing.

This connection to mental health and other providers allowed the adherence program nurses to keep accurate and complete records of clients' needs.

## Study Limitations

The results of this evaluation represent the views of those who participated in the client focus groups and the staff interviews. Randomization of participants was not done because of the small number of clients enrolled in the programs and the difficulty of recruiting for the focus groups. In any research study with human participants, the results are limited to those who self-select to participate, as their participation is always voluntary. This does not cause the results in this study to be any less valid than in other studies; however, it means that these results should be understood to reflect only the views of those who participated. Therefore, the recommendations discussed next should be considered preliminary and need to be adapted to the specific needs of HIV medication adherence clients in other programs.

## Discussion and Recommendations for Practice

Overall, there was high staff and client satisfaction with the current state-funded HIV medication adherence programs reviewed in this process evaluation. Current and future programs should continue to employ licensed staffs (i.e., Registered, Licensed Practical, and Advanced Practice Registered Nurses) to administer the adherence intervention to clients. The adherence program nursing staff person was key, which was clearly stated in the client focus groups. These models were unique in their approach to adherence in that they had staff employed to follow up with and provide support to clients. The evaluation findings supported literature in HIV medication adherence and showed the importance of social support and how it positively affects HIV medication adherence (Holzemer et al., 1999; Power et al., 2002).

Our evaluation results highlight the importance of social support from both family and friends and, even more important, the relationship between the client and the adherence nurse. Clinician factors that contributed to increased adherence included having a consistent provider, the existence of a positive relationship between clinician and client, a knowledge of clinical regimens, and prior treatment experience (Frank & Miramontes, 1999; Friedland & Williams, 1999). Consistent with these findings, Golin et al. (2002) found that clients reported that a continuing and honest communication with their medical practitioner had a positive impact on their ability to follow their medication regimen. This was also true in our evaluation, in particular with regard to the communication between the client and the adherence nurse.

Although the client-provider relationship is critical in the adherence process, the clinician (in this case, the adherence program nurse) must be able to assess the client for readiness in starting a medication regimen, and the client should be involved in the decision-making process (Frank & Miramontes, 1999). Nurses should use effective communication techniques to establish a positive relationship with the patient, show facilitative body language, and create a clinical setting that fits the patient's needs both culturally and logistically (Chesney et al., 2000).

Use of the transtheoretical model stages of change would assist nurses in assessing the willingness of their clients to begin a medication regimen. The transtheoretical model is a model of behavior change that focuses on individual decision making and the internal and external influences that impact a decision to change a behavior and actions taken based on that decision (Prochaska, Redding, & Evers, 1997). The model conceptualizes the decision to change as a series of steps an individual must pass through including pre-contemplation, contemplation, preparation, action, and maintenance. The use of this theory allows practitioners to start where their clients are and help them to adopt a new behavior through a process of change.

On the basis of our results and the supporting literature, several recommendations for future and current HIV medication adherence programs were developed. They include the following:

1. Program goals should be expanded to include outcome measures beyond adherence and behavior changes, increases in knowledge, and other aspects of adherence based on adherence program methods.

2. Program impact objectives should continue to include client viral loads, CD4 counts, and missed appointments and doses. Increases in self-esteem, self-efficacy, and knowledge of medications can also be added measures. The use of behavior change theories to inform the development of these interventions should help nurses and other staff to determine the level of commitment and readiness to change among their clients. The use of behavior change theories, such as the transtheoretical model stages of change, will also assist staff in the evaluation of program outcomes.

3. Staff must be able to promote trust with their clients and facilitate social support. As stated previously, social support is seen as a reciprocal support system that is initiated through social and interpersonal relationships and which can be given in the form of informational and emotional support. Hence, providing support that was not only effective but also instructive was clearly a strength of the visiting nurse programs and an expression of satisfaction among focus group participants.

4. The adherence nurse, and her relationship with clients, is essential in increasing adherence to HIV medications. Adherence programs should continue to include the hiring of a staff nurse to be the contact and support person for all clients.

From the review of the literature, interviews with practitioners, and firsthand experiences, it is clear that evaluation of HIV medication adherence programs is not an exact science. Through definition of the primary goals of the programs, measurable process objectives should be formulated to help planners identify how a program is successful. The objectives of the program should consider that HIV viral load and increases in CD4 counts are measures of adherence. Further, objectives should include nonbiological factors that influence patient's adherence behaviors, including skills and self-efficacy to take their medications and social support. Through the development of individualized program objectives, it is possible that more time-efficient and user-friendly reporting tools can be constructed. Most important, a considerate and caring staff is crucial to adherence through the mechanism of social support.

## References

Chesney, M. A. (2003). Adherence to HAART regimens. *AIDS Patient Care and STDs, 17,* 169–177.

Chesney, M. A., Morin, M., & Sherr, L. (2000). Adherence to HIV combination therapy. *Social Science and Medicine, 50,* 1599–1605.

Frank, L., & Miramontes, H. (1999). AIDS Education and Training Center adherence curriculum. HIV InSite. Retrieved January 22, 2001, from http://hivinsite.ucsf.edu/topics/adherence/209.4504.htm

Friedland, G., & Williams, A. (1999). Attaining higher goals in HIV treatment: The central importance of adherence. *AIDS, 13*(Suppl 1), S61–S71.

Golin, C., Isasi, F., Breny Bontempi, J. M., & Eng, E. (2002). Secret pills: HIV positive patients' perceptions of the stigma and barriers associated with antiretroviral use. *AIDS Education and Prevention, 14,* 318–329.

Holzemer, W., Corless, I., Nokes, K., Turner, J., Brown, M., Powell-Cope, G., et al. (1999). Predictors of self-reported adherence in persons living with HIV disease. *AIDS Patient Care and STDs, 13,* 185–189.

More, M. E. (2002). *HIV medication adherence program: An evaluation report 2002.* New Haven, CT: Urban Policy Strategies.

Power, R., Koopman, C., Volk, J., Israelski, D. M., Stone, L., Chesney, M. A., et al. (2002). Social support, substance use, and denial in relationship to antiretroviral treatment adherence. *AIDS Patient Care and STDs, 17,* 245–252.

Prochaska, J., Redding, C., & Evers, K. (1997). The transtheoretical model and stages of change. In K. Glanz, F. M. Lewis, & B. Rimer (Eds.), *Health behavior and health education: Theory, research, and practice* (pp. 60–84). San Francisco: Jossey-Bass.

Steckler, A., & Linnan, L. (2002). *Process evaluation for public health interventions and research.* San Francisco: Jossey-Bass.

**Acknowledgments**: This evaluation was made possible by funding from the Connecticut Department of Public Health and the U.S. Health Resources and Services Administration.

**Address correspondence to**: Jean M. Breny Bontempi, Southern Connecticut State University, Department of Public Health, 144 Farnham Avenue, New Haven, CT 06515. E-mail: brenybontejl@southernct.edu

# Exercise for Article 23

## Factual Questions

1. According to the authors, a process evaluation can answer what question?

2. Are "Atlas," "Crossroads," and "La Familia" the real names of the programs?

3. The researchers had three aims. Two of them were to explore and compare the goals and modalities of each program, and provide recommendations for the improvement of current programs. What was the other aim?

4. What was the note taker's role in the focus groups?

5. Approximately what percentage of program clients participated in the focus groups?

6. According to the researchers, was there high overall staff and client satisfaction with the programs?

## Questions for Discussion

7. The researchers state that to ensure accuracy in the content analysis, the transcripts were read and coded separately by the three coders, who then compared and revised the coding scheme. (See lines 188–191.) In your opinion, how important is it to code separately (i.e., without consulting with each other)? Explain.

8. In your opinion, are the semistructured focus group guides described in sufficient detail? (See lines 163–166.)

9. The description of the "Human Participants' Approval" in lines 196–207 is more detailed than it is in many research articles. In your opinion, is it desirable for researchers to discuss this matter in detail? Explain.

10. Do you agree with the "Study Limitations" discussed in lines 411–426? Explain.

11. This process evaluation was qualitative. In your opinion, would a quantitative process evaluation with objective instruments and statistical analyses also be desirable? Explain.

## Quality Ratings

Directions: Indicate your level of agreement with each of the following statements by circling a number from 5 for strongly agree (SA) to 1 for strongly disagree (SD). If you believe an item is not applicable to this research article, leave it blank. Be prepared to explain your ratings. When responding to criteria A and B, keep in mind that brief titles and abstracts are conventional in published research.

A. The title of the article is appropriate.

SA 5 4 3 2 1 SD

B. The abstract provides an effective overview of the research article.

SA 5 4 3 2 1 SD

C. The introduction establishes the importance of the study.

SA 5 4 3 2 1 SD

D. The literature review establishes the context for the study.

SA 5 4 3 2 1 SD

E. The research purpose, question, or hypothesis is clearly stated.

SA 5 4 3 2 1 SD

F. The method of sampling is sound.

SA 5 4 3 2 1 SD

G. Relevant demographics (for example, age, gender, and ethnicity) are described.

SA 5 4 3 2 1 SD

H. Measurement procedures are adequate.

SA 5 4 3 2 1 SD

I. All procedures have been described in sufficient detail to permit a replication of the study.

SA 5 4 3 2 1 SD

J. The participants have been adequately protected from potential harm.

SA 5 4 3 2 1 SD

K. The results are clearly described.

SA 5 4 3 2 1 SD

L. The discussion/conclusion is appropriate.

SA 5 4 3 2 1 SD

M.  Despite any flaws, the report is worthy of publication.

            SA   5   4   3   2   1   SD

# Article 24

# Subsequent Childbirth After a Previous Traumatic Birth

**Cheryl Tatano Beck**, DNSc, CNM, FAAN, **Sue Watson**[*]

## ABSTRACT

*Background*: Nine percent of new mothers in the United States who participated in the Listening to Mothers II Postpartum Survey screened positive for meeting the *Diagnostic and Statistical Manual of Mental Disorders, Fourth Edition* criteria for posttraumatic stress disorder after childbirth. Women who have had a traumatic birth experience report fewer subsequent children and a longer length of time before their second baby. Childbirth-related posttraumatic stress disorder impacts couples' physical relationship, communication, conflict, emotions, and bonding with their children.

*Objective*: The purpose of this study was to describe the meaning of women's experiences of a subsequent childbirth after a previous traumatic birth.

*Methods*: Phenomenology was the research design used. An international sample of 35 women participated in this Internet study. Women were asked, "Please describe in as much detail as you can remember your subsequent pregnancy, labor, and delivery following your previous traumatic birth." Colaizzi's phenomenological data analysis approach was used to analyze the stories of the 35 women.

*Results*: Data analysis yielded four themes: (a) riding the turbulent wave of panic during pregnancy; (b) strategizing: attempts to reclaim their body and complete the journey to motherhood; (c) bringing reverence to the birthing process and empowering women; and (d) still elusive: the longed-for healing birth experience.

*Discussion*: Subsequent childbirth after a previous birth trauma has the potential to either heal or retraumatize women. During pregnancy, women need permission and encouragement to grieve their prior traumatic births to help remove the burden of their invisible pain.

From *Nursing Research*, 59, 241–249. Copyright © 2010 by Lippincott Williams & Wilkins. Reprinted with permission.

In the United States, 9% of new mothers who participated in the Listening to Mothers II Postpartum Follow-Up Survey screened positive for meeting the *Diagnostic and Statistical Manual of Mental Disorders, Fourth Edition* (American Psychiatric Associa-
5
tion, 2000) criteria for posttraumatic stress disorder (PTSD) after childbirth (Declercq, Sakala, Corry, & Applebaum, 2008). In this survey, the mothers' voices revealed a troubling pattern of maternity care. A large
10
percentage of women giving birth in the United States experienced hospital care that did not reflect the best evidence for practice nor for women's preferences. The Institute of Medicine (2003) identified childbirth as a national healthcare priority for quality improvement. A
15
maternity care quality chasm still exists (Sakala & Corry, 2007).

Researchers and healthcare professionals at an international meeting on current issues regarding PTSD after childbirth recommended the need for research
20
focusing on women's subjective birth experiences (Ayers, Joseph, McKenzie-McHarg, Slade, & Wijma, 2008). Olde, van der Hart, Kleber, and van Son (2006) called for examining the chronic nature of childbirth-related posttraumatic stress lasting longer than 6
25
months after birth.

The purpose of the current study was to help fill the knowledge gap of one aspect of the chronicity of birth trauma: women's subjective experiences of the subsequent pregnancy, labor, and delivery after a traumatic
30
childbirth.

## Review of Literature

Traumatic childbirth is defined as "an event occurring during the labor and delivery process that involves actual or threatened serious injury or death to the mother or her infant. The birthing woman experiences
35
intense fear, helplessness, loss of control, and horror" (Beck, 2004a, p. 28). For some women, a traumatic birth also involves perceiving their birthing experience as dehumanizing and stripping them of their dignity (Beck, 2004a, 2004b, 2006). After a traumatic child-
40
birth, 2% to 21% of women meet the diagnostic criteria for PTSD (Ayers, 2004; Ayers, Harris, Sawyer, Parfitt, & Ford, 2009), involving the development of three characteristic symptoms stemming from the exposure to the trauma: persistent reexperiencing of the trau-
45
matic event, persistent avoiding of reminders of the trauma and a numbing of general responsiveness, and

[*]*Cheryl Tatano Beck*, DNSc, CNM, FAAN, is distinguished professor, School of Nursing, University of Connecticut, Storrs. *Sue Watson* is chairperson, Trauma and Birth Stress, Auckland, New Zealand.

persistent increased arousal (American Psychiatric Association, 2000).

*Risk Factors*

50  Risk factors contributing to women perceiving their childbirth as traumatic can be divided into three categories: prenatal factors, nature and circumstances of the delivery, and subjective factors during childbirth (van Son, Verkerk, van der Hart, Komproe, & Pop,
55  2005). Under the prenatal category are factors such as histories of previous traumatic births, prenatal PTSD (Onoye, Goebert, Morland, Matsu, & Wright, 2009), child sexual abuse, and psychiatric counseling. Factors included in the category of nature and circumstances of the delivery include a high level of medical interven-
60  tion, extremely painful labor and delivery, and delivery type (Ayers et al., 2009). Subjective risk factors during childbirth can include feelings of powerlessness, lack of caring and support from labor and delivery staff, and fear of dying (Thomson & Downe, 2008).

*Long-Term Impact of Traumatic Childbirth*

65  Researchers are uncovering an unsettling gamut of long-term detrimental effects of traumatic childbirth not only on the mothers themselves but also on their relationships with infants and other family members. Mothers' breastfeeding experiences and the yearly an-
70  niversary of their birth trauma can also be negatively impacted.

Impaired mother-infant relationships after traumatic childbirth are being confirmed in the literature. For example, in the study of Ayers, Wright, and Wells
75  (2007) of mothers who experienced birth trauma in the United Kingdom, women described themselves as feeling detached and having feelings of rejection toward their infants. Nicholls and Ayers (2007) reported two different types of mother-infant bonding in couples
80  who shared that PTSD after childbirth affected their relationships with their children; they became anxious/overprotective or avoidant/rejecting. Childbirth-related PTSD also impacted their relationships with their partners, including their physical relationship,
85  communication, conflict, emotions, support, and coping.

Long-term detrimental effects of traumatic childbirth can extend also into women's breastfeeding experiences. In their Internet study, Beck and Watson
90  (2008) explored the impact of birth trauma on the breastfeeding experiences of 52 mothers. For some mothers, their traumatic childbirth led to distressing impediments that curtailed their breast-feeding attempts, such as feeling that their breasts were just one
95  more thing to be violated.

Another aspect of the chronic effect of birth trauma was identified in Beck's (2006) Internet study of the anniversary of traumatic childbirth, an invisible phenomenon that mothers struggled with. Thirty-seven
100  women comprised this international sample of mothers from the United States, New Zealand, Australia, United Kingdom, and Canada. Beck concluded that a failure to rescue occurred for women as the anniversary approached, and all others focused on the celebration of
105  the children's birthdays. This failure to rescue led to unnecessary emotional or physical suffering or both.

Catherall (1998) warned of secondary trauma in families living with trauma survivors. The entire family is vulnerable to becoming secondarily traumatized. The
110  long-term impact of trauma does not result necessarily in PTSD symptoms in family members. Catherall stated that it can have a more insidious effect of a disturbing milieu in the family. The members of the family may be close physically, but their ability to express
115  emotions is limited. True closeness in the family is missing, and their problem solving is impaired. Abrams (1999) identified one of the central clinical characteristics of intergenerational transmission of trauma is the silence that happens in families regarding traumatic
120  experiences. Abrams pleaded that the multigenerational impact of trauma should not be underestimated.

*Posttraumatic Growth*

Researchers are reporting that traumatic experiences can have positive benefits in a person's life.
125  Posttraumatic growth has been documented in a wide range of people who faced traumatic experiences such as bereaved parents (Engelkemeyer & Marwit, 2008), human immunodeficiency virus caregivers (Cadell, 2007), and homeless women with histories of traumatic
130  experiences (Stump & Smith, 2008). "Posttraumatic growth describes the experience of individuals whose development, at least in some areas, has surpassed what was present before the struggle with the crisis occurred. The individual has not only survived, but has
135  experienced changes that are viewed as important, and that go beyond what was the previous status quo" (Tedeschi & Calhoun, 2004, p. 4). It is not the actual trauma that is responsible for posttraumatic growth but what happens after the trauma. Tedeschi and Calhoun
140  (2004, p. 6) proposed five domains of posttraumatic growth: "greater appreciation of life and changed sense of priorities; warmer, more intimate relationships with others; a greater sense of personal strength; recognition of new possibilities or paths for one's life; and spiritual
145  development."

Childbirth can have an enormous potential to help change how a woman feels about herself and can impact her transition to motherhood (Levy, 2006). Attias and Goodwin (1999, p. 299) noted that a woman who
150  survives a traumatic experience may be able to rebuild her wounded inner self "by having a child, transforming her body from a container of ashes to a container for a new human life." A positive childbirth has the potential to empower a traumatized woman and help
155  her reclaim her life.

One study was located that touched on the positive growth of women after a previous negative birthing

170

experience. In Cheyney's (2008) qualitative study of women in the United States who chose home births
160 after experiencing a negative birth, three integrated conceptual themes emerged from their home birth narratives: knowledge, power, and intimacy. The power of their home births helped heal scars of their past hospital births. Positive growth after birth trauma has yet to
165 be investigated systematically by researchers.

One of the knowledge gaps identified in this literature review focused on an aspect of the long-term effects of birth trauma: mothers' subsequent childbirth. This phenomenological study was designed to answer
170 the research question: What is the meaning of women's experiences of a subsequent childbirth following a previous traumatic birth?

**Methods**

*Research Design*

The term *phenomenology* is derived from the Greek word phenomenon, which means "to show itself." The
175 goal of phenomenology is to describe human experiences as they are experienced consciously without theories about their cause and as free as possible from the researchers' unexamined presuppositions about the phenomenon under study. In phenomenology, re-
180 searchers "borrow" other individuals' experiences to better understand the deeper meaning of the phenomenon (Van Manen, 1984).

The existential phenomenological method developed by Colaizzi (1973, 1978) was used in this Internet
185 study. His method is designed to uncover the fundamental structure of a phenomenon, that is, the essence of an experience. An assumption of phenomenology is that for any phenomenon, there are essential structures that comprise that human experience. Only by examin-
190 ing specific experiences of the phenomenon being studied can their essential structures be uncovered.

Colaizzi's (1973, 1978) method includes features of Husserl's and Heidegger's philosophies. Colaizzi maintains that description is the key to discovering the
195 essence and the meaning of a phenomenon and that phenomenology is presuppositionless (Husserl, 1954). Colaizzi, however, holds a Heideggerian view of reduction, the process of researchers bracketing presuppositions and their natural attitude about the phenome-
200 non being studied. For Colaizzi (1978, p. 58), researchers identify their presuppositions regarding the phenomenon under study not to bracket them off to the side but instead to use them to "interrogate" one's "beliefs, hypotheses, attitudes, and hunches" about the
205 phenomenon to help formulate research questions. Colaizzi agrees with Merleau-Ponty (1956, p. 64) that "the greatest lesson of reduction is the impossibility of a complete reduction." Individual phenomenological reflection about the phenomenon being studied is one
210 approach Colaizzi (1973) offers for assisting researchers to decrease the coloring of their presuppositions and biases on their research activity.

Because the phenomenon of subsequent childbirth after a previous traumatic birth had not been examined
215 systematically before this current study, description of the meaning of women's experiences was the focus of this study. Before the start of the study, the researchers undertook an individual phenomenological reflection. They questioned themselves regarding their presuppo-
220 sitions about the phenomenon of subsequent childbirth after a traumatic birth and how these might influence what and how they conducted their research.

*Sample*

Thirty-five women participated in the study (Table 1). Saturation of data was achieved easily with this
225 sample size. Their mean age was 33 years (range = 27 to 51 years). All the participants were Caucasian and had two to four children. The length of time since their previous birth trauma to the subsequent birth ranged from 1 to 13 years. Eight of the 35 women (23%) opted
230 for a home birth for their subsequent births. Of these 8 mothers who gave birth at home, 4 lived in Australia, 3 in the United States, and 1 in the United Kingdom. Fourteen mothers (40%) had been diagnosed with PTSD after childbirth.

Table 1
*Demographic and Obstetric Characteristics*

|  | n | % |
| --- | --- | --- |
| Country |  |  |
| United States | 15 | 43 |
| United Kingdom | 8 | 23 |
| New Zealand | 6 | 17 |
| Australia | 5 | 14 |
| Canada | 1 | 3 |
| Marital status |  |  |
| Married | 34 | 98 |
| Divorced | 1 | 2 |
| Single | 0 | 0 |
| Education |  |  |
| High school | 3 | 9 |
| Some college | 5 | 15 |
| College degree | 13 | 38 |
| Graduate | 7 | 19 |
| Missing | 7 | 19 |
| Delivery |  |  |
| Vaginal | 25 | 72 |
| Cesarean | 10 | 29 |
| Diagnosed PTSD |  |  |
| Yes | 14 | 40 |
| No | 19 | 55 |
| Missing | 2 | 5 |
| Currently under care of therapist |  |  |
| Yes | 8 | 23 |
| No | 22 | 63 |
| Missing | 5 | 15 |

*Note.* PTSD = posttraumatic stress disorder

235 All the birth traumas were self-defined. Women were not asked if they had experienced other traumas before their birth traumas. Therefore, this was not an exclusionary criterion. The most frequently identified traumatic births focused on emergency cesarean deliv-
240 eries; postpartum hemorrhage; severe preeclampsia;

171

preterm labor; high level of medical interventions (i.e., forceps, vacuum extraction, induction); infant in the neonatal intensive care unit; feeling violated; lack of respectful treatment; unsympathetic, nonsupportive
245 labor and delivery staff; and "emotional torture."

*Procedure*

Once institutional review board approval was obtained from the university, recruitment began. Data collection continued for 2 years and 2 months. Women were recruited by means of a notice placed on the Web
250 site of Trauma and Birth Stress (TABS; www.tabs.org.nz), a charitable trust located in New Zealand. The mission of TABS is to support women who have experienced traumatic childbirth and PTSD because of their birth trauma. The sample criteria required that the
255 mother had experienced a traumatic childbirth with a previous labor and delivery, that she was willing to articulate her experience, and that she could read and write English. This international representation of participants was a strength of this recruitment method. A
260 disadvantage, however, was that only women who had access to the Internet and who used TABS for support participated in this study.

Women who were interested in participating in this Internet study contacted the first author at her univer-
265 sity e-mail address, which was listed on the recruitment notice. An information sheet and directions for the study were sent by attachment to interested mothers. After reading these two documents, women could e-mail the researcher if they had any questions concern-
270 ing the study.

Women were asked, "Please describe in as much detail as you can remember your subsequent pregnancy, labor, and delivery following your previous traumatic birth." Women sent their descriptions of their
275 experiences as e-mail attachments to the researcher. The sending of their story implied their informed consent. The length of time varied from when a mother first e-mailed about her interest in the study to when she sent her completed story to the researchers. The

280 shortest turnaround time was 2 days, whereas the longest was 9 months. If women did not respond within a certain period, the researchers did not recontact them. The women's wish not to follow through on participation in the study was respected. Throughout this proce-
285 dure, the first author kept a reflexive journal.

*Data Analysis*

Colaizzi's (1978) method of data analysis was used. The order of his steps is as follows: written protocols, significant statements, formulated meanings, clusters of themes, exhaustive description, and fundamental struc-
290 ture. It should be noted, however, that these steps do overlap. From each participant's description of the phenomenon, significant statements, which are phrases or sentences that directly describe the phenomenon, are extracted (Table 2). For each significant statement, the
295 researcher formulates its meaning. Here, creative insight is called into play. Colaizzi cautioned that in this step of data analysis, the researcher must take a precarious leap from what the participants said to what they mean. Formulated meanings should never sever
300 all connections from the original transcripts. It is in this step of formulating meanings that Colaizzi's connection to Heidegger can be seen. The next step entails organizing all the formulated meanings into clusters of themes. At this point, all the results to date are com-
305 bined into an exhaustive description. This step is followed by revising the exhaustive description into a more condensed statement of the identification of the fundamental structure of the phenomenon being studied. The fundamental structure can be shared with the
310 participants to validate how well it captured aspects of their experiences. If any participants share new data, they are integrated into the final description of the phenomenon. Member checking was done with one participant who reviewed the themes and totally agreed
315 with them. In addition, one mother who had not participated in the study but had experienced the phenomenon being studied reviewed the findings and also agreed with them.

Table 2
*Example of Extracting Significant Statements*

| No. | Significant statements |
| --- | --- |
| 1 | One thing that I'd noticed when I was a child was that when my parents got together with other adults, the talk eventually turned to two things: for my father (a Vietnam veteran) and the other men, the talk turned to the war and interestingly, to me as a small child, for my mother and the other women the talk always turned to childbirth. |
| 2 | It was as if, from a young age, for me, the connections between the two were drawn. A man is tested through war, a woman is tested through childbirth. |
| 3 | My dad, as abusive as he was, was considered a "good man" because he'd been a good soldier and so, I reasoned forward with a child's intelligence, that all that really mattered for a woman was to be strong and capable in childbirth. |
| 4 | And I failed. In the past, with the previous two births (particularly with the one that resulted in PTSD)—that's what it felt like. I failed at being a woman. |
| 5 | I don't think that I am alone in [this] feeling. I have a sneaking suspicion that this is pretty universal. |

*Continued →*

Table 2 (*continued*)

| No. | Significant statements |
| --- | --- |
| 6 | Just as a man who "talks" under torture in a POW situation feels as though he's failed, a woman who can't "handle" tortuous situations during childbirth feels like she's failed. It is not true. But it feels true. |
| 7 | My dad received two Purple Hearts and a Bronze Star during Vietnam. He, by most standards, would be considered a hero. Where are my Purple Hearts? My Bronze Star? I've fought a war, no less terrifying, no less destroying but there are no accolades. At least that's what it feels like. |
| 8 | I am viewed as flawed if not downright strange that I find L & D so terrifying. |
| 9 | The medical establishment thinks that I am "mental" and I have no common ground on which to discuss my childbirth experiences with "normal" women. |
| 10 | I know, I've tried. And that makes me feel isolated and inferior. |

*Note.* PTSD = posttraumatic stress disorder

## Results

The researchers reflected on the written descriptions provided by the 35 women to explicate the phenomenon of their experiences of subsequent childbirth after a previous traumatic birth. These reflections yielded 274 significant statements that were clustered into four themes and finally into the fundamental structure that identified the essence of this phenomenon (Table 3).

Table 3
*Fundamental Structure of the Phenomenon*

Subsequent childbirth after a previous traumatic birth far exceeds the confines of the actual labor and delivery. During the 9 months of pregnancy, women ride turbulent waves of panic, terror, and fear that the looming birth could be a repeat of the emotional and/or physical torture they had endured with their previous labor and delivery. Women strategized during pregnancy how they could reclaim their bodies that had been violated and traumatized by their previous childbirth. Women vowed to themselves that things would be different and that this time they would complete their journey to motherhood. Mothers employed strategies to try to bring a reverence to the birthing process and rectify all that had gone so wrong with their prior childbirth. The array of various strategies entailed such actions as hiring doulas for support during labor and delivery, becoming avid readers of childbirth books, writing a detailed birth plan, learning birth hypnosis, interviewing obstetricians and midwives about their philosophy of birth, doing yoga, and drawing birthing art. All these well-designed strategies did not ensure that all women would experience the healing childbirth they desperately longed for. For the mothers whose subsequent childbirth was a healing experience, they reclaimed their bodies, had a strong sense of control, and their birth became an empowering experience. The role of caring supporters was crucial in their labor and delivery. Women were treated with respect, dignity, and compassion. Although their subsequent birth was positive and empowering, women were quick to note that it could never change the past. Still elusive for some women was their longed-for healing subsequent birth.

### Theme I: Riding the Turbulent Wave of Panic During Pregnancy

Fear, terror, anxiety, panic, dread, and denial were the most frequent terms used to describe the world women lived in during their pregnancy after a previous traumatic birth.

I remember the exact moment I realized what was happening. I was on my lunch break at work, sitting under a large oak tree, watching cars go by my office, talking with my husband. I suddenly knew...I am pregnant again! I remember the exact angle of the sun, the shading of the objects around me. I remember looking into the sun, at that tree, at the windows to the office thinking, "NO! God PLEASE NO!" I felt my chest at once sink inward on me and take on the weight of 1000 bricks. I was short of breath, my head seared. All I could think of was "NOOOOOOOOO!"

Another woman described in detail the day she took her pregnancy test.

I took the test and crumpled over the edge of our bed, sobbing and retching hysterically for hours. I was dizzy. I was nauseous. I was sick. I could not breathe. I thought my chest would implode. I had a terrible migraine. I could not move from the spot where I had crumpled. I could not talk to my husband or see our daughter. I felt torn to pieces, shredded as shards of glass. I spent the next 2 trimesters hanging on for my life with suicidal thoughts but no real desire to carry them out though. I wanted to see my little girl. It was hell on earth.

Some women went into denial during the first trimester of their pregnancy to cope. Throughout her pregnancy, one woman revealed that she "felt numb to my baby." Some women described how they turned their denial of pregnancy into something positive. One multipara explained that after she was in denial for a few months, she then became determined to make things different this next time, and right at the end of her pregnancy she felt empowered by all that she had learned: "After 3 months of ignoring the fact that I was going to have to go through birth again, I decided I would treat my next labor and delivery as a healing and empowering experience."

Other mothers remained in a heightened state of anxiety throughout their pregnancy, and for some this anxiety escalated to panic and terror. Knowing she may have to go through the same "emotional torture" she endured with her previous traumatic birth, one woman shared, "My 9 months of pregnancy were an anxiety-filled abyss which was completely marred as an experience due to the terror that was continually in my

375 mind from my experience 8 years earlier." As the delivery date got closer, some mothers reported having panic attacks.

### Theme 2: Strategizing: Attempts to Reclaim Their Body and Complete the Journey to Motherhood

"Well, this time; I told myself *things would be different.* I actually started planning for this birth literally
380 while they were stitching me up from the traumatic first birth." During pregnancy, women described a number of different strategies they used to help them survive the 9 months of pregnancy while waiting for what they were dreading: labor and delivery (Table 4).
385 Some women spent time nurturing themselves by swimming, walking, going to yoga classes, and spending time outdoors.

Table 4
*Strategies Used to Cope with Pregnancy and Looming Labor and Delivery*

- Writing a detailed birth plan
- Mentally preparing for birth
- Learning birth hypnosis
- Doing birth art
- Writing positive affirmations
- Preparing for birthing at home
- Hiring a doula for labor and delivery
- Celebrating upcoming birth
- Avoiding ultrasounds
- Trying not to think about upcoming birth
- Reading books on healthy pregnancy and birth
- Mapping out your pelvis
- Learning birthing positions to open up the pelvis
- Practicing hypnosis for labor
- Researching birth centers and scheduling tours
- Interviewing obstetricians and midwives
- Exercising to help baby get in the correct position
- Using Internet support group
- Hiring a life coach
- Painting previous birth experience
- Creating "what if" sheet with all possible concerns and then solutions for them
- Creating "Yes, if necessary No" sheet for labor of what the mother wanted to happen
- Determining role of supporters during birth
- Researching homeopathic remedies to prepare body for labor and birth
- Developing a tool kit to help cope in labor
- Developing trust with healthcare provider

Keeping a journal throughout the pregnancy helped mothers because they had somewhere to write things
390 down, especially if they felt that family and friends did not understand just how difficult this pregnancy, subsequent to their prior traumatic delivery, was. Inspirational quotes were placed around the house to read and motivate women.
395 Figure 1 is an illustration of one mother's poster that she put up in her home.

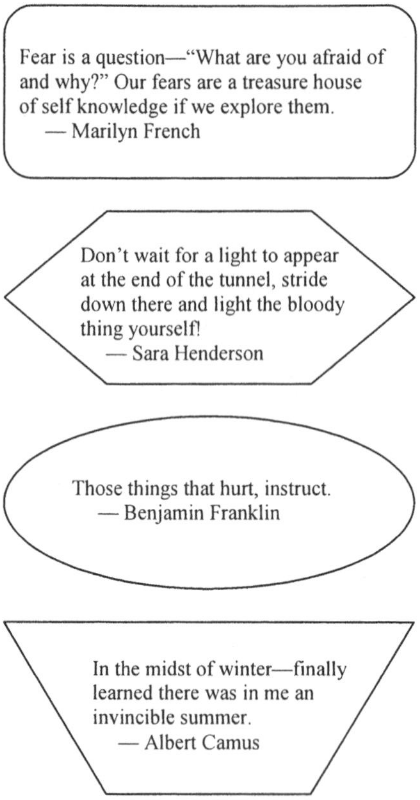

*Figure 1.* A poster of inspirational quotes by one mother.

Women strategized how to ensure that their looming labor and delivery was not another traumatic one. As one multipara explained, "I need to bring a rever-
400 ence to the process so I won't feel like a piece of meat lost in the system." Attempts were made to put into place a plan that would attempt to rectify all that had gone wrong with the previous childbirth. Some women turned to doulas in hopes of being supported during
405 their subsequent labor and delivery. Hypnobirthing was a plan used by some women to keep the first traumatic birth from being repeated.

Women reported reading avidly to understand the birth process fully. The most frequently cited books
410 were *Rebounding from Childbirth* (Madsen, 1994), *Birthing from Within* (England & Horowitz, 1998), and *Birth and Beyond* (Gordon, 2002). Mothers often engaged in birth art exercises.

Toward the end of pregnancy I did the birth art exercises
415 out of the book *Birthing from Within*...I began to trust myself. That will stay with me forever. That is more than just what I needed to birth the way I wanted to. That is what I needed to become a real woman.

Opening up to their healthcare providers about their
420 previous traumatic births was helpful for some mothers. Once clinicians knew of their history, they would address the mothers' concerns during each prenatal visit. Also sharing with their partners their fears and insecurities around pregnancy and birth helped wom-
425 en's emotional preparedness.

*Theme 3: Bringing Reverence to the Birthing Process and Empowering Women*

Three-quarters of the women who participated in this Internet study reported that their subsequent labor and delivery was either a "healing experience" or at least "a lot better" than their previous traumatic birth. Women became more confident in themselves as women and as mothers in that they really did know what was best for their babies and themselves. The role of supporters throughout labor and delivery was crucial. What was it that made a subsequent birth a healing experience? In the mothers' own words:

> I was treated with respect; my wishes and those of my husband were listened to. I wasn't made to feel like a piece of meat this time but instead like a woman experiencing one of nature's most wonderful events.

> Pain relief was taken seriously. First time around I was ignored. I begged and pleaded for pain relief. Second time it was offered but because I was made to feel in control, I was able to decline.

> I wasn't rushed! My baby was allowed to arrive when she was ready. When my first was born, I was told "5 minutes or I get the forceps" by the doctor on call. I pushed so hard that I tore badly.

> Communication with labor and delivery staff was so much better the second time. The first time the emergency cord was pulled but no one told me why. I thought my baby was dead and no one would elaborate.

Women reclaimed their bodies, had a strong sense of control, and birth became an empowering experience. Only essential fetal monitoring and minimal medical intervention occurred. Women were allowed to start labor on their own and not be induced. Under gentle supervision of caring and supportive healthcare professionals, women were reassured to just do what their body felt like doing and to follow their body's lead. The number of vaginal examinations was kept at a minimum, and women were permitted to walk around and choose the position they felt best laboring in. One mother described her healing birth:

> I pushed my baby into the world and I was shocked. I had never dared to dream for such a perfect delivery. They let me push spontaneously and my baby was delivered into my arms. My husband and I both cried with utter relief that I had given birth exactly how I wanted to and my trauma was healed.

For some women, the birth plan they had prepared during their pregnancy was honored by the labor and delivery staff, which helped them feel like they had some control and were a part of the birth and not just a witness.

Eight women opted for home births after their previous traumatic births, and for six of them, it did end in fulfilling their dream.

> It was as healing and empowering as I had always hoped for. I did not want any high-tech management. My home birth was the proudest day of my life and the victory was sweeter because I overcame so very much to come to it.

Another mother who had a successful home birth labored mostly in her bedroom under candlelight and music playing. She described it as very peaceful being at home surrounded by all her things. Her dog kept vigil by her side. She shared how it was such a gentle way for her baby to be born.

> My baby cried for a minute or two as if telling me his birth story and crawled up my body and found my heart and left breast. My heart swelled with so many emotions—love, joy, happiness, pride, relief, and wonderment.

A couple of women explained that their subsequent birth was healing, but at the same time they mourned what they had missed out with their prior birth. The following quote illustrates this.

> Even though it was an enormously healing experience, the expectations I had were unrealistic. What I went through during and after my first delivery cannot be erased from memory. If anything with this second birth being so wonderful, it makes dealing with my first birth harder. It makes it sadder and me angrier as before I had nothing to compare it to. I didn't know how different it could be or how special those first few moments are. I didn't fully understand what I had missed out on. So now 3 years later I find myself grieving again for what we went through, how I was treated and what I missed out on.

Other mothers admitted that although their subsequent births were healing, they could never change the past.

> All the positive, empowering births in the world won't ever change what happened with my first baby and me. Our relationship is forever built around his birth experience. The second birth was so wonderful I would go through it all again, but it can never change the past.

*Theme 4: Still Elusive: The Longed-for Healing Birth Experience*

Sadly, some mothers did not experience the healing subsequent birth they had hoped for. Two women chose to try a home birth after their previous traumatic birth but did not end up with the healing experience they longed for. One mother did deliver at home, but because of postpartum hemorrhage, she was transported by ambulance to the hospital, terrified she would not live to raise her baby. After laboring at home, another multipara who attempted a vaginal birth after cesarean needed to be transported by ambulance for a repeat cesarean birth after she failed to progress.

> When the ambulance arrived I felt rescued. I have never been so grateful that hospitals exist. The blue light ambulance journey was terrifying and I was in excruciating pain. By this point I was trying to detach my head from my body, as I had done years earlier when I was being raped.

175

She went on to vividly describe that as she lay on the operating table:

> ...with my legs held in the air by 2 strangers while a third mopped the blood between my legs I felt raped all over again. I wanted to die. I had failed as a woman. My privacy had been invaded again. I felt sick.

One multipara shared that although this birth had been a better experience, she would not say it was healing in relation to her first birth that had been so traumatic. "The contrast in the way I was treated just emphasized how bad the first one was. I had no sense of healing until 30 years later when I received counseling for PTSD."

## Discussion

Healthcare professionals' failure to rescue women during their previous traumatic childbirth can result in a troubling effect on mothers as they courageously face another pregnancy, labor, and delivery. Subsequent childbirth after a previous birth trauma provides clinicians with not only a golden opportunity but also a professional responsibility to help these traumatized women reclaim their bodies and complete their journey to motherhood.

To help women prepare for a subsequent childbirth after a previous traumatic birth, clinicians first need to identify who these women are. There are instruments available to screen women for posttraurtuatic stress symptoms due to birth trauma. An essential part of initial prenatal visits should be taking time to discuss with women their previous births. Traumatized women need permission and encouragement to grieve their prior traumatic births to help remove the burden of their invisible pain. Pregnancy is a valuable time for healthcare professionals to help women recognize and deal with unresolved, buried, or traumatic issues. Women should be asked about their hopes and fears for their impending labor and delivery and how they envision this birth. If a woman is exploring the possibility of a home birth, clinicians should question the mother about her previous births. Opting for a home birth may be an indication of a prior traumatic birth (Cheyney, 2008). If women need mental health follow-up during their pregnancy, cognitive behavior therapy and eye movement desensitization reprocessing treatment are two options for PTSD because of birth trauma. Treatment can be given in conjunction with a woman's family members to address secondary effects of PTSD.

Strategies can be employed to help mothers heal and increase their confidence before labor and delivery. Clinicians can share with mothers the Web site for TABS (www.tabs.org.nz), a charitable trust in New Zealand that provides support for women who have suffered through a traumatic birth. Obstetric care providers can suggest to the women some of the numerous strategies that mothers in this study described using during their pregnancies. Women can be encouraged to write down their previous traumatic birth stories.

Mothers can share their written stories with their current obstetric care providers so that they understand these women. Some women who participated in this study revealed that birthing artwork definitely helped them prepare for their subsequent labor and delivery after a traumatic childbirth.

Some women in this study touched on one of Tedeschi and Calhoun's (2004) domains of posttraumatic growth, a sense of personal growth. These women revealed feelings of empowerment and of reclaiming their bodies with their subsequent childbirths. Future research needs to be focused specifically on examining the five domains of posttraumatic growth in women who have experienced a subsequent childbirth after a previous birth trauma.

When women are traumatized during childbirth, this can leave a lasting imprint on their lives. If subsequent childbirth has the potential to either heal or retraumatize women, healthcare professionals need to be carefully aware of the consequences their words and actions during labor and delivery can have (Levy, 2006).

## References

Abrams, M. S. (1999). Intergenerational transmission of trauma: Recent contributions from the literature of family systems approaches to treatment. *American Journal of Psychotherapy, 53*(2), 225–231.

American Psychiatric Association. (2000). *Diagnostic and Statistical Manual of Mental Disorders–text revision.* Washington, DC: Author.

Attias, R., & Goodwin, J. M. (1999). A place to begin: Images of the body in transformation (pp. 287–303). In J. M. Goodwin & R. Attias (Eds.). *Splintered reflections.* New York: Basic Books.

Ayers, S. (2004). Delivery as a traumatic event: Prevalence, risk factors, and treatment for postnatal posttraumatic stress disorder. *Clinical Obstetrics and Gynecology, 47*(3), 552–567.

Ayers, S., Harris, R., Sawyer, A., Parfitt, Y., & Ford, E. (2009). Posttraumatic stress disorder after childbirth: Analysis of symptom presentation and sampling. *Journal of Affective Disorders, 119*(1–3), 200–204.

Ayers, S., Joseph, S., McKenzie-McHarg, K., Slade, P., & Wijma, K. (2008). Post-traumatic stress disorder following childbirth: Current issues and recommendations for future research. *Journal of Psychosomatic Obstetrics and Gynaecology, 29*(4), 240–250.

Ayers, S., Wright, D. B., & Wells, N. (2007). Symptoms of post-traumatic stress disorder in couples after birth: Association with the couple's relationship and parent-baby bond. *Journal of Reproductive and Infant Psychology, 25*(1), 40–50.

Beck, C. T. (2004a). Birth trauma: In the eye of the beholder. *Nursing Research, 53*(1), 28–35.

Beck, C. T. (2004b). Posttraumatic stress disorder due to childbirth: The aftermath. *Nursing Research, 53*(4), 216–224.

Beck, C. T. (2006). The anniversary of birth trauma: Failure to rescue. *Nursing Research, 55*(6), 381–390.

Beck, C. T., & Watson, S. (2008). Impact of birth trauma on breast-feeding: A tale of two pathways. *Nursing Research, 57*(4), 228–236.

Cadell, S. (2007). The sun always comes out after it rains: Understanding posttraumatic growth in HIV caregivers. *Health & Social Work, 32*(3), 169–176.

Catherall, D. R. (1998). Treating traumatized families. In C. R. Figley (Ed.). *Burnout in families: The systematic costs of caring* (pp. 187–215). Boca Raton, FL: CRC Press.

Cheyney, M. J. (2008). Homebirth as systems-challenging praxis: Knowledge, power, and intimacy in the birthplace. *Qualitative Health Research, 18*(2), 254–267.

Colaizzi, P. F. (1973). *Reflection and research in psychology: A phenomenological study of learning.* Dubuque, IA; Kendall/Hunt Publishing Company.

Colaizzi, P. F. (1978). Psychological research as the phenomenologist views it. In R. Valle & M. King (Eds.). *Existential phenomenological alternatives for psychology* (pp. 48–71). New York: Oxford University Press.

Declercq, E. R., Sakala, C., Corry, M. P., & Applebaum, S. (2008). *New mothers speak out: National survey results highlight women's postpartum experience.* New York: Childbirth Connection.

Engelkemeyer, S. M., & Marwit, S. J. (2008). Posttraumatic growth in bereaved parents. *Journal of Traumatic Stress, 21*(3), 344–346.

England, P., & Horowitz, R. (1998). *Birthing from within.* Albuquerque, NM: Partera Press.

Gordon, Y. (2002). *Birth and beyond.* London: Vermilion.

Husserl, E. (1954). *The crisis of European sciences and transcendental phenomenology.* The Hague: Martinus Nijhoff.

Institute of Medicine. (2003). *Board on Health Care Services Committee on identifying priority areas for quality improvements.* Washington, DC: National Academy Press.

Levy, M. (2006). Maternity in the wake of terrorism: Rebirth or retraumatization? *Journal of Prenatal and Perinatal Psychology and Health, 20*(3), 221–249.

Madsen, L. (1994). *Rebounding from childbirth: Toward emotional recovery.* Westport, CT: Bergin & Garvey.

Merleau-Ponty, M. (1956). What is phenomenology? *Crosscurrents, 6,* 59–70.

Nicholls, K., & Ayers, S. (2007). Childbirth-related post-traumatic stress disorder in couples: A qualitative study. *British Journal of Health Psychology, 12*(Pt. 4), 491–509.

Olde, E., van der Hart, O., Kleber, R., & van Son, M. (2006). Post-traumatic stress following childbirth: A review. *Clinical Psychology Review, 26*(l), 1–16.

Onoye, J. M., Goebert, D., Morland, L., Matsu, C., & Wright, T. (2009). PTSD and postpartum mental health in a sample of Caucasian, Asian, and Pacific Islander women. *Archives of Women's Mental Health, 12*(6), 393–400.

Sakala, C., & Corry, M. P. (2007). Listening to Mothers II reveals maternity care quality chasm. *Journal of Midwifery & Women's Health, 52*(3), 183–185.

Stump, M. J., & Smith, J. E. (2008). The relationship between post-traumatic growth and substance use in homeless women with histories of traumatic experience. *American Journal on Addictions, 17*(6), 478–487.

Tedeschi, R. G., & Calhoun, L. G. (2004). Posttraumatic growth: Conceptual foundations and empirical evidence. *Psychological Inquiry, 15*(l), 1–18.

Thomson, G., & Downe, S. (2008). Widening the trauma discourse: The link between childbirth and experiences of abuse. *Journal of Psychosomatic Obstetrics and Gynaecology, 29*(4), 268–273.

Van Manen, M. (1984). Practicing phenomenological writing. *Phenomenology + Pedagogy, 2*(1), 36–69.

van Son, M., Verkerk, G., van der Hart, O., Komproe, I., & Pop, V. (2005). Prenatal depression, mode of delivery and perinatal dissociation as predictors of postpartum posttraumatic stress: An empirical study. *Clinical Psychology & Psychotherapy, 12*(4), 297–312.

**Acknowledgments**: To all the courageous women who shared their most personal and powerful stories of their subsequent childbirth after a previous traumatic birth, the authors are forever indebted.

**Address correspondence to**: Cheryl Tatano Beck, DNSc, CNM, FAAN, School of Nursing, University of Connecticut, 231 Glenbrook Road, Storrs, CT 06269-2026. E-mail: cheryl.beck@uconn.edu

# Exercise for Article 24

## Factual Questions

1. According to the literature review, can traumatic experiences have positive benefits?

2. What is the explicitly stated research question for this research?

3. How many of the participants were Caucasian?

4. How many of the participants had vaginal deliveries?

5. To participate in this study, the women needed to be able to read and write in what language?

6. The reflections yielded how many "significant statements" that were subsequently clustered into four themes?

## Questions for Discussion

7. Before reading this article, how familiar were you with the term "phenomenology"? Does the discussion of phenomenology in lines 173–212 improve your understanding of this term? Explain.

8. What is your opinion on the use of the Internet to collect the data for this study? Was it a good idea to use the Internet? Explain. (See lines 246–285.)

9. What is your opinion on the use of implied consent in this study? (See lines 276–277.)

10. In your opinion, is the method of analysis described in sufficient detail? Explain. (See lines 286–318.)

11. Did the direct quotations from participants help you understand the results of this study? Explain. (See lines 319–546.)

12. If you were to conduct a study on the same topic, what changes in the research methodology would you make?

## Quality Ratings

Directions: Indicate your level of agreement with each of the following statements by circling a number from 5 for strongly agree (SA) to 1 for strongly disagree (SD). If you believe an item is not applicable to this research article, leave it blank. Be prepared to explain your ratings. When responding to criteria A and B, keep in mind that brief titles and abstracts are conventional in published research.

A. The title of the article is appropriate.

SA  5  4  3  2  1  SD

B. The abstract provides an effective overview of the research article.

SA  5  4  3  2  1  SD

C. The introduction establishes the importance of the study.

SA  5  4  3  2  1  SD

D. The literature review establishes the context for the study.

SA  5  4  3  2  1  SD

E. The research purpose, question, or hypothesis is clearly stated.

SA  5  4  3  2  1  SD

F. The method of sampling is sound.

SA  5  4  3  2  1  SD

G. Relevant demographics (for example, age, gender, and ethnicity) are described.

SA   5   4   3   2   1   SD

H. Measurement procedures are adequate.

SA   5   4   3   2   1   SD

I. All procedures have been described in sufficient detail to permit a replication of the study.

SA   5   4   3   2   1   SD

J. The participants have been adequately protected from potential harm.

SA   5   4   3   2   1   SD

K. The results are clearly described.

SA   5   4   3   2   1   SD

L. The discussion/conclusion is appropriate.

SA   5   4   3   2   1   SD

M. Despite any flaws, the report is worthy of publication.

SA   5   4   3   2   1   SD

# Article 25

# Barriers in Providing Psychosocial Support for Patients With Cancer

**Mari Botti**, RN, RM, BN, PhD, MRCNA, **Ruth Endacott**, RN, DipN, MA, PhD,
**Rosemary Watts**, RN, RM, Crit Care Cert, BN, Grad Dip in Adv Nurs (Ed), MHSc, PhD,
**Julie Cairns**, RN, BN, Cert Cancer Nursing, Master of Bioethics,
**Katrina Lewis**, RN, **Amanda Kenny**, RN, RM, PhD[*]

ABSTRACT. There is sound evidence to support the notion that the provision of effective psychosocial care improves the outcomes of patients with cancer. Central to the implementation of this care is that health professionals have the necessary communication and assessment skills. This study aimed to identify key issues related to providing effective psychosocial care for adult patients admitted with hematological cancer, as perceived by registered nurses with 3 or more years of clinical experience. An exploratory qualitative design was used for this study. Two focus group interviews were conducted with 15 experienced cancer nurses. The provision of psychosocial care for patients with cancer is a dynamic process that has a professional and personal impact on the nurse. The 5 analytic themes to emerge from the data were as follows: when is it a good time to talk?; building relationships; being drawn into the emotional world; providing support throughout the patient's journey; and breakdown in communication processes. The findings from this study indicate an urgent need to develop a framework to provide nurses with both skill development and ongoing support in order to improve nurses' ability to integrate psychosocial aspects of care and optimize patient outcomes.

## Introduction

There is growing evidence that the provision of effective psychosocial care improves the outcomes of patients with cancer.[1,2] However, providing psychosocial care for patients with cancer can place specific
5 burdens on health professionals. The effectiveness of the care provided is dependent on the training, skills, attitudes, and beliefs of staff. The *Clinical practice guidelines for the psychosocial care of adults with cancer* have been developed by the National Breast Cancer
10 Centre and the National Cancer Control Initiative in Australia as a benchmark for the psychosocial needs of patients with cancer. These evidence-based guidelines are designed for use by all health professionals who care for people during the course of cancer diagnosis
15 and treatment. Central to the successful implementation of these guidelines is the ability for health professionals to exercise the necessary assessment and communication skills, for example, discuss prognosis and treatment options available with the patient or the move
20 from curative to palliative treatments. We know that health professionals can have low confidence in exercising these skills that can result in a failure by health professionals to provide effective psychosocial care to patients with cancer.

25 The purpose of this paper is to elicit the key issues perceived by registered nurses that arise when caring for adults with hematological cancer to enable the development of a framework to assist nurses to provide optimal evidence-based psychosocial care. In addition,
30 such a framework will assist nurses to recognize the point at which psychosocial and emotional responses to patients' needs require specialist intervention.

### Background

Approximately 350,000 Australians are diagnosed with cancer each year[3] and, as a consequence, experi-
35 ence a variety of psychosocial and emotional responses. People with cancer suffer significant emotional morbidity and psychological distress and face physical issues related to their cancer and treatment, end-of-life issues, and survival issues. According to the
40 few available estimates, the prevalence of psychological distress in patients ranges from 20% to 60%,[4] and evidence suggests that 12% to 30% will experience clinically significant anxiety problems.[5] Clinical depression has been reported in up to 40% of patients in
45 palliative care[6] but is also prevalent in patients undergoing surgery for cancer[7,8] and in patients receiving

[*]*Mari Botti* and *Rosemary Watts*, the Centre for Clinical Nursing Research, Epworth/Deakin Nursing Research Centre, Richmond Vic 3121, Australia. *Ruth Endacott*, La Trobe/The Alfred Clinical School, The Alfred Hospital, Prahran Vic 3121, Australia; and School of Nursing and Community Studies, University of Plymouth, Exeter EX2 6AS, England. *Julie Cairns* and *Katrina Lewis*, The Alfred, Commercial Road, Prahran Vic 3121, Australia. *Amanda Kenny*, School of Nursing, LaTrobe University, Bendigo Vic 3550, Australia.

chemotherapy, adjuvant therapy, or radiation therapy.[9–11] These psychological responses can have impact on the persons and their family, affecting day-to-day functioning and capacity to cope with the burden of the disease, and may reduce adherence to recommended treatments.

The provision of optimal care for patients with cancer involves both effective physical and psychosocial care. According to the *Clinical practice guidelines for the psychosocial care of adults with cancer*,[12] the psychosocial care of a person with cancer "...begins from the time of initial diagnosis, through treatment, recovery and survival, or through the move from curative to non-curative aims of treatment, initiation of palliative care, death and bereavement" (p.37) and involves all members of the treatment team, family, friends, and careers. Health professionals can help reduce patient and family distress through interventions that strengthen the patient's own coping resources. Evidence based on meta-analyses and systematic reviews of randomized controlled trials have shown that the provision of information, psychological interventions, and emotional and social support improves patient outcomes. For example, rates of anxiety, depression, mood disturbances, nausea, vomiting, and pain[1] have been shown to decrease, and emotional adjustment and overall quality of life[2] have been shown to improve.

Nurses provide 24-hour care for patients and families and often provide psychosocial support while meeting patients' physical needs and providing symptomatic support. Providing psychosocial care for patients with cancer can place specific burdens on health professionals, and the effectiveness of the care provided is dependent on the training, skills, attitudes, and beliefs of staff. There is evidence of high stress levels among oncology nursing staff[13] and that a common source of stress is associated with the provision of emotional support for patients and their families.[14,15] Kent et al.[16] reported that a potential source of stress for health professionals is associated with caring for the dying patient and the perceived inability to relieve the patients' and/or the families' suffering. Communication in the context of cancer care includes general interactional skills to convey empathy and support and to provide medical information that is understood and retained. A failure to communicate well often seems to result from a lack of confidence or a perceived lack of knowledge.[17] Health professionals who feel insufficiently prepared in communication skills are reported to have a higher level of stress.[18]

Although it is recognized that the provision of psychosocial care is a multiprofessional process, this study uncovers psychosocial issues that arise from a nursing perspective in the context of the 24-hour management of the patient.

## The Study

### Aim

This study aimed to identify key issues related to providing effective psychosocial care for adult patients admitted with hematological cancer, as perceived by registered nurses with 3 or more years of clinical experience.

## Methods

### Design

A descriptive qualitative design was used for this study. A qualitative approach was selected because rich descriptive data, not available through quantitative methods, were desired to document the nurses' experiences. Focus groups were chosen because of their added benefits above individual interviews, in particular the synergy generated between group members,[19] their naturalistic approach in tapping into everyday social processes of communication,[20] and their "permissive" and peer support function in encouraging participants to divulge opinions and beliefs that might not emerge through an individual interview.[21] Approval for this study was granted by the Deakin University Ethics Committee and the ethics committee of the participating tertiary referral hospital.

### Participants

Participants were purposively selected based on their role in providing psychosocial care. Although it is recognized that psychosocial care is a multiprofessional process, this study aimed to uncover psychosocial care in the context of the 24-hour management of the patient. The rationale for selecting experienced registered nurses was that there was an expectation they would carry the burden of providing complex psychosocial care in the ward environment. In Australia, registered nurses usually have a degree qualification. It was considered that these nurses would be role models and coaches for inexperienced nurses. Hence, the study sample was limited to experienced registered nurses. Nurses who had been working on the cancer ward at a major Melbourne tertiary level hospital, a key center in the provision of oncology services in Victoria and Australia, for 3 years or more were approached to participate in the study. A total of 15 experienced nurses participated.

The participants work on a busy hematology/oncology/radiotherapy and bone marrow transplant ward that has a complex patient acuity and associated significant morbidity. The nurses face a range of complex psychosocial issues related to patients' diagnoses and associated treatments and their personal circumstances. The 30-bed ward admits approximately 640 oncology patients, 50 bone marrow transplant patients, and more than 100 radiotherapy patients each year. At the time of the study, the ward had just commenced a Nursing Care Delivery system pilot project that was a modification of the previous Primary Nursing model utilized by the ward.

### Procedure

Two focus groups, 8 participants and 7 participants, respectively, in each group, were conducted in October 2003. One member of the research team who had experience in facilitating focus group interviews conducted the sessions. At both sessions, an observer was present to take notes pertinent to each session. Before commencing each interview, introductions were made between the participants and the researchers present. The facilitator [R.E.] gave an overview of the purpose of the interview, followed by outlining the ground rules that apply to the conduct of focus group interviews, and consent was then requested to audiotape the session. A statement was made relating to maintaining confidentiality of individual group members' perceptions at the conclusion of the session. Participants were also reminded of their right to withdraw from the study. The facilitator circulated written details to participants of whom to contact should they require any emotional support after the interview.

A brief biographical form was circulated to capture data such as the qualifications, experience, and role configuration of the individual participants. Before commencing the interview, the facilitator encouraged the participants to use "real life" examples to identify situations in which psychosocial support for patients and families was considered effective or could have been enhanced.

During both sessions, the facilitator used a guide consisting of open-ended questions and probes drawn from the relevant literature and existing clinical guidelines regarding the psychosocial needs of patients with life-threatening diseases. The guide was designed to allow participants to talk freely about their experiences of caring for patients with hematological cancer and their family members. The focus group sessions lasted 1 hour; both were tape-recorded and transcribed verbatim.

### Ethical Considerations

Participants were invited to participate in the study based on their experience; they were informed that they did not have to take part in the study and that nonparticipation would not affect their position within the ward. Once the nurses agreed to participate in the study, they were asked to sign a consent form. Although there was no perceived inherent risk to participants, before commencing the sessions, the facilitator circulated written details of a psychologist available to them should they require emotional support at the conclusion of the session. Individual participant data have not been reported.

### Data Analysis

The data were coded and analytic themes developed using content analysis. The transcripts were initially read by one member of the research team. This took some time and required the text to be understood as a whole. Notes taken by the observer during each of the focus group interviews were also read at this time to provide a context for the interview transcript. Common themes within the context of each interview were identified resulting in the identification of 5 major themes. Validation of themes occurred in 2 ways. The coding of the themes was reviewed between the project research fellow who had initially coded the data and 2 other members of the research team: one academic and one clinician. All members were in agreement with the themes. A presentation of the study findings was given to participants, further validating the findings.

## Results

### Demographic Characteristics

All participants were female and were registered Division 1 nurses; 20% ($n = 3$) had hospital registration with 80% ($n = 13$) having completed a Diploma of Nursing. One participant had completed an Honors degree, 2 had completed a Postgraduate Diploma in Nursing. Most participants (53%, $n = 8$) had had greater than 9 years of experience in nursing; however, the majority (53%, $n = 8$) had been in their current position for between 1 and 3 years.

Five themes were identified: when is it a good time to talk?, building relationships, being drawn into the emotional world, providing support throughout the patient's journey, and breakdown in communication processes.

*When is it a good time to talk?* The participants recognized that there was a need to first gain entry to the patient's environment in order to provide psychosocial care. The nurses reported that they were often able to gain such entry in a discrete and nonthreatening manner by carrying out what they termed "nursing tasks"; such tasks included meeting the patient's hygiene needs or making the patient's bed, as illustrated by the following comments:

> You know, tasks are a good excuse to get into the patient's room and talk…doing those tasks gives you permission to enter their room without them actually knowing. (focus group 1)

> …giving them a wash and because you are doing something and not looking at them directly they'll talk because it seems safe, there's something that's happening between the two of you and they start speaking. (focus group 1)

However, the participants identified workload as a potential barrier to their ability to provide psychosocial care. Interestingly, although the participants perceived their own workload as a barrier, they also felt that patients also considered their workload as an impediment to asking for care as demonstrated by the following quotes:

> Lots of patients say you're too busy…. (focus group 1)

Even if you are busy we like to be honest with people and just say I can't right now but I will come back because sometimes we just can't and that's a reality. (focus group 1)

The impact of workload and the provision of psychosocial care were considered to be further exaggerated when the nurse was perceived as "inexperienced" in caring for patients with cancer. This affected the ability to engage with the patient at the required level:

...before you feel comfortable providing social support you need to feel comfortable knowing what is going on with them medically and until you can discuss that with them at the same time, I think it's very hard to engage them. (focus group 2)

It was also acknowledged that when the nurse considered it a good time to talk to the patient, it did not always coincide with when the patient wanted to talk. A good time to talk from the patient's perspective could occur anywhere—24 hours a day, 7 days a week—and the need to provide psychosocial care during the night shift was a common scenario participants reported, as the following quote illustrates:

So much happens at night, like people have so much time to think. (focus group 1)

To provide psychosocial care to patients admitted with hematological cancer, the participants reported that they often entered the patient's environment using the need to perform tasks to establish and engage in dialogue with patients about other issues. However, the time available to participants was related to workload issues. Workload, number of years of experience as a nurse, and the timing of the patient's need were all cited as potential barriers to the ability of the nurse to provide adequate psychosocial care.

*Building relationships.* To provide effective psychosocial care, there was a requirement to build a relationship with the patient. To build this relationship, there was a need to first gain the patient's trust, and it was not until this trust had been gained that psychosocial care could be provided. A key factor that participants considered assisted them to gain the trust of the patient was working as their primary nurse; this was often associated with one-to-one access to the patient discussed in terms of continuity of care. Other factors cited were the ability to demonstrate competency when carrying out routine care and the ability to demonstrate an understanding of the patient's complex medical history.

There was a general agreement among the participants that it was a quicker process to engage with patients and hence gain their trust when working in a full-time capacity as opposed to working part-time, as the following illustrations show:

...I only work two days a week now, so I find even though a patient tends to be long-term it takes a bit longer to build up rapport, you just can't go in there. (focus group 2)

...I only work one day a week.... I feel like I do my work and then I go home because they don't know me to kind of open up.... (focus group 2)

Participants, in both a positive and negative manner, discussed the relationship between primary nursing and continuity of care extensively. Although the primary nurse had the ability to deliver improved continuity of care to patients that allowed the establishment of a relationship with the patient, the primary nursing role was only available to those staff who worked full-time. This meant that relatively inexperienced nurses who worked full-time could work as primary nurses; however, it was considered by the participants that they often struggled to provide psychosocial care within this role:

If you are full-time you get the reward of primary nursing I think but if you are not full-time...you're a bandaid fill-in basically for the shift.... (focus group 1)

I think when you first start becoming a primary nurse after your grad year [graduate year]...and everybody thinks that you have enough experience and have your first patient and you barely cope with the complexity of their sickness...the psychosocial aspects just, you don't even think about it until much, much too late. (focus group 1)

The participants considered that an understanding of the patient's history was important in 2 significant ways in relation to building a relationship with the patient. First, this information would be relevant to any subsequent psychosocial care that the patient received, and second, it was perceived that nurses needed to be able to demonstrate such an understanding if they were to gain the patient's trust:

...until you gain their trust as their nurse you're not going to be able to really help them. (focus group 2)

Although the participants generally considered the care delivery modality of primary nursing facilitated continuity of care and thus enabled them to build a relationship with the patient and their significant others, they felt alone and stated that there was a void of professional dialogue with other nurses regarding the patient's plan of care. This lack of professional dialogue actually resulted in increasing the amount of stress felt by the participants. The only time nominated by participants when they considered that there was an opportunity to discuss the patient's plan of care with another nurse was at handover:

Everybody starts to work alone in primary nursing and you only talk about that patient at handover. (focus group 1)

It was important to first gain the patient's trust in order to establish a rapport with the patient, and being the patient's primary nurse was considered an important vehicle to achieve this as was the need to demonstrate an understanding of the complexity of the patient's medical history and treatment.

*Being drawn into the emotional world.* For nurses working with patients diagnosed with hematological cancer, there was a recognized need to protect oneself from being taken on the emotional journey that these patients travel, as the following comments demonstrate:

> ...it's very easy to be drawn in emotionally.... (focus group 1)

> How incredibly difficult it is not to be drawn into their emotional world.... (focus group 2)

To avoid being drawn into the emotional world, it was a common scenario for participants to report that they had set personal boundaries with regard to the amount of personal information they were willing to disclose. The participants reflected that they felt especially vulnerable to being drawn into the patient's emotional world when faced with the following situations: being new to the ward or lacking clinical experience in providing care to this cohort of patients:

> It's probably only this year that I've felt really comfortable sort of branching into that care [psychosocial care] more in depth...I set boundaries for myself...when I first started on the ward I found I gave everything and I'd come home and I'd feel completely drained and I wasn't coping and I was really upset and very involved.... (focus group 2)

Interestingly, some participants reflected that although they had boundaries in place to protect themselves against becoming too involved with patients and these barriers had proved effective for a considerable period of time, occasions still arose when patients were able to get "under" these barriers and invade their personal space. Participants were undecided if this was an intentional or unintentional act by the patient; however, this invasion still caught the participants by surprise:

> Participant: You care for them emotionally as well, that's the thing you...give some [information about yourself] away and then you feel like you've given too much.

> R.E.: So does it come as a bit of a shock when a particular patient does, as you say, get under the barrier?

> Participant: We think we are really good at it, I can go for three years and then someone will just sneak in and I get really annoyed with myself because I'm smarter than that person.... (focus group 2)

In summary, nurses working with patients admitted with hematological cancer recognized that they were vulnerable to being emotionally drained by being drawn into the patient's emotional world. Participants reported they had set personal boundaries for 3 key reasons: to prevent becoming too involved with patients, to prevent excessive personal disclosure, and to prevent becoming emotionally drained. The unresolved question for the participants was: How can I help the patient and their family and still look after myself?

*Providing support throughout the patient's journey.* The analogy of describing the patient as being on a journey when admitted to hospital for treatment after the diagnosis of hematological cancer was used. Participants considered that there were key times on this journey when patients needed or demanded more psychosocial care and times when they needed less care. Key times nominated by the participants when more psychosocial care would be needed or demanded were times when they found it difficult to provide the appropriate care. Times nominated were when the provision of care changed from being aggressive to palliative, the end of the patient's life, and for others the interim period "...the interim period is really difficult because no-one makes a decision." Other participants nominated when the patient's perception of their illness changed from a state of denial to one of acceptance, and for other participants, it was simply related to the length of time the patient was hospitalized, as demonstrated by the following quotes:

> I find the hardest thing in nursing, the first acute [presentation] you are busy because you know that they are going to usually get better, you know they're got fevers, you can treat it...but when they come in chronic it's like throwing your hands up and saying I'm sorry there's nothing I can do. (focus group 2)

> And that's a really hard swing for us too because you push and push and give drugs and then it can be a matter of hours. We have to turn around and change the way that we provide care and that could be in a palliative nature. Perhaps you're not even ready for that and the family are not ready...I find that really challenging. (focus group 2)

The patient's journey is dynamic. At certain points of this journey, the patient requires more psychosocial care and participants recognized these times as difficult times not only for the patient and their significant other but also for themselves.

*Breakdown in communication processes.* The communication process was considered to be ineffective by participants on 2 levels. The participants reported that they considered ineffective communication occurred between the ward nurses and ward doctors in relation to the timing of communication. The participants cited 2 main perceived problems. First, medical staff often communicated with the patient in isolation from the nursing staff, in particular when telling the patient their diagnosis and then failing to consider any of the possible ramifications of such action. Second, the nurse would be aware of sensitive information regarding the patient's diagnosis for a period of time before the patient being told. This placed the nurse in a very uncomfortable position when having to care for the patient:

> ...I think the doctors...shouldn't just say I'm going to tell the patient, I think you need to actually be there because the patients don't hear.... (focus group 1)

> I've known for days before a patient...that they've got terminal cancer and you just have to go in there and you just have to lie. (focus group 1)

Participants reported that they felt they received little information from doctors regarding patient progress both during the period of hospitalization and after their discharge from hospital. Participants reported, for example, that if they happened to meet a patient in the hospital corridor during an outpatient's visit, they could find out how the patient was managing postdischarge. Participants reported that working solely in the ward environment was isolating, citing that this was exacerbated by not having the opportunity to rotate to the outpatients department, and as such, ongoing knowledge of patient progress was further restricted.

Ineffective communication was also reported as existing between the ward nurses themselves, and there was a general feeling among the participants that they worked in isolation from one another. As previously discussed, this feeling of isolation was partly attributed to the model of primary nursing. Handover was cited as the one time that allowed some professional dialogue to take place.

## Discussion

The nurses in this study reported that they constantly faced a number of professional and personal issues when addressing the practical, emotional, and psychological demands of patients with cancer. There was a general recognition of the uniqueness of each patient's needs and that these needs could change over time, whether it be the timing of the provision of information or assisting the move from curative to palliative treatment. It appeared, however, that the issues faced in constantly meeting these needs had the ability, at times, to deeply affect the nurses' level of contentment with their personal lives.

The findings from this study suggest that professional support is an area that may be improved in an effort to improve job satisfaction, particularly in responding to the expressed feeling of not working as a team member. As in Barrett and Yates' study[22] that found over one-third of nurses indicated dissatisfaction in the degree to which they felt like part of a team, nurses in this study also did not feel like team members. This was voiced in 2 ways: a feeling of working in isolation, and not being included in the communication processes. The support offered to nurses working as primary nurses may need to improve to counteract the current feeling of working in isolation. However, it should be remembered that at the time of the study, the ward had just commenced the Nursing Care Delivery System pilot project. Providing feedback to nursing staff regarding the progress of patients after discharge from hospital provides not only information about patient progress but also reinforces their contribution to the interdisciplinary team, and this may be beneficial because it can then foster a sense of unity among staff members.[23]

There is a recognized deficit in the literature concerning the effects of providing care to patients with cancer on the quality of life of nursing professionals.[22,24] The findings suggested in this study support those of Ergun et al.,[24] who found that providing care to patients with cancer has a negative impact on the quality of life of oncology nurses. An Australia study, conducted by Barrett and Yates,[22] found that emotional exhaustion is a very real concern among oncology/hematology nurses with more than 70% ($n = 243$) of their sample experiencing moderate to high levels of stress.

High workload and a lack of available time were both cited by the participants as potential barriers that limited their ability to sit down and engage in conversation with patients to elicit their specific needs. These findings are supported by Barrett and Yates'[22] findings where dissatisfaction with workloads was found to be a major concern: nearly 40% of the nurses in their study perceived their workloads to be excessive. The workload issue is exacerbated by an overall reduction in nursing supply. In Australia, between 1995 and 1999, there was an overall decrease in full-time equivalent nurses per 100,000 population. This reduction in full-time equivalency is thought to be associated with an overall decrease in the level of nursing supply. Over the past 10 years, there has also been the trend for registered nurses to become part-time workers with national figures showing that the majority (53.7%) are working part-time.[25]

Findings from this study in relation to ineffective communication processes are similar to McCaughan and Parahoo's[26] findings. They found that nurses' self-perceived educational needs in caring for patients with cancer included the need for more knowledge and skills in providing psychosocial care and communication. Interestingly, the nurses in their study reported higher competence in providing physical care than in psychosocial care.

The development of effective strategies to assist clinicians to use communication skills in the provision of care is fundamental to achieving optimal psychosocial outcomes for patients. Such communication is vital to enable the provision of appropriate, accurate, and detailed information to the patient at key stages relating to the pathological process of the disease. Because this information has the potential to affect the patient's decision-making process, the provision of information must be appropriate, accurate, and detailed. Hematology is a dynamic specialty that incorporates the implementation of new and rapidly changing treatment regimens. Consideration must be given to the timing of the information. To successfully meet these demands, effective communication skills are required. Wilkinson[19] believes that in general, nurses' communication skills are inadequate and have not improved over the past 20 years. Training in communication skills can assist clinicians to improve,[27–30] and continuing training in the appropriate clinical setting may be beneficial, given that skills need to be reinforced and consolidated over time.[27,29,31]

These findings do support the development of a framework that addresses the personal and professional issues reported by experienced registered nurses as barriers to the delivery of psychosocial care. Clinical supervision is well recognized in the literature as an effective strategy for enhancing professional development, promoting self-awareness, and providing support[32–34] and has been used extensively across professional groups.[33,35–37] Clinical supervision has the potential to assist nurses with finding creative solutions to patient problems.[38] This potential can be realized through using an action learning approach to clinical supervision. Action learning uses a group process of learning and reflection, with an emphasis on getting things done.[39] A key feature of action learning is the focus on challenging assumptions but also legitimizing the reflection that is a necessary part of the process.[39] By incorporating group process into an action learning model means that nurses will find their own way to address specific issues encountered. The combination of these 2 approaches holds the potential to inform the knowledge, skills, and attitudes of nurses providing psychosocial care to patients with cancer.

A clinical supervision and action learning model is proposed by the authors. The proposed clinical supervision and action learning model is an interactive approach designed to enhance the communication skills of nurses and as such will assist nurses to manage difficult events[40] and to reduce their stress[41,42] through structured learning and reflective practice. It is proposed that individuals will learn with and from their peers by reflecting on real experiences and working on real problems. Data from this study have highlighted the need to include opportunity for nurses to discuss their own difficulties with patients; hence, such an approach was deemed preferable to a didactic teaching approach. The research team is currently giving further consideration to the implementation process of the proposed model.

## Limitations

Participants were selected based on their role with patients with cancer, enhancing the trustworthiness of the data in relation to study aims. This study used a small number of participants to enable in-depth clarification and exploration. Although this limits the generalizability of the findings, the diverse patient mix to which the participants were exposed provided them with a rich source of psychosocial care opportunities and challenges. This increases the credibility of the findings and representativeness to a wider population.[43]

The participants of each focus group worked within the same setting. This serves as both a strength and a limitation as it will enhance the relevance of the findings for that particular setting but perhaps limit applicability to other settings.

## Conclusion

It is clear from the findings of this study that the psychosocial needs of patients with cancer are dynamic. At present, a number of barriers are perceived to exist that impedes delivery of care to address these needs. In addition, there is clearly a professional and personal impact upon the nurse. However, for nurses to be effective in this area of care delivery and to improve patient outcomes, they must have the necessary skills and support. Therefore, a clinical supervision and action learning model with management, education, and support functions has been proposed. Such a model needs to address both the skill needs and support needs of registered nurses through the use of available evidence.

## References

1. Devine EC, Westlake SK. The effects of psychoeducational care provided to adults with cancer: Meta-analysis of 116 studies. *Oncol Nurs Forum.* 1995;22:1369–1381.
2. Meyer TJ, Mark M. Effects of psychosocial interventions with adult cancer patients: A meta-analysis of randomized experiments. *Health Psychol.* 1995;14(2):101–108.
3. Australian Institute of Health and Welfare, Registries. Cancer in Australia 1998: Incidence and Mortality Data for 1998. Cancer Series; 2001 (No. 17).
4. Zabora J, Brintzenhofeszoc H, Curbow B, Hooker C, Piantadosi S. The prevalence of psychological distress by cancer site. *Psychooncology.* 2001;10:19–28.
5. Bodurka-Bevers D, Basen-Engquist K, Carmack CL, et al. Depression, anxiety, and quality of life in patients with epithelial ovarian cancer. *Gynaecol Oncol.* 2000;78:302–308.
6. Bukberg J, Penman D, Holland JC. Depression in hospitalized cancer patients. *Psychosom Med.* 1984;46:199–212.
7. Fallowfield L, Hall A, Maguire GP, Baun M. Psychological outcomes of different treatment policies in women with early breast cancer outside a clinical trial. *BMJ.* 1990;301:575–580.
8. Royak-Schaler R. Psychological processes in breast cancer: A review of selected research. *J Psychosoc Oncol.* 1991;9(4):71–89.
9. Jenkins C, Carmody TJ, Rush AJ. Depression in radiation oncology patients: A preliminary evaluation. *J Affect Disord.* 1998;50:17–21.
10. Jacobsen PB, Bovberg DH, Redd WH. Anticipatory anxiety in women receiving chemotherapy for breast cancer. *Health Psychol.* 1998;12:469–475.
11. Dean C. Psychiatric morbidity following mastectomy: Preoperative predictors and type of illness. *J Psychosom Res.* 1987;31:385–392.
12. National Breast Cancer Centre and National Cancer Control Initiative. Clinical Practice Guidelines for the Psychological Care of Adults with Cancer. Camperdown, NSW: National Breast Cancer Centre; 2003.
13. Kelly B, Varghese F. The emotional hazards of medical practice. In: Sanders MR, Mitchell C, Byrne GJA, eds. *Medical Consultation Skills.* Melbourne: Addison-Wesley; 1997:472–488.
14. Herschbach P. Work-related stress specific to physicians and nurses working with cancer patients. *J Psychosoc Nurs.* 1992;10:79–99.
15. Catalan J, Burgess A, Pergami A, Hulme N, Gazzard B, Phillips R. The psychosocial impact on staff caring for people with serious diseases: The case of HIV infection and oncology. *J Psychosom Res.* 1996;40:425–435.
16. Kent G, Wills G, Faulkner A, Parry G, Whipp M, Coleman R. The professional and personal needs of oncology staff: The effects of perceived success and failure in helping patients on levels of personal stress and distress. *J Cancer Nurs.* 1994;3:153–158.
17. Ley P. Communicating with patients. Improving communication, satisfaction and compliance. London: Croom Helm; 1988.
18. Ramirez AJ, Graham J, Richards MA, et al. Burnout and psychiatric disorder among cancer clinicians. *Br J Cancer.* 1995;71:1263–1269.
19. Wilkinson S. Focus groups in feminist research: Power, interaction and the construction of meaning. *Womens Stud Int Forum.* 1998;21(1):111–125.
20. Wilkinson S, Bailey K, Aldridge J, Roberts A. A longitudinal evaluation of a communication skills programme. *Palliat Med.* 1999;13:341–348.
21. Kreuger RA. *Focus Groups: A Practical Guide for Applied Research.* 2nd ed. Thousand Oaks: Sage Publications; 1994.
22. Barrett L, Yates P. Oncology/haematology nurses: A study of job satisfaction, burnout, and intention to leave the specialty. *Aust Health Rev.* 2002;25(3):109–121.

23. Gullante MM, Levine NM. Recruitment and retention of oncology nurses. *Oncol Nurs Forum*. 1990;17(3):419–423.

24. Ergun FS, Oran NT, Bender CM. Quality of life of oncology nurses. *Cancer Nurs*. 2005;28(3):193–199.

25. Australian Institute of Health and Welfare. Labour forces-nurses. Australian Government; 2005. Available at: http://www.aihw.gov.au/publications/hwl/nurslfo2/nurs/fo2-col. Accessed August, 2005.

26. McCaughan E, Parahoo K. Medical and surgical nurses' perceptions of their level of competence and educational needs in caring for patients with cancer. *J Clin Nurs*. 2000;9:420–428.

27. Maguire P. Can communication skills by taught? *Br J Hosp Med*. 1990; 43:215–216.

28. Razavi D, Delvaux N, Marchal S, Bredart A, Farvaques C, Paesmans M. The effects of a 24-hour psychological training program on attitudes, communication and occupational stress in oncology: A randomised study. *Eur J Cancer*. 1993;29A:1858–1863.

29. Bird J, Hall A, Maguire P, Heavy A. Workshops for consultations on teaching of clinical communication skills. *Med Educ*. 1993;27:181–185.

30. Baile WF, Lenzi R, Kudelka AP, et al. Improving patient–physician communication in cancer care: Outcome of a workshop for oncologists. *J Cancer Educ*. 1997;12:166–173.

31. Girgis A, Sanson-Fisher RW. How to Break Bad News. An Interaction Skills Training Manual for General Practitioners, Junior Medical Officers, Nurses and Surgeons. Woolloomooloo: NSW Cancer Council; 1997.

32. Lyth G. Clinical supervision: A concept analysis. *J Adv Nurs*. 2000;31(3): 722–729.

33. Scaife J. *Supervision in the mental health professionals: A practitioners guide*. East Sussex: Brunner-Routledge; 2001.

34. Jones A. Possible influences on clinical supervision. *Nurs Stand*. 2001;16(1):38–42.

35. Crowe F, Wilkes C. Clinical supervision for specialist nurses. *Prof Nurse*. 1998;13(5):284–287.

36. Burke P. Risk and supervision: Social work responses to referred user problems. *Br J Soc Work*. 1997;25:115–129.

37. Gennis VM, Gennis MA. Supervision in the outpatient clinic: Effects on teaching and patient care. *J Gen Intern Med*. 1993;8(7):378–380.

38. Ayer S, Knight S, Joyce L, Nightingale V. Practice led education and development project: Developing styles in clinical supervision. *Nurse Educ Today*. 1997;17(5):347–358.

39. McGill I, Beaty L. Action Learning: A Guide for Professional, Management and Educational Development. London: Kogan Page; 1995.

40. Teasdale K, Brocklehurst N, Thom N. Clinical supervision and support for nurses: An evaluation study. *J Adv Nurs*. 2001;33:216–224.

41. Williamson GM, Dodds S. The effectiveness of a group approach to clinical supervision in reducing stress: A review of the literature. *J Clin Nurs*. 1999;8:338–344.

42. Severinsson E, Kamaker D. Clinical nursing supervision in the workplace–effects on moral stress and job satisfaction. *J Nurs Manag*. 1999;7(2): 81–90.

43. Daly J, Lumley J. Bias in qualitative research designs. *Aust N Z J Public Health*. 2002;26:299–300.

**Acknowledgment**: This study was supported by The Alfred Research Trusts Small Project Grant.

**Address correspondence to**: Mari Botti, RN, RM, BN, PhD, MRCNA, Centre for Clinical Nursing Research, Epworth/Deakin Nursing Research Centre, 89 Bridge Road, Richmond Vic 3121, Australia. E-mail: mari.botti@deakin.edu.au

# Exercise for Article 25

## Factual Questions

1. The ward where this study was conducted admits approximately how many oncology patients each year?

2. There were 8 participants in one focus group. How many were in the other one?

3. Were participants free to withdraw from the study?

4. Did the participants sign a consent form?

5. The researchers state that the themes were validated in two ways. What was the second way?

6. The researchers state that they used a small number of participants to enable what?

## Questions for Discussion

7. Do you agree with the researchers that it was a good idea to study only experienced nurses? Explain. (See lines 127–140.)

8. While 15 nurses participated, it is not clear how many were approached. Would it be of interest to know how many were approached? Explain. (See lines 135–140.)

9. Are the focus group discussions described in sufficient detail? Explain. (See lines 175–190.)

10. Did any of the results surprise you? Were any of the results especially interesting? Explain. (See lines 219–503.)

11. Do you agree that the fact that all participants worked within the same setting is a potential limitation? Explain. (See lines 648–652.)

12. If you were planning a follow-up study to explore the topic of this research further, would you plan an additional qualitative study or a quantitative study? Explain.

## Quality Ratings

Directions: Indicate your level of agreement with each of the following statements by circling a number from 5 for strongly agree (SA) to 1 for strongly disagree (SD). If you believe an item is not applicable to this research article, leave it blank. Be prepared to explain your ratings. When responding to criteria A and B, keep in mind that brief titles and abstracts are conventional in published research.

A. The title of the article is appropriate.

    SA   5   4   3   2   1   SD

B. The abstract provides an effective overview of the research article.

    SA   5   4   3   2   1   SD

C. The introduction establishes the importance of the study.

    SA   5   4   3   2   1   SD

D. The literature review establishes the context for the study.

      SA   5   4   3   2   1   SD

E. The research purpose, question, or hypothesis is clearly stated.

      SA   5   4   3   2   1   SD

F. The method of sampling is sound.

      SA   5   4   3   2   1   SD

G. Relevant demographics (for example, age, gender, and ethnicity) are described.

      SA   5   4   3   2   1   SD

H. Measurement procedures are adequate.

      SA   5   4   3   2   1   SD

I. All procedures have been described in sufficient detail to permit a replication of the study.

      SA   5   4   3   2   1   SD

J. The participants have been adequately protected from potential harm.

      SA   5   4   3   2   1   SD

K. The results are clearly described.

      SA   5   4   3   2   1   SD

L. The discussion/conclusion is appropriate.

      SA   5   4   3   2   1   SD

M. Despite any flaws, the report is worthy of publication.

      SA   5   4   3   2   1   SD

# Article 26

# What Adolescents With Type I Diabetes and Their Parents Want From Testing Technology

**Aaron E. Carroll**, MD, MS, **Stephen M. Downs**, MD, MS, **David G. Marrero**, PhD[*]

ABSTRACT. The presence of diabetes in an adolescent can significantly affect his/her normal development. Mobile technology may offer the ability to lessen this negative impact. We wished to learn from adolescents with diabetes and their parents how monitoring systems that incorporated mobile communication technology could potentially help to reduce hassles associated with testing, improve compliance, and ease adolescent-parent conflict about testing behavior. We recruited adolescents between the ages of 13 and 18 years, living with type 1 diabetes mellitus, and their parents for focus groups. Qualitative analysis of the focus group data followed a set procedure. From the discussions, the following themes were identified: *issues with blood glucose monitoring* and *desired technology*. Elements of *desired technology* included *hardware requirements, software requirements, communication,* and *miscellaneous requirements*. The reported needs of this end-user group can help others to leverage maximally the capabilities of new and existing technology to care for children managing chronic disease.

From *CIN: Computers, Informatics, Nursing*, 25, 23–29. Copyright © 2007 by Lippincott Williams & Wilkins. Reprinted with permission.

## Introduction

Adolescence can be a difficult time for young people and their families. In this developmental stage, a child is seeking to form a personal identity, requiring ongoing renegotiation between themselves and their
5 parents regarding norms and values. In particular, there is a redefining of what is appropriate behavior. The presence of diabetes in an adolescent can have a significant effect on this developmental process.[1-4] Parents, concerned about their child's well-being, often try
10 to dictate or enforce therapeutic behavior to their child, who is expected to "be responsible" for his/her diabetes self-care.[4-6] This is particularly evident when considering self-monitoring of blood glucose. In focus group studies conducted by our group, adolescents often re-
15 ported that they do not test as much as they were supposed to. This apparent lack of responsibility resulted in great anxiety in parents, who worry that failure to

achieve strict glycemic control will result in long-term complications associated with the disease. The result-
20 ing conflicts between parent and child created key points of stress in their relationship because many of the parents thought they were put in the position of having to constantly "nag" their children to test their blood glucose.

25 We are interested in whether mobile technology might be used to help address these issues. Specifically, we explored if a device that contained a glucose meter and was capable of transmitting glucose values to either a parent or provider could reduce adolescent-
30 parent conflict over self-management.

Mobile technology could help adolescents to work through complex information that must be processed to make good decisions. Home monitoring data can be transmitted to providers who can react to values indi-
35 cating need for therapeutic response. Because this "assistance" comes from medical professionals, it may help reduce parents' concerns, thus reducing problems associated with parental hypervigilance and manipulation of the regimen to avoid problems of hypoglyce-
40 mia. Children are usually required to check their blood sugar several times each day and make decisions about their insulin dose based upon the results and their meals. Many parents worry about giving their children the freedom to make these decisions. For this to be
45 successful, parents need to be properly informed of the technology's capabilities and convinced that their children will be more competent at managing their diabetes. In addition, using a device's ability to upload information to a provider might mitigate parental stress
50 because parents might feel that a health professional is watching out for their child. Conversely, such a device could also provide an adolescent with the means to contact the healthcare team without having to go through his or her parents. This could provide a sense
55 of empowerment by enabling an adolescent to take corrective action outside of parental awareness. Mobile technology may present an opportunity to build on past experiences and successes to give adolescents a tool

[*]*Aaron E. Carroll* and *Stephen M. Downs*, Children's Health Services Research, Indiana School of Medicine, The Regenstrief Institute for Health Care; and Diabetes Prevention and Control Center, Indiana University School of Medicine, Indianapolis, Indiana. *David G. Marrero*, Diabetes Prevention and Control Center, Indiana University School of Medicine, Indianapolis, Indiana.

that they can use at the point of care to improve their diabetes management, while reducing family stress and concern.

However, there is a danger in assuming that new technology will always be better. Independent consultants estimate that 25% to 50% of information technology (IT) costs are paying for redundant work processes and are therefore unnecessary.[7] Some believe that new IT is as likely to decrease efficiency as it is to increase it.[8] For instance, recent reports in the media have shown a significant backlash against previously validated physician order entry systems and electronic medical record systems in general.[9] This is not to say that the potential does not exist for the success of IT, particularly among adolescents. Adolescents as a group have been consistently more likely to accept technology as an adjunct to care. They have trusted computers to report high-risk behaviors directly to their providers more often and more accurately than they would otherwise.[10–12] Computers have also been used with some success to help with the monitoring and management of adolescent diabetes.[13–15] More novel uses of technology have also met with some success. An educational diabetes video game was used to improve some management-related skills in a relatively well-controlled population.[16] Telephonic contact and automated transmission of blood sugar data resulted in improvement in some measures of care.[17]

Unfortunately, many of the new technologies often discussed for use in patients with diabetes have been around for some time, yet have not been adopted widely. One methodology that could be used to optimize adoption and minimize later problems is that of qualitative research. Qualitative inquiry offers great potential for us to understand better the needs and desires of our end users.[18–20] Therefore, the purpose of this study was to use focus group methodology to learn from adolescents with diabetes and their parents whether mobile monitoring technology could help to reduce hassles associated with testing, improve compliance, and ease adolescent-parent conflict about testing behavior.

## Methods

### Sample

Adolescents with type 1 diabetes and their parents were recruited from a diabetes clinic in Indianapolis, IN. Ten focus groups were conducted with a total of 59 participants (23 males and 36 females); five groups consisted of adolescents with diabetes ($n = 31$) and five groups consisted of their parents ($n = 28$). The parents and the adolescents met separately, and the content of each group was not revealed to the other. This study was approved by the Institutional Review Board of Indiana University, and all subjects provided informed consent. Subjects were paid $40 to participate.

### Focus Group Methodology

The purpose of these focus groups was to gather information from adolescents with type 1 diabetes and their parents related to blood glucose monitoring and the use of mobile technology to improve compliance with diabetes management. The focus group leader was a professional facilitator trained and experienced in working with healthcare populations. She used a prepared set of open-ended qualitative questions to facilitate the 2-hour sessions (e.g., "What do you like about your testing equipment and what do you not like? How can we use technology to improve the way your children manage their diabetes? Design what you think would be the ideal testing device."). Participants were then shown a prototype of a mobile technology that combines the benefits of blood glucose testing with that of a mobile phone.[21] Participants were asked to verbalize their thoughts about the device, suggest any relevant changes to it that would increase their use of this technology, and speculate how this technology might influence parent-child relations regarding self-monitoring behavior. The focus groups were all tape-recorded and later transcribed. Efforts were made to elicit responses from all participants.

### Qualitative Analysis

Qualitative analysis of the data was conducted using a set procedure: (1) review of the audiotapes, (2) review of the tape transcriptions, (3) discussions among investigators regarding key elements of subjects' statements, (4) determination of conceptual themes, and (5) assignment of relevant responses to appropriate thematic constructs.[22] A pediatrician, a social ecologist, and a nurse practitioner with training in medical sociology, all of whom have experience with qualitative methods, were the study team. In particular, the social ecologist (DGM) has experience with focus group methodology and has published a number of studies using the quantitative methods reported here. All of the research team members had experience with the target population through clinical work and research efforts. A group consisting of eight clinicians and two experienced qualitative researchers worked in conjunction with the research team to contribute to the development of the group questions used by the facilitator (see Acknowledgments). The pediatrician attended the focus group sessions, contributed appropriate additional questions, and took detailed notes. Transcriptions were available within a week or two of each focus group, and audiotapes were reviewed within 1 week of session completion.

## Results

The five adolescent focus groups had 31 participants; the five parent focus groups had 28 participants. The numbers of males and females were about equal. Adolescents were between 13 and 18 years (mean, 14.9 years) and had been living with diabetes for between 6 months and 14 years (mean, 6.6 years). Demographic data on the focus group participants are presented in Table 1.

Table 1
*Demographic Data of Focus Group Participants*

|  | Parents (*n* = 28) | Adolescents (*n* = 31) |
|---|---|---|
| Gender |  |  |
| Female | 23 | 13 |
| Male | 5 | 18 |
| Child's age |  |  |
| 13–14 y | 15 | 14 |
| 15–16 y | 8 | 11 |
| 17–18 y | 5 | 6 |
| Ethnicity |  |  |
| White | 26 | 28 |
| African American | 2 | 3 |
| Parent employment status |  |  |
| Working | 19 (68%) |  |
| Not working | 9 (32%) |  |
| Child's duration of diabetes (y) |  |  |
| 0–3 | 6 (21%) |  |
| 3–6 | 11 (39%) |  |
| 6–9 | 3 (11%) |  |
| 10 or more | 8 (29%) |  |

The themes that emerged were *issues with blood glucose monitoring* and *desired technology*. Elements of *desired technology* included *hardware requirements, software requirements,* and *communication.*

### Issues with Blood Glucose Monitoring

Blood glucose monitoring was a contentious issue for the focus group participants: Parents struggled with controlling their adolescents' blood glucose at a time when the teenagers themselves wanted to assert more control over their lives. Discussions related to blood glucose monitoring within the adolescent groups and the parent groups clustered into the same categories: compliance with the diabetic regimen and parent-child relationships.

### Compliance with the Diabetic Regimen

Self-monitoring was viewed by many of the teens as the most inconvenient, disruptive, and least favorite aspect of having diabetes. Several stated that they do not like to test and admitted that they tested less often than advised. For some, there is a social discomfort in testing in front of friends. This may explain why most participants who acknowledged skipping testing did so before lunch at school.

Parents in all groups noted that as their children hit adolescence, it became more difficult to control their children's blood glucose monitoring. Testing behavior was noted by parents and adolescents to be influenced by several forces: school, peer influences, and social stigma. Several participants stated that they frequently forgot to test at various times throughout the day or week, and some of the teens did not test if they thought their levels were high or low because they expected a negative parental reaction.

### Parent-Child Relationships

Parents noted that it was difficult to determine when to step in versus when to give up control of the management of diabetes to their children. In general, as the adolescents neared adulthood, most parents felt the need to relinquish some control of managing the diabetes to their children.

Parents expressed frustration and felt they were constantly "nagging" children about testing because they were worried about irreversible damage that can occur to their children's bodies. Parents across all groups wanted to know their teenagers were testing, without being perceived negatively by their children. There was clearly tension between the desire to "let go and trust" that the adolescents would be responsible and the need to "just be sure" that they were, in fact, managing their diabetic regimen.

The adolescents stated that their parents' behaviors as a result of this concern could be overbearing or "annoying," "stressful," "controlling," "nagging," and "overprotective." Trust was discussed across the groups in that it was important for the teens to feel that their parents trusted their diabetic management. They acknowledge that it was scary for parents to let go of control and suggested keeping lines of communication open so that diabetes management could be discussed in a way that was not punitive or "blaming."

### Desired Technology

Teenagers and their parents were asked to design the ultimate testing equipment (i.e., a system that would best work for their lifestyle). Although the basic technology discussed was fairly similar across groups, the suggestions of what to do with the data once the values were collected were very different between parents and adolescents.

*Hardware requirements.* Participants in all groups were asked to design the ideal testing device as a component of the self-management routine, without prompting from the moderator. Discussion in the adolescent focus groups initially centered on the actual method of testing. They came up with ideas for an implantable or wearable device that would test blood glucose, calculate insulin dosage, and deliver the appropriate insulin dose. This was especially popular among the teenagers because it would require no intervention by the teens themselves. Comments included:

> It would be inserted somewhere, so that every couple of hours it would just test by itself.

> I just had something that is permanently inside of you that send[s] the reading to your pump and tells you what to do.

The teenage participants then quickly moved away from the actual test into how technology could be used for all other aspects of their care. They initially focused on technology with which they were already familiar:

190

personal digital assistants (PDAs) and cell phones. One of the participants suggested the following:

> It is the size of a PDA—a little smaller. It would have a calendar on it so when it tests your blood it records the level to the calendar. It would also have a thing that would automatically e-mail your doctor. Then it would have a part that would prick your finger and suck blood out, so that you would not have to squeeze it out. When it was done checking the blood sugar, it would read out and spit the old tester out. It would have a number like a beeper so that you could call it from phones [in case it was misplaced]. It could be washer safe, so if it got left in your clothes it could go through the washer.

Other teenagers jumped immediately to the idea of using their cell phones as a tester. They explained that their cell phone was with them at all times, looked like everyone else's cell phone, and combining the two technologies would prevent them from having to carry both a phone and a tester. This idea was especially popular with the older teenagers (17–18 years old); it was moderately popular with those 15 to 16 years old and only slightly popular with those 13 to 14 years old. This may be indicative of the more common use of cell phones as the participants aged.

Parents also quickly discussed the idea of using a cell phone as a tester. They felt that most adolescents had cell phones and that they almost always carried them. Some of their comments included:

> I think it would be cool because all kids have phones, so they would still look like a normal kid.

> I'm thinking that kids don't forget cell phones. So if you can put it in there somehow, that would work.

However, it should be noted that parents of the younger adolescents were less excited about the idea of a cell phone. There were concerns about responsibility for having a cell phone at the age of 13 or 14 years; the parents of those 17 to 18 years old did not share those concerns. Again, this seems to be an indication that the average age for cell phone use is likely somewhat older than 13 or 14 years.

After the groups discussed their designs, the facilitator focused on the cell phone/glucose meter option, explaining that this type of device was available as a prototype. Reactions to this prototype were extremely positive across all groups, including participants who had not been overly enthusiastic when they thought they were discussing a concept rather than a reality. Discussions about the prototype in the parent and adolescent groups clustered into the following categories: (1) software requirements, and (2) communication.

*Software requirements.* Participants were asked to identify what functions the tester and/or the phone would need to excite them about this product. There were three primary functions that parents and adolescents identified: (1) calculations, (2) data capture/upload/storage, and (3) alarms.

*Calculations.* There was one primary analytic capability that was considered essential across all groups: calculating the amount of insulin required for a given blood glucose level, based on an individual's management plan. Insulin dose calculation was seen as a burden by the adolescents and their parents; it was complicated by orders changing frequently so that memorization of dosages is nearly impossible.

*Data capture/upload/storage.* One of the most interesting features for both the parents and the adolescents was the idea of blood glucose levels being automatically uploaded onto a Web site that parents, healthcare providers, and the teens could access at any time. Some of the teenagers saw this as a positive feature because they felt that it would decrease the "constant nagging" by their parents regarding their test results. Parents also liked the idea because it would be automatic, the teenagers would be unable to lie about their results, and they could not adjust or change the results to appear normal. Some of the comments about this feature included:

> You wouldn't have to always call your parents and tell them what you got. They could just look on the computer.

> I want it to go to some type of document where they can record their readings and you can hook it up to the computer and the doctor can see all the test readings when you go. That way they won't have to write everything down.

> I think that if you are going to spend all this money then my doctor should see the results at least every 2 weeks because that is how often he wants to see them now.

*Alarms.* The idea of an alarm that would sound when it was time to test elicited a strong negative response from most of the teens but was a positive feature for the majority of the parents. The teenagers stated that alarms during class or when friends were around were embarrassing and called attention to them. Others stated that they tended to ignore the alarms if they had them, so they did not see them as a helpful feature.

During the initial discussion, many parents saw the alarm feature as extremely important; some even felt it was a necessity. There was discussion as to whether or not it would be a "deal breaker"—that if the alarm was not an option, it would stop parents from purchasing the phone. It is of importance that the parents of the younger teenagers, the 13- to 14-year-olds, felt this was a more important function than did the parents of the teenagers 15 to 18 years. However, after additional discussion among themselves, none of the parents felt it was essential; they would purchase the phone even if it did not have an alarm function.

### Communication

Four primary themes centered on communication: (1) parent notification of test results, (2) physician notification of test results, (3) communication between provider and adolescent, and (4) emergency assistance.

*Parent notification of test results.* Perhaps the most contentious issue between the parents and their teenagers was whether the self-monitoring results should be communicated directly to the parents. As the adolescents aged, they found this feature to be more offensive. The group with participants 13 to 14 years old was the most accepting of this communication; not surprisingly, the group with those 17 to 18 years old had the most negative reaction to this feature. Some of the comments from the teens regarding automatic notifications included:

> It should only tell my parents if it went really low.

> Why would you tell your parents? We are going to be adults very soon.

> If I tested and my sugar is 400 and it goes to my mom immediately, I don't want her calling and bitching me out because my sugar is high. I already know that it is high. I don't need to hear it from you, too.

> Seriously, if it sent it to my parents every time then they would just call me all the time.

During the initial discussions, this issue was a deal breaker for many of the parents. However, as discussion continued, it became apparent that the primary goal of the parents was to encourage compliance with testing; they were willing to accept anything that would increase the likelihood of testing, even if it meant that they did not get immediate feedback on test results. Some of the other parent comments concluded:

> It's not so much of us having control but giving us information so that if we need to take control we can.

> It is letting them take responsibility and letting us feel that we can oversee it.

> Text message results to the parents. See, then we wouldn't have to nag them because we would know that they are testing and we would know that they are alive.

> I would prefer to be notified just when they are out of range.

After discussion, the pediatrician told the parents that this feature was sometimes not well received by the adolescents. If the teenagers would not use the meter because of this feature, the parents were willing to omit it. They noted that they would still have access to the numbers via the Internet, or by accessing the teenagers' phone tester directly. This gave them more comfort because they would still be able to access the data and track their children's progress. One mother may have summed up the basic concern of the parents when she stated: "I don't need control. I need access."

*Physician notification of test results.* In contrast to the concerns raised with parental notification, the teenagers had no issue with directly providing their physicians with testing data. Indeed, they admitted that they would be more likely to test as they were supposed to and be more careful with their diabetes management because they would know their clinics would be getting the whole picture. There were no negative responses to this feature of the testing device; positive comments from the teenagers included:

> I think that kids would be healthier because they will know that they couldn't cheat.

> There would be better compliance because you don't want your doctor to yell at you.

> That would be cool. It would really be convenient.

Parents also had positive reactions about this feature, and it allowed them to be somewhat more comfortable with the idea of not directly receiving the results. In fact, it was seen as a way to decrease the burden of diabetes on their children because the results would automatically flow to the clinic. This would relieve the children of the need to keep logs of their test results.

*Communication between provider and adolescent.* Participants were queried about how they would feel if communication regarding regimen changes occurred directly between the adolescents and their providers, with parents receiving e-mail or text messages summarizing the communication. Teenagers had an overall positive reaction to this idea. However, there was some difference regarding how communication would take place: speaking with the provider versus receiving a text message with the regimen changes.

Parents of the younger teenagers were somewhat skeptical of their children's ability to understand the changes in regimen unless the physicians were more careful about how they explained the changes. However, the parents' overall responses were positive as long as the parents were "kept in the loop." Some of their comments included:

> At this age he should start taking on the responsibility, but I would like to know what happens.

> Or just store it on a Web site where I can access it. She is my little girl, and I want to be able to keep track. I don't want to be a nag; I just want to say, "Hey, your regimen changed" or "Do you need any help?"

> It would be great! It would take the monkey off our backs. Who wouldn't like that?

> I am comfortable with that because I know this is where it has to head.

*Emergency assistance.* One feature identified by both the teenagers and their parents as essential was some sort of emergency notification of parents, emergency personnel, or other identified individuals in the event that a blood sugar reading was dangerously high or low. Some of the recommendations included:

> It would be nice if it would contact somebody if you were really high or really low.

The phone would have to have GPS. That way if there is a situation where they are comatose, then we know where the hell they are.

475 I want it to beep me if his sugar is too high or too low. Also if it is really high or low maybe even have it contact the ER.

Can this phone have an, "I am diabetic" thing that will tell people in case they get into a car accident? Well, they won't wear a bracelet.

## Discussion

480 This study used qualitative research techniques to conduct an investigation into the needs of an end-user group to leverage maximally the capabilities of new and existing technology to care for children managing chronic disease. Type 1 diabetes is a disease in which 485 information management is imperative; there are multiple checks every day and many decisions that must be made correctly based not only on the most recent information, but also information gathered in the past. In the adolescent population, this difficult task is compli-490 cated by the teens' desire to accept greater responsibility while still needing assistance from adults. Ideally, technology should help them to make this transition more easily.

Adolescents want their testing equipment to inte-495 grate into the social realm in which they live. They want their devices to be "cool," to mimic devices already ubiquitous in their peer groups. They don't mind such devices acting as a safety net for their excessively high or low blood sugar readings, but they do not want 500 their parents getting real-time values as they are checked. Interestingly, they are not opposed to the health system, including their physicians, receiving real-time values. They desire an interaction with the healthcare system that is empowering and developmen-505 tally appropriate. Any device that seeks to capitalize on these desires and make a real difference must also account for the behavioral and relationship difficulties among adolescents, their parents, peers, and school. It must help to ease the age-old conflict between devel-510 opmental norms of independence and the appearance of rebellion. Furthermore, developers and users must be sensitive to developmental needs across the ages of the adolescent spectrum. Prior research has shown that the safety net provided by some forms of mobile technol-515 ogy can have an impact on these relationships. Advances in technology have made the ability to collect and transmit data more sophisticated and synchronous.

There are several limitations to this study. Some include the focus group methodology itself: small con-520 venience samples limit the generalizability of the findings; group consensus may inhibit an individual from stating his/her differing opinion; introverted individuals may be more apt to keep silent about their opinions.

The current study provides an opportunity to under-525 stand the potential impact of new testing technology on type 1 diabetes through the eyes of adolescents aged 13 to 18 years and their parents. Novel testing technology should set a new norm for the way adolescents interact with the healthcare system. It should introduce them to 530 the fact that it is appropriate to have a relationship with their providers without their parents' involvement. It should open lines of communication and allow for the transmission of data to parties who can make use of it. Most important, it should help to reduce the burden felt 535 by parents to enforce proper testing and management. Diabetes can be a crucible for family problems, enmeshment, and dysfunctional behavior; advances in technology should seek to lessen its impact.

Cell phones appear to be an excellent vehicle for 540 meeting the needs and desires of adolescents with diabetes and their parents. Such phones already are used by a large number of adolescents and would draw no attention to their users; in fact, it might be seen as an attractive addition to many users. The devices have the 545 ability to [set] house alarms, if desired, and transmit text messages and more detailed information. Cell phones with glucose meters embedded within them could meet most of the needs expressed by subjects in this study. Such devices are under development by a 550 number of companies. However, they must be coupled with new systems of care that leverage these abilities to change behavior and the actions of all parties involved.

## References

1. Anderson BJ. Children with diabetes mellitus and family functioning: translating research into practice. *J Pediatr Endocrinol Metab.* 2001;14(Suppl 1):645–652.
2. Gowers SG, Jones JC, Kiana S, North CD, Price DA. Family functioning: A correlate of diabetic control? *J Child Psychol Psychiatry.* 1995;36(6):993–1001.
3. Daneman D, Wolfson DH, Becker DJ, Drash AL. Factors affecting glycosylated hemoglobin values in children with insulin-dependent diabetes. *J Pediatr.* 1981;99(6):847–853.
4. Anderson BJ, Brackett J, Ho J, Laffel LM. An office-based intervention to maintain parent-adolescent teamwork in diabetes management. Impact on parent involvement, family conflict, and subsequent glycemic control. *Diabetes Care.* 1999;22(5):713–721.
5. Miller-Johnson S, Emery RE, Marvin RS, Clarke W, Lovinger R, Martin M. Parent–child relationships and the management of insulin-dependent diabetes mellitus. *J Consult Clin Psychol.* 1994;62(3):603–610.
6. Coyne JC, Anderson BJ. The 'psychosomatic family' reconsidered: diabetes in context. *J Marital Fam Ther.* 1988;14:113–123.
7. Dorenfest S. The decade of the '90s: Poor use of IT investment contributes to the growing healthcare crisis. *Healthc Inform.* 2000;17(8):64–67.
8. Gibbs WW. Taking computers to task. *Sci Am.* 1997;277(1):82–89.
9. Langberg ML. Challenges to implementing CPOE: A case study of a work in progress at Cedars-Sinai. *Modern Physician.* 2003; February 1; 21.
10. Turner CF, Ku L, Rogers SM, Lindberg LD, Pleck JH, Sonenstein FL. Adolescent sexual behavior, drug use, and violence: Increased reporting with computer survey technology. *Science.* 1998;280(5365):867–873.
11. Millstein SG, Irwin CE Jr. Acceptability of computer-acquired sexual histories in adolescent girls. *J Pediatr.* 1983;103(5):815–819.
12. Paperny DM, Aono JY, Lehman RM, Hammar SL, Risser J. Computer-assisted detection and intervention in adolescent high-risk health behaviors. *J Pediatr.* 1990;116(3):456–462.
13. Rosenfalck AM, Bendtson I. The Diva System, a computerized diary, used in young type 1 diabetic patients. *Diabetes Metab.* 1993;19(1):25–29.
14. Horan PP, Yarborough MC, Besigel G, Carlson DR. Computer-assisted self-control of diabetes by adolescents. *Diabetes Educ.* 1990;16(3):205–211.
15. Marrero DG, Kronz KK, Golden MP, Wright JC, Orr DP, Fineberg NS. Clinical evaluation of computer-assisted self-monitoring of blood glucose system. *Diabetes Care.* 1989;12(5):345–350.

16. Brown SJ, Lieberman DA, Germeny BA, Fan YC, Wilson DM, Pasta DJ. Educational video game for juvenile diabetes: Results of a controlled trial. *Med Inform (Lond)*. 1997;22(1):77–89.
17. Marrero DG, Vandagriff JL, Kronz K, et al. Using telecommunication technology to manage children with diabetes: The Computer-Linked Outpatient Clinic (CLOC) Study. *Diabetes Educ*. 1995;21(4):313–319.
18. Leys M. Health technology assessment: The contribution of qualitative research. *Int J Technol Assess Health Care*. 2003;19(2):317–329.
19. Ash JS, Sittig DF, Seshadri V, Dykstra RH, Carpenter JD, Stavri PZ. Adding insight: A qualitative cross-site study of physician order entry. *Int J Med Inform*. 2005;74(7–8):623–628.
20. May C, Harrison R, Finch T, MacFarlane A, Mair F, Wallace P. Understanding the normalization of telemedicine services through qualitative evaluation. *J Am Med Inform Assoc*. 2003;10(6):596–604.
21. HealthPia America. http://www.healthpia.us
22. Morgan DL. *Focus Groups as Qualitative Research*. Beverly Hills, CA: Sage Publications; 1988.

**Acknowledgments**: The authors thank the adolescents, their parents, and the physician offices that referred them to our study. We are especially grateful to the adolescents who were willing to share with us their experiences of living with diabetes so that we can better understand and provide care for them. We also thank Terri Matousek of Matousek and Associates for conducting all of the focus groups, and Heather Herdman, RN, PhD, for her assistance with data analysis.

**Funding**: This research was funded by grants from the NIH to AEC (1 K23 DK067879-01), and from Clarian Health Partners to AEC (VFR-190).

**Address correspondence to**: Aaron E. Carroll MD, MS, Riley Research 330, 699 West Drive, Indianapolis, IN 46202 E-mail: aaecarro@iupui.edu

# Exercise for Article 26

## Factual Questions

1. What was the total number of participants?

2. How much were the participants paid for their participation?

3. Were the proceedings of the focus groups tape-recorded?

4. The study team consisted of a pediatrician, a social ecologist, and who else?

5. How many of the adolescents were African American?

6. How many of the parents had children between 13 and 14 years of age?

## Questions for Discussion

7. Do you think it was a good idea to have the parents and adolescents meet separately? (See lines 107–108.)

8. Do you think the method of qualitative analysis is described in sufficient detail? (See lines 136–160.)

9. To what extent do the quotations from participants interspersed throughout the Results section help you understand the results of this study? (See lines 161–480.)

10. Do you think that the use of a small convenience sample greatly limits the generalizability of the results of this study? (See lines 519–522.)

11. Do you agree that the focus group methodology may have inhibited some participants from stating differing opinions? (See lines 522–524.)

12. If you were planning a follow-up study to explore the topic of this research further, would you plan an additional qualitative study or a quantitative study? Explain.

## Quality Ratings

Directions: Indicate your level of agreement with each of the following statements by circling a number from 5 for strongly agree (SA) to 1 for strongly disagree (SD). If you believe an item is not applicable to this research article, leave it blank. Be prepared to explain your ratings. When responding to criteria A and B, keep in mind that brief titles and abstracts are conventional in published research.

A. The title of the article is appropriate.

    SA   5   4   3   2   1   SD

B. The abstract provides an effective overview of the research article.

    SA   5   4   3   2   1   SD

C. The introduction establishes the importance of the study.

    SA   5   4   3   2   1   SD

D. The literature review establishes the context for the study.

    SA   5   4   3   2   1   SD

E. The research purpose, question, or hypothesis is clearly stated.

    SA   5   4   3   2   1   SD

F. The method of sampling is sound.

    SA   5   4   3   2   1   SD

G. Relevant demographics (for example, age, gender, and ethnicity) are described.

    SA   5   4   3   2   1   SD

H. Measurement procedures are adequate.

    SA   5   4   3   2   1   SD

I. All procedures have been described in sufficient detail to permit a replication of the study.

    SA   5   4   3   2   1   SD

J. The participants have been adequately protected from potential harm.

    SA   5   4   3   2   1   SD

K. The results are clearly described.

    SA   5   4   3   2   1   SD

L. The discussion/conclusion is appropriate.

    SA   5   4   3   2   1   SD

M. Despite any flaws, the report is worthy of publication.

    SA   5   4   3   2   1   SD

# Article 27

# One Breath at a Time: Living With Cystic Fibrosis

**Dona Rinaldi Carpenter,** EdD, RN, CS, **Georgia L. Narsavage,** PhD, RN, CS[*]

### ABSTRACT

The purpose of this qualitative investigation was to describe the lived experiences of families caring for a child with cystic fibrosis at the time of initial diagnosis. Phenomenological research methodology as described by Colaizzi (1978) was used to guide the investigation. A purposive sample of 9 family members voluntarily participated in the study. Data were gathered through focus groups and written narratives.

Data analysis yielded 3 essential theme clusters with subthemes: *Falling Apart, Pulling Together,* and *Moving Beyond.* Within the theme of *Falling Apart,* the subthemes of Devastation of Diagnosis, An All-Encompassing Sense of Fear and Isolation, and An Overwhelming Sense of Guilt and Powerlessness are described. The theme of *Pulling Together* included the subthemes of Perpetual Vigilance and Returning to Normalcy, and the third theme of *Moving Beyond* included the subtheme of An Optimal Unfolding of a New Kind of Consciousness. This article describes in detail the themes and subthemes identified during data analysis and the fluid nature of the relationship that exists within the essential structure of caring for a family member with cystic fibrosis.

The diagnosis of cystic fibrosis most often comes as a life-shattering experience to families. Lifestyle readjustments are made in an attempt to return to some sense of family normalcy. In order to achieve stability in their daily lives, families are vigilant in the care and monitoring of the health of a child with cystic fibrosis. Ongoing support from health care professionals that is grounded in the realities of living with cystic fibrosis is critical. This study describes how families develop their own unique way of controlling the experience of living with cystic fibrosis, one day and one breath at a time.

From *Journal of Pediatric Nursing: Nursing Care of Children and Families, 19,* 25–32. Copyright © 2004 by Elsevier, Inc. Reprinted with permission.

Until recently, cystic fibrosis (CF) was classified as a terminal childhood disease. New information and treatment protocols have changed this perception. A short lifespan is no longer the norm for individuals with CF (White, Munro, & Boyle, 1996). Advances in research along with newer treatment protocols have increased life expectancy (Fiel, 1993). Many patients with CF live high-quality lives well into adulthood, often into their 40s. With increased life expectancy, patients and their families are given new hope that scientists will find a cure within their lifetimes.

Despite the multitude of research studies related to CF, the nature and essence of the family caregiving experience for a child with CF is not known. The purpose of this qualitative research study was to describe the life experience of individuals caring for a family member with cystic fibrosis. A phenomenological approach to studying the caregiver experience provides a means to describe, in depth, the lived experience of providing care for a child with CF. The research question guiding the study was, "*What is the lived experience of caring for a family member with cystic fibrosis?*"

### Related Literature

CF is a genetic disease caused by mutations in a single gene that encodes the cystic fibrosis transmembrane conductance regulator (Hopkins, 1996). Clinical manifestations of CF vary widely and are characterized by abnormal secretions of the respiratory, gastrointestinal, and reproductive tracts and the sweat glands (Wilmott & Fiedler, 1994). The severity of the disease varies considerably as well. Some patients experience mild gastrointestinal or pulmonary problems, whereas others experience severe malabsorption problems and fatal pulmonary complications. The gastrointestinal manifestations of cystic fibrosis are not as typical of the disease as are the pulmonary complications, but family members must understand the potential impact of the disease on the child's overall growth and development (Duffield, 1996). After the discovery of the CF gene in 1989, treatment for cystic fibrosis changed as research related to CF gathered momentum. Although a cure is still unavailable, scientists have made progress in identification and early treatment of exacerbations, thus extending life expectancy in this often devastating illness.

---

[*]*Dona Rinaldi Carpenter* currently teaches medical-surgical nursing as well as undergraduate and graduate research for the Department of Nursing, University of Scranton. *Georgia L. Narsavage* is associate professor of nursing; associate dean of academic programs; and director, ND program; Frances Payne Bolton School of Nursing, Case Western Reserve University.

Most patients with CF live at home and incorporate a variety of treatments into their daily lives. Family members are most often the primary caregivers, and they interact with providers from multiple disciplines as episodic care is needed (Reed, 1990; Sawyer, 1992; Tracy, 1997). Treatment generally focuses on control of symptoms using regimens of physiotherapy to loosen secretions, medications to prevent and cure infections, and enzymes as nutritional supplements for support of gastrointestinal functioning (Fiel, 1993; Hopkins, 1995). New approaches to treatment are being developed, but until a cure is achieved, pulmonary infection and inflammation that lead to respiratory failure and premature death remain the focus of therapy.

Living with CF involves changes in identities, roles, relationship abilities, and patterns of behavior for all family members (Brown & Powell-Cope, 1991). Routine therapies that are required of the CF family are rigorous, complex, and time consuming. Dealing with complex drug and therapy regimens at home can prove to be very stressful for parents and other family members. Helping families understand the purpose and effective implementation of therapies as well as what to expect when living with a family member who has a chronic disease can be effective in helping them cope with the situation.

Clearly, the medical aspects of CF and the effectiveness of medications used to manage the disease have been studied extensively using quantitative methodology (Hopkins, 1996). However, quantitative studies are, by their very nature, restricted to examining a limited number of variables. There are relatively few qualitative research studies on family care giving related to cystic fibrosis that can provide a window into the experience of living with this extremely complex multivariate disease.

What is known is that the routine stresses in caring for a child with CF can become overwhelming for everyone in the family (Eiser, Zprotch, Hiller, Havermans, & Billig, 1995). A Scottish ethnographic study of 4 families living with family members who had CF described the crisis experience and the continuing care burden. The emotional devastation felt was placed within the context of needing to share the experience with other families in an attempt to make lifestyle adjustments (Whyte, 1992). Baine, Rosenbaum, and King (1995) surveyed families living with a child with a chronic illness (diabetes or CF). The researchers identified knowing about the illness, what to expect, continuity and accessibility of care, and involvement of the family in care as being the highest priority in terms of family preparatory needs. The sense of fear and isolation expressed by the participants in a study by Baine et al. (1995) was further described in a 22-week telephone support intervention study that improved life quality for parents of children with CF (Ritchie et al., 2000). Geiss et al. (1992) described a significant relationship between perceived compliance with CF treatment and the mother's decreased social contacts. Mothers of children with chronic illness experienced stressful interactions with partners and professionals as they tried to manage the child's disease and keep daily life as "normal" as possible (Stewart, Ritchie, McGrath, Thompson, & Bruce, 1994). Similarly, D'Auria, Christian, and Richardson (1997), in a grounded theory study of 20 children living with CF, found that "keeping up" or leading as normal a life as possible was a theme central to the experience of those in middle childhood. Siblings of children with CF reported being worried, jealous, and frustrated as activities were restricted for everyone in the family, and conversely, they noted "positive" outcomes of the impact of CF on the family—strengthened relationships, enhanced independence, and feelings of satisfaction as the child with CF improves (Derouin & Jessee, 1996). Coping with stress can be both positive and negative.

Interventions that can assist families in coping with the stress of CF have also been studied. Ryan and Williams (1996), describing the use of a cystic fibrosis handbook shared by parents with the children's teachers, found that this written information could enhance knowledge of the disease, support communication to overcome the sense of powerlessness that parents experience, and help the child return to a less abnormal school experience. Additionally, a pilot intervention study (Williams et al., 1997) for 22 siblings of children with CF, cancer, diabetes, and spina bifida found that an educational intervention could increase knowledge about the chronic illness, but support sessions were equally as important to the intervention. Bartholomew et al. (1997) used a CF Family Education Program intervention for 104 families and compared it with 94 "usual care" families living with CF. Knowledge and self-efficacy scores had a significant interaction effect on short-term disease management outcomes for both caregivers and children with CF.

Although the research on identified stressors and interventions is valuable in understanding coping in families who have lived with CF for extended periods of time, these studies do not explain experiences of living with a family member who has CF at the time of diagnosis. Relating the pathophysiology of the diagnosis to the coping issues, Reed (1990) has proposed possible family responses to a diagnosis of CF from a theoretical perspective. Reed (1990) described the potential for "altered family process" as families learn to live with the need to recognize problems and assist the child in a timely manner. Nevertheless, this theoretical approach to the family experience when the diagnosis is first known has not been tested or developed from a real-world perspective.

In summary, there is a large body of quantitative research related to the medical aspects surrounding the care of individuals with CF. Understanding the perspective of families caring for a child with CF at the time of diagnosis has not been studied. Qualitative research approaches are best suited to describing the phenomena of living with and adapting to CF at this critical point in time.

## Method

165 The study design was descriptive and grounded in phenomenological research methodology. The anticipated outcome was to describe the essential information needed by individuals with family members who have cystic fibrosis by developing rich descriptions of 170 the life experiences of families caring for a child with cystic fibrosis. Families who are actively involved in the caring process were sought as an expert source of how to live with and care for a child with CF.

### Sample

A purposive sample of 9 family members voluntar175 ily participated in data collection. Participants were selected based on their firsthand experience with the phenomenon of interest to allow for development of rich descriptions of the life experiences of families caring for a child with cystic fibrosis. Family members 180 involved in support groups for children with cystic fibrosis from 3 metropolitan areas participated in the study. Institutional review board (IRB) approval was obtained.

### Procedures for Generation and Treatment of Data

Although the researchers intended to collect all data 185 using focus group technique, only 3 family members agreeing to participate in the study were able to attend a focus group. Parents caring for children with CF expressed great interest in participating in the research; however, family caregiving responsibilities left little 190 time for any activity that required time away from home. Therefore, the remaining 6 participants contributed to the study via written narratives. Detailed written responses to the same open-ended questions used with the focus groups were completed, providing com195 parable data to that collected in the focus group.

Anderson and Hatton (2000) noted that time and energy are limited in vulnerable populations, such as families living with illness. Sensitivity to issues of vulnerability is critical, and in this particular instance, data 200 collection methods required modification. Responding to the questions used for the first focus group provided an opportunity for parents to participate without leaving their family. Participants completing written narratives were asked to write in as much detail as possible 205 to ensure full and rich descriptions.

IRB approval for the study was obtained from the University of Scranton, and written informed consent for participation and audiotaping was obtained from all participants. The focus group was conducted using a 210 semistructured interview process, and it took place in a seminar setting suitable for audiotaping. Consent forms were distributed along with a brief demographic data sheet and questionnaire. The moderator (first author) used an interview guide (see Table 1) consisting of

215 open-ended questions. Questions for the interview were generated in advance to guide and elicit rich descriptions of the experience of caring for a child with cystic fibrosis. The focus group was audiotaped and transcribed verbatim by a department assistant. Detailed 220 field notes were kept as well by the second researcher/author. Upon conclusion of the interview, participants were encouraged to contact the researchers by phone or in writing if additional information relevant to the study became evident.

Table 1
*Questions Guiding Data Collection*

1. What comes to mind when you hear the words cystic fibrosis?
2. What is the meaning of caring for someone with cystic fibrosis?
3. What aspects of care have proven to be most beneficial?
4. What aspects of care have you found most manageable?
5. What do you wish you had been told when you first had to care for your child at home?
6. What additional problems have occurred that you have had to deal with at home?
7. If you were to give another person a video to help them, what information do you think it should include?

225 Participants who responded in narrative format were requested to answer the same questions used to guide the focus group, to write in as much detail as possible, and to continue writing until no new ideas came to mind. The first author contacted participants 230 by phone to clarify questions that emerged from the written narratives. Data were gathered until no new themes emerged and significant repetition of themes reflecting data saturation was established.

Data were generated and analyzed from a phe235 nomenological perspective using the procedures identified by Colaizzi (1978). The steps used to guide this were (1) describe the phenomenon of interest; (2) collect participants' description of the phenomena through the use of focus groups and narrative written responses; 240 (3) transcribe audiotaped interviews and written narratives; (4) return to the original transcripts and extract significant statements; (5) describe the meaning of each significant statement; (6) organize the aggregate formalized meanings into clusters of themes; (7) write an 245 exhaustive description; (8) return the exhaustive description to the subjects for validation; and (9) incorporate new data revealed during the validation into an exhaustive description.

The transcripts from the focus group and written 250 narratives were read and reread in their entirety by the first author. Significant statements related to families' experiences caring for a child with cystic fibrosis were extracted, followed by description of the formulated meaning. Clusters of themes were organized from ag-

Table 2
*Selected Examples of Significant Statements and Corresponding Formulated Meanings*

| Significant statement | Formulated meaning |
| --- | --- |
| **Theme cluster**: "Falling Apart" | |
| …it's really overwhelming when you first find out your child has cystic fibrosis. | The diagnosis of CF is a life-shattering experience. |
| …it is easy to fall apart very quickly. | The experience is so devastating the presentation of new and unfamiliar stressors can result in a very sudden sense of losing control over what one knows as normal or routine. |
| …when you are initially diagnosed, you think that this only happened to you. | The diagnosis of CF brings with it a sense of isolation. |
| …we were afraid to leave the house…afraid we might go around someone that might have an infection or a cold. | Fear directs life choices immediately following diagnosis. |
| …to do percussions on 2 children two to three times a day is sometimes physically impossible. | Fitting everything that is required into each day is sometimes unrealistic, yet parents feel guilty and experience a sense of powerlessness. |
| **Theme cluster**: "Pulling Together" | |
| …how do you put it all together to make a life that makes sense? | Living with CF means putting the requirements of care for a child with CF together with the requirements of daily living. |
| …we tried to get CF to be part of the fabric of our lives. | CF becomes a part of everything in the lives of the patient and family. |
| …your whole life changes to make living with CF manageable. It changes because it has to change. | Lifestyle adaptations are ongoing and in response to new stressors as they present themselves. Continuous adaptation is required to promote and maintain health. |
| **Theme cluster**: "Moving Beyond" | |
| …live for now and focus on the present. | Living with CF requires patients and families to live in the moment and hope for a cure. |
| …we remain conscious of everything we do. | Remain tuned in to CF at all times. |

255 gregated formulated meanings. Table 2 depicts examples of significant statements and corresponding formulated meanings. Original raw data from the transcripts and narratives were examined for each theme cluster. The researchers then integrated results, and an
260 exhaustive description was prepared describing the life experience of families caring for a child with cystic fibrosis.

*Authenticity and Trustworthiness of Data*

Techniques to enhance the rigor of this work as described by Guba and Lincoln (1994) include credibil-
265 ity, dependability, confirmability, and transferability. These evaluative criteria for qualitative research have been discussed at length in the literature (Beck, 1993; Guba & Lincoln, 1985, 1994; Sandelowski, 1986; Yonge and Stewin, 1988).
270 Participants reviewed the final exhaustive description to verify that it was representative and true to their life experiences. Dependability and credibility do not occur in isolation. Results are considered dependable if they are found to be credible. Participants reported to
275 the researchers that they recognized the exhaustive description as being true to their life experiences, thus establishing credibility and dependability. Confirmability was achieved through the use of an audit trail and review of raw data by the second researcher. Transfer-
280 ability or fittingness refers to the probability that the study findings have meaning to others in similar situa-

tions (Streubert, 2003). This criterion will be evaluated through additional research.

**Results**

Learning that a child has cystic fibrosis is an all-
285 encompassing, life-shattering experience that requires a continuous series of family adjustments as unfamiliar stressors present themselves. Data analysis revealed 3 essential theme clusters or stages related to the diagnosis of cystic fibrosis within a family. The 3 main theme
290 clusters were *Falling Apart*, *Pulling Together*, and *Moving Beyond*. Subthemes were identified as being connected to the 3 essential theme clusters. A detailed discussion of the relationships among the essential themes and subthemes follows. Relationships among
295 the major themes and subthemes are illustrated in Figure 1.

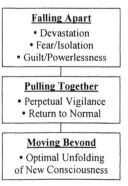

*Figure 1.* Initial diagnosis of cystic fibrosis.

Once a family learns that a child has cystic fibrosis, there is a sense of *Falling Apart* within the context of what the family has always known to be their normal or routine lifestyle. Within this theme, there were 3 subthemes: *The Devastation of Diagnosis, An All-Encompassing Sense of Fear and Isolation,* and *An Overwhelming Sense of Guilt and Powerlessness.* The initial diagnosis of CF was described as a life-shattering experience. Parents reported feeling that their life had fallen apart and that what had been routine or normal was forever changed. Parents, family members, and friends were devastated by the diagnosis, setting in motion a continuous series of family adjustments in response to new and unfamiliar stressors. One parent stated, "In the beginning we were completely devastated...every single day you face the fact that this is not going to change...not tomorrow, or the next day, or the next year." Further, families felt afraid. They experienced a sense of isolation and became overwhelmed with feelings of guilt and powerlessness. These emotions were reflected in one parent's comment: "When you first learn that your child has cystic fibrosis, they tell you all the negative information so that even when your child is doing well, there is always a cloud." Another parent similarly noted: "The hardest part is all the negativeness. I don't think the actual physical care was ever really a concern...it was the emotional aspect that seemed more important to us."

This first theme cluster or stage of *Falling Apart* is followed by a sense of *Pulling Together* as a family makes the necessary lifestyle adjustments required to care for the child with CF and to return to a routine that brings with it some sense of family normalcy. Subthemes of this second theme or stage include the need for *Perpetual Vigilance* and developing *Lifestyle Adaptations That Bring a Sense of Normalcy.* Moving to the stage of pulling together requires families to be perpetually vigilant in caring for the child with CF, keeping daily routines, finding ways to do things better or more efficiently, and constantly adjusting and adapting to new and different stressors as they present themselves. One participant said, "Everything with CF becomes manageable, simply because it is a requirement to getting and staying healthy. Your entire lifestyle has to change, and you make many sacrifices. You continually try to get CF to be part of the fabric of your life." Identifying lifestyle adaptations that bring a sense of normalcy is also critical as families "pull together." Comments from this participant reflect the need to regain control and some sense of normalcy: "You must become really well-educated and informed. Get a basic routine...and be consistent. Being consistent helps the child realize that this is going to be a way of life, for the rest of their life."

*Moving Beyond* is the third essential theme or stage and includes the subtheme of an *Optimal Unfolding of a New Kind of Consciousness.* Within this stage, families move beyond the fear, beyond the guilt, and beyond the sense of powerlessness. Identification of new ways of coping facilitates achievement of a positive view and sense of control or normalcy. As one participant noted, "You live for now, focus on the present, and realize that missing one treatment won't kill anyone." To "move beyond," patients and families find new ways to cope and new ways to be in life that are reflective of living a life that holds an optimal level of quality. One participant vividly describes the final theme cluster of moving beyond in the following comment: "All of this living helps me to believe that CF won't stop me from my dreams. I am learning to take life one breath at a time, living for today, trying not to worry about tomorrow, and looking to God for strength and guidance."

Although the 3 essential themes are presented as separate entities, families describe a process where they move back and forth through the 3 stages. When and how they move among these stages of adjustment seems to be directly influenced by how the child is doing in terms of health and well-being. For example, a family that has adjusted and *"Moved Beyond"* might be thrown very quickly back to the stage of *"Falling Apart"* should the child have a serious setback related to his or her health. Or perhaps new treatments or medication might require a return to *"Pulling Together"* as lifestyle is once again readjusted in an attempt to achieve a state of family normalcy.

## Discussion

The experience of families caring for a child with cystic fibrosis involves the fluid nature of 3 essential themes or stages related to (a) *Falling Apart*, (b) *Pulling Together*, and (c) *Moving Beyond*. The themes, as well as subthemes, are consistent with Reed's theory (1990) and research in the area of chronic illness in children and adults as well as family responses to living with a child with a chronic, life-threatening disease. For example, the themes can be identified in clinical case findings that examine the benefits and burdens of those living with chronic genetic diseases such as CF (Geller, 1995). Geller concludes that quality of life for CF children will depend both on the severity of their disease and the ongoing care and attention they receive. Nurses in research and practice need to understand patient and families' experiences and to use their expert voice to assist families in providing the needed care and attention.

Published research can also be related to the theme and associated subthemes of Falling Apart. The *Devastation of the Diagnosis* has been reported in other chronic childhood diseases, such as asthma (Englund, Rydstrom, & Norberg, 2001). The *Sense of Fear and Isolation* was described by participants in the telephone support intervention study (Ritchie et al., 2000). *Powerlessness* has been described by mothers of children with chronic illness as stressful interactions with partners and professionals (Stewart et al., 1994).

The *Perpetual Vigilance* theme was identified as a component of the use of the cystic fibrosis handbook that parents shared with the children's teachers (Ryan & Williams, 1996). Adaptation that *Brings a Sense of Normalcy* was reported by D'Auria, Christian, and Richardson (1997) in their grounded theory study of 20 children living with CF, wherein leading as normal a life as possible was a theme central to the experience of those in middle childhood.

In the third theme of *Moving Beyond*, the subtheme of *An Optimal Unfolding of a New Kind of Consciousness* emerged. Tracy (1997) described similar aspects of the experience of growing up with CF in qualitative interviews with 10 adults. This study provided support for the theme of "faith" as a new consciousness of the meaning of living with chronic illness. *Moving Beyond* could also be argued as increasing self-efficacy of the family and its members seen in the CF Family Education Program comparative study (Bartholomew et al., 1997). The ability of families to move beyond the experience of devastation was seen as caregivers and children with CF worked together to optimize their lives.

Clinical implications can be derived from the descriptions of families living with CF. Detailed descriptions of their experiences provide recognition of the dynamic nature of CF and the vigilance required to attain a sense of family normalcy and to promote and maintain optimal health.

The qualitative data gathered in this study reflect the physical and emotional roller coaster that parents and families experience when caring for a child with cystic fibrosis. At the time of initial diagnosis, parents clearly need information on how to care for their child. The physical aspects of care, however, seem to be less of a concern at the time of initial diagnosis than the emotional aspects. Helping parents and patients develop a sense of control, and a belief that the ride will not always be bumpy, is a key component to care at the time of initial diagnosis.

Additional research is needed to examine how patients and families cope with cystic fibrosis over the long term. Adults living with cystic fibrosis face new challenges, such as issues surrounding marriage and childbirth. Studies addressing the transition to adulthood and the life experience of adults with cystic fibrosis can add significant information to the research literature and will be important as more and more individuals with cystic fibrosis live longer lives. Understanding the life experiences of family members caring for a child with CF will provide the empirical underpinnings for appropriate clinical interventions.

## References

Anderson, D. G., & Hatton, D. C. (2000). Accessing vulnerable populations for research. *Western Journal of Nursing Research, 22*, 244–251.

Baine, S., Rosenbaum, P., & King, S. (1995). Chronic childhood illnesses: What aspects of caregiving do parents value? *Child Care Health and Development, 21*, 291–304.

Bartholomew, L. K., Vzyzewski, D. I., Parcel, G. S., Swank, P. R., Sockrider, M. M., Mariotto, M. J., Schidlow, D. V., Fink, R. H., & Seilheimer, D. K. (1997). Self-management of cystic fibrosis: Short-term outcomes of the Cystic Fibrosis Family Education Program. *Health Education and Behavior, 24*, 652–666.

Beck, C. T. (1993). Qualitative research: The evaluation of its credibility, fittingness, and audit ability. *Western Journal of Nursing Research, 15*, 263–265.

Brown, M. A., & Powell-Cope, G. M. (1991). AIDS family caregiving: Transitions through uncertainty. *Nursing Research, 40*, 338–345.

CF Foundation. (1998). Pseudomonas Genome Project. Available at: http:///www.pseudomonas.com/cystic-fibrosis.html, Accessed.

Colaizzi, P. F. (1978). Psychological research as the phenomenologist views it. In R. Valle & M. Kings (Eds.), *Existential phenomenological alternatives for psychology.* New York: Oxford University Press.

Cystic Fibrosis. (1997). NIH Publication 97-4200. Bethesda, Maryland. Available at: http://www.esiason.org

D'Auria, J. P., Christian, B. J., & Richardson, L. F. (1997). Through the looking glass: Children's perceptions of growing up with cystic fibrosis. *Canadian Journal of Nursing Research, 29*, 99–122.

Derouin, D., & Jessee, P. O. (1996). Impact of chronic illness in childhood: Siblings' perceptions. *Issues in Comprehensive Pediatric Nursing, 19*, 135–147.

Duffield, R. A. (1996). Cystic fibrosis and the gastrointestinal tract. *Journal of Pediatric Health Care, 10*, 51–57.

Eiser, C., Zprotch, B., Hiller, J., Havermans, T., & Billig, S. (1995). Routine stresses in caring for a child with cystic fibrosis. *Journal of Psychosomatic Research, 39*, 641–646.

Englund, A. D., Rydstrom, I., & Norberg, A. (2001). Being the parent of a child with asthma. *Pediatric Nursing, 27*, 365–373.

Fiel, S. B. (1993). Clinical management of pulmonary disease in cystic fibrosis. *Lancet, 341*, 1070–1074.

Geiss, S. K., Hobbs, S. A., Hammersley-Maercklein, G., Kramer, J. C., & Henley, M. (1992). Psychosocial factors related to perceived compliance with cystic fibrosis treatment. *Journal of Clinical Psychology, 48*, 99–103.

Geller, G. (1995). Cystic fibrosis and the pediatric caregiver: Benefits and burdens of genetic technology. *Pediatric Nursing, 21*, 57–61.

Guba, E. G., & Lincoln, Y. S. (1994). Competing paradigms in qualitative research. In N. K. Denzin & Y. S. Lincoln (Eds.), *Handbook of qualitative research* (pp. 105–117). Thousand Oaks, CA: Sage.

Hopkins, S. (1995). Advances in the treatment of cystic fibrosis. *Nursing Times, 91*, 40–41.

Hopkins, K. (1996). Cystic fibrosis: Approaching treatment from multiple directions. *The Journal of NIH Research, 8*, 40–43.

Lincoln, Y. S., & Guba, E. G. (1985). *Naturalistic inquiry.* Beverly Hills, CA: Sage.

Myers, M. F., Bernhardt, B. A., Tamoor, E. S., & Holtzman, N. A. (1994). Involving consumers in the development of an educational program for cystic fibrosis carrier screening. *American Journal of Human Genetics, 54*, 719–726.

Pickler, R. H., & Munro, C. L. (1995). Gene therapy for inherited disorders. *Journal of Pediatric Nursing: Nursing Care of Children and Families, 10*, 40–47.

Reed, S. B. (1990). Potential for alterations in family process: When a family has a child with cystic fibrosis. *Issues in Comprehensive Pediatric Nursing, 13*, 15–23.

Ritchie, J., Stewart, M., Ellerton, M., Thompsons, D., Meade, D., & Viscount, P. W. (2000). Parents' perceptions of the impact of a telephone support group intervention. *Journal of Family Nursing, 6*, 25–45.

Ryan, L. L., & Williams, J. K. (1996). A cystic fibrosis handbook for teachers. *Journal of Pediatric Nursing, 7*, 304–311.

Sandelowski, M. (1986). The problem of rigor in qualitative research. *Advances in Nursing Science, 8*, 27–37.

Sawyer, E. H. (1992). Family functioning when children have cystic fibrosis. *Journal of Pediatric Nursing, 7*, 304–311.

Stewart, M. J., Ritchie, J. A., McGrath, P., Thompson, D., & Bruce, B. (1994). Mothers of children with chronic conditions: Supportive and stressful interactions with partners and professionals regarding caregiving burdens. *Canadian Journal of Nursing Research, 26*, 61–82.

Streubert, H. J. (2003). The conduct of qualitative research: Common essential themes. In Streubert H. J. & Carpenter D. R. (Eds.) *Qualitative research in nursing: Advancing the humanistic imperative* (3rd ed.). Philadelphia: Lippincott Williams & Wilkins.

Tracy, J. P. (1997). Growing up with chronic illness: The experience of growing up with cystic fibrosis. *Holistic Nursing Practice, 12*, 27–35.

White, K. R., Munro, C. L., & Boyle, A. H. (1996). Nursing management of adults who have cystic fibrosis. *MedSurg Nursing, 5*, 163–167.

Whyte, D. A. (1992). A family nursing approach to the care of a child with a chronic illness. *Journal of Advanced Nursing, 17*, 317–327.

Williams, J. L. (1995). Genetics and cystic fibrosis: A focus on carrier testing. *Pediatric Nursing, 21*, 444–448.

Williams, P. D., Hanson, S., Karlin, R., Ridder, L., Liebergrn, A., Olson, J., Barnard, M. U., & Tobin-Rommerlhart, S. (1997). Outcomes of a nursing intervention for siblings of chronically ill children: A pilot study. *Journal of the Society of Pediatric Nurses, 2,* 127–137.

Wilmott, R. W., & Fiedler, M. A. (1994). Recent advances in the treatment of cystic fibrosis. *Pediatric Clinics of North America, 41,* 431–451.

Yonge, O., & Stewin, L. (1988). Reliability and validity: Misnomers for qualitative research. *The Canadian Journal of Nursing Research, 20,* 61–67.

**Acknowledgments**: The authors wish to thank Mary Harvey, MSW, for her assistance contacting participants, and Dr. John Sanko, University of Scranton, for his work on the project. An internal research grant from the University of Scranton, Panuska College of Professional Studies, and a grant from The Edward R. Leahy Jr. Center for Faculty Research and Development provided additional support.

**Address correspondence to**: Dona Rinaldi Carpenter, EdD, RN, CS, Department of Nursing, University of Scranton, Scranton, PA 18510-4595. E-mail: carpenterd1@tiger.uofs.edu

# Exercise for Article 27

## Factual Questions

1. What is the research question that guided this study?

2. Have any of the research studies discussed in the related literature section of this article explained experiences of living with a family member who has CF at the time of diagnosis?

3. The family members who participated in this study were drawn from how many metropolitan areas?

4. How many of the participants in this study were not able to attend a focus group?

5. How did the first author contact participants to clarify questions that emerged from the written narratives?

6. Participants reviewed the final exhaustive description to verify what?

## Questions for Discussion

7. The researchers state that "Qualitative research approaches are best suited to describing the phenomena of living with and adapting to CF at this critical point in time." If you had planned to study the topic of this research, would you have planned to conduct qualitative research *or* quantitative research? Explain. (See lines 161–164.)

8. The researchers state that the study design was descriptive and grounded in "phenomenological research methodology." If you have a research methods textbook, examine it to see if "phenomenological research" is covered. If so, how is it defined in the textbook? How is "phenomenology" defined in a dictionary? (See lines 165–166.)

9. The researchers state that they used a "purposive sample." What is your understanding of the meaning of this term? (See lines 174–175.)

10. Some of the data for this study were collected through focus group discussions and some were collected by having participants provide written answers to open-ended questions. In your opinion, are both methods equally good for collecting the type of data needed for this study? Explain. (See lines 184–195.)

11. How important are the "significant statements" (i.e., quotations) in Table 2 in helping you understand the results of this study?

12. The main analysis was conducted by the first author of this study. How important is it to know that the raw data were reviewed by the second author? Would it have been sufficient to have the data examined by only one researcher? Explain. (See lines 277–279.)

## Quality Ratings

Directions: Indicate your level of agreement with each of the following statements by circling a number from 5 for strongly agree (SA) to 1 for strongly disagree (SD). If you believe an item is not applicable to this research article, leave it blank. Be prepared to explain your ratings. When responding to criteria A and B, keep in mind that brief titles and abstracts are conventional in published research.

A. The title of the article is appropriate.
SA   5   4   3   2   1   SD

B. The abstract provides an effective overview of the research article.
SA   5   4   3   2   1   SD

C. The introduction establishes the importance of the study.
SA   5   4   3   2   1   SD

D. The literature review establishes the context for the study.
SA   5   4   3   2   1   SD

E. The research purpose, question, or hypothesis is clearly stated.
SA   5   4   3   2   1   SD

F. The method of sampling is sound.
SA   5   4   3   2   1   SD

G.  Relevant demographics (for example, age, gender, and ethnicity) are described.

      SA   5   4   3   2   1   SD

H.  Measurement procedures are adequate.

      SA   5   4   3   2   1   SD

I.  All procedures have been described in sufficient detail to permit a replication of the study.

      SA   5   4   3   2   1   SD

J.  The participants have been adequately protected from potential harm.

      SA   5   4   3   2   1   SD

K.  The results are clearly described.

      SA   5   4   3   2   1   SD

L.  The discussion/conclusion is appropriate.

      SA   5   4   3   2   1   SD

M.  Despite any flaws, the report is worthy of publication.

      SA   5   4   3   2   1   SD

# Article 28

# Weighing the Consequences:
# Self-Disclosure of HIV-Positive Status Among
# African American Injection Drug Users

**Maribel Valle**, PhD, **Judith Levy**, PhD[*]

ABSTRACT. Theorists posit that personal decisions to disclose being HIV positive are made based on the perceived consequences of that disclosure. This study examines the perceived costs and benefits of self-disclosure among African American injection drug users (IDUs). A total of 80 African American IDUs were interviewed in-depth subsequent to testing HIV positive. Participants reported that interpersonal costs of self-disclosure included stigma, loss of sexual/romantic partners, emotional harming of family/friends, shattering of privacy, physical isolation, blame, and loss of income. The benefits of disclosure included social support, emotional catharsis, and income. Four factors that help to tip the scales in either direction were identified. Study findings have implications for the delivery of counseling, testing, and partner notification services to African American IDUs living with HIV.

From *Health Education & Behavior, 36*, 155–166. Copyright © 2009 by SOPHE. Reprinted with permission.

For many people living with HIV, revealing their serostatus to others is a difficult task that raises issues of vulnerability, privacy, and stigmatization. Because the consequences of being known as HIV positive can
5 be harsh, the legal protocols in medicine that surround confidentiality in HIV counseling and diagnostic testing are among the most stringent of all disorders (Cline & McKenzie, 2000).

Fearing possible negative consequences, individu-
10 als often choose to disclose their status late in the process of coming to terms with their infection or not to disclose at all (Mansergh, Marks, & Simoni, 1995). Although this choice protects the individual from consequences, maintaining secrecy about having contracted the virus
15 tracted the virus can interfere with gaining access to social support, obtaining medical services, and may result in social isolation (Rao, Kekwaletswe, Hosek, Martinez, & Rodriguez, 2007; Vance, 2006).

The decision to disclose one's HIV status often oc-
20 curs after examining the consequences of disclosure in the context of a particular relationship (Mayfield Arnold, Rice, Flannery, & Rotheram-Borus, 2008). Hays et al. (1993), for example, found that gay men told their partners of their positive HIV serostatus only after
25 weighing the costs and benefits of the act. In the end, they chose to tell only those individuals whom they thought would react most helpfully, and some men chose not to disclose to others at all for fear of rejection and the disruption of social relationships. It appears
30 that for disclosure to occur, the discloser must believe that he or she will benefit in some way that outweighs the costs.

Disclosing HIV status has been found to be an acute and recurrent stressor for those who test HIV
35 positive. In a sample of 40 gay men, Holt et al. (1998) found that their informants were unlikely to disclose immediately postdiagnosis. They disclosed when disclosure was perceived to increase practical and emotional support, as a means to share responsibility for
40 sex, and/or to facilitate self-acceptance.

Disclosure plays a dual role in HIV infection as a stressor and as a mechanism by which individuals can come to terms with their infection. Telling others can exert a therapeutic effect, particularly in terms of ac-
45 cessing social support (Hays et al., 1993). At the same time, HIV disclosure can create stigma and other negative consequences (Weiner, Battles, & Heilman, 2000).

Research on HIV disclosure has focused primarily on White men who have sex with men (MSM). Conse-
50 quently, we know little about disclosure of HIV status among injection drug users. Some research indicates that although the process of weighing the costs and benefits is similar to MSMs, the factors that are considered are slightly different. Parsons, Missildine et al.
55 (2004) and Parsons, VanOra, Missildine, Purcell, and Gomez (2004) examined the positive and negative consequences of disclosure among an ethnically diverse sample of seropositive injection drug users (IDUs) and found that in addition to assessing the negative and
60 positive consequences of disclosure, feeling personal

[*]*Maribel Valle*, School of Nursing and Health Studies, Northern Illinois, DeKalb. *Judith Levy*, School of Public Health, University of Illinois at Chicago.

responsibility for others played a major function in decision-making regarding disclosure. No current study, however, examines the process of self-disclosure exclusively among African American IDUs.

65   According to the latest surveillance data from the Centers for Disease Control and Prevention (2005), although African Americans account for approximately 13% of the population, they comprise approximately 55% of new HIV cases. Furthermore, since the beginning of the epidemic, injection drug use has directly or indirectly accounted for approximately 38% of estimated AIDS cases diagnosed in the United States. In 2003, injection drug use accounted for 25% of all AIDS cases diagnosed in Black men and women, compared with 16% of AIDS cases diagnosed overall.

This study examines HIV disclosure and adds to the limited body of knowledge concerning how African American IDUs confront the challenges of telling others. The analysis focuses on the costs and the benefits of such disclosure and also identifies the factors that help tip the scales in one direction or another.

## Method

This research draws on data from the Partners in Community Health Project (R01-DA092321) that examined HIV partner notification among IDUs on the west side of Chicago. Using snowball sampling techniques and a monetary incentive to compensate for time spent being interviewed, street outreach workers recruited 839 African American IDUs and their sex and/or needle partners for HIV counseling, testing, and partner notification. To qualify for the study, prospective participants must have tested HIV negative at their last testing or be unaware of their serostatus. Of the 839 IDUs who were recruited for testing and a baseline interview, 167 (20%) subsequently tested HIV positive. Of these, 164 (98%) returned for a second structured interview and 121 (76%) returned for a third.

Participants who tested HIV positive were asked during the third quantitative interview if they would be willing to be interviewed in-depth concerning their experience with receiving a positive test result. The sample for analysis was drawn from those who agreed. Following criteria set out by Glaser and Strauss (1967), interviewing stopped at 80 individuals because saturation had been reached and no new answers to the study's research questions or properties of the categories were emerging from the data.

To examine the possibility of selection bias, the 80 participants who were interviewed qualitatively were compared with the 41 who were not, using the following variables: gender, age, education, having a significant other, time at current residence, total injection drug use, and rock cocaine use. No significant differences were found between the two groups ($p > .05$).

### Sample Characteristics

Of the 80 individuals who were interviewed, 64% were male and 36% were female. Participants' age ranged from 24 to 67 years, with more than 50% being between the ages of 40 and 49. About half were at least high school graduates, 20% having had some college education, and 46% had never finished high school. Sixty-three percent of males had significant others, and 62% of females had significant others. All were African American.

### Data Collection and Analysis

The data were collected using an interview guide and subsequently audiotaped and transcribed. Transcripts of the interviews were coded using ATLAS-ti (Muhr, 2001), a qualitative analysis software package. Preliminary analysis focused on finding common themes throughout the interviews and was guided by two questions: (a) How did participants disclose their status to others? (b) How did they decide how and when to disclose?

Using a constant comparison methodology (Glaser & Strauss, 1967), it became clear that study participants believed there were both positive and negative consequences to disclosing their positive HIV status, and they weighed the perceived costs and benefits when deciding whether or not to disclose this information. Participants' perception of the costs and benefits of disclosing formed the basis for this analysis.

## Results

Many reasons exist for not letting others know about the private and secret parts of ourselves. How people manage the challenge of self-disclosure is an essential part of everyday life (Rosenfeld, 2000). We begin this analysis by examining the perceived costs of disclosure as reported by the study's participants.

### The Costs of HIV Disclosure

*Stigma.* Study participants discussed incurring stigma as the greatest impediment to revealing their HIV-positive serostatus. Concern centered on fear of negative reactions. Sara, a 39-year-old woman, experienced the stigmatizing effects of HIV when a family member revealed Sara's status to others in the neighborhood. She recounts, "When I first found out, and people found out, they threw bottles at me, and they looked at me, and stayed away from me. It was like I was dirt."

For the IDU, the discrediting aspects of testing HIV positive can further compromise an identity already socially compromised by substance abuse. Moreover, in disclosing their HIV status, IDUs who have kept their drug use secret run the risk of inadvertently revealing their use to unknowing family and friends. After 30 years of successfully hiding his drug dependency from his mother, Calvin explains why at age 42 he also chose to keep his HIV test results hidden.

I live with my moms now, and she don't know I use. She knows I drink and she's always after me. If she knew I was shooting up, I'd find my ass back on the street lickity split. I don't need that shit. What she don't know don't hurt her. I gots no reason to tell her I'm HIV.

170     Of course, whether or not Calvin's mother is, in fact, unaware of his drug use is open to speculation. Families often collude with the user to ignore or deny a serious substance abuse problem (Rotunda, West, & O'Farrell. 2004). Revealing an HIV diagnosis forces

175     confrontation with the question of how the virus was acquired, and the answer can reveal secrets that one or more parties wish to maintain.

*Loss of Sexual/Romantic Partners.* The possible loss of current and future sexual partners is another

180     perceived cost of disclosure. Not only did informants fear that a current partner might abandon them on learning their serostatus, they also worried that future prospects might shun them. Participants judged that opportunities for romantic involvement would lessen or

185     end if their serostatus became widely known. Wanda, who at age 50 was without a partner at the time of the interview, kept her serostatus secret for this reason.

Who's going to want an old woman with HIV? I don't want to be alone.... When I meet someone, I sure ain't

190     going to tell him. I'm talking to a couple of gentlemen. Maybe one of those will get more serious. I don't know. But until it does, I'm not going to tell them. It ain't none of their business.

Such strategies of concealment or gradual disclo-

195     sure postpone rather than obviate the costs. Should her search for a partner prove successful, Wanda may discover that tactical covertness at the onset of a relationship has compounded the problems of disclosure at a later date by raising issues of omission or deceit.

200     One way to escape the costs of disclosing to a sexual or romantic partner is to reject having a partner at all. Informants explained that fear of the consequences of disclosure could prevent them from entering into or maintaining intimate relationships. Daunted by the

205     prospect of knowing when and/or how to disclose their status within an interpersonal context, they preferred to avoid these problems altogether. This was the case with Tammy, a 38-year-old woman who had recently been diagnosed with HIV.

210     I don't want to get involved in some relationship, because I will have to let them know what's happening with me and that could be too hard. I don't know how far this relationship might go, and I think it would cause a lot of pain, or it could have a profound effect on someone else's

215     life.

For Tammy, becoming sexually involved necessitated protecting the well-being of an intimate partner by not burdening him with her serostatus. Uncertain as to how to do this, she preferred to side-step the prob-

220     lems of disclosure entirely.

*Emotionally Harming Relatives and Friends.* Nondisclosure also may occur to protect others from what is perceived as potentially devastating information. Informants reported reluctance to tell friends and fam-

225     ily members for fear of causing them pain. Parents often are the most difficult to tell (Gard, 1990). Theresa felt this emotion so strongly that she decided never to tell her mother.

My mother is 70. She'll never know if it is up to me. I'm

230     her only daughter and I know what it will do to her. So, for her sake and mine, I'm not going to tell her because I'm not going to kill her. I'm not going to do that to her. It don't even cross my mind. No. It would kill her.

As can happen when maintaining a secret, however,

235     Theresa's adherence to silence exerted a toll on her other relationships. The only way to ensure that no one else told her mother was not to tell anyone at all.

*Shattering of Privacy.* Participants consistently asserted that some personal information belongs to the

240     public domain, whereas other information belongs solely to the person involved. Opinions varied as to how private they considered health information. Philip was among those who believed that his status was no one's concern but his own.

245     It ain't no one's business that I'm positive. No one needs to know. I'm not putting anyone at risk and I ain't going to. It's private, it's personal information. Would you want people to know? I ain't telling no one.

As was common among informants, Philip bal-

250     anced the personal costs of disclosure against the benefits of others knowing his status. Because he perceived that his silence carried no adverse effects and that no one would benefit from knowing his status, he saw no reason to tell anyone.

255     *Physical Isolation.* Participants reported wanting to maintain the status quo of their relationships, and they feared that family members, friends, and society in general would physically recoil from them on hearing that they were living with HIV. They perceived that

260     they might be considered contagious and that people would avoid physical contact with them or things they had touched. Sara recalls a particularly painful experience.

One day I remember cutting my finger almost off, and

265     my mama grabbed me and threw my hands in the tub and the blood flowed into the water. She said. "Oh, should I put my hand in that AIDS shit?! Get away from me, girl! Get away from me!"

Maggie, a 55-year-old woman who encountered

270     similar reactions from friends, explains, "You got some people that be just so ignorant to the facts about HIV. They be washing dishes behind you, throwing them away too, not wanting you to use their toilet."

*Loss of Personal Safety.* Disclosure of being sero-

275     positive also carried the risk of incurring physical violence or other types of retribution, especially from those with whom they shared exposure to the virus. Daphne, a 36-year-old transsexual, greatly feared revealing her HIV status to her sexual partner, who had

280     been released recently from prison for assault.

I don't know what kind of effect it may have on him, cause like I said, a lot of people blow up if they found out they been with a positive. He could be one of those. I don't know if he'll have a crazy attitude and hurt me. Plus he asked me, and I told him no. I lied to him.

For Daphne, the price of safety was being forced to lie or prevaricate about her status.

*Blame.* Since the beginning of the AIDS epidemic, HIV-positive IDUs and men who have sex with men have been castigated and blamed for their behavior, which was perceived to place themselves and others at risk for the virus (Herek, Capitanio, & Widaman, 2002). Sara shared being told by her mother,

I hate you cause you gave it to my grandson. Terrance born with the virus and he never had sex and he never knew nothin' about life. You know, you wrong for giving it to Terrance. And that's, that's something to think about, alright. An innocent child born, an innocent child born with the disease, for no reason.

These words illustrate a pervasive attitude of moral judgment surrounding HIV infection. As is true of the sick role in general (Parsons, 1951), children and adults who acquire the virus through no fault of their own are subject to greater compassion and support than those held personally responsible. In disclosing their status, IDUs risk being blamed for their condition based on others' moral judgments. For some, this may be too great a price to pay.

*Loss of Income.* After being diagnosed with HIV, individuals may encounter job discrimination and the loss of employment (Conyers, Boomer, & McMahon, 2005). Among IDUs, the costs of disclosure can affect both legal employment and also income obtained through illicit activities. For example, some IDUs trade sex for money and/or drugs. Whether they do so professionally as sex workers or more discreetly through favors conferred on acquaintances, testing HIV positive is commonly believed to lessen sexual marketability. Tracy, a 29-year-old woman who has been HIV positive for 2 years, explains,

I don't like telling dates anymore I got HIV cause the ones I like, the ones that are handsome, do not date me once I tell them. I tell them, admit it, and they don't want to anymore. Not even with a rubber. They say, "No rubber. No, no, no. Even with a rubber, no I can't take the chance the condom might bust." They was kind too, before I told them.

Given such treatment, it is not surprising that women in Tracy's situation may opt to remain silent about their status with clients.

### The Benefits of HIV Disclosure

The costs of disclosure of a positive HIV status can be both extensive and sufficiently severe to warrant keeping the information secret. Yet two-thirds of all injectors in this study at the time of their interview had informed at least one other person that they were HIV positive. This section explores the benefits of disclosure that they perceived.

*Social Support.* Increased social support was the most commonly cited benefit of disclosure. Carl, for example, chose to disclose his HIV serostatus to his wife and, in doing so, gained both sympathy and her continued support.

I told Glory I was positive. I'm real glad I did. She's right there for me. Thank God, she's negative. We never really did do a lot of sex, and she never shot up. But, she is there for me. 110%. That woman's got a heart of gold. She's just there for me, whatever I want. If I need to talk, or whatever. She's got my back, and I'm crazy about her for it. It makes me feel real good to be able to talk to her, to know she understands what I'm going through. It makes me feel like I'm not alone. Someone cares. God's got a special place in heaven for women like that.

His disclosure also affirmed the strength of his marital bond in the face of adversity.

Sharing the information that they had contracted the virus could pave the way to reconnect with family members and others with whom prior relationships had dwindled or ceased due to the IDU's drug use. Estrangements could be successfully bridged when concern for the IDU's well-being outweighed the resentments of past grievances. This was true for Philip, a 39-year-old injector, who revealed his HIV status to his family after being admitted to the hospital for pneumonia.

I was there in the hospital, all these IVs and shit, hooked up like you see on TV. And I thought, I could really die here. This could be it. I just had to let someone know how bad it was. I didn't want to die by myself. I called my mom and told her I was HIV positive. She got real quiet. She hadn't heard from me in over a year, since she kicked me out of the house. She didn't believe me at first, then I told her I was at UIC [a university teaching hospital] if she wanted to come and see me. She came by, with my sister, and she's been there for me ever since. Only good thing came out of this shit, that's for sure.

Philip was fortunate in that he was able to reestablish connections with his mother and sister that had been strained through years of chronic substance abuse. Not all IDUs, of course, experience such rebonding, as some relationships are too damaged to successfully resurrect.

*Emotional Catharsis.* Informants reported gaining feelings of emotional release after disclosing their HIV status to others. They often spoke of feeling that a burden had been lifted from their shoulders after disclosing their status. Denise describes her experience:

I'd been carrying that around with me, for months. Feeling like I had some sort of deep secret and no one else knew. Once I told my friend, who is HIV positive himself, it felt like I could breathe again. I wondered what had taken me so long to talk about it.

As her words indicate, Denise's confidant was also HIV positive. Perhaps the possibility of reciprocal in-

terpersonal exchange based on shared circumstance
395 helped to smooth the way for disclosure and a positive
response. Yet as informants report, intimate partners
and friends irrespective of serostatus can serve as em-
pathetic listeners.

*Income.* In 1996, after the Social Security Admini-
400 stration tightened its eligibility criteria for receiving
disability benefits, many injectors found themselves
unable to qualify for medical treatment and other social
service programs based solely on their drug use. Nonetheless, informants found that disclosure of being HIV
405 positive could open alternative doors to income transfer
and third-party payment through Ryan White funding,
Social Security, and Medicaid. They also discovered
that substance abuse treatment programs with long
waiting lists might accord them priority based on their
410 HIV status.

Willingness to disclose being HIV positive also
could help in generating income earned through society's underground economy. When panhandling, for
example, disclosure of illness can evoke sympathy that
415 increases the dole (Higgins, 1980). Calvin, the 42-year-
old who lives with his mother but is unwilling to tell
her his status, is not above discussing his infection
when trying to make money on the streets.

> People can be real good to you if you handle the situation
420 right. See, what I'll do is, I'll go to Oak Park. I gots a li-
cense to sell the *Streetwise* newspaper in Oak Park. Go to
the same spots all the time. People gets to know me. You
know, they sitting there waiting on a ride or something. I
starts to talk to them. Introduce myself. Talk about what a
425 nice day it is, the weather, whatever. Tell them I just got
out of the joint. Build up to it. Finally, I tell em I'm positive. That I'm trying to get myself together by selling
these papers. They more likely to buy then, sometimes
give me $5 or $10 for one paper, or not take a paper at
430 all. You just gotta be careful. You gotta be smart. But it
can make you some money, sure can. I know some people say it, and I don't even think it's true.

### Tipping the Scales

We have seen that our informants perceive that disclosing a positive HIV status carries the potential for
435 both positive and negative outcomes. Given that remaining silent offers both advantages and disadvantages, what factors tip the scale in favor of either maintaining silence or choosing disclosure? Four factors
appeared discernible in the data.

440 The need to disclose constitutes one tipping factor.
As long as no compelling reason exists to tell others,
maintaining silence may appear the more persuasive
course. Wayne explains this reasoning in terms of informing his girlfriend.

445 > There is just no way I'm going to tell Celia I have HIV.
We ain't been together that long. We always use con-
doms anyway. Don't want no more kids. She don't need
to know no way. I tell her, she's gonna be afraid to leave
her kids with me, and I can't give 'em nothing anyway.

450 > This way, everyone's happy. Don't need to rock the boat
now.

Should Wayne's health worsen, his life situation
change, or suppression of the information become too
burdensome to maintain, however, the need to tell
455 Celia or others may outweigh the advantages of silence. Thus, the boundaries of personal privacy, including information about having the virus, can shift with
time and circumstance. As HIV/AIDS becomes more
of a chronic disease through new treatment options, the
460 window of personal privacy may widen (Petronio,
2000).

The influence of personal values constitutes a second tipping factor. People differ in the weight that they
accord to such human values as friendship, privacy,
465 morality, social support, and sexual intimacy. Philip,
for example, explains the moral code to which he sub-
scribes in not disclosing his diagnosis.

> I think you should have the freedom. I think you should
have the liberty to keep things like this private, if that's
470 what you decide to do.

Other data indicate that not all informants agree
with Philip's reasoning. Weighing the costs and benefits of disclosure involves calculations that are intrinsic
to the value structure of the person making the deci-
475 sion. This framework differs by individual and may
change with time, circumstance, disease trajectory, or a
revision of thinking. Such weighing of values can
prove a repeated and dynamic process as new people
enter the person's social network, others become
480 knowledgeable about the person's status, and/or circumstances change.

A third tipping factor is the anticipated reaction of
the person who will receive the information. Informants reported trying to anticipate how others would
485 react to being told. Whether or not they chose to tell or
remain silent was influenced by the reaction that they
expected. Michelle, a 32-year-old mother of two, explains,

> When I was using, I didn't care about no one but me. My
490 life was all about scoring and getting high. When DCFS
got my kids, it hurt like hell. But it was kind of a relief,
ya know? Now I'm straight, I'm clean. I want my kids
back. But I'm scared to tell the caseworker I gots the virus. Is she going to say, "She's gonna die anyway" and
495 leave my kids where they are now? I know the right thing
to do is to tell them. But I'm scared.

As Michelle's worries indicate, one dilemma of
HIV disclosure is determining who is safe to tell. Michelle is afraid of the reaction from the Department of
500 Children and Family Services caseworker and this
keeps her silent about her status.

The fourth tipping factor lies in the person's self-
perceived ability to control the dissemination of the
information. Telling the wrong person, for example,
505 can have disastrous results when it comes to controlling who knows what about one's serostatus. Steve

committed a serious error in judgment by disclosing his HIV status to his father who, in turn, betrayed his confidence by telling others.

510    About 5 years ago, I tell my Daddy that I got this and he said "Man, bla, bla, bla," and he went back and told everybody that I got; you know in the neighborhood, went to the job. A guy lives down the street that owns a few buses I used to drive. So I kind of like shy away from
515    them, you know. I tell him that I was so sick and man he slipped. Yeah. Shit. He told the neighborhood a lot of shit, you know; tell them my heart.

As Steve discovered, keeping silent may have little payoff for individuals once the information about their
520    infection has been made public.

### Conclusions

As a communicable disease, HIV raises moral and legal questions about the rights of individuals to personal privacy versus the benefits of disclosure for public good. The public health perspective focuses on the
525    dynamics of the epidemic and strategies to control it. Disclosing to sexual partners and others at risk often is encouraged as a way to curb further transmission and also to identify possible undiagnosed cases. For the informants in this study, however, HIV/AIDS is a per-
530    sonal experience rather than a matter of public domain. To tell others about their infection entails some loss of personal privacy and control over the information that has been shared. Thus, disclosure of a positive HIV status carries a set of personal and social risks for IDUs
535    that compete for attention with those of drug use and managing HIV/AIDS as a life-threatening illness.

At present, HIV/AIDS is a treatable but incurable condition. Consequently, as our data suggest, the weighing of costs and benefits of HIV disclosure likely
540    continues throughout life as new people enter the IDU's social circle. Deciding whom to tell and when to tell is a recurring dilemma for the person living with the virus, and the perceived need of others to know figures heavily into the calculations. For example, the
545    anticipated cost of disclosing to a casual acquaintance may outweigh the perceived benefits of such disclosure. Disclosure to a sexual partner, however, may be worth the potential increased costs due to the important benefit of engaging in safer sex and reducing the risk
550    of HIV transmission.

*Implications for Practitioners*

The findings of this study have implications for the delivery of HIV counseling, testing, and partner notification services. First, as service providers guide their HIV-positive clients through the process of deciding
555    whom to tell, providers should be aware that the outcomes of such deliberations are based in part on the client's assessment of the costs and benefits of disclosure. Service providers can assist IDUs in this process by helping them arrive at a realistic assessment and
560    also by developing strategies to minimize the costs and maximize the benefits to the chosen course of action.

Second, the data show that decisions to disclose rest in part on the HIV-positive person's perception of how the recipient of the information will respond. Couple
565    and family counseling that addresses HIV concerns and alleviates unnecessary fears should be available to support and assist clients in the decision to disclose. Third, a growing body of research, including findings from this study, indicates that the maintenance and rules of
570    personal privacy differ by gender, race/ethnicity, and age (Dindia, 2000; Rubin, Yang, & Porte, 2000). Thus, to be effective, HIV counseling must be specifically tailored to the norms and beliefs of the population being served. Fourth, as our informants report, telling
575    others about having become HIV infected can be an emotionally stressful experience that sometimes yields unexpected outcomes. Role-play and counseling about how to disclose may help to reduce some of the emotional stress.

*Limitations of the Study*

580    Disclosure of HIV status can be distressing, even during the privacy of a research interview. Consequently, participants may not have been fully forthcoming. To encourage openness, efforts were made to build rapport. The interviews were conducted in a
585    community-based field station where study participants were welcome to drop in for coffee, HIV prevention supplies, and referral for services by a trained staff of former drug users. The interviewer was a certified addictions therapist who was comfortable with eliciting
590    confidential information. Moreover, this was the fourth in a series of interviews by which time trust between interviewer and participant likely had been well established.

The data from this study are drawn from interviews
595    with African American IDUs living on the west side of Chicago. Therefore, the findings must be generalized with caution. As Hastings (2000) has shown, the social norms governing revelation of personal information differ by culture and circumstance. Having experienced
600    a long history of social disadvantage and misuse by others of their personal information, African Americans and low-income groups such as IDUs tend to be wary of self-disclosure that carries possible stigma or censure (Parrott, Duncan, & Duggan, 2000). Thus, the
605    study's findings may not apply to individuals who are IDUs from other racial/ethnic groups or individuals who are not substance abusers. Further study with other populations would help determine whether or not these findings are generalizable. The current study, however,
610    is valuable given the importance of understanding the disclosure process in this very high-risk population.

This investigation focused on the perceived costs and benefits that our informants believe must be considered when disclosing positive HIV status. We also
615    found that disclosure rests on an interactive process in which the informant and informed play a reciprocal role in delivering or suppressing the information. Fu-

ture research might do well to focus on the personal strategies used to disclose or withhold information about HIV status and on how the recipient of HIV disclosure affects the disclosure process. Also normatively, those who are told of infection are expected to assume some degree of responsibility for appropriately handling the information (Petronio, 2000). Future research may elucidate how recipients manage this role and the costs and benefits of the joint ownership that are experienced in being privy to this information.

### References

Centers for Disease Control and Prevention. (2005). *HIV prevention in the third decade: Activities of CDC's division of HIV/AIDS prevention.* Retrieved October 12, 2007, from www.cdc.gov/hiv/resources/reports/hiv3rddecade/

Cline, R. J., & McKenzie, N. J. (2000). Dilemmas of disclosure in the age of HIV/AIDS: Balancing privacy and protection in the health care context. In S. Petronio (Ed.), *Balancing the secrets of private disclosures* (pp. 71–82). Mahwah, NJ: Lawrence Erlbaum.

Conyers, L., Boomer, K., & McMahon, B. (2005).Workplace discrimination and HIV/AIDS: The National EEOC ADA Research Project. *Work, 25*(1), 37–48.

Dindia, K. (2000). Sex differences in self-disclosure, reciprocity of self-disclosure, and self-disclosure and liking: Three meta-analyses revised. In S. Petronio (Ed.), *Balancing the secrets of private disclosure* (pp. 21–35). Mahwah, NJ: Lawrence Erlbaum.

Gard, L. (1990). Patient disclosure of HIV to parents: Clinical considerations. *Professional Psychology, Research, and Practice, 21*, 252–256.

Glaser, B., & Strauss, A. (1967). *Discovery of grounded theory.* Chicago: Aldine.

Hastings, S. O. (2000). "Egocasting" in the avoidance of disclosure. In S. Petronio (Ed.), *Balancing the secrets of private disclosures* (pp. 235–248). Mahwah, NJ: Lawrence Erlbaum.

Hays, R. B., Mckusick, L., Pollack, L., Hilliard, R., Hoff, C., & Coates, T. J. (1993). Disclosing HIV seropositivity to significant others. *AIDS, 7*, 425–431.

Herek, G., Capitanio, J., & Widaman, K. (2002). HIV-related stigma and knowledge in the United States: Prevalence and trends, 1991–1999. *American Journal of Public Health, 92*, 371–377.

Higgins, P. C. (1980). *Outsiders in a hearing world: A sociology of deafness.* Beverly Hills, CA: Sage.

Holt, R., Court, P., Vedhara, K., Nott, K. H., Holmes, J., & Snow, M. H. (1998). The role of disclosure in coping with HIV infection. *AIDS Care, 110,* 49–60.

Mansergh, G., Marks, G., & Simoni, J. M. (1995). Self-disclosure of HIV infection among men who vary in time since seropositive diagnosis and symptomatic status. *AIDS, 9*, 639–644.

Mayfield Arnold, E., Rice, E., Flannery, D., & Rotheram-Borus, M. J. (2008). HIV disclosure among adults living with HIV. *AIDS Care, 20*(1), 80–92.

Muhr, T. (2001). Atlas.ti (version 4.1) [Computer software]. Released August 4, 2000. Berlin, Germany: Scientific Software Development.

Parrott, R., Duncan, V., & Duggan, A. (2000). Promoting patients' full and honest disclosure during conversations with health caregivers. In S. Petronio (Ed.), *Balancing the secrets of private disclosure* (pp. 137–147). Mahwah, NJ: Lawrence Erlbaum.

Parsons, J. T., Missildine, W., VanOra, J., Purcell, D. W., Gomez, C. A., & the Seropositive Urban Injector's Study. (2004). HIV serostatus disclosure to sexual partners among HIV positive injection drug users. *AIDS Patient Care and STDs, 18*, 457–469.

Parsons, J. T., VanOra, J., Missildine, W., Purcell, D. W., & Gomez, C. A. (2004). Positive and negative consequences of HIV disclosure among seropositive injection drug users. *AIDS Education and Prevention, 16*, 459–475.

Parsons, T. (1951). *The social system.* Glencoe, IL: Free Press.

Petronio, S. (2000). The boundaries of privacy: Praxis of everyday life. In S. Petronio (Ed.), *Balancing the secrets of private disclosure* (pp. 37–39). Mahwah, NJ: Lawrence Erlbaum.

Rao, D., Kekwaletswe, T. C., Hosek, S., Martinez, J., & Rodriguez, F. (2007). Stigma and social barriers to medication adherence with urban youth living with HIV. *AIDS Care, 19*(1), 28–33.

Rosenfeld, L. B. (2000). Overview of the ways privacy, secrecy, and disclosure are balanced in today's society. In S. Petronio (Ed.), *Balancing the secrets of private disclosure* (pp. 3–17). Mahwah, NJ: Lawrence Erlbaum.

Rotunda, R., West, L., & O'Farrell, T. (2004). Enabling behavior in a clinical sample of alcohol-dependent clients and their partners. *Journal of Substance Abuse Treatment, 26*, 269–276.

Rubin, D. L., Yang, H., & Porte, M. (2000). A comparison of self-reported self-disclosure among Chinese and North Americans. In S. Petronio (Ed.),

*Balancing the secrets of private disclosure* (pp. 215–234). Mahwah, NJ: Lawrence Erlbaum.

Vance, D. (2006). The relationship between HIV disclosure and adjustment. *Psychological Reports, 99*, 659–663.

Weiner, L. S., Battles, H. B., & Heilman, N. (2000). Public disclosure of a child's HIV infection: Impact on children and families. *AIDS Patient Care and STDs, 14*, 485–496.

**Address correspondence to**: Maribel Valle, PhD, School of Nursing and Health Studies, Northern Illinois University, 250 Wirtz Hall, DeKalb, IL 60112. E-mail: mvalle@niu.edu

# Exercise for Article 28

## *Factual Questions*

1. What kind of sampling technique did the recruiters use to select the 839 African American IDUs and their sex and/or needle partners?

2. How many of the 839 IDUs who were recruited for testing and a baseline interview subsequently tested HIV positive?

3. How many participants were selected for the study following criteria set out by Glaser and Strauss (1967) regarding saturation?

4. Of the 80 selected participants for the study, what percentage were males?

5. What percentage of the selected participants for the study never finished high school?

6. Do the researchers believe it is likely that trust between interviewers and participants had been established?

## *Questions for Discussion*

7. Do you think it was a good idea to use a monetary incentive? Explain. (See lines 85–90.)

8. Do you think the data collection and analysis are described in sufficient detail? Explain. (See lines 123–139.)

9. In your opinion, do the results of this study have important practical implications? Explain. (See lines 551–579.)

10. The researchers suggest that further study with other populations would help determine whether or not their results are generalizable. Do you agree with their suggestion? Explain. (See lines 607–609.)

11. In your opinion, how important are the limitations described in lines 580–611? Explain.

12. If you were conducting a study on the same topic, would you use a qualitative approach *or* a quantitative approach? Explain.

## *Quality Ratings*

Directions: Indicate your level of agreement with each of the following statements by circling a number from 5 for strongly agree (SA) to 1 for strongly disagree (SD). If you believe an item is not applicable to this research article, leave it blank. Be prepared to explain your ratings. When responding to criteria A and B, keep in mind that brief titles and abstracts are conventional in published research.

A.   The title of the article is appropriate.

SA   5   4   3   2   1   SD

B.   The abstract provides an effective overview of the research article.

SA   5   4   3   2   1   SD

C.   The introduction establishes the importance of the study.

SA   5   4   3   2   1   SD

D.   The literature review establishes the context for the study.

SA   5   4   3   2   1   SD

E.   The research purpose, question, or hypothesis is clearly stated.

SA   5   4   3   2   1   SD

F.   The method of sampling is sound.

SA   5   4   3   2   1   SD

G.   Relevant demographics (for example, age, gender, and ethnicity) are described.

SA   5   4   3   2   1   SD

H.   Measurement procedures are adequate.

SA   5   4   3   2   1   SD

I.   All procedures have been described in sufficient detail to permit a replication of the study.

SA   5   4   3   2   1   SD

J.   The participants have been adequately protected from potential harm.

SA   5   4   3   2   1   SD

K.   The results are clearly described.

SA   5   4   3   2   1   SD

L.   The discussion/conclusion is appropriate.

SA   5   4   3   2   1   SD

M.   Despite any flaws, the report is worthy of publication.

SA   5   4   3   2   1   SD

# Article 29

# The Contribution of Research Knowledge and Skills to Practice: An Exploration of the Views and Experiences of Newly Qualified Nurses

**Gill Hek**, MA, RGN, NDN, Cert. Ed. (FE), **Alison Shaw**, PhD, MSc[*]

ABSTRACT. The question of how best to equip nurses with research knowledge and skills has been explored in a number of studies. This paper contributes to growing evidence about how research is perceived in practice, as part of the overall preparedness of a newly qualified nurse. Taking a longitudinal qualitative approach, this study found when interviewing nurses at 3 months, newly qualified nurses felt that they had received too much teaching about research, were not interested in the subject and struggled to see its relevance to clinical practice. However, at 12 months, about half of the 58 newly qualified nurses who participated in this study felt that research was "embedded" in the practice of their ward/work area, and were able to give examples such as research activity on the ward, research folders, notice boards, and conference feedback. In some areas, the newly qualified nurses were teaching students using evidence-based materials and said that research was often talked about. In the struggle to improve the use of research in everyday nursing practice, this study provides some evidence that newly qualified nurses feel they are engaging in relevant research activities.

## Introduction

Over the last two decades, there have been major changes in the provision of preregistration and continuing professional education for nurses in the United Kingdom, and substantial changes in healthcare policy
5 and delivery. At the centre of many debates is the fundamental questioning of the extent to which educational developments have given newly qualified nurses greater knowledge, skills, and confidence to function in the modern healthcare workplace.

10 One area of debate is the expectation that newly qualified nurses need to develop research knowledge and skills during their training and to use these to provide better patient care. The research presented in this paper was designed to explore newly qualified nurses'

15 perceptions of how prepared they were for practice. Specifically, the paper focuses on newly qualified nurses' views about their research knowledge and skills at 3 months and 12 months postqualifying.

### Background and Literature Review

The impact of changes in the UK curricula, such
20 as Project 2000 and the subsequent outcomes of the preregistration nursing programs, have been evaluated by many (Bedford et al., 1993; While et al., 1995; Bartlett et al., 1998, 2000; Parahoo, 1999). In particular, the relative merits of moving nursing education into higher
25 education has been rigorously debated in the United Kingdom (UK), and significant policy changes impinging on the education and practice of nurses have been seen in government proposals, such as Making a Difference (Department of Health, 1999), the NHS Plan
30 (Department of Health, 2000), and Liberating the Talents (Department of Health, 2002). The report from the then-UK nursing statutory body, Fitness for Practice (UKCC, 1999), provided a new term of reference for the education of nurses. Specifically the report empha-
35 sized the need to provide preregistration education that enabled "fitness for practice based on health care need" (UKCC, 1999:2). This was specified through core-learning outcomes and competencies at the end of the common foundation program, and at the point of regis-
40 tration by the UK nursing statutory body as requirements for preregistration nursing programs across the UK (UKCC, 2000). The standards for the education of preregistration nursing programs and the standards of proficiency required for entry to the nursing register
45 are given in "Standards of proficiency for preregistration nursing education" (NMC, 2004) and are guided by four principles: fitness for practice, fitness for purpose, fitness for award, and fitness for professional standing.

50 Across Europe, and particularly in the UK, the drive toward evidence-based nursing practice has led to greater clarity about research education in the preregis-

---

[*]*Gill Hek*, reader in nursing research, Faculty of Health and Social Care, University of the West of England, Bristol. *Alison Shaw*, lecturer in primary care research, Academic Unit of Primary Health Care, Department of Community Based Medicine, University of Bristol (University of the West of England during the study).

tration nursing curriculum. Over the past 10 years, there has been general acceptance about what newly qualified nurses should know and be able to do in relation to research. The strategy for nursing Making a Difference (Department of Health, 1999) stressed the importance of ensuring that nursing practice is "evidence-based" and that nurses have the knowledge and skills to enable them to translate research findings into practice. This is generally accepted as being able to read research critically, have a basic understanding of the research process, identify areas of practice that need researching, and to use research to improve patient care (Parahoo, 1999). Furthermore, the NMC standards (NMC, 2004) identify the need and use for research and evidence to be incorporated into practice, and that evidence-based knowledge should be used to individualize nursing interventions as a standard of proficiency for entry to the nursing register. The recent StLaR project (Butterworth, 2004:4) reiterates the need for a workforce that is "educated to understand the benefits and the pitfalls in the outcomes of the research process" and is "research aware," while the Quality Assurance Agency nursing academic and professional standards, used to assess higher-education provision, include for nursing awards that award holders should be able to "use appropriate research and other evidence to underpin nursing decisions…" (QAA, 2001).

A number of studies have explored how best to equip nurses with research skills and which teaching strategies and techniques to use (Clark & Sleep, 1991; Harrison et al., 1991; Reed, 1995; Dyson, 1997; Mulhall et al., 2000; Blenkinsop, 2003). Some studies have focused on specific groups of students (Lacey, 1996; Burrows and Baillie, 1997; Parahoo, 1999) or qualified staff (Veeramah, 1995; Meah et al., 1996). Many have studied the barriers to using research (e.g., McSherry 1997; Dunn et al., 1997; Retsas & Nolan, 1999; Kajermo et al., 2000; Parahoo & McCaughan, 2001; French, 2005) and two large postal surveys, one in Northern Ireland (Parahoo, 1999) and one in the southeast of England (Veeramah, 2004) both reported perceived barriers to using research following qualification, and shortfalls in training. However, the researchers found generally positive attitudes toward research. Similar findings were reported from a Swedish survey of nursing standards (Bjorkstrom et al., 2003).

Overall, the literature is inconclusive on the role of education and how best to prepare nurses with regard to research. There is also limited work done on how research knowledge and skills contribute to the overall preparedness for practice of nurses. This paper considers one aspect of "preparedness for practice"—research knowledge and skills—and how newly qualified nurses feel this contributes to their practice and their experiences.

## The Study

### Purpose and Aims

The Regional Workforce Development Confederation commissioned the two-year research project with the aim of facilitating a greater shared understanding between NHS service providers and nursing education providers regarding the preparedness for practice of newly qualified nurses.

Set against the national context and recent research, the need was identified for a longitudinal qualitative study within the region, looking in-depth at issues from a range of perspectives (educationalists, senior practitioners, nurse managers, newly qualified nurses), across all the branches of nursing (adult, child, mental health and learning disabilities) and including a range of clinical areas entered by newly qualified practitioners.

The data collected and analyzed in the study yielded a substantial dataset covering a wide variety of issues that have been reported elsewhere (Shaw & Hek, 2003). The findings reported here relate specifically to the views of newly qualified nurses of their research knowledge and skills.

### Methods

A longitudinal qualitative approach was employed with data collected from newly qualified nurses at three months and 12 months postqualification to enable comparison over time.

### Ethical Issues and Approval

The study was approved by the UK South-West Multi-Centre Research Ethics Committee and the University Ethics Committee. The seven NHS Trusts participating in the study gave management approval.

The usual procedures for ensuring ethical research practice were followed. Letters and information sheets were provided to all potential participants prior to obtaining written consent. Care was taken to conduct the research in a way that respected the views and experiences of participants and ensured the anonymity and confidentiality of any information they provided. All information on participants (e.g., names and addresses) was stored separately from a list of identifying codes to prevent identification. All interview tapes, transcripts and data used in research reports were anonymized and tapes were destroyed at the end of the study. The researchers were not directly involved in the students' education and no major ethical issues emerged during the course of the research.

### Sample Selection

The sampling strategy involved several stages: First, seven NHS Trusts employing newly qualified nurses exiting from the university from each branch of nursing were identified. Second, a maximum-variation strategy (Patton, 2002) was used to identify nursing students from each branch of the preregistration nursing programs (adult, child, mental health, and learning disabilities) and each award (diploma and degree) who were about to enter practice in one of the seven participating NHS Trusts. The sampling strategy also aimed to include a proportional reflection of the differing numbers of students in each branch program. Nursing students from the degree and diploma cohorts exiting the preregistration nursing programs in 2001/2002 were approached and given information about the research at tutorial sessions at each campus for each branch just prior to their qualification.

The students who were planning to take up posts in one of the selected Trusts participating in the research were identified. They provided contact details and indicated the Trust and ward/unit where they would take up their first (usually D grade) post after qualifying. Once qualified, the potential participants were approached and invited for interview. Some were not contactable, others had not taken up their planned posts, and others had moved away from the region. The final sample included 43 diploma nurses and 15 degree nurses from the two cohorts. The numbers of participants proportionally reflected the numbers of students in each branch program/award (see Table 1).

Table 1
*Newly Qualified Nurses: Participants by Award/Campus/Branch*

| Award/campus | Branch | Total number of students in cohort | Number of newly qualified nurses participating in study |
|---|---|---|---|
| **DipHE** | | | |
| Campus A | Adult | 46 | 16 |
| | Child | 14 | 3 |
| | M'Health | 10 | 5 |
| | L'Disabilities | 6 | 3 |
| Campus B | Adult | 24 | 10 |
| Campus C | Adult | 11 | 6 |
| Campus D | Adult | 21 | 0 |
| | | | (not included as hospital not in study) |
| **Total DipHE** | | | **43** |
| **BSc** | Adult | 30 | 15 |
| **Total BSc** | | | **15** |
| **Grand total** | | **162** | **58** |

## Data Collection

Two data-collection methods were used: in-depth face-to-face interviews in the clinical setting at three months postqualifying, and telephone interviews at 12 months postqualifying. For the first interviews, a topic guide was used to ensure some comparability between interviews through coverage of the same broad issues. The initial topic guide was based on the literature and on data from interviews with nursing education providers and service providers early in the study (Shaw & Hek, 2003). However, the interviews also included considerable flexibility in order to allow the participants to pursue their own lines of thought and introduce new topics that were of importance to them. This approach followed the twin principles of control and

flexibility that are central to the in-depth interview method (Burgess, 1991). The interviews explored their early experiences as newly qualified staff nurses, examining the extent to which they felt that their nursing education had prepared them for practice, and their experiences of support and preceptorship provided by the NHS Trust. Specific areas of practice where difficulties or successes had been experienced were investigated. Throughout the interviews, attention was given to the specific area of nursing and the clinical setting that the person had entered, exploring the role of the particular work environment in shaping their experiences.

At the first face-to-face interview at three months, questions focused generally on perceived knowledge and skills and areas of practice where they felt confident/unconfident and competent/not competent. They were also asked the extent to which they felt their education had prepared them and whether their prior expectations about working as a qualified nurse had been met. However, following analysis of the early data when research emerged as a theme, questions were framed to explore the topic further at 12 months in the telephone interviews. These tended to focus on the extent to which research is used in practice, and whether they would like to be able to use research in their practice, both now and in the future.

Each face-to-face interview lasted from 45 minutes to one hour and took place at a convenient time for the participant—often during or shortly after the "handover" period when there were greater numbers of staff present on the ward to free up the newly qualified nurse. The telephone interviews were usually shorter, at around 30 minutes, and were arranged mostly for when the nurse was at home or at a convenient time at work.

## Data Analysis

All the transcripts from the first interviews with the newly qualified nurses were audiotaped and fully transcribed. This process generated a large volume of qualitative data, which were managed and analyzed with the assistance of the software package "AT-LASti." Detailed notes from the follow-up semistructured telephone interviews were made for the purposes of thematic analysis.

As is common in all qualitative research, data collection and analysis were not separate stages of the research, but were closely interwoven throughout. Insights from analysis of the data gathered earlier in the process shaped the topics and questions covered during later data collection. This iterative process allowed reflection on the data and the generation of themes and ideas for further exploration. Throughout, the aim was to produce "thick description" (Fetterman, 1989) of the area under investigation, using the words of the participants.

Throughout the research process, analysis of the qualitative data involved coding interview transcripts for key issues and emerging themes. Analysis drew on the principles of constant comparison (Strauss & Corbin, 1998), elements of data continually being compared with other elements to allow the development of core categories. Throughout this process, the principal researcher cross-checked the developing coding strategy and categories with the other researcher on the team, to ensure that the emerging themes were trustworthy and credible (Mays & Pope, 1995).

The data from the first interviews with newly qualified nurses were examined for key categories and themes relating to their views and experiences of the preregistration nurse training and their own preparedness for practice during the early weeks/months postqualifying. The data from the follow-up telephone interviews were examined for changes in views and experiences since the first interviews.

## Findings

### Research in the Curriculum

Research was a key theme within newly qualified nurses' accounts of the preregistration course. At three months, the majority of diploma nurses felt that they had received too much teaching on research during their training and struggled to see the relevance to their own nursing practice. While acknowledging that research did have its place, many were not personally interested in the subject and did not seem to have engaged with the research teaching they had received.

While recognizing the broad principle of evidence-based practice, the newly qualified nurses tended to see research as a peripheral subject within the work of a newly qualified practitioner. The majority seemed to view it as something that some people may choose to pursue at a later stage of their nursing career, but they did not necessarily see it as particularly relevant for new nurses. However, some of the degree nurses expressed a more positive view of the research teaching and reflected on the value of undertaking a research dissertation for improving their understanding of the research process—including the process of ethical review at the university and Trusts. This experience seemed to have increased their confidence to undertake research, if such an opportunity should arise in their nursing practice.

A lot of research, how to carry out your research, the different types of research, and I think yes you need to know it but at the time I was there thinking well as a D grade I won't really be involved in running that myself, I might be putting it into practice or helping put it into practice...but it's probably more something you could do maybe as a qualified if you wanted to go into that sort of field rather than actually during our training.

(NQA05 Child branch)

I think it was good to have to do [research]. I chose to come out to the hospital. I did my research here with the nurses in A & E, which was a lot more difficult with the ethics approval. I had to go through [the university] and the Trust, which was a pain, but at least I have done that so if I wanted to do it again, I would know what I was doing filling in all the forms.... It was good; at least I know what I am doing now, and I understand the whole process so if I had to do something, I am sure I would be able to do it.

(NQD07 Adult branch)

...research during training didn't help...a fake trial where everyone did a bit...would be better.

(NQB09 Adult branch)

At 12 months some of the nurses perceived a greater relevance of the research component of their preregistration education for their current and future practice. Specifically it helped them to think about research, have a basic overview of issues, and they felt they knew how to find out more about research:

...the preparation for thinking about research during the training helped me think about research now.

(NQB08 Adult branch)

...course gave me basic knowledge to do research...feel confident and competent to do it...big values of the training...didn't so much give us knowledge but taught us how to find that knowledge.

(NQB07 Child branch)

### Research and Clinical Practice

At 12 months, about half the nurses felt that "research" was "embedded" in the practice of the ward. The examples they gave included conference feedback to staff and research activity on wards such as collecting data, project work, auditing, and research folders and notice boards. In some clinical areas the nurses had got involved in teaching students and care staff using evidence-based material and they said that research was often "talked about." However, only a few of the nurses read or subscribed to nursing journals, or regularly consulted books regarding clinical issues that emerged from their practice.

Research is talked about and used on the wards.... I haven't been involved in any big projects, but if I hear about things, I like to go and find the information for myself.... I'm always on the Internet at home.

(NQC05 Adult branch)

...research on the ward is quite important, and they like staff to have the knowledge.

(NQD03 Adult branch)

I get the learning disability journal and take it into work, and the unit takes a few journals now, and people can look at these for the latest research.

(NQH01 Learning disabilities branch)

Although the majority of nurses at 12 months expressed a general awareness of research, there was little direct experience, and it was still often seen as something for certain interested nurses in the future.

*Barriers to Using Research*

360   Although not asked specifically, the nurses identified some "barriers" to using research in practice at 12 months. There were resource issues, such as lack of access to a computer on the ward or the library not being close to the workplace. Also, there was felt to be

365   expectations that this sort of work should take place in the nurses' own time:

> ...don't have time and I'm too tired to do it in my own time.
>
> (NQA07 Adult branch)

370   It was felt by some to be quicker to ask other members of the nursing staff rather than find out through consulting research information, and there was a criticism that the link between audit and research had not been taught on their preregistration course.

375   I haven't done any research, but lots of people are doing audits on everything...not portrayed all that well through the university...never really mentioned how audits were done...[didn't] recognize the link between research and audit.

380   (NQA05 Adult branch)

A small number of nurses were not interested in research and felt that this was made more difficult because research was never talked about within their clinical area.

385   ...no formal essays to write...haven't done research.

(NQA04 Adult branch)

...not used research at all. Research is not something that's really talked about.

(NQA09 Adult branch)

## Discussion

390   The findings in this qualitative study add to the growing amount of research in the field of research education and utilization of research findings in practice. There is some evidence that research is embedded in nursing practice in certain clinical areas, with some

395   participants in this study able to give examples of research activity in their area of practice. The findings are not generalizable, but they do provide insight from a fairly large qualitative longitudinal study, and there may be some transferability of the findings to other

400   similar settings or participants. They also make a contribution by placing research knowledge and skills within the overall context of being a newly qualified nurse, and the study does provide some understanding about how nurses feel over time about research as part

405   of their overall preparedness for practice. Similar to other studies, the barriers to using research in practice are still evident.

The diploma nurses in this study had received two discrete research modules about sources of evidence

410   and using research in practice, and the degree nurses additionally had a module to prepare them to undertake a small research project and write a dissertation. It is not possible to determine whether the degree students

415   had more positive feelings about research, nor if they had more experience of research in their clinical practice once qualified. This would be an interesting line to pursue in further studies, as would research that examined the purpose of research education and skills in the curriculum, and what difference this makes to clinical

420   practice.

There is a body of literature about the outcomes of preregistration nursing programs, and emerging research about how best to equip nurses with research skills, particularly in terms of learning strategies and

425   teaching techniques to provide them with a general understanding of research. However, there is a need for more longitudinal research that follows students and newly qualified nurses over extended periods of time to see how research education in the formative years is

430   translated into knowledge and skills in experienced practitioners.

## References

Bartlett, H., Simonite, V., Westcott, E., & Taylor, H. (2000). A comparison of the nursing competence of graduates and diplomates from UK nursing programmes. *Journal of Clinical Nursing, 9,* 369–381.

Bartlett, H., Westcott, L., Hind, P., & Taylor, H. (1998). *An evaluation of preregistration nursing education: A literature review and comparative study of graduate outcomes,* Report no. 4, Oxford Centre for Health Care Research and Development, Oxford Brookes University.

Bedford, H., Phillips, T., Robinson, J., & Schostak, J. (1993). *Assessing competencies in nursing and midwifery education,* Final Report, English National Board for Nursing and Midwifery, London.

Bjorkstrom, M. E., Hamrin, E. K. F., & Athlin, E. E. (2003). Swedish nursing students' attitudes to aid awareness of research and development within nursing. *Journal of Advanced Nursing, 41,* 393–402.

Blenkinsop, C. (2003). Research: An essential skill of a graduate nurse. *Nurse Education Today, 23,* 83–88.

Burgess, R. G. (1991). The unstructured interview as conversation. In Burgess, R.G. (ed.) *Field research: A sourcebook and field manual.* London: Routledge.

Burrows, D. E., & Baillie, L. (1997). A strategy for teaching research to adult branch diploma students. *Nurse Education Today, 17,* 115–120.

Butterworth, T. (2004). *The StLaR HR Plan Project.* London: Department for Education and Skills, Department of Health, NHSU.

Clark, E. H., & Sleep, J. (1991). The what and how of teaching research. *Nurse Education Today, 11,* 172–178.

Department of Health (1999). *Making a difference: Strengthening the nursing, midwifery and health visiting contribution to health and healthcare.* London: Department of Health.

Department of Health (2000). *The NHS Plan: A plan for investment, a plan for reform.* London: Department of Health.

Department of Health (2002). *Liberating the talents.* London: Department of Health.

Dunn, Y., & Crighton, N., Roe, B., Seers, K., & Williams, K. (1997). Using research for practice: A UK experience of the BARRIERS scale. *Journal of Advanced Nursing, 27,* 1203–1210.

Dyson, J. (1997). Research: Promoting positive attitudes through education. *Journal of Advanced Nursing, 26,* 608–612.

Fetterman, D.M. (1989). *Ethnography: Step by step.* London: Sage.

French, B. (2005). The process of research use in nursing. *Journal of Advanced Nursing, 49,* 125–134.

Harrison, L. L., Lowery, B., & Bailey, P. (1991). Changes in nursing students' knowledge about and attitudes toward research following an undergraduate research course. *Journal of Advanced Nursing, 16,* 807–812.

Kajermo, K. N., Nordstrom, G., Krusebrant, A., & Bjorvell, H. (2000). Perceptions of research utilization: Comparisons between health care professionals, nursing students and a reference group of nurse clinicians. *Journal of Advanced Nursing, 31,* 99–109.

Lacey, A. E. (1996). Facilitating research-based practice by educational intervention. *Nurse Education Today, 16,* 96–30.

McSherry, R. (1997). What do registered nurses and midwives feel and know about research? *Journal of Advanced Nursing, 25,* 985–998.

Mays, N., & Pope, C. (1995). Rigour and qualitative research. *British Medical Journal, 311,* 109–112.

Meah, S., Luker, K. A., & Cullum, N. A. (1996). An exploration of midwives' attitudes to research and perceived barriers to research utilisation. *Midwifery, 12,* 73–84.

Mulhall, A., Le-May, A., & Alexander, C. (2000). Research-based nursing practice: An evaluation of an educational programme. *Nurse Education Today, 20,* 435–443.

Nursing and Midwifery Council (2004). *Standards of proficiency for pre-registration nursing education.* London: Nursing and Midwifery Council.

Parahoo, K. (1999). A comparison of pre-Project 2000 and Project 2000 nurses' perceptions of their research training, research needs, and of their use of research in clinical areas. *Journal of Advanced Nursing, 29,* 237–245.

Parahoo, K., & McCaughan, E. M. (2001). Research utilization among medical and surgical nurses: A comparison of their self-reports of barriers and facilitators. *Journal of Nursing Management, 9,* 21–30.

Patton, M. Q. (2002). *Qualitative research and evaluation methods. 3rd edition.* London: Sage.

Quality Assurance Agency for Higher Education (2001). *Benchmark statement: Health care programmes, nursing.* Gloucester: Quality Assurance Agency for Higher Education.

Reed, J. (1995). Using a group project to teach research methods. *Nurse Education Today, 15,* 56–60.

Retsas, A., & Nolan, M. (1999). Barriers to nurses' use of research: An Australian hospital study. *International Journal of Nursing Studies, 36,* 335–343.

Shaw, A. & Hek, G. (2003). *Preparedness for practice: A longitudinal Qualitative study of newly qualified nurses, trust stakeholders and educationalists.* Bristol: University of the West of England.

Strauss, A., & Corbin, J. (eds) (1998). *Basics of qualitative research, second edition.* London: Sage.

UKCC (1999). *Fitness for practice: the UKCC Commission for Nursing and Midwifery Education.* London: UKCC.

UKCC (2000). Requirements for preregistration nursing programmes. London: UKCC.

Veeramah, V. (1995). A study to identify the attitudes and needs of qualified staff concerning the use of research findings in clinical practice within mental health settings. *Journal of Advanced Nursing, 22,* 855–861.

Veeramah, V. (2004). Utilization of research findings by graduate nurses and midwives. *Journal of Advanced Nursing, 47,* 183–191.

While, A., Roberts, J., & Fitzpatrick, J. (1995). *A comparative study of outcomes of preregistration nurse education programmes.* London: English National Board for Nursing, Midwifery and Health Visiting.

**Acknowledgments**: The study was funded by the Avon, Gloucestershire and Wiltshire Workforce Development Confederation. We would like to acknowledge the support of nurses within the local NHS Trusts who participated and facilitated access for the research and members of the Project Steering Group who guided and supported the researchers. Some of the findings were presented at the Workgroup of European Research Nurses Conference in Lisbon 2004.

**Address correspondence to**: Gill Hek, University of the West of England, Faculty of Health and Social Care, Glenside, Blackberry Hill, Stapleton, Bristol, BS16 1DD. E-mail: Gill.Hek@uwe.ac.uk

# Exercise for Article 29

## Factual Questions

1. Were the researchers able to contact all of the potential participants who were qualified?

2. How many of the participants in the final sample were degree nurses?

3. Were face-to-face interviews *or* telephone interviews used at three months postqualifying?

4. The researchers characterized what feature of their research as "common in all qualitative research"?

5. Did the researchers cross check with each other when developing coding strategy and themes?

6. At 12 months, about what percentage of the participants felt that research was embedded in the practice of the ward?

## Questions for Discussion

7. Is the section on ethical issues and approval an important element of this research report? Explain. (See lines 133–151.)

8. Is the use of flexible interviews a strength of this study? Explain. (See lines 191–197.)

9. Is the use of "thick description" (i.e., using the words of participants) an important part of this study? Explain. (See lines 247–250 and the quotations interspersed in lines 295–389.)

10. How important is it to know that the principal researcher cross-checked with the other researcher? (See lines 257–261.)

11. Does this research convince you that there was a change in the perceptions of the relevance of research from 3 months to 12 months? (See lines 270–330.)

12. If you were planning a follow-up study to explore the topic of this research further, would you plan an additional qualitative study or a quantitative study? Explain.

## Quality Ratings

Directions: Indicate your level of agreement with each of the following statements by circling a number from 5 for strongly agree (SA) to 1 for strongly disagree (SD). If you believe an item is not applicable to this research article, leave it blank. Be prepared to explain your ratings. When responding to criteria A and B, keep in mind that brief titles and abstracts are conventional in published research.

A. The title of the article is appropriate.

SA   5   4   3   2   1   SD

B. The abstract provides an effective overview of the research article.

SA   5   4   3   2   1   SD

C. The introduction establishes the importance of the study.

SA   5   4   3   2   1   SD

D.  The literature review establishes the context for
    the study.

    SA   5   4   3   2   1   SD

E.  The research purpose, question, or hypothesis is
    clearly stated.

    SA   5   4   3   2   1   SD

F.  The method of sampling is sound.

    SA   5   4   3   2   1   SD

G.  Relevant demographics (for example, age, gender,
    and ethnicity) are described.

    SA   5   4   3   2   1   SD

H.  Measurement procedures are adequate.

    SA   5   4   3   2   1   SD

I.  All procedures have been described in sufficient
    detail to permit a replication of the study.

    SA   5   4   3   2   1   SD

J.  The participants have been adequately protected
    from potential harm.

    SA   5   4   3   2   1   SD

K.  The results are clearly described.

    SA   5   4   3   2   1   SD

L.  The discussion/conclusion is appropriate.

    SA   5   4   3   2   1   SD

M.  Despite any flaws, the report is worthy of publica-
    tion.

    SA   5   4   3   2   1   SD

# Article 30

# Student Nurses' Perceptions of Alternative and Allopathic Medicine

**Ron Joudrey**, MA, **Sheila McKay**, RN, MN, **Jim Gough**, PhD[*]

ABSTRACT. This exploratory study of student nurses is based on the results of the responses to one question on an open-ended questionnaire: How would you define the relationship between alternative medicine and allopathic (conventional) medicine? A specific goal of the study was to find out how the surveyed respondents conceptualized the relationship between allopathic and alternative medicine. Three themes were identified: (a) "They are not at all alike," (b) "The two can or should be used together," and (c) "Those who practice alternative medicine and those who practice allopathic do not get along very well." The discussion suggests some reasons for these perceptions and considers some implications for future health care.

From *Western Journal of Nursing Research, 26,* 356–366. Copyright © 2004 by Sage Publications. Reprinted with permission.

The long-standing hegemony of allopathic medicine has been challenged by the increasing popularity of alternative medicine. The reaction of mainstream health care providers to the growth of alternative medi-
5  cine has been given much attention in professional medical and nursing journals. Although the perceptions of those already practicing in the health care system are certainly worthy of research interest, there is also a need to investigate the views of health care practitio-
10  ners in training. The extent to which alternative and allopathic therapies become integrated will depend somewhat on how the future generation of health care workers conceptualizes the relationship between the conventional and alternative modes of health care. The
15  present study examines how student nurses perceive this relationship.

### Nurses, Physicians, and the Rise of Alternative Medicine

In recent times, health care professionals working within the dominant allopathic tradition have become aware that many of their clients are utilizing various
20  forms of alternative or complementary therapies. Research in a number of countries, including the United States (Eisenberg et al., 1998; Eisenberg et al., 1993) and Canada (McClennon-Leong & Kerr, 1999), has

clearly demonstrated such use. In response to large
25  consumer demand, a number of nursing researchers (Hayes & Alexander, 2000; McClennon-Leong & Kerr, 1999; Melland & Clayburgh, 2000; Reed, Pettigrew, & King, 2000) have called for the need to include alternative therapies in the nursing curricula. King, Pettigrew,
30  and Reed (1999) presented one practical rationale for nurses to increase their interest in such therapies: "If significantly more Americans are using some form of complementary therapy, it is imperative that nurses have a knowledge base of a variety of therapies in or-
35  der to assist clients with decision making related to therapies" (p. 250).

We contend that health care practitioners' perceptions of complementary and alternative therapies will influence the future direction of health care. Writers
40  from the sociological tradition known as symbolic interactionism have agreed that meanings held by social actors influence behavior (Stryker, 1980). Whether nurses and other health care professionals have favorable or unfavorable views of alternative therapies will
45  likely influence the extent to which these therapies are integrated into health care practice. The relationship between the two systems of health care (allopathic and alternative) has changed somewhat over time. Budrys (2001) argued that allopathic medicine had established
50  itself as the dominant form of health care by the turn of the 20th century. With this hegemony came the tendency for those working within this tradition to relegate other forms of therapy to a subordinate status. Therapies offered outside the allopathic domain were
55  viewed as quackery, unscientific, and dangerous (Budrys, 2001; Goldstein, 2000). There are, however, recent indications of increasing acceptance of some alternative and complementary therapies by physicians and nurses. For example, a Canadian study of general
60  practitioners found that 54% perceived some benefits from the use of alternative therapies and were sometimes willing to recommend their patients use these therapies (Verhoef & Sutherland, 1995). Other studies (Hayes & Alexander, 2000; King et al., 1999) found
65  evidence of favorable opinions toward alternative and

---

[*]*Ron Joudrey* is a sociology instructor at Red Deer College. *Sheila McKay* is nursing department chair at Red Deer College. *Jim Gough* is a philosophy instructor at Red Deer College.

complementary therapies on the part of practicing nurses. The Hayes and Alexander (2000) study of nurse practitioners found that "almost two-thirds (65%) indicated that they had recommended or referred clients for one or more alternative modalities" (p. 52). To our knowledge there have been few, if any, extant studies on how future generations of health care professionals view alternative and complementary therapies. There is a need to investigate how groups, such as student nurses, make sense of the relationship between alternative therapies and allopathic therapies because their perceptions will undoubtedly have some influence on whether the two previously hostile systems of health care will reach some sort of rapprochement in future.

Many writers, including Budrys (2001), Clarke (2000), and Goldstein (2000), have pointed out the difficulty in finding an agreed-on definition to encompass the eclectic range of therapies variously labeled as alternative, complementary, unconventional, and more recently, complementary and alternative medicine (CAM). Goldstein (2000) suggested that residual definitions of the phenomena are common. An example of a residual definition would be the following from Matcha (2000): "Alternative medicine refers to medical treatments that are not taught or offered in Western medical practice" (p. 299). This type of definition is perhaps too restrictive because there are a growing number of such therapies that are offered by allopathic practitioners (Clarke, 2000).

Finding acceptable terminology to use in this area is also problematic. Although the label "complementary and alternative medicine (CAM)" has become more common, many writers such as Budrys (2001), Clarke (2000), Goldstein (2000), and Hayes and Alexander (2000) have not used this term consistently. The tendency has often been to acknowledge the newer, more encompassing label, while also continuing to employ terms such as "complementary," "alternative," or "unconventional" in a synonymous fashion. A cover story in *Newsweek* (Cowley et al., 2002) was titled "Inside the Science of Alternative Medicine," even though the writers referred to CAM throughout the story. We decided to use the designation "alternative medicine" because this term is still employed in common parlance.

## Purpose

The aim of the present study was to explore student nurses' perceptions of the relationship between allopathic and alternative medicine.

## Method

### Design

A qualitative, cross-sectional descriptive design was used for this exploratory survey of student nurses' perceptions.

### Sample

A convenience sample was used to study student nurses at a community college in Alberta, Canada. Students in this program have the option of completing a 3-year diploma or a 4-year degree. The intent was to sample as many student nurses as possible out of the 250 enrolled in the program. A total of 81 students completed the survey for a return rate of 30.86%. A breakdown of study participants by year of program was the following: 1st year, $N = 9$; 2nd year, $N = 28$; 3rd year, $N = 11$; and 4th year, $N = 33$. No information was obtained as to whether the respondents in the first 3 years were degree or diploma students because this was not regarded by the researchers as important to the study. Among the respondents, 96.3% were women, and 3.7% were men. They ranged in age from 18 to 45 years, with a mean age of 22.7. Most participants (74%) reported being single, and 26% were married. The majority were residents of Alberta (71.6%), and the remainder resided elsewhere prior to entering the program.

### Procedures

The researchers first obtained permission from the college Research Ethics Committee to carry out this study. A seven-item, open-ended questionnaire was used to survey student nurses' perceptions of alternative medicine (see the Appendix). The findings discussed in this article are the responses to one question from the larger study: How would you define the relationship between alternative medicine and allopathic medicine?

Various nursing instructors distributed the questionnaire in their classes between January and December 2000. A cover letter to potential respondents stressed that participation was voluntary and anonymous and was not a required component of their program.

### Data Analysis

Responses to the study question were analyzed using schema analysis as described by Ryan and Bernard (2000). Two of the study authors compared and coded the responses in an effort to find common themes. These themes were developed inductively by carefully reading and comparing the responses, looking for repetitions of words and phrases. Responses that were judged similar and frequently mentioned formed the basis for the content of major themes. The themes discussed are illustrated with direct quotes from study participants in an effort to faithfully represent their discourse (Stryker, 1980).

The researchers initially intended to do a year-by-year comparison of student responses; however, after a careful reading of the data, no major differences were detected between those in different phases of the program. The findings presented herein are based on analysis of the collective groups of respondents.

As a means of testing the trustworthiness of the themes, the technique of member checking was used. Discussion with several study participants indicated the analysis was recognizable to them. Lincoln and Guba (1985) recommended member checking as an important technique for establishing credibility of analysis.

## Results

Based on analysis of responses to the question "How do you define the relationship between alternative and allopathic medicine?" we identified three themes: (a) "They are not at all alike," (b) "The two can or should be used together," and (c) "Those who practice alternative medicine and those who practice allopathic do not get along well." The findings of the study are presented with these themes.

### "They Are Not At All Alike"

A total of 15 study participants mentioned differences between the two therapeutic modes. One respondent simply stated, "They are not at all alike." Others delineated the differences more specifically. The perception of alternative medicine as being more natural, whereas allopathic is otherwise, was voiced by a few students: "Alternative medicine draws on the body's natural, innate healing forces, while conventional medicine is more synthetic, complex, and highly technological."

And, "Alternative medicine is more natural without using chemicals and invasive procedures while allopathic is the opposite."

In a few cases, the natural noninvasive nature of alternative medicine was extolled as a virtue, as illustrated by a 3rd-year student: "I don't think the two therapies are similar at all. I'd rather do the alternative first, especially if it's noninvasive, before I let someone decide that I need to be cut open. I think everything can be cured/controlled by what we eat and natural methods."

A second contrast was to perceive alternative medicine as more holistic and allopathic as more specific: "Alternative medicine deals more with the person as a whole human being, whereas conventional medicine focuses only on the physical ailment."

And in a similar vein: "Alternative medicine allows for the possibility of a mind/body connection which [sic] allopathic medicine focuses only on the physical body."

Evaluation of the two types of medicine was also noted: "I feel that it is harder to evaluate alternative medicine's effects compared to the other type"; and "Conventional therapies may be more reliable as there are more studies that prove their effectiveness but this may change as more people research alternative medicine."

### "The Two Can or Should Be Used Together"

The second theme suggesting complementarity was voiced by 23 respondents. One 2nd-year student commented, "The two can or should be used together because both types of therapies can be beneficial."

One perception was that allopathic and alternative have similar goals. Consider the following statements as illustrative: "Both have the intention and purpose of improving one's health" and "They both should be working together to restore or maintain health."

Others perceived that both approaches have strengths and limitations: "Often conventional medicine can be augmented by alternative medicine or vice versa. Both therapies have strengths and limitations so a combination of the two would likely prove more effective than one used in isolation"; "I think they can complement one another. There are certainly benefits and hindrances to both types, but they each have their place in treatment of patients."

### "Those Who Practice Alternative Medicine and Those Who Practice Allopathic Do Not Get Along Well"

In this theme, the focus was on the practitioners. Many spoke of the tension between allopathic and alternative practitioners using adjectives such as "shaky," "poor," "tense," "strained," and "competing" to describe the relationship. Of the respondents, 43 spoke of the opposition between allopathic and alternative practitioners, making this the most common theme. Of these student nurses, 20 attributed the conflicts to the attitudes of allopathic practitioners: "Those who practice conventional medicine are not receptive to other treatments. One reason that could be plausible is that they are defending their territory"; "There is a lot of misinformation and misunderstanding by doctors over alternative medicine"; "I think that conventional doctors and nurses do not see the positive effects that alternative medicine can have"; and "Conventional medicine is threatened by the success of alternative medicine."

Only one respondent perceived alternative practitioners as responsible for the conflict: "I think that those people who practice alternative medicine often extol the virtues of 'natural remedies' and discourage patients from seeking advice from doctors."

Several respondents (15) expressed that although present relationships are strained, the situation seems to be improving: "Alternative medicine is just beginning to be accepted by conventional health practitioners" and "I think that at this time (despite a history of conflict) that [sic] physicians and other medical practitioners like nurses are starting to insert more alternative medicine into their practices. They are still fairly focused on conventional medicine but do use alternative medicine a bit."

Some (19) hoped that the relationship would improve in the future as shown in these examples: "The time for fighting and animosity is over. They need to work more together"; "There needs to be more respect for each other between doctors, nurses, and those who practice alternative medicine. This would be in the best interest of clients."

We must note that, in most cases, particular responses could be filtered into one category. There were five responses that overlapped categories. For example, one respondent mentioned the complementarity between the therapies but also referred to conflict between the practitioners.

## Discussion

This exploratory study found that although student nurses' perceptions about alternative and allopathic medicine varied, these perceptions did appear to cluster around three themes. These different conceptualizations might be a reflection of the amorphous and fluctuating relationship between the two modes of health care.

The first theme identified was "They are not at all alike." The use of the term *alternative* may have predisposed some respondents to concentrate on differences, although this was not the case with many others in the sample.

One specific difference mentioned was that alternative therapies are more holistic, whereas allopathic therapies focus only on the physical ailment. Some writers, including Clarke (2000) and Goldstein (2000), have suggested that holism is one feature that distinguishes alternative medicine from the allopathic mode. This rather common perception might have also influenced some of the study participants to notice differences. Students enrolled in this particular nursing program are also extensively exposed to the seminal work on nursing philosophy by Watson (1985) who emphasized the importance of a holistic emphasis.

Some alternative practitioners have made the claim that their therapies are superior to conventional ones because the former are more natural and noninvasive. A few of our respondents echoed this sentiment. The perception that natural is better needs more careful scrutiny because clearly some natural substances can be harmful.

The second theme was "The two can or should be used together." Those who expressed this view demonstrated a more current awareness of the efforts under way to promote more integration of the previously separate medical systems, although there was no mention of which types of therapies might be complementary. Certainly not all types of alternative medicine are likely to be integrated with conventional medical practice. We believe it is important that these students learn to make more critical distinctions between different types of alternative therapies, distinguishing those that may be harmful from those that may be beneficial. Some of these students did, however, demonstrate evidence of critical thinking by recognizing that both types of therapies have strengths and limitations.

The most common theme identified was "Those who practice alternative medicine and those who practice allopathic do not get along very well." This perception does not fit with recent evidence showing that physicians and nurses sometimes recommended their clients to alternative practitioners (Hayes & Alexander, 2000; Verhoef & Sutherland, 1995). Perhaps these students had not witnessed any examples of such crossover in their own experiences to date. As they enter practice situations, this perception may very well change, particularly if they work with physicians and nurses who are open to the use of some alternative therapies.

The tendency for several study respondents to attribute strained relationships between allopathic and alternative practitioners mostly to the nonacceptance of alternative medicine by those nurses and physicians practicing within the conventional (allopathic) tradition is worthy of comment. Clarke (2000) suggested that nurses in their efforts to achieve professional status have adopted an antitechnology ideology that rejects the medical model and advocates a model based on holistic care. If this is true, it may account for some of the accusations leveled against the allopathic practitioners by some student nurses in the present study.

In holding allopathic nurses and physicians responsible for the animosity between the two types of medicine, there seemed to be almost a carte blanche acceptance of alternative medicine and its practitioners. With a few exceptions, study participants did not hold the same critical stance toward alternative medicine as they did toward allopathic medicine. There may be some dangers in the wholesale and uncritical acceptance of alternative medicine. As the results of clinical trials investigating the safety and effectiveness of various alternative therapies become more available, this should enable nurses and other health care practitioners to discern which alternative therapies are useful and safe for clinical practice.

In a more positive vein, some of the student nurses perceived an improvement toward better relationships between allopathic and alternative practitioners, and some expressed the hope that this would continue for the best interest of clients.

The sources of these various perceptions just discussed are unclear. This particular nursing program has paid some attention to the topic of alternative medicine. Conversations with nursing instructors and students revealed there were one or two lectures devoted to this area, and the topic has been discussed in some of the scenarios the students dealt with in tutorials.

There are many other sources of information that may have influenced the respondents' perceptions: mass media, Internet, personal experiences, hearsay, testimonials, advertisements from alternative practitioners, and so on. How these other sources juxtaposed with professional socialization is an empirical question but one that should be addressed.

This small study of student nurses uncovered a variety of perceptions about how alternative medicine relates to allopathic medicine. The findings demonstrate a general receptiveness toward the integration of alternative and conventional therapies. As new generations of nurses continue to be socialized into a more holistic emphasis on health care, we believe this will contribute to the increasing integration of two previously separate systems of health care. Medical sociologists such as Northcott (2002) argued that there is an increasing similarity and convergence between alternative and conventional medicine. Such a rapprochement is reflected in the perceptions of student nurses in the present study. The future direction of health care will be influenced by the perceptions of various categories of health care practitioners. This study contributes to our knowledge of these perceptions by concentrating on a previously neglected group of study participants, student nurses. The study is obviously limited by the relatively small sample size, and we do not claim the perceptions are representative of student nurses in general.

### APPENDIX
### Survey Questions

1. How do you define alternative medicine?
2. Have you ever used any type of alternative medicine? If so, which type did you use? Were you satisfied with the results?
3. If you have never used any form of alternative medicine, would you be willing to? Under what conditions?
4. How would you define the relationship between alternative medicine and allopathic medicine?
5. Does your nursing program give any consideration to alternative medicine? If yes, how is the topic dealt with?
6. Describe your perceptions of the effectiveness of alternative medicine.
7. What factors do you feel account for the increasing popularity of alternative medicine?

### References

Budrys, G. (2001). *Our unsystematic health care system.* Lanham, MD: Rowman & Littlefield.

Clarke, J. N. (2000). *Health, illness, and medicine in Canada* (3rd ed.). Don Mills, ONT: Oxford University Press.

Cowley, G., Eisenberg, D., Kalb, C., Kaptchuk, T., Komaroff, A., Nonnan, D., et al. (2002, December 2). Health for life: Inside the science of alternative medicine. *Newsweek*, pp. 45–75.

Eisenberg, D. M., Davis, R. B., Ettner, S. L., Appel, S., Wilkey, J., Van Rompay, M., et al. (1998). Trends in alternative medicine use in the United States, 1990–1997: Results of a follow-up national survey. *Journal of the American Medical Association, 280,* 1569–1575.

Eisenberg, D. M., Kessler, R. C., Foster, C., Norlock, F. E., Calkins, D., & Delbanco, L. (1993). Unconventional medicine in the United States: Prevalence, costs, and patterns of use. *New England Journal of Medicine, 328,* 246–252.

Goldstein, M. S. (2000). The growing acceptance of complementary and alternative medicine. In C. E. Bird, P. Conrad, & A. M. Fremont (Eds.), *Handbook of medical sociology* (5th ed., pp. 284–297). Upper Saddle River, NJ: Prentice Hall.

Hayes, K. M., & Alexander, I. M. (2000). Alternative therapies and nurse practitioners: Knowledge, professional experience, and personal use. *Holistic Nurse Practitioner, 14,* 49–58.

King, M., Pettigrew, A., & Reed, F. (1999). Complementary, alternative, integrative: Have nurses kept pace with their clients? *Medsurg Nursing, 8,* 249–256.

Lincoln, Y. S., & Guba, E. G. (1985). *Naturalistic inquiry.* Beverly Hills, CA: Sage.

Matcha, D. A. (2000). *Medical sociology.* Boston: Allyn & Bacon.

McClennon-Leong, J., & Kerr, J. R. (1999). Alternative health care options in Canada. *Canadian Nurse, 95,* 26–30.

Melland, H. I., & Clayburgh, T. L. (2000). Complementary therapies: Introduction into a nursing curriculum. *Nurse Educator, 25,* 247–250.

Northcott, H. C. (2002). Health care restructuring and alternative approaches to health and medicine. In B. S. Bolaria & H. D. Dickinson (Eds.), *Health, illness, and health care in Canada* (3rd ed., pp. 460–474). Scarborough, ONT: Nelson.

Reed, F., Pettigrew, A., & King, M. (2000). Alternative and complementary therapies in nursing curricula. *Journal of Nursing Education, 39,* 133–139.

Ryan, G. W., & Bernard, H. R. (2000). Data management and analysis methods. In N. K. Denzin & Y. S. Lincoln (Eds.), *Handbook of qualitative research* (2nd ed., pp. 769–802). Thousand Oaks, CA: Sage.

Stryker, S. (1980). *Symbolic interactionism.* Menlo Park, CA: Benjamin-Cummings.

Verhoef, M. J., & Sutherland, L. R. (1995). Alternative medicine and general practitioners. *Canadian Family Physician, 41,* 1004–1012.

Watson, J. (1985). *Nursing: The philosophy and science of caring.* Boulder: Colorado Associated University Press.

**Acknowledgments**: We wish to express our appreciation to the nursing students of Red Deer College who participated in this study; to the nursing faculty who supported this project, especially nursing instructor Sandy MacGregor; administrative assistants Ida Murray and Patricia Couture; and Dr. Herbert C. Northcott for commenting on the revised version of this article.

**Address correspondence to**: Ron Joudrey, Red Deer College, Department of Sociology, 100 College Boulevard, Alberta, Canada, T4N 5H5.

# Exercise for Article 30

## Factual Questions

1. The acronym "CAM" stands for what words?

2. What percentage of the respondents were women?

3. Before conducting the study, the researchers obtained permission from whom?

4. Who distributed the questionnaire?

5. How many of the study authors compared and coded the responses?

6. "Member checking" (i.e., discussing the findings with the participants) was used in order to test what?

## Questions for Discussion

7. The researchers had a return rate of 30.86% (see lines 122–123). In your opinion, how does this return rate affect the quality of the study?

8. If you were approached to participate in a replication of this study (as a student nurse), would you have agreed to participate? Why? Why not?

9. In your opinion, is the method of data analysis presented in lines 152–175 described in sufficient detail? Explain.

10. In your opinion, what are the practical implications of the results of this study?

11. Do you agree with the last sentence in the article (see lines 407–410)? Explain.

## *Quality Ratings*

Directions: Indicate your level of agreement with each of the following statements by circling a number from 5 for strongly agree (SA) to 1 for strongly disagree (SD). If you believe an item is not applicable to this research article, leave it blank. Be prepared to explain your ratings. When responding to criteria A and B, keep in mind that brief titles and abstracts are conventional in published research.

A. The title of the article is appropriate.

    SA   5   4   3   2   1   SD

B. The abstract provides an effective overview of the research article.

    SA   5   4   3   2   1   SD

C. The introduction establishes the importance of the study.

    SA   5   4   3   2   1   SD

D. The literature review establishes the context for the study.

    SA   5   4   3   2   1   SD

E. The research purpose, question, or hypothesis is clearly stated.

    SA   5   4   3   2   1   SD

F. The method of sampling is sound.

    SA   5   4   3   2   1   SD

G. Relevant demographics (for example, age, gender, and ethnicity) are described.

    SA   5   4   3   2   1   SD

H. Measurement procedures are adequate.

    SA   5   4   3   2   1   SD

I. All procedures have been described in sufficient detail to permit a replication of the study.

    SA   5   4   3   2   1   SD

J. The participants have been adequately protected from potential harm.

    SA   5   4   3   2   1   SD

K. The results are clearly described.

    SA   5   4   3   2   1   SD

L. The discussion/conclusion is appropriate.

    SA   5   4   3   2   1   SD

M. Despite any flaws, the report is worthy of publication.

    SA   5   4   3   2   1   SD

# Article 31

# The Use of Music to Promote
# Sleep in Older Women

**Julie E. Johnson**, PhD, RN, FAAN[*]

ABSTRACT. Fifty-two women over the age of 70 participated in a study to investigate the use of an individualized music protocol to promote sleep onset and maintenance. They were recruited from the practices of physicians and nurse practitioners and met the inclusion and exclusion criteria of the *International Classification of Sleep Disorders* (1990), and the *Diagnostic and Statistical Manual of Mental Disorders* (1994). Results indicated that the use of music decreased time to sleep onset and the number of nighttime awakenings. Consequently, it increased satisfaction with sleep. Nurses may wish to recommend the use of music at bedtime to older women with insomnia.

From *Journal of Community Health Nursing*, 20, 27–35. Copyright © 2003 by Lawrence Erlbaum Associates, Inc. (www.erlbaum.com). Reprinted with permission.

More than 50% of adults over the age of 65 experience some problem with sleep (National Commission of Sleep Disorders Research, 1993). Women report greater problems than men. Their most common com-
5 plaint is insomnia or difficulty in initiating and maintaining sleep (Tabloski, Cooke, & Thoman, 1998). As insomnia worsens, individuals seek assistance from a health care provider. The typical response of the provider is to prescribe a sedative hypnotic, usually a ben-
10 zodiazepine (Walsh & Engelhardt, 1992). As tolerance to the medication develops, a parallel worsening of insomnia occurs and medication dosage is increased. With prolonged use of the drug, dependence and impaired psychomotor and cognitive functioning result
15 (Ashton, 1994). Consequently, these elders are at much greater risk for car accidents (Ray, Fought, & Decker, 1992), as well as falls, hip fractures, and admission to long-term care (Ray, Griffin, & Downey, 1989).

Music has been shown to decrease anxiety, stress,
20 and tension in a variety of populations (Davis & Thaut, 1989), including surgical patients (Moss, 1988; Kaempf & Amodei, 1989) and individuals admitted to the coronary care unit (Guzzetta, 1989). Other investigators have found that the use of music significantly
25 reduces pain in cancer patients (Zimmerman, Pozehl, Duncan, & Schmitz, 1989) and agitation in elders with Alzheimer's disease (Gerdner, 1999). Because music

can reduce muscular energy, heart and respiratory rates, blood pressure, and alleviate psychological dis-
30 tress (Kartman, 1984), its use at bedtime to promote relaxation and decrease insomnia may be a viable, cost-effective, and nonaddictive alternative to sedative hypnotics for older women. Yet, there is little research available to validate this assumption.

## Purpose
35 The purpose of this study was to describe the impact of an individualized music protocol on the sleep of older women experiencing chronic insomnia. The guiding research questions (RQ) were:

RQ1: Does the use of an individualized music pro-
40 tocol decrease time to sleep onset in older women experiencing chronic insomnia?

RQ2: Do older women using an individualized music protocol report fewer nighttime awakenings following sleep onset?

45 RQ3: Does the use of an individualized music protocol influence older women's satisfaction with their sleep experience?

The term *individualized music protocol* is defined as "music that has been integrated into the person's life
50 and is based on personal preferences" (Gerdner, 1999). Such an approach is preferred because individuals may respond differently to the same piece of music. What is enjoyable and relaxing to one person may be distasteful and stressful to another.

## Method
*Sample Selection*
55 The names of potential participants for this study were obtained from three family practice physicians and five family nurse practitioners. Inclusion and exclusion criteria for chronic insomnia were established using the *International Classification of Sleep Disorders* (American Sleep Disorders Association, 1990)
60 and the *Diagnostic and Statistical Manual of Mental Disorders* (4th ed. [DSM-IV]; American Psychiatric Association, 1994). Inclusion criteria included:

---
[*]*Julie E. Johnson* is a dean and professor at the College of Nursing, Kent State University.

225

65

1. Subjective complaints of difficulty initiating and/ or maintaining sleep at least 3 times a week for more than 6 months.
2. Seventy years of age or over.
3. Alert and oriented.

70

4. Able to read, write, and communicate verbally in English.
5. Living in their own homes.

Exclusion criteria included:

1. Use of sedative-hypnotics within 3 months of the study.

75

2. Significant neurological (e.g., dementia) or medical disorders (e.g., cancer).
3. Presence of other sleep disorders (e.g., sleep apnea, periodic limb movements).
4. Use of medications known to disturb sleep (e.g.,

80

psychotropics, beta-blockers).
5. A score lower than 27 on the Mini-Mental State Exam (MMST; Folstein, Folstein, & McHugh, 1975).
6. A score higher than 16 on the Center for Epide-

85

miologic Studies Depression Scale (CES-D; Radloff, 1977).
7. An affirmative response to two or more questions on CAGE (Ewing, 1984) to determine alcohol abuse.

90

According to the initial screening by the primary health care provider, 113 women met the inclusion criteria for participation in this study. Following a telephone interview conducted by two trained research assistants in which the study was explained and verbal

95

consent was obtained to assess potential participants for the presence of any exclusion criteria, arrangements were made to screen them in their health care practitioner's office. The same two research assistants questioned the potential participants for their use of pre-

100

scribed and over-the-counter medications to promote sleep within the previous three months; reviewed their medical records for the presence of prohibited medical and neurological diagnoses, sleep disorders, and medications known to interfere with sleep; and administered

105

the CES-D (Radloff, 1977) to determine the presence of depression, the MMST (Folstein, Folstein, & McHugh, 1975) to determine cognitive function, and the CAGE (Ewing, 1984) to assess for alcohol abuse. Ultimately, 61 (54%) of the potential participants were

110

eliminated (see Table 1). The remaining 52 (46%) gave informed consent to continue in the study.

### Sample

The final sample consisted of 52 participants. They ranged in age from 71 to 87 years old, with a mean of 80.5 years. Nineteen (37%) were married and 33 (63%)

115

were widowed. Thirty-seven (71%) were high school graduates, 11 (21%) were college graduates, and 4 (8%) had a graduate degree. All lived in their own

homes and were alert, oriented, and able to read, speak, and communicate verbally in English. They com-

120

plained of prolonged initial sleep onset at least three times per week ($M = 49$ min, $R = 27$–69 min) for over 6 months.

Table 1
*Reasons for Exclusion from Participation*

| Exclusion criteria | $n$ | % |
| --- | --- | --- |
| Sedative/hypnotic use | 49 | 80 |
| Use of medication interfering with sleep | 38 | 63 |
| Depression | 37 | 61 |
| Alcohol abuse | 33 | 54 |
| Prohibited medical diagnosis | 31 | 51 |
| Decreased cognitive function | 25 | 41 |
| Neurological disorders | 19 | 31 |
| Presence of other sleep disorders | 12 | 20 |

*Note.* $N = 61$; may exceed 61 due to the presence of more than one exclusionary criterion.

### Procedure

Data were collected for 10 nights before the use of music and for 10 nights during its use with the Stanford

125

Sleepiness Scale (Hoddes, Dement, & Zarcone, 1972) and a sleep log. An investigator-constructed tool was used to interview participants after they had completed 10 nights of music use.

The Stanford Sleepiness Scale is a single item

130

measure of the subjective perception of sleepiness. The individual is asked to rate her level of sleepiness-alertness on a scale ranging from 1 (*feeling active and alert*) to 7 (*lost the struggle to stay awake*). It has been used to determine sleepiness in shift workers (Paley &

135

Tepas, 1994) and in those suffering from sleep deprivation (Dinges, Whitehouse, Orne, & Orne, 1988) and sleep fragmentation (Bonnet, 1986).

A sleep log requires that the individual write down specific information regarding the sleep experience.

140

For this study, participants were instructed to specify the time they got into bed. In the morning they were asked to indicate the estimated length of time it took to fall asleep, number of awakenings during the night, and the time of final awakening.

145

The investigator-constructed interview tool was used only after the use of music for 10 nights. Participants were asked to respond to questions that described their sleep before and after the use of music and to indicate how satisfied they were with use of music to

150

help them sleep. All interviews were audiotaped for later transcription and analysis.

Participants were instructed to select their own music for bedtime use, and selections could vary nightly providing they remained in the same category, such as

155

classical. The majority of participants ($n = 33$, 64%) selected soothing classical music, such as Pachelbel's *Canon in D* or compact discs like *Bach at Bedtime*. The remainder selected sacred music ($n = 10$, 19%) or new age music ($n = 9$, 17%). If a participant did not own or

160

have access to a compact disc or tape player with an automatic shut-off, one was provided for her.

During the pretest phase of the study, participants were instructed to go to bed at night when they felt sleepy, indicate their level of sleepiness using the Stan-
165   ford Sleepiness Scale, and note the time they got into bed in their sleep log. In the morning, they recorded the length of time it took to fall asleep, the number of times they awakened at night, the time they awoke in the morning, and their level of satisfaction with the
170   night's sleep. They followed the same routine for the 10 nights they used music, with the added directive to turn the music on as soon as they got into bed.

## Results

Data from the Stanford Sleepiness Scale and sleep log were analyzed by computing means and standard
175   deviations of pre- and posttest scores. Differences between means were analyzed with $t$ tests for correlated samples. Interview data were analyzed using conceptual coding and Strauss' (1987) constant comparative method. To validate the data, themes that emerged
180   were discussed with the participants. From the identified and validated themes, categories were developed.

Table 2
*Sleep Characteristics Before Music*

| Sleep characteristic | $n$ | % |
| --- | --- | --- |
| Bedtime sleepiness | | |
| "Foggy, losing interest in staying awake" | 30 | 58 |
| "Sleepy, woozy" | 22 | 42 |
| Minutes to sleep onset | | |
| 27–31 | 3 | 5 |
| 32–36 | 7 | 14 |
| 37–41 | 9 | 17 |
| 42–46 | 9 | 17 |
| 47–51 | 10 | 19 |
| 52–56 | 2 | 4 |
| 57–61 | 5 | 10 |
| 62–66 | 2 | 4 |
| 67–69 | 5 | 10 |
| Number of awakenings | | |
| 5 | 13 | 25 |
| 6 | 17 | 33 |
| 7 | 12 | 23 |
| 8 | 10 | 19 |

*Note. N* = 52.

Table 3
*Sleep Characteristics with Music*

| Sleep characteristic | $n$ | % |
| --- | --- | --- |
| Bedtime sleepiness | | |
| "No longer fighting sleep" | 52 | 100 |
| Minutes to sleep onset | | |
| 6–7 | 17 | 37 |
| 8–9 | 11 | 21 |
| 10–11 | 18 | 35 |
| 11–12 | 3 | 6 |
| 12–13 | 3 | 6 |
| Number of awakenings | | |
| 1 | 23 | 44 |
| 2 | 19 | 37 |
| 3 | 10 | 19 |

*Note. N* = 52.

Results showed that there was a significant increase in level of sleepiness at bedtime ($t = 3.72$, $p < .01$) and a significant decrease in time to sleep onset ($t = 3.12$, $p$
185   $< .01$) and number of nighttime awakenings ($t = 2.30$, $p < .05$) from pre- to posttest (Tables 2 and 3). Prior to the use of music, all the participants rated themselves as 5 ("foggy; losing interest in remaining awake; slowed down") or 6 ("sleepy, woozy, fighting sleep;
190   prefer to lie down") on the Stanford Sleepiness Scale. However, they experienced prolonged sleep onsets ranging from 27 to 69 min ($M = 49$ min) and frequent nighttime awakenings ranging from five to eight *(M = 6)*. With the use of music, the participants rated them-
195   selves as 7 ("no longer fighting sleep, sleep onset soon; having dream-like thoughts") on the Stanford Sleepiness Scale. Time to sleep onset ranged from 6 to 13 min ($M = 10$ min) and the number of nighttime awakenings ranged from one to three ($M = 2$). Music be-
200   came more effective with each night it was used, with a peak effect reached on the fifth night and maintained thereafter. There was no significant difference for time of morning awakening from pre- to posttest.

These categories emerged from the interview data:
205   pure frustration, restless and exhausting, a world of difference, no more dread, and very satisfied. All the women expressed a great deal of frustration with their bedtime experience before the introduction of music. These comments were representative of that feeling:

210   > I dreaded going to bed at night. It was the most frustrating time of the day for me. I was sleepy, but just couldn't get to sleep.

> It was just awful! I was SO frustrated. I was SO tired, but I didn't even really want to try to sleep 'cause I
215   > just got more frustrated and my nerves was on edge. I'd just be in that bed worryin' about sleepin'.

In addition to the frustration of being unable to fall asleep, the participants noted that their efforts to do so were exhausting. As this 73-year-old woman said,

220   > I'd just roll 'n roll around trying to fall asleep. I did all the stuff you hear about, you know, counting sheep backwards and forwards, thinking about nice things, stuff like that. None of it worth a tinker's darn and the time would pass and I'd just roll on more. I'd
225   > just wear myself out. I was exhausted after a few hours.

This comment by an 83-year-old was also typical:

> I was so darn tired when I'd go to the bed, I was just sure I could fall asleep. But, oh no! My head hit the
230   > pillow and I'd be rollin' all over the place. I was as restless as a dog without a bone. It was plum sad. I just plain wore myself out trying to get some decent sleep.

Participants noted a remarkable difference in their
235   ability to fall and remain asleep with the use of music. These remarks were representative:

240 I can't believe the difference falling asleep to music made. I wasn't a believer when all this started, but I am now! It relaxes me and I just drift off. It's made a world of difference about how I feel about going to bed!

I don't believe the difference music has made in the way I fall asleep. It's so much better than before. I do think it could be one of those miracles.

245 The use of music also lessened the sense of dread that these women felt at bedtime. As this 71-year-old stated,

I used to hate going to bed. It was a dreadful thing to do. But now that I've tried music to help me sleep 250 better, it's not so bad to go to bed. I don't dread it now.

This 80-year-old woman agreed,

It was awful, I just dreaded getting into bed. Not now. This has really made a big difference! I actually 255 fall asleep! And if I wake up during the night, I just turn it on and go back to sleep.

Not surprisingly, the ability to fall asleep and return to sleep led to satisfaction with the use of music and the total sleep experience. These comments were repre-260 sentative:

I'm just flat out amazed at the way music helps me relax and fall asleep. It's a wonderful thing. I wish I'd known about it years ago. My sleep is just plain better with it.

265 The music is just great. I'm so satisfied with the way I fall asleep now, so when all's said and done, I'm also very satisfied with the music.

## Discussion and Implications

Due to the size of the sample, the findings of this study should be interpreted with caution. However, 270 they support those of previous research (Tabloski, Cooke, & Thoman, 1998) indicating that older women experience difficulty in initiating and maintaining sleep. It was not particularly surprising that the women in this study experienced prolonged sleep onset and 275 frequent awakenings in the pretest phase of the investigation. Consequently, they were frustrated with their sleep, dreaded going to bed, and were restless sleepers. Nurses may wish to place greater emphasis on the assessment of their older, female clients' sleep patterns. 280 If problems are identified early, appropriate treatment can be provided so that such frustration and dread are minimized or avoided altogether.

The finding that the use of an individualized music protocol improved insomnia in this study's participants 285 is encouraging. As others (Davis & Thaut, 1989; Guzzeta, 1989) have noted, music decreases stress, tension, and anxiety. Insomnia may have multiple causes including age, stress, tension, and anxiety. Unfortunately, when individuals have continued difficulty 290 falling and remaining asleep, anxiety and tension may be exacerbated to the point that frustration and dread make relaxation impossible. This study shows that music is effective in decreasing the frustration and dread associated with insomnia, while increasing the ability 295 to relax. Nurses can use these findings to suggest that older women with insomnia use music to help them fall asleep. They should instruct their clients to select a piece of music that is soothing to them and/or evokes pleasant memories and feelings, get into bed, turn the 300 music on and the lights out, and close their eyes. It is important to encourage them to use music for at least five nights before assuming it does not work. They may also alter their nightly music selection if they wish.

305 Participants also noted that the use of music helped them return to sleep following nighttime awakenings. Nurses can use this information to suggest that music may promote relaxation and return to sleep in their older clients who have difficulty maintaining sleep due 310 to frequent awakenings.

A serendipitous finding of concern was the number of older women who were disqualified from participating in this study due to the habitual use of sedative-hypnotics and/or alcohol. In addition, a significant 315 number of potential participants were clinically depressed. These findings deserve further investigation, not only for their influence on sleep, but for the impact they may have on the functional and cognitive status of older women living in their own homes.

## References

American Psychiatric Association. (1994). *Diagnostic and statistical manual of mental disorders* (4th ed.). Washington, DC: Author.

American Sleep Disorders Association. (1990). *International classification of sleep disorders (ICSD): Diagnostic and coding manual*. Rochester, MN: Author.

Ashton, H. (1994). Guidelines for the rational use of benzodiazepines: When and what to use. *Drugs, 48*, 25–40.

Bonnet, M. H. (1986). Performance and sleepiness following moderate sleep disruption and slow wave sleep deprivation. *Physiological Behavior, 37*, 915–918.

Davis, W. B., & Thaut, M. H. (1989). The influence of preferred relaxing music on measures of state anxiety, relaxation, and physiological responses. *Journal of Music Therapy, 26*, 168–187.

Dinges, D. F., Whitehouse, W. G., Orne, E. C., & Orne, M. T. (1988). The benefits of a nap during prolonged work and wakefulness. *Work & Stress, 2*, 139–153.

Ewing, J. A. (1984). Detecting alcoholism: The CAGE questionnaire. *Journal of the American Medical Association, 252*, 1905–1907.

Folstein, M. F., Folstein, S. E., & McHugh, M. R. (1975). "Mini-Mental State." A practical method for grading the cognitive state of patients for the clinician. *Journal of Psychiatric Research, 12*, 189–198.

Gerdner, L. A. (1999). Individualized music intervention protocol. *Journal of Gerontological Nursing, 25*, 10–16.

Guzzetta, C. (1989). Effects of relaxation and music therapy on patients in a coronary care unit with presumptive acute myocardial infarction. *Heart & Lung, 18*, 609–616.

Hoddes, E., Dement, W., & Zarcone, V. (1972). The history and use of the Stanford Sleepiness Scale. *Psychophysiology, 9*, 150–152.

Kaempf, G., & Amodei, M. E. (1989). The effect of music on anxiety. *AORN Journal, 50*, 112–118.

Kartman, L. L. (1984). Music hath charms. *Journal of Gerontological Nursing, 10*, 20–24.

Moss, V. A. (1988). Music and the surgical patient. *AORN Journal, 48*, 64–69.

National Commission of Sleep Disorders Research (1993). *Wake up America: A national sleep alert: Vol. 1. executive summary and executive report*.

Paley, M., & Tepas, D. I. (1994). Fatigue and the shiftworker: Firefighters working on a rotating shift schedule. *Human Factors, 36*, 269–284.

Radloff, L. S. (1977). The CES-D Scale: A self-report depression scale for research in the general population. *Journal of Applied Psychological Measurement, 1*, 385–401.

Ray, W. A., Fought, R. L., & Decker, M. D. (1992). Psychoactive drugs and the risk of injurious motor vehicle crashes in the elderly drivers. *American Journal of Epidemiology, 136*, 873–883.

Ray, W. A., Griffin, M. R., & Downey, W. (1989). Benzodiazepines of long and short elimination half-life and the risk of hip fracture. *Journal of the American Medical Association, 262*, 3303–3307.

Strauss, A. (1987). *Qualitative analysis for social scientists.* New York: Cambridge University Press.

Tabloski, P. A., Cooke, K. M., & Thoman, E. B. (1998). A procedure for withdrawal of sleep medication in elderly women who have been long-term users. *Journal of Gerontological Nursing, 24*, 20–28.

Walsh, J. K., & Engelhardt, C. L. (1992). Trends in the pharmacologic treatment of insomnia. *Journal of Clinical Psychiatry, 53*(Suppl.12), 10–18.

Zimmerman, L., Pozehl, B., Duncan, K., & Schmitz, R. (1989). Effects of music in patients who had chronic cancer pain. *Western Journal of Nursing Research, 11*, 298–309.

**Address correspondence to:** Julie E. Johnson, dean and professor, College of Nursing, Kent State University, P.O. Box 5190, Kent, OH 44242.

# Exercise for Article 31

## Factual Questions

1. How is the term *individualized music protocol* defined?

2. The names of potential participants for this study were obtained from how many health care professionals?

3. What was the mean age of the participants?

4. Differences between means were analyzed with what significance test?

5. Was there a significant increase in level of sleepiness at bedtime from pre- to posttest? If yes, at what probability level?

6. What was the "serendipitous finding of concern" reported by the researcher?

## Questions for Discussion

7. The exclusion criteria are listed in lines 72–89 and Table 1. If you had conducted this study, would you have excluded individuals with these characteristics? Explain.

8. The researcher points out that the Stanford Sleepiness Scale has been used in three previously published studies. In your opinion, is it important to know that it has been used in other studies? Explain. (See lines 129–137.)

9. The researcher used three outcome measures (the Stanford Sleepiness Scale, a sleep log, and an investigator-constructed interview tool). Is the use of three measures instead of only one a special strength of this study? Explain. (See lines 123–128.)

10. There was no control group in this study. In your opinion, would it be desirable to use a control group in future studies on this topic? Why? Why not?

11. In your opinion, are the quantitative *or* qualitative results more important? Are they equally important? Explain.

12. Do you agree that these findings deserve further investigation? Explain. (See lines 316–319.)

## Quality Ratings

Directions: Indicate your level of agreement with each of the following statements by circling a number from 5 for strongly agree (SA) to 1 for strongly disagree (SD). If you believe an item is not applicable to this research article, leave it blank. Be prepared to explain your ratings. When responding to criteria A and B, keep in mind that brief titles and abstracts are conventional in published research.

A. The title of the article is appropriate.

   SA   5   4   3   2   1   SD

B. The abstract provides an effective overview of the research article.

   SA   5   4   3   2   1   SD

C. The introduction establishes the importance of the study.

   SA   5   4   3   2   1   SD

D. The literature review establishes the context for the study.

   SA   5   4   3   2   1   SD

E. The research purpose, question, or hypothesis is clearly stated.

   SA   5   4   3   2   1   SD

F. The method of sampling is sound.

   SA   5   4   3   2   1   SD

G. Relevant demographics (for example, age, gender, and ethnicity) are described.

   SA   5   4   3   2   1   SD

H. Measurement procedures are adequate.

   SA   5   4   3   2   1   SD

I.  All procedures have been described in sufficient detail to permit a replication of the study.

SA   5   4   3   2   1   SD

J.  The participants have been adequately protected from potential harm.

SA   5   4   3   2   1   SD

K.  The results are clearly described.

SA   5   4   3   2   1   SD

L.  The discussion/conclusion is appropriate.

SA   5   4   3   2   1   SD

M.  Despite any flaws, the report is worthy of publication.

SA   5   4   3   2   1   SD

# Article 32

# Factors Which Influence Latino Community Members to Self-Prescribe Antibiotics

**Elaine L. Larson**, RN, PhD, CIC, FAAN, **Joann Dilone,**
**Magaly Garcia**, MD, **Janice Smolowitz**, RN, EdD, DrNP [*]

## ABSTRACT

*Background*: Although there is consistent evidence of a link between antibiotic use and increasing antimicrobial resistance in the community, inappropriate use of antimicrobials continues to be a global problem.

*Objective*: To describe knowledge, attitudes, and practices of Latino community members in upper Manhattan regarding use of antibiotics.

*Methods*: Written questionnaires and eight focus groups comprised of Hispanic community members (three groups), bodega employees, and healthcare providers (one group) in a Latino neighborhood in New York City.

*Results*: There were major knowledge deficits regarding use of antibiotics. Informants reported taking antibiotics for pain or other conditions as well as for symptoms of infection. Antibiotics were frequently obtained from bodegas without prescription, but generally only for adults, not for children.

*Discussion*: Interventions to improve antibiotic use that are focused on the formal healthcare system (e.g., clinicians, pharmacists, persons with health insurance) are unlikely to be effective with recently immigrated Latino community members. Successful interventions for this population should include targeted messages to bodega employees, community organizations, and children and their parents.

From *Nursing Research, 55*, 94–102. Copyright © 2006 by Lippincott Williams & Wilkins. Reprinted with permission.

There is consistent evidence of a link between antibiotic use and increasing antimicrobial resistance in the community (Diekema, Brueggemann, & Doern, 2000; Levy, 2002; Melander, Ekdahl, Jonsson, & Molstad, 2000). Nevertheless, inappropriate use of antimicrobials continues to be a global problem. Reasons for this include public expectations and demand for medication, lack of understanding about the ineffectiveness of antibiotics against viral illness, and the ease of access to antibiotics without prescription in many parts of the world (Mainous, Hueston, & Clark, 1996; McKee, Mills, & Mainous, 1999; Metlay, Shea, Crossette, & Asch, 2002).

Antibiotic misuse and resistance are more common in countries such as those in Latin America in which antibiotics are available over the counter and in which cultural patterns regarding medication use and beliefs about medication effectiveness differ (Corbett et al., 2005; Garfield, Broe, & Albano, 1995). If successful strategies to reduce misuse of antibiotics (and other medications) in the Latino population are to be developed, it is essential to understand the cultural norms regarding antibiotic use that characterize this group. The aim of this study was to describe the knowledge, attitudes, beliefs, and practices of Latino community members in northern Manhattan regarding use of antibiotics. The ultimate goal is to use this information to develop a culturally relevant and effective intervention to improve the judicious use of antibiotics among Latino community members.

## Background

Antibiotic use patterns among Latinos are important because Latinos represent the fastest growing minority population in the United States (United States Census Bureau, 2001), and they have generally immigrated from countries in which antibiotics are available without prescription. In a recent survey, 39% of 631 Latino households ($n$ = 2,840 individuals) in northern Manhattan reported that one or more persons had taken antibiotics in the previous 30 days, a rate even higher than that reported in a prevalence survey almost a decade ago in Mexico (Calva & Bojalil, 1996; Larson, Lin, & Gomez-Duarte, 2003). In a study of shigellosis in Oregon, Latinos had the highest prevalence of antimicrobial resistant strains (Replogle, Fleming, & Cieslak, 2000).

Multiple private and public agencies, in particular the Centers for Disease Control and Prevention (CDC) (Weissman & Besser, 2004), have undertaken public and provider campaigns and other educational and policy interventions to reduce inappropriate use of antibiotics. While many interventions have reported positive

[*]*Elaine L. Larson* is a professor; *Joann Dilone* is a research assistant, School of Nursing; *Magaly Garcia*, Hispanic Resource Center; and *Janice Smolowitz* is associate professor of clinical nursing, School of Nursing, Columbia University, New York, NY.

results (Gonzales, Steiner, Lum, & Barrett, 1999; Hennessy et al., 2002; Perz et al., 2002; Trepka, Belongia, Chyou, Davis, & Schwartz, 2001), they have been focused primarily on prescribing patterns in the "majority" population. Such interventions, however, have not been evaluated among recent immigrants or subgroups of the population.

Some previous research about factors which enable, predispose, or reinforce antibiotic use patterns among Latino members of the community has been conducted. Corbett et al. (2005) have reported that knowledge deficits are more common among Spanish-speaking Latinos as compared with non-Latino White people and English-language Latino people. In several studies, less knowledge has been associated with a greater demand for antibiotics (Finkelstein et al., 2003; Kuzujanakis, Kleinman, Rifas-Shiman, & Finkelstein, 2003). Braun and Fowles (2000) reported that parents who believed that antibiotics were helpful for treating colds were significantly more likely to request antibiotics from a provider. In a large survey of 543 parents from 38 managed care pediatric practices in Los Angeles, Asian and Latino parents were 17% more likely to state that antibiotics were needed than non-Latino White parents (Mangione-Smith et al., 2004). Also several studies have confirmed that many Latinos obtain antibiotics from Latin America where they are considerably cheaper and available without prescription from pharmacies and bodegas (Macias & Morales, 2001; Weinberg et al., 2003). Even in the United States, however, patients have often expressed the opinion that they can decide for themselves whether an antibiotic is needed without consulting a healthcare provider (Belongia, Naimi, Gale, & Besser, 2002).

Blanchard and Lurie (2004) have reported that significantly more Latino people when compared with non-Latino White people felt disrespected in the healthcare setting. Further, those persons who thought that they would receive better care if they were a different ethnicity or race were significantly less likely to seek care or follow the clinician's advice. Patients have indicated that even if they did not get an antibiotic prescription, they would be satisfied if they received an explanation, a contingency plan, or both (Barden, Dowell, Schwartz, & Lackey, 1998; Mangione-Smith et al., 2001). In one study, however, pamphlets regarding antibiotic use which were passively placed in waiting rooms of pediatric practices were not read (Wheeler et al., 2001).

In addition to increased direct provider-patient interactions (Mangione-Smith, Stivers, Elliott, McDonald, & Heritage, 2003), computer-based information resources have been shown to be a potentially valuable vehicle for providing high quality, accurate health information, and could be one mechanism to reinforce recommendations provided during short face-to-face visits (D'Alessandro, Kreiter, Kinzer, & Peterson, 2004). Informational messages can be tailored as appropriate to the recipient; Krueter, Farrell, Olevitch, and Brennan (2000) described a nine-step tailoring process, and Witte, Meyer, and Martell (2001) have developed a framework for developing culturally specific messages. Such information resources might be helpful within the Latino community if they have access to and use computers, but the extent to which recent immigrants from Latin America have access to computers has not been previously described.

## Methods

This was an exploratory, descriptive study using focus group interviews and questionnaires.

### Sample and Setting

A purposive sample of three different groups participated in this study. One group ($n = 6$) was composed of community members who were not linked into the formal healthcare system (i.e., did not have a designated primary care provider or health insurance), and a second group ($n = 19$) who had some type of health insurance. Participants in these groups were as follows: (a) women of Latino origin, born either in the United States or elsewhere, but with Spanish as their first language; (b) members of households that included at least one preschool child; and (c) residents of northern Manhattan. The rationale for including households with preschool children was that antibiotic use and resistance are more likely to occur when there are children in the household (Chiou et al., 1998; Mangione-Smith, McGlynn, Elliott, Krogstad, & Brook, 1999; McCaig, Besser, & Hughes, 2002).

The third group ($n = 5$) included two local small-business employees of independent stores which sell food and toiletry items (bodegas) and three healthcare professionals with extensive experience providing services for Latino adults from the same neighborhood. This group was convened to determine whether their perspective on community use of antibiotics differed from the community members themselves.

Community participants were recruited by posting flyers in local stores, churches, day care centers, and community organizations. Bodega employees and healthcare professionals were recruited by direct contact in their place of work.

### Procedures

Approval of the university institutional review board was obtained and participants signed a written Spanish-language consent form. This study was guided by the educational and environmental approach to health promotion planning espoused by Green and Kreuter (1991), the precede-proceed model, in which an educational and organizational diagnosis is the first step in planning health promotion activities. This stage of the diagnosis requires identification of factors which predispose, enable, and reinforce healthy behaviors (Figure 1), in this case antibiotic practices, as a prerequisite for planning relevant interventions to improve behavior. Focus group discussions were designed to elicit information about these three factors.

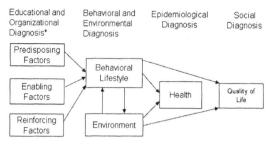

*This project was undertaken to conduct the Educational and Organizational Diagnosis

*Figure 1.* The Green precede-proceed model (Green & Kreuter, 1991) used as conceptual underpinnings.

165    The community member focus groups were conducted in Spanish in a lounge at the study institution by a trained Latina facilitator at times convenient for participants. The facilitator (Garcia) was a native Spanish-speaking psychiatrist born in Latin America with for-
170    mal training in the conduct of focus groups. The three community member focus groups each met on two occasions—once for about 2 hr and a second time 2–3 weeks later for about 1 hr to review a summary of their previous discussion. The bodega employees and
175    healthcare professionals met in two separate groups, one conducted in Spanish and the other in English, and these two groups met only one time each. Because selling antibiotics over the counter is illegal, bodega employees were asked not to discuss whether or not they
180    sold them, but rather to respond by discussing what they thought their customers expected. These participants individually validated the summary of the focus group discussion 2–3 weeks later.

The focus groups were conducted according to the
185    methodology described by Morgan and Krueger (1998). Participants and investigators introduced themselves and the facilitator reviewed the consent form and purpose of the study. The facilitator also described the precede-proceed model and informed the group that
190    they would be discussing their use of antibiotics with regard to predisposing, enabling, and reinforcing factors. Then a short Spanish-language questionnaire (see Instruments section) was administered to introduce the topic and obtain baseline data on participants' knowl-
195    edge, attitudes, and practices regarding antibiotic use. The questionnaires were completed individually by participants without discussion with each other.

After the questionnaires were collected, the discussions were initiated by the facilitator, who began with
200    open-ended general statements such as "Tell us about when your family uses antibiotics" and "The last time you used an antibiotic, describe what your symptoms were." Discussions were based on a written guide that included the three concepts of predisposing, enabling,
205    and reinforcing factors associated with antibiotic use.

Scenarios were also presented to elicit specific practices. For example, "It is 4 am and your 2 year old is crying in pain and hitting her ear. You know that she has another ear infection. Let's discuss what actions
210    you would take and why." The group also discussed current sources of their health information, their computer literacy, and how health communications could be targeted to them in the most credible ways. At the end of the discussion about each of the three concepts
215    of the model, the facilitator provided a general summary and asked the group for validation and clarification.

A second 1-hr debriefing session was held after responses from the initial focus groups were summarized
220    and collated. The facilitator provided a summary of the discussion so that group members could add comments and clarifications. The themes and issues that emerged were reviewed with participants to assess credibility (i.e., that the input of the participants had been accu-
225    rately captured) and to provide an opportunity for participants to clarify, amplify, and correct the summaries. In addition, any opinions that were not expressed in the focus groups but that were raised in the written questionnaires were presented in this second session. Dur-
230    ing each session, a Spanish-speaking research assistant took extensive notes and all sessions were audiotaped.

*Instruments*

A short questionnaire provided quantitative data for comparative analysis with the qualitative data gener-
235    ated by the focus groups. The questionnaire was adapted from that used in a community intervention study to assess knowledge and awareness of antibiotic resistance and appropriate antibiotic use (Trepka et al., 2001). It was used to gather factual information about antibiotic use in each household within the previous 3
240    months, knowledge and attitudes (i.e., predisposing factors) about appropriate use and types of antibiotics (Tables 1 and 2), and information regarding where respondents obtained antibiotics and health information (i.e., enabling and reinforcing factors). The question-
245    naire and consent forms were translated into Spanish by a professional translator in the Hispanic Research and Recruitment Center, Columbia University Medical Center, and then back-translated by the focus group facilitator to assure accuracy of the meaning of all
250    words and phrases. Lay language and, when appropriate, "street" names for medications were used. The instrument was then pilot tested with five Spanish-speaking members of the community for readability, time required to complete, and clarity. As noted above,
255    the focus group discussions were used to confirm, correct, or expand on information reported in the written questionnaire.

*Data Analysis*

Responses from the questionnaire were summarized using SPSS (Chicago, IL). Focus group data were ex-
260    amined using tape-based analysis as described by Mor-

gan and Kreuger (1998). About 1 week after each focus group, three of the investigators listened to the audiotape, took extensive notes, and independently identified common themes and factors related to attitudes, beliefs,
265 and practices in the context of precede-proceed model. Each investigator categorized these factors as predisposing, reinforcing, or enabling for appropriate antibiotic use. Then the investigators compared their notes and the field notes for congruence, and agreement was
270 reached on emerging themes by consensus. Data from the taped focus group discussions were also examined to assure that all common themes had been fully identified and explored (i.e., that saturation had been reached). The focus group facilitator then indepen-
275 dently reviewed the audiotapes, field notes, and investigator analysis to validate the developing themes. Audiotapes were reviewed at least three times and themes were confirmed by consensus of the four investigators with feedback from participants to affirm trustworthi-
280 ness of the finding.

### Results

*Participants*

Twenty-five Latina women participated in the two community focus groups. Their mean age was 35.7 years (22–47 years); the majority of participants (92%)
were born in the Dominican Republic, one in El Salva-
285 dor, and two in New York City. The average family size was 4.7 members (3–8 members). All but one participant (96%) had high school or less education. The bodega employees and one of the healthcare professionals were born in the Dominican Republic; the other
290 healthcare professionals were born in the United States. All bodega employees had a high school education.

*Questionnaire*

Twelve informants (44.4%) reported that they had taken an antibiotic within the past 3 months, and 13 (48.1%) reported that at least one other person in their
295 household had taken an antibiotic. Antibiotics named included ampicillin, amoxicillin, erythromycin, amoxicillin/clavulanate potassium (Augmentin), and penicillin and were taken for a mean of 12 doses (1–28). While most reported taking an antibiotic for symptoms
300 of infection (sore throat, ear infection, and fever), one-third (5/15) of reasons given for taking antibiotics were for other symptoms, including nausea, pain, itching, and allergies.

*Predisposing factors: knowledge and attitudes.*
305 There were a number of factual misconceptions among respondents (Table 1). For example, 56% thought that antibiotics would help cure a cold and would kill both viruses and bacteria, and only 36% reported that antibiotics could be harmful to one's health. The propor-
310 tion of those able to correctly identify antibiotics from a list of commonly used drugs ranged 12–92%. While the majority (56%) reported that they stopped antibiotics because the prescribed duration was complete, 48%

315 also reported stopping antibiotics when they felt better (Table 2).

Table 1
*Predisposing Factors (Knowledge) Regarding Antibiotic Use (n = 25 community focus group respondents)*

| Item | Agree n (%) | |
|---|---|---|
| Antibiotics help cure a cold | 14 | (56) |
| Treating a cold with antibiotics will help prevent an ear infection | 18 | (72) |
| Antibiotics should be stopped as soon as the person feels better | 6 | (24) |
| Antibiotics are usually needed if there is yellow drainage in the nose | 4 | (16) |
| Some germs are becoming harder to treat with antibiotics | 11 | (44) |
| If there is excessive use of antibiotics, they will not be as effective in treating infections | 14 | (56) |
| Bacteria can become resistant to antibiotics if they are taken in inadequate doses | 15 | (60) |
| Antibiotics work to kill viruses and bacteria | 14 | (56) |
| If antibiotics are taken for fewer or more than the days indicated, bacteria can become resistant | 12 | (48) |
| Antibiotics can be harmful to one's health | 9 | (36) |

| Is this an antibiotic? | Correct response n (%) | | Do not know n (%) | |
|---|---|---|---|---|
| Amoxicillin | 23 | (92) | 1 | (4) |
| Aspirin | 21 | (84) | 3 | (12) |
| Chloramphenicol | 3 | (12) | 13 | (52) |
| Cough medicine | 20 | (80) | 4 | (16) |
| Acetaminophen (e.g., Tylenol) | 18 | (72) | 4 | (16) |
| Erythromycin | 11 | (44) | 11 | (44) |
| Albuterol | 13 | (52) | 8 | (32) |
| Epinephrine | 8 | (32) | 14 | (56) |
| Ampicillin | 22 | (88) | 1 | (4) |
| Theophylline | 5 | (20) | 13 | (52) |
| Tetracycline | 18 | (72) | 4 | (16) |
| Sulfa (Bactrim) | 5 | (20) | 14 | (56) |
| Penicillin | 20 | (80) | 3 | (12) |

*Enabling factors: economic and access issues.* Most community informants (84%) had either no insurance or received Medicaid. While most (72%) respondents reported getting antibiotics from a pharmacy
320 with a prescription, they also reported buying them without prescription from pharmacies (24%), bodegas (32%), or from outside the United States (20%), or obtaining them from friends or leftover from previous uses.

325 *Reinforcing factors.* When asked to name their most reliable source of information about medicines, respondents named the physician, books, and family members in rank order. Most (68%, 17/25) community participants had access to a computer, but 20% (5/25)
330 reported never using a computer (Table 3).

*Focus Group Findings for Adults*

*Predisposing factors.* Across focus groups, participants described how knowledge toward symptom treatment and cultural attitudes about antibiotics (predisposing factors) provided the basis for self-prescribed

Table 2
*Predisposing Factors (Attitudes) Regarding Antibiotic Use (n = 25 community focus group respondents)*

| How often do you think antibiotics should be used for the following conditions? | Always n (%) | Sometimes n (%) | Never n (%) | Do not know n (%) |
|---|---|---|---|---|
| Ear infection | 15 (40) | 15 (60) | 0 | 0 |
| Bronchitis | 12 (48) | 5 (20) | 4 (16) | 4 (16) |
| Cold | 0 | 17 (68) | 1 (4) | 7 (28) |
| Dry cough without fever | 0 | 3 (12) | 10 (40) | 11 (44) |
| Cold with cough and body aches | 1 (4) | 7 (28) | 9 (36) | 6 (24) |
| Sinusitis | 5 (20) | 6 (24) | 5 (20) | 8 (32) |
| Throat inflammation (tonsillitis) | 16 (64) | 6 (24) | 1 (4) | 1 (4) |
| Sore throat | 6 (24) | 14 (56) | 4 (16) | 0 |
| Diarrhea | 4 (16) | 5 (20) | 10 (40) | 5 (20) |
| Nasal discharge or secretion | 0 | 7 (28) | 9 (36) | 8 (32) |
| Vomiting | 0 | 5 (20) | 11 (44) | 8 (32) |
| Conjunctivitis | 3 (12) | 9 (36) | 8 (32) | 5 (20) |
| Boils | 2 (8) | 10 (40) | 6 (24) | 7 (28) |
| Pain or burning sensation when urinating | 5 (20) | 15 (60) | 2 (8) | 2 (8) |
| Wounds | 2 (8) | 13 (52) | 4 (16) | 4 (16) |
| Tightness in chest (asthma) | 2 (8) | 8 (32) | 8 (32) | 6 (24) |

| Indicate reasons you have decided to stop taking an antibiotic | |
|---|---|
| I felt better | 12 (48) |
| I had side effects | 3 (12) |
| My prescription expired | 6 (24) |
| It was too problematic to take | 3 (12) |
| Cost too much | 3 (12) |
| Did not have a prescription | 3 (12) |
| The indicated time of treatment had expired | 14 (56) |

medication: "We use it there (in our country) until symptoms go away. That is the tradition." "It is a sign of friendship when you go to the pharmacist and he provides you with medicine."

Easy access to antibiotics through bodegas and other independent stores in northern Manhattan continued a tradition of care from the country of origin as did the practice of treating family and friends. Family members shared antibiotic prescriptions when they developed similar symptoms. Family members living in the country of origin routinely sent antibiotics to relatives and friends in northern Manhattan. Focus group discussions among the community members identified novel uses of antibiotics based on traditional home remedies. "In the Dominican Republic as well as here, we prepare a deodorant called Deporte. We add penicillin and oil and use it for burns, bruises or cuts on the skin."

*Enabling factors.* Enabling factors identified during the focus group discussions included socioeconomic and access issues. Lack of insurance, monetary constraints, and legal status had financial implications that affected treatment choice. "Some people don't have citizenship or medical insurance to go to the doctor." "Antibiotics should be more accessible to the public, the ones that are not strong. There are a lot of people who don't have any medical insurance." "My dad would tell me in my country (I suffered from my throat) that it's too much money to take me to the doc-

tor every time. It's better to keep antibiotics in the fridge, in case."

Based on contextual factors and the perception that antibiotics were necessary to treat symptoms, participants reported purchasing one or two pills of penicillin or other antibiotic at local independent pharmacies and bodegas or obtaining antibiotics from family members. "Well, I will be the first to admit it, when any person I know comes to me and tells me that they have a toothache I tell them to buy two penicillin and that will make them feel better." "If you come in with any pain they will give it to you. If you have a cold they will sell it to you. Here they become a doctor." "Antibiotics in my country you can get anywhere. They sell them to you without any prescription. When my sister-in-law came back not too long ago, she brought me back a bag full of antibiotics for different things: for the cold, in a cream for any type of burns." "It is easier and one does not have time to go to the doctor." "It's much easier with the kids, work, and business of life. We don't have time to spend the night in the hospital."

Community focus group members expressed positive, negative, and ambivalent feelings regarding sale of antibiotics in bodegas. Despite the fact that few reported in the written questionnaire that they thought antibiotics should be sold in bodegas, all informants verbally reported that they did buy them there. Because of their perception that bodegas would continue to sell antibiotics without prescription, participants recommended that bodega staff members receive education about what to sell for various symptoms.

Table 3
*Enabling and Reinforcing Factors in Obtaining Antibiotics and Health Information (Written Responses Only)*

| Item | Affirmative Response | |
| --- | --- | --- |
| | *n* | (%) |
| Where do you regularly get antibiotics? | | |
|     Pharmacy with a prescription | 18 | (72) |
|     Bodega | 8 | (32) |
|     Pharmacy without a prescription | 6 | (24) |
|     A friend | 6 | (24) |
|     Outside the United States | 5 | (20) |
|     Left over from previous prescription | 3 | (12) |
| Do you generally store antibiotics at home for when they are needed? | 6 | (24) |
| Do you think antibiotics should be sold without a prescription? | 9 | (36) |
| Is it useful for bodegas to sell antibiotics? | 6 | (16) |
| | | |
| When you want information on medicines, what is the most reliable source of information for you? | | |
|     Doctor | 17 | (68) |
|     Books | 11 | (44) |
|     Family or friends | 9 | (36) |
|     Internet | 2 | (8) |
| Do you have access to a computer? | 17 | (68) |
| How often do you use the Internet? | | |
|     Never | 5 | (20) |
|     1–2 times/week | 7 | (28) |
|     Almost daily | 13 | (52) |

*Reinforcing factors.* When symptom relief was obtained, the practice of self-prescribing was reinforced and repeated with each episode of illness: "We take the medication 2–3 times. When we feel better we stop taking it."

Participants also described experience with two types of problems associated with antibiotic use. In the first scenario, the antibiotic had secondary effects. Temporary effects included diarrhea, vomiting, and allergic reactions; permanent effects included anemia, ulcers, and liver problems. "Frequent use of antibiotics can cause anemia. Yes, my friend took antibiotics frequently and she became anemic. The doctor had to prescribe some vitamins to balance it out for her." "The antibiotics eat red blood cells." "Antibiotics can cause paleness of the skin." "Antibiotics cure one thing and destroy another."

In the second scenario, individuals perceived that resistance to the antibiotic had developed. Participants defined resistance: "It is when antibiotics have no effect on the body because of frequent use, they have to use a different antibiotic or a stronger one." "He became resistant to an antibiotic; that is why they gave him a stronger antibiotic." "The prescribed medication was not the sufficient dosage."

When symptoms were not relieved or when side effects occurred, participants reported seeking care from physicians. Despite the fact that participants reported that physicians provided a full course of treatment with an antibiotic as well as educational material, the experience in the mainstream healthcare system did not change their self-prescribing practices; that is, this reinforcing factor was not sufficient to change behavior. Cultural and contextual factors weighed heavily in the decision process and self-prescription continued with the next episode of illness.

The predisposing, enabling, and reinforcing factors that justified self-prescription by adults are summarized in Figure 2A.

### Focus Group Findings for Children

Universally, participants reported that they did not self-prescribe antibiotics for their children. Initially, parents might provide common symptomatic treatments. If symptoms did not resolve, children were taken immediately to the clinician. Parents expressed concern about harming their children by purchasing over-the-counter antibiotics without consulting a physician. They were concerned also that city agencies would intervene with regard to their children's welfare. The predisposing, enabling, and reinforcing factors described in the treatment of children are summarized in Figure 2B.

### Focus Group Findings from the Healthcare Community

Responses from bodega employees showed the same level of knowledge as the community members and reflected similar attitudes. Bodega employees did not voice opposition to over-the-counter sale of antibiotics but were reluctant to discuss specifics. Responses from other healthcare professionals providing services to the Latino community confirmed information obtained from the community members. Unlike bodega employees, however, healthcare professionals voiced strong opposition to the sale of antibiotics in bodegas. They also voiced concern about antibiotic resistance in the community. Discussion focused on the difficulty of enforcing the current law because of the large number of bodegas and the community's cultural expectations.

### Discussion

Based on results of the questionnaire and focus group discussions, the implications of the predisposing, enabling, and reinforcing factors associated with antibiotic self-prescribing are examined below.

### Predisposing Factors

Knowledge deficits about antibiotics were prevalent and of concern in this population—for example, many reported that antibiotics can be used to treat viral infections and even headaches. Of particular concern was the fact that one-third of reported reasons for taking antibiotics were for symptoms such as pain, allergy, or asthma. As has been reported by others (Belongia et al., 2002), many of our participants expressed the opinion that they could decide for themselves whether an antibiotic was needed. Clearly, effective interventions

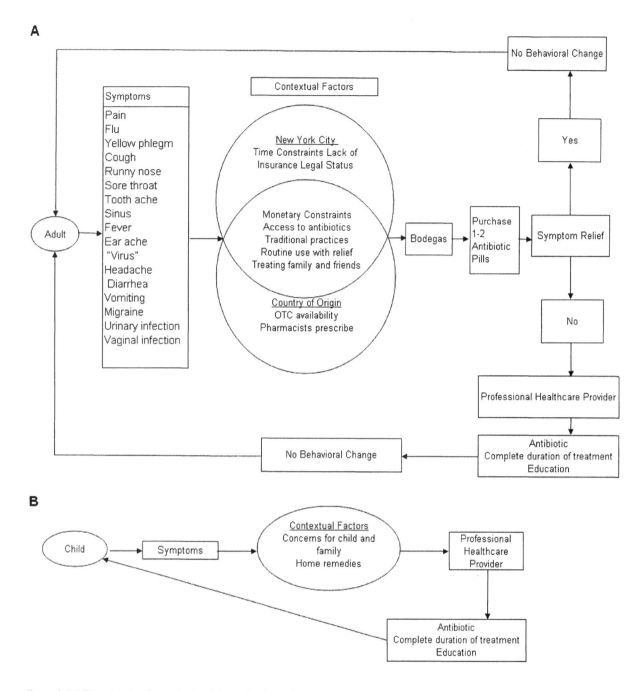

*Figure 2.* (A) Educational and organizational diagnosis of precede-proceed model: Latino community members' description of predisposing, enabling, and reinforcing factors associated with antibiotic use for adults. (B) Educational and organizational diagnosis of precede-proceed model. Latino community members' description of predisposing, enabling, and reinforcing factors associated with antibiotic use for children.

475  for this population would need to include Spanish-language educational materials, such as those available through CDC's Get Smart program (National Center for Infectious Diseases, 2005). While such materials may be necessary, however, they are certainly not sufficient unless provided in ways meaningful and rele-
480  vant to this group (Wheeler et al., 2001).

*Enabling Factors*

One of the most important enabling factors for this population was the availability of antibiotics inexpen-

sively from bodegas. Access was important to this group. While only about a third of participants in the
485  written questionnaire reported buying antibiotics from a bodega, every participant then verbally confirmed during the discussion that they did indeed regularly do so. They noted that the necessity for waiting in a clinic or waiting room to see a healthcare provider was a ma-
490  jor deterrent. Consistent with previous literature (Macias & Morales, 2001; Weinberg et al., 2003), our informants reported that they obtain antibiotics from

237

Latin America where they are cheaper and available without prescription.

In this culture, community participants reported that the bodega employee and the pharmacist are important and respected sources of health information. Both community members and the healthcare professionals confirmed that interventions to improve appropriate antibiotic use in the Latino population would have to include bodega staff. As respected members of the community and longstanding, traditional sources of antibiotics, bodega employees could serve as important sources of information. Providing educational materials to be distributed in bodegas would be consistent with their established role in the community. There have been no known attempts to include the sellers of antibiotics in educational interventions to improve their use.

*Reinforcing Factors*

Respondents named "doctors" as their major source of health information in the written survey, and yet they also reported that receiving care from a health professional did not change their self-prescribing patterns. Although this seems to be contradictory, there may be great potential for a positive influence of the healthcare provider if a meaningful relationship is established. Since the participants in our study also identified that they often received their health information from family and friends and self-medicated with antibiotics obtained from bodegas, traditional interventions such as pamphlets in clinic waiting rooms are unlikely to meet with success in this population (Wheeler et al., 2001).

Of interest among our informants was that while adults self-prescribed antibiotics, they stated that they would be unlikely to do so for their children. One potentially effective strategy among the Latino population would be to include the child as well as parents and Latino community organizations directly in educational efforts.

Based on information provided by our participants, being told by even respected healthcare providers not to self-prescribe antibiotics was insufficient as a reinforcing factor. Such health messages must be delivered in respectful and culturally sensitive ways and must be accompanied by alternative suggestions for what can or should be done (Weissman & Besser, 2004). Despite the fact that the participants in our focus groups were not highly educated, many reported using a computer almost daily. Innovative and tailored Spanish-language messages delivered electronically might also be one promising component of a multifactorial, culturally relevant intervention to reduce the self-prescribing of antibiotics in this important segment of the population.

## Summary and Recommendations

Described earlier are predisposing, enabling, and reinforcing factors that influence Latino community members to self-prescribe antibiotics. Some factors (e.g., time and money constraints, long waiting periods in clinics, and language barriers) will require long-term policy and systems change. Other proximal determinants that might be promising targets as immediate intervention strategies are recommended:

1. Include small-business owners who sell antibiotics in educational interventions. This would involve (a) suggesting alternatives to antibiotics that they might offer customers so that they would not risk losing income or customers, (b) providing small-business owners and employees with Spanish language, culturally appropriate educational materials for dissemination to customers, and (c) working collaboratively with the Bodega Association of America (Asociacion de Bodegueros de los Estados Unidos, Inc.). Since there are about 14,000 bodegas in New York alone and > 22,000 nationally (Bodega Association of the United States, 2005), such a partnership would seem an essential component of an effective and sustainable community-wide intervention.

2. Include lay community workers (*promotores*) and children in educational messages regarding antibiotic use and resistance through public schools or other community organizations. Community groups directed toward assisting immigrants could be good partners in providing education in basic healthcare and care of minor infections.

3. Develop informational messages through the Spanish-speaking media and Internet, which are tailored to be culturally specific and relevant.

Clearly, interventions targeted solely to traditional, mainstream clinicians and the English-speaking population will fail to reach a large segment of the population, which may serve as one reservoir for antibiotic resistance in the community.

## References

Barden, L. S., Dowell, S. F., Schwartz, B., & Lackey, C. (1998). Current attitudes regarding use of antimicrobial agents: Results from physician's and parents' focus group discussions. *Clinical Pediatrics, 37,* 665–671.

Belongia, E. A., Naimi, T. S., Gale, C. M., & Besser, R. E. (2002). Antibiotic use and upper respiratory infections: A survey of knowledge, attitudes, and experience in Wisconsin and Minnesota. *Preventive Medicine, 34,* 346–352.

Blanchard, J., & Lurie, N. (2004). R-E-S-P-E-C-T: Patient reports of disrespect in the healthcare setting and its impact on care. *Journal of Family Practice, 53,* 721–730.

Bodega Association of the United States. (2005). Retrieved August 31, 2005, from http://www.bodegaassociation.org/

Braun, B. L., & Fowles, J. B. (2000). Characteristics and experiences of parents and adults who want antibiotics for cold symptoms. *Archives of Family Medicine, 9,* 589–595.

Calva, J., & Bojalil, R. (1996). Antibiotic use in a periurban community in Mexico: A household and drugstore survey. *Social Science & Medicine, 42,* 1121–1128.

Chiou, C. C., Liu, Y. C., Huang, T. S., Hwang, T. K., Wang, J. H., Lin, H. H., et al. (1998). Extremely high prevalence of nasopharyngeal carriage of penicillin-resistant Streptococcus pneumoniae among children in Kaohsiung, Taiwan. *Journal of Clinical Microbiology, 36,* 1933–1937.

Corbett, K. K., Gonzales, R., Leeman-Castillo, B. A., Flores, E., Maselli, J., & Kafadar, K. (2005). Appropriate antibiotic use: Variation in knowledge and awareness by Hispanic ethnicity and language. *Preventive Medicine, 40,* 162–169.

D'Alessandro, D. M., Kreiter, C. D., Kinzer, S. L., & Peterson, M. W. (2004). A randomized controlled trial of an information prescription for pediatric patient education on the Internet. *Archives of Pediatric & Adolescent Medicine, 158*, 857–862.

Diekema, D. J., Brueggemann, A. B., & Doern, G. V. (2000). Antimicrobial-drug use and changes in resistance in Streptococcus pneumoniae. *Emerging Infectious Diseases, 6*, 552–556.

Finkelstein, J. A., Stille, C., Nordin, J., Davis, R., Raebel, M. A., Roblin, D., et al. (2003). Reduction in antibiotic use among US children, 1996–2000. *Pediatrics, 112*, 620–627.

Garfield, R., Broe, D., & Albano, B. (1995). The role of academic medical centers in delivery of primary care: An urban study. *Academic Medicine, 70*, 405–409.

Gonzales, R., Steiner, J. F., Lum, A., & Barrett, P. H. Jr. (1999). Decreasing antibiotic use in ambulatory practice: Impact of a multidimensional intervention on the treatment of uncomplicated acute bronchitis in adults. *Journal of the American Medical Association, 281*, 1512–1519.

Green, L., & Kreuter, M. (1991). *Health promotion planning: An educational and environmental approach* (2nd ed.). Mountain View, CA: Mayfield.

Hennessy, T. W., Petersen, K. M., Bruden, D., Parkinson, A. J., Hurlburt, D., Getty, M., et al. (2002). Changes in antibiotic-prescribing practices and carriage of penicillin-resistant Streptococcus pneumoniae: A controlled intervention trial in rural Alaska. *Clinical Infectious Diseases, 34*, 1543–1550.

Kreuter, M., Farrell, D., Olevitch, L., & Brennan, L. (2000). *Tailoring health messages: Customizing communication with computer technology.* Mahwah, NJ: Erlbaum.

Kuzujanakis, M., Kleinman, K., Rifas-Shiman, S., & Finkelstein, J. A. (2003). Correlates of parental antibiotic knowledge, demand, and reported use. *Ambulatory Pediatrics, 3*, 203–210.

Larson, E., Lin, S. X., & Gomez-Duarte, C. (2003). Antibiotic use in Hispanic households, New York city. *Emerging Infectious Diseases, 9*, 1096–1102.

Levy, S. B. (2002). The 2000 Garrod lecture. Factors impacting on the problem of antibiotic resistance. *Journal of Antimicrobial Chemotherapy, 49*, 25–30.

Macias, E. P., & Morales, L. S. (2001). Crossing the border for healthcare. *Journal of Health Care for the Poor and Under-served, 12*, 77–87.

Mainous, A. G., 3rd, Hueston, W. J., & Clark, J. R. (1996). Antibiotics and upper respiratory infection: Do some folks think there is a cure for the common cold? *Journal of Family Practice, 42*, 357–361.

Mangione-Smith, R., Elliott, M. N., Stivers, T., McDonald, L., Heritage, J., & McGlynn, E. A. (2004). Racial/ethnic variation in parent expectations for antibiotics: Implications for public health campaigns. *Pediatrics, 113*, e385–e394.

Mangione-Smith, R., McGlynn, E. A., Elliott, M. N., Krogstad, P., & Brook, R. H. (1999). The relationship between perceived parental expectations and pediatrician antimicrobial prescribing behavior. *Pediatrics, 103*, 711–718.

Mangione-Smith, R., McGlynn, E. A., Elliott, M. N., McDonald, L., Franz, C. E., & Kravitz, R. L. (2001). Parent expectations for antibiotics, physician-parent communication, and satisfaction. *Archives of Pediatric & Adolescent Medicine, 155*, 800–806.

Mangione-Smith, R., Stivers, T., Elliott, M., McDonald, L., & Heritage, J. (2003). Online commentary during the physical examination: A communication tool for avoiding inappropriate antibiotic prescribing? *Social Science & Medicine, 56*, 313–320.

McCaig, L. F., Besser, R. E., & Hughes, J. M. (2002). Trends in antimicrobial prescribing rates for children and adolescents. *Journal of the American Medical Association, 287*, 3096–3102.

McKee, M. D., Mills, L., & Mainous, A. G. 3rd. (1999). Antibiotic use for the treatment of upper respiratory infections in a diverse community. *Journal of Family Practice, 48*, 993–996.

Melander, E., Ekdahl, K., Jonsson, G., & Molstad, S. (2000). Frequency of penicillin-resistant pneumococci in children is correlated to community utilization of antibiotics. *Pediatric Infectious Disease Journal, 19*, 1172–1177.

Metlay, J. P., Shea, J. A., Crossette, L. B., & Asch, D. A. (2002). Tensions in antibiotic prescribing: Pitting social concerns against the interests of individual patients. *Journal of General Internal Medicine, 17*, 87–94.

Morgan D. L., & Krueger, R. A. (1998). *The focus group kit.* Thousand Oaks: Sage.

National Center for Infectious Diseases. (2005). Retrieved August 31, 2005, from http://www.cdc.gov/drugresistance/community/

Perz, J. F., Craig, A. S., Coffey, C. S., Jorgensen, D. M., Mitchel, E., Hall, S., et al. (2002). Changes in antibiotic prescribing for children after a community-wide campaign. *Journal of the American Medical Association, 287*, 3103–3109.

Replogle, M. L., Fleming, D. W., & Cieslak, P. R. (2000). Emergence of antimicrobial-resistant shigellosis in Oregon. *Clinical Infectious Diseases, 30*, 515–519.

Trepka, M. J., Belongia, E. A., Chyou, P. H., Davis, J. P., & Schwartz, B. (2001). The effect of a community intervention trial on parental knowledge and awareness of antibiotic resistance and appropriate antibiotic use in children. *Pediatrics, 107*, E6.

United States Census Bureau. (2001). Census 2000 Briefs and Special Reports. Retrieved August 31, 2005, from http://www.census.gov/prod/2001pubs/c2kbr01-3.pdf

Weinberg, M., Waterman, S., Lucas, C. A., Falcon, V. C., Morales, P. K., Lopez, L. A., et al. (2003). The U.S.-Mexico Border Infectious Disease Surveillance project: Establishing bi-national border surveillance. *Emerging Infectious Diseases, 9*, 97–102.

Weissman, J., & Besser, R. E. (2004). Promoting appropriate antibiotic use for pediatric patients: A social ecological framework. *Seminars in Pediatric Infectious Diseases, 15*, 41–51.

Wheeler, J. G., Fair, M., Simpson, P. M., Rowlands, L. A., Aitken, M. E., & Jacobs, R. F. (2001). Impact of a waiting room videotape message on parent attitudes toward pediatric antibiotic use. *Pediatrics, 108*, 591–596.

Witte, K., Meyer, G., & Martell, D. (2001). *Effective health risk messages: A step-by-step guide.* Thousand Oaks, CA: Sage.

**Acknowledgments:** This study was funded in part by a pilot grant from Center for Evidence-based Practice in the Underserved (P20NR007799), National Institutes of Health. The authors express their gratitude to focus group participants and to Maria Cornelio, Director, Hispanic Resource Center, Columbia University Medical Center, and Mary Byrne, NP, PhD, professor of Clinical Nursing, for their support.

**Address correspondence to:** Elaine L. Larson, RN, PhD, CIC, FAAN, Columbia University School of Nursing, 630 West 168th Street, New York, NY 10032. E-mail: ell23@columbia.edu

# Exercise for Article 32

## *Factual Questions*

1. How were community participants recruited?

2. Why didn't the researchers ask the bodega employees to discuss whether they sold antibiotics over the counter?

3. Was the questionnaire administered before *or* after the focus group discussions?

4. The focus group discussions were based on a written guide that included what three concepts?

5. The questionnaire was pilot tested for what three characteristics?

6. Did many of the informants report buying antibiotics in bodegas?

## *Questions for Discussion*

7. The researchers refer to the sample as a "purposive sample." Speculate on the meaning of this term. (See lines 121–122.)

8. Does the fact that the researchers conducted a debriefing session increase your confidence in the results of this study? (See lines 218–231.)

9. Is it important to know that the data analysis was initially conducted "independently"? Explain. (See lines 261–265 and 274–276.)

10. To what extent did Figure 2 help you understand the rationale and results of this study? Explain.

11. The researchers used both qualitative and quantitative methods in this study. In your opinion, did both methods contribute important information? Would this study have been as informative if only one of the methods had been used? Explain.

12. If you were to conduct a follow-up study on the same topic, what changes, if any, would you make in the research methodology?

## Quality Ratings

Directions: Indicate your level of agreement with each of the following statements by circling a number from 5 for strongly agree (SA) to 1 for strongly disagree (SD). If you believe an item is not applicable to this research article, leave it blank. Be prepared to explain your ratings. When responding to criteria A and B, keep in mind that brief titles and abstracts are conventional in published research.

A. The title of the article is appropriate.

SA   5   4   3   2   1   SD

B. The abstract provides an effective overview of the research article.

SA   5   4   3   2   1   SD

C. The introduction establishes the importance of the study.

SA   5   4   3   2   1   SD

D. The literature review establishes the context for the study.

SA   5   4   3   2   1   SD

E. The research purpose, question, or hypothesis is clearly stated.

SA   5   4   3   2   1   SD

F. The method of sampling is sound.

SA   5   4   3   2   1   SD

G. Relevant demographics (for example, age, gender, and ethnicity) are described.

SA   5   4   3   2   1   SD

H. Measurement procedures are adequate.

SA   5   4   3   2   1   SD

I. All procedures have been described in sufficient detail to permit a replication of the study.

SA   5   4   3   2   1   SD

J. The participants have been adequately protected from potential harm.

SA   5   4   3   2   1   SD

K. The results are clearly described.

SA   5   4   3   2   1   SD

L. The discussion/conclusion is appropriate.

SA   5   4   3   2   1   SD

M. Despite any flaws, the report is worthy of publication.

SA   5   4   3   2   1   SD

# Article 33

# Computer-Mediated Support Group Use Among Parents of Children With Cancer: An Exploratory Study

Hae-Ra Han, PhD, RN, **Anne E. Belcher**, PhD, RN, AOCN, FAAN[*]

ABSTRACT. This study describes aspects of computer group use as a vehicle for self-help by parents of children with cancer. Using an electronic mail system, data were gathered from 73 parents who had participated in online support groups. Most participants were Caucasian, well educated, and reported annual incomes of more than $50,000. The perceived benefits of the computer group involvement were getting information, sharing experiences, receiving general support, venting feelings, gaining accessibility, and using writing. The disadvantages included "noise," negative emotions, large volume of mail, and lack of physical contact and proximity. The findings indicate that computer group use is more common in parents with relatively high socioeconomic status. There are certain advantages and disadvantages of computer group use that need to be recognized and addressed by health professionals and users.

From *Computers in Nursing*, *19*, 27–33. Copyright © 2001 by Lippincott Williams & Wilkins. Reprinted with permission.

## Background

Cancer is the second leading cause of death in children ages 5 to 15 years in the United States,[1] but approximately 70% of children diagnosed with cancer today will have a five-year or more disease-free survival.[2] The life-threatening and often chronic nature of cancer is a major stressor for children and their parents.[3–9]

Remarkable advances have been made in cancer diagnosis and treatment since the 1930s, and care for chronically ill children has shifted from the hospital to the home setting. An increasing number of children with cancer and their families cope with problems in day-to-day living at home.[10] As a result, not only are parents responsible for providing physical care, but they also must become skilled in clinical assessment, clinical decision making, and coordination of care.[11] Furthermore, the needs of the child with cancer demand constant parental vigilance. How parents cope with their child's cancer diagnosis and its treatment has been found to impact on the child's treatment-related morbidity, quality of life, and even treatment outcome.[8,12–14]

Evidence points to the central role of social support in alleviating the impact of illness so that the individual can achieve better coping outcomes.[15–17] Support groups, as a form of social support, have long been recognized as an effective intervention, producing positive psychological outcomes in cancer patients and their families.[18] Even for individuals with strong familial and interpersonal networks, support groups have been found to bridge the gap between information giving and social support.[19] According to Yalom,[20] there are 11 therapeutic factors existing in support groups: instillation of hope, universality, imparting information, altruism, the corrective recapitulation of the primary family group, development of socialization techniques, imitative behavior, interpersonal learning, group cohesiveness, catharsis, and existential factors.

Thoits[21] states that the effective provision of support is likely to arise from people who are socially similar to the support recipient and who have experienced similar stressors or situations. Self-help groups are experiential mutual-support, peer-support groups and recognized as an important part of the social support system for parents of children with cancer.[22] Self-help groups differ from counseling groups, which are structured as a formal part of the therapeutic process. The peer-support group approach has demonstrated its value in enhancing the ability of parents to cope with their child's chronic conditions.[23] However, researchers have reported that transportation, distance,[10] and time restrictions[24] are major barriers to attending face-to-face support groups.

Computers are becoming more accessible to the general public, and computer use for self-help has become a more common vehicle to connect to resources, obtain information, and gain support.[25] In a study that investigated computer-mediated support group use among six breast cancer patients, Weinberg et al.[26]

[*]*Hae-Ra Han* was a doctoral candidate at the University of Maryland School of Nursing at the time of the study. *Anne E. Belcher* is the director of the undergraduate program at the Thomas Jefferson University College of Health Professions.

60  found that the patients discussed their medical conditions, shared personal concerns, and offered support to one another. Brennan et al.[27] investigated subjects' uses of ComputerLink, a computer-mediated support group for caregivers of persons with Alzheimer's disease,
65  during a one-week period. The researchers reported that subjects used ComputerLink as an opportunity for contact with other caregivers who were experiencing similar caregiving problems and stresses. Eaglesham[25] conducted a study to examine the implications of using
70  computers as a vehicle for self-help groups. Shared experiences were often cited as a reason why people joined a computer group. Klemm et al.[28,29] reported exchange of personal experiences as one of the major categories of responses in such groups.

75  Computer-mediated self-help groups have also been reported to overcome the limitations of face-to-face support groups and to provide 24-hour availability, selective participation, anonymity, and privacy.[26,30,31] According to Finn,[30] there are more than 500,000
80  computer-mediated support groups in the United States that are accessed by more than 15 million people. Computer groups are used by individuals with such diverse problems as cancer, diabetes, mental illness, alcohol or drug addiction, disability, bereavement, do-
85  mestic violence, and divorce.[25,30]

Despite their proliferation, little information is available about parents of children with cancer who belong to computer-mediated support groups. Furthermore, no study has examined the advantages and dis-
90  advantages of computer group use from the perspective of parent users. The exploratory nature of this study enabled researchers to collect basic information about the parent participants, as well as the perceived benefits and disadvantages of computer group use.

## Methods

### Settings and Sample

95  The online settings were three support groups for family members of children with cancer: N-BLASTOMA, PED-ALL, and PED-ONC. They are part of more than 70 online cancer support groups hosted by the Association of Cancer On-line Re-
100  sources, Inc. (ACOR), a nonprofit organization incorporated in New York in 1996 to create, produce, host, and manage a number of specific online resources for cancer patients, caregivers, healthcare professionals, and basic research scientists.[32] ACOR provides support
105  to more than 30,000 patients, family members, and caregivers.[32] The three online support groups for families of children with cancer post more than 100 messages per day about diagnosis, self-care skills, life stories, and encouragement as well as postings about the
110  children (i.e., how the sick children are doing). General types of messages (e.g., fund-raising activities, humor, and requests for specific medical information) are also posted to the groups. There were 222, 162, and 224

members on N-BLASTOMA, PED-ALL, and PED-
115  ONC, respectively, at the time of data collection.[33]

Seventy-three parents (55 mothers and 18 fathers) participated in the study (17 from N-BLASTOMA, 28 from PED-ALL, and 28 from PED-ONC). Selection criteria for the convenience sample were as follows: (1)
120  age 18 years or older, (2) parent of a child diagnosed with cancer, and (3) participant in a computer-mediated support group. The sample ranged in age from 25 to 55 years, with a mean age of 38. Most participants were Caucasian, well educated, and reported annual incomes
125  of more than $50,000. Diagnoses of the children included leukemia (57.5%), neuroblastoma (24.7%), and other forms of childhood cancer (17.8%). Time since diagnosis of the child's cancer varied, ranging from 2 months to 13 years ($M = 29.6$ months, $SD = 27.8$). The
130  demographic characteristics of the sample are presented in Table 1.

Table 1
*Demographics of Study Participants**

| Characteristic | $n$ | $\%$ |
|---|---|---|
| Gender | | |
| Female | 55 | 75.3 |
| Male | 18 | 24.7 |
| Ethnicity | | |
| Caucasian | 65 | 89.0 |
| Asian | 2 | 2.7 |
| Native American | 1 | 1.4 |
| Unknown | 5 | 6.8 |
| Educational level | | |
| 9–12th grade | 4 | 5.5 |
| Vocational and/or some college | 12 | 16.4 |
| College graduate | 26 | 35.6 |
| Graduate and/or professional school | 26 | 35.6 |
| Unknown | 5 | 6.8 |
| Annual income | | |
| Less than $24,999 | 7 | 9.6 |
| $25,000–$29,999 | 9 | 12.3 |
| $30,000–$39,999 | 6 | 8.2 |
| $40,000–$49,999 | 7 | 9.6 |
| $50,000–$99,999 | 24 | 32.9 |
| $100,000 or more | 13 | 17.8 |
| Unknown | 7 | 9.6 |
| Child's cancer diagnosis | | |
| Leukemia | 42 | 57.5 |
| Neuroblastoma | 18 | 24.7 |
| Brain tumor | 4 | 5.5 |
| Wilms tumor | 2 | 2.7 |
| Non-Hodgkins lymphoma | 2 | 2.7 |
| Rhabdomyosarcoma | 2 | 2.7 |
| Germ cell tumor | 1 | 1.4 |
| Osteosarcoma | 1 | 1.4 |
| Sinonasal carcinoma | 1 | 1.4 |

| | $M$ | $SD$ |
|---|---|---|
| Age | 38.1 | 6.5 |
| Time since child's diagnosis (months) | 29.6 | 27.8 |

*$N = 73$.

*Instrumentation*

A survey was developed for the purpose of the study. The survey contained eight questions that focused on demographic data and six questions on the use of computers for support. Examples of these questions were: "Has connecting to the group been helpful to you? If so, please describe how it has been helpful to you" and "What are disadvantages of the group (if any)?"

*Procedure*

Using search engines on the Internet, the three data collection sites were identified. N-BLASTOMA and PED-ALL are online lists devoted to issues pertaining to neuroblastoma and acute lymphoblastic leukemia in children, respectively. PED-ONC focuses on issues that are related to various types of childhood cancer. After approval of the university's Institutional Review Board, an electronic mail message requesting approval for data collection was sent to the list of owners. Once approved, an introductory letter explaining the purpose of the study and criteria for participation was posted twice to each list within a two-week period. A consent form and the survey were then sent via electronic mail to parents who requested one from the primary investigator. Parents who participated were directed to send completed questionnaires and the consent form to the electronic mail address of the researcher. As each questionnaire was received, it was assigned a number and all identifying information was deleted as a means of maintaining anonymity and protecting confidentiality. A hard copy of each response was printed out for analysis.

*Data Analysis*

Frequencies and descriptive statistics were obtained for demographic characteristics of participants using the Statistical Package for the Social Sciences (SPSS) 10.0 for Windows. The subjects' descriptions of advantages and disadvantages of computer-mediated support group use were categorized by the primary investigator who is master's-prepared and has expertise in pediatric oncology nursing. The categorization of every response was reviewed by the second author who is a doctorally prepared, certified oncology nurse. Interrater reliability was 95%.

## Results

Most parents (75.3%) reported that they had learned about the computer groups through an Internet search, and 12.3% replied that the group was recommended by others (e.g., relative, chat-room member, oncologist, social worker, or other parent at the hospital). Four parents read about the groups in books or newsletters. Approximately two-thirds of the participants accessed the computer groups from home. The parents reported that they had been connecting to the computer groups from two weeks to three years ($M = 13.3$ months, $SD = 11.0$). Most participants (85%) connected daily to the group, while 10.9% connected between one and three times a week. Overall, the participants spent an average of five hours a week connected to the computer groups ($SD = 6.1$), with a range from 30 minutes to 40 hours (Table 2).

Table 2
*Participants' Usage of the Computer Groups*

|  | n | % |
|---|---|---|
| How parent learned about the computer groups | | |
| Internet search | 55 | 75.3 |
| Recommended by others | 9 | 12.3 |
| Books and newsletters | 4 | 5.5 |
| Unknown | 5 | 6.9 |
| Place of computer group use | | |
| Home | 46 | 63.0 |
| Work | 12 | 16.4 |
| Home and work | 10 | 13.7 |
| Unknown | 5 | 6.8 |
| Frequency of computer group use | | |
| Daily | 62 | 85.0 |
| 2–3 times a week | 6 | 8.2 |
| Once a week | 2 | 2.7 |
| Unknown | 3 | 4.1 |
|  | M | SD |
| Time since being connected to the computer groups (months) | 13.3 | 11.0 |
| Length of computer group use per week (hours) | 5.0 | 6.1 |

*Advantages of Computer Group Use*

The participants' responses are summarized in Table 3. Benefits of the computer group use included getting information, sharing experiences, receiving general support, venting feelings, gaining accessibility, and using writing. The most frequently cited benefit of the computer group use was information giving and receiving (76.7%).

Table 3
*Perceived Advantages and Disadvantages of the Computer Group Use*

| Category | n | % |
|---|---|---|
| Advantages | | |
| Getting information | 56 | 76.7 |
| Sharing experiences | 49 | 67.1 |
| General support | 21 | 28.8 |
| Venting of feelings | 10 | 13.7 |
| Accessibility | 6 | 8.2 |
| Use of text | 2 | 2.7 |
| Disadvantages | | |
| "Noise" | 36 | 49.3 |
| Negative emotions | 19 | 26.0 |
| Large volume of mail | 15 | 20.5 |
| Lack of physical contact | 8 | 11.0 |

It is a forum to ask questions about treatment options and side effects that maybe an oncologist hasn't explained. It stops the panic in the middle of the night when you sud-

denly think some symptom must be abnormal. Then you
ask someone in the group and you find that his or her
child has had that happen and it was OK.

I joined the group to gather as much medical information
as I could in a short period of time. This is a highly educated group of people who have researched much of their
children's treatment protocol. I took their combined expertise.

The information obtained from the list appears to
serve parents in a variety of ways, one of which includes the development of informed decision making.
One mother stated "... recently we [list members] discussed the pros and cons of a new testing procedure; it
helped me to make an informed decision about my
daughter's participation with the test."

About two-thirds (67.1%) of the participants listed
a number of benefits related to the issue of shared experiences. When confronted with circumstances that
seem to alienate the parent from the normal world, the
parent may feel that people do not understand what the
family of a child with cancer is dealing with every day.
The computer group gives the parent assurance that he
or she is not alone.

Through this group, I have discovered that I am not
alone. I have found that the fears I face are common to all
cancer parents. I have found people who understand what
I face emotionally every single day. There aren't words
to describe how much support I receive from this group.

To find a group of people that understand the incredible
pressures of trying to live with this disease, is a great relief. Most people [who have not experienced it] just don't
understand. It functions like a family. I couldn't live
without it.

Twenty-one (28.8%) parents described receiving
general support from the computer group use. One father stated that the group had been immensely helpful
by being generally supportive of each other, as they all
go through what is basically a pretty rough time. Another comment about the supportive nature of the computer group was "Some of the people in the group are
so inspiring that I feel I have grown spiritually and
emotionally just reading their posts."

Venting feelings refers to expression of emotion.[29]
Ten (13.7%) parents reported that the computer group
provided an outlet for emotional disturbances. One
participant described it in the following way:

The group has saved my sanity. In the area in which I
live, there are no other parents of kids with cancer close
by. The hospital clinic is an hour away. Plus, you have to
spend a lot of time with your child, and cannot leave
them for long to go to meetings. Thus, there is no one I
can really talk to about this in person. Having others to
talk to on-line about treatment and especially about their
feelings makes me know that my feelings are normal, and
therefore I feel a lot better.

Gaining accessibility to the group regardless of
time and place is another unique advantage of the computer group use recognized by six parents (8.2%). The
advantage of 24-hour availability and easy access from
most places is seen in the following excerpts:

I can access these people any time. [It is] not like going
to a physical parent support group that is time-
consuming....

Getting out of the house to be involved with local support
groups is just about impossible [as] I have seven children.
The Internet allows me to interact with others going
through similar difficulties on my own time.

Computer groups are unique because they take
place solely through the medium of written text. This
creates some benefits for participants, as recognized by
two parents (2.7%) in this study. One parent stated:

I recognize my thoughts and put words to them. I learn
more about my own thoughts [by writing them down].
Also, I believe it's easier to say what you really think in
words, I'd probably chicken out in a face-to-face encounter. Plus, in-person encounters are so affected by facial
and body expressions, by the way someone looks, and by
the way they respond when one starts to say something.
Plus you can get interrupted and lose your train of
thought. Yes, I like the written word. I can go back over
and read things again, posts that are too good to be read
just one time, and things I wrote a few months back to recall how I was thinking then.

*Disadvantages of Computer Group Use*

Four disadvantages of the computer group use were
identified. They included "noise," negative emotions,
large volume of mail, and lack of physical contact.
"Noise," which refers to posts that are not of interest,
off topic, or are vapid,[25] was the most frequently
(49.3%) perceived disadvantage of the computer group
use.

People who send full copies of the message they are re-
plying to within their own e-mail is a disadvantage of the
computer group use.

Occasionally I get bogged down in trivia, and sometimes,
too many prayers are flying around.

"Noise" sometimes leads to a rather devastating result as depicted in the following:

The group consists of people who hold a variety of opinions on many subjects. We are bound together by our
children's fight with cancer. Sometimes a fringe subject
will come up and some people use the list as a sounding
board for something totally unrelated to cancer. Often
feelings are hurt and we lose members.

Nineteen (26%) parents stated that they sometimes
received a lot of news about other children losing the
battle that was frightening and depressing.

You hear how each child fights the beast and yet sometimes it takes over and wins. You share your life with
these people and they become friends, so it hurts and
takes a piece of you when you hear the bad news.

A large volume of mail is another disadvantage of
the computer group, indicated by fifteen parents
(20.5%). Parents reported that they dealt with the prob-

lem by saving messages for less busy times or sorting out messages.

The lack of physical contact and physical proximity was perceived as a drawback of the computer group use by eight parents (11%): "You can't touch and hug people when you want." In this way, another participant pointed out that "... you are never sure who is listening to your conversation." Sometimes the lack of physical closeness may increase difficulties in understanding between list members: "... [It is] hard to express humor without being face to face or hearing tone of voice!"

## Discussion

The findings indicate that computer group use is more common among parents with relatively high socioeconomic status. They also suggest that there are certain advantages and disadvantages of computer group use which health professionals and potential users need to recognize.

While computer users were commonly thought to be young, well-educated men with a high socioeconomic status,[34] more recent evidence indicates that the demographics of computer group users have been diversifying, with an increasing number of women [35] as well as elderly users.[36] Even though the demographic data collected may not be representative of parents participating in computer-mediated support groups, the results of this study seem to support the diversifying demographics of computer group users, especially in terms of gender. The current sample represented both genders; 55 (75.3%) of the 73 participants were women. In a study of 75 participants in computer-mediated support groups for various problems (e.g., sexual abuse, adoption, parenting, and alcoholism), Eaglesham [25] reported that approximately 60% of the sample was women, 90% of the subjects were Caucasian, 95% had some tertiary education, and the mean age was 36.7 (range of 20 to 56 years). Klemm et al.[29] content-analyzed messages posted on an online colorectal cancer support group. Of the 97 people who posted messages during the study period, 47.4% were women.

Various aspects of the computer-mediated support group for parents of children with cancer were described and appear to be of potential benefit to participants. The parents identified advantages as being able to get information, share experiences, get general support, vent feelings, access the group, and use writing. These results corroborate those of previous studies [25–29] that documented a list of advantages of computer group use, including sharing concerns and information and offering support. These results suggest that computer-mediated support groups may offer participants many of the therapeutic features of face-to-face groups in the comfort and privacy of their own homes at any time. The identified perceived benefits of the computer groups match some of Yalom's therapeutic factors [20]

that exist in face-to-face support groups and indicate that a computer group can be used as a source of support and information.

The advantages of online support groups are not, however, without certain limitations. The parents identified the disadvantages of participating in the computer groups, including "noise," negative emotions, heavy volume of mail, and lack of physical contact and proximity. In Eaglesham's study,[25] participants perceived "noise," negative messages, physical distance among participants, concerns about confidentiality, financial and legal issues, and problem behaviors as disadvantages of computer group use. It is important to note that even though the parents participating in this study generally reported positive experiences, less is known about parents having negative experiences with the computer group.

Although information giving and receiving were recognized as advantages of computer group use in the study, there is a concern that members may receive misinformation and not have it corrected due to the time delay in computer communication. Information that these parents obtain from the list may significantly influence their decisions on the child's treatment. Smith [37] also points out that by sharing experiences and referring each other to print articles and Web sites, patients (and their families) have become more aware of issues and options regarding diagnosis, treatment, and recovery. Nurses and health professionals should be aware of the full range of available supportive resources, including computer groups, and be able to inform clients of the potential risks of computer group use.

The methodological implications of this study may need to be addressed. Even though it lacks the interaction of face-to-face interviews and nonverbal cues, using e-mail as a way of data collection may be less time-consuming and more cost-effective than other data collection methods. The costs of posting messages to e-mail lists may be only a few cents compared with the hundreds of dollars required to mail questionnaires to a similar number of subjects or to interview them directly. Furthermore, written e-mail may provide a rich source of communication. The electronic data obtained from the parents in this study showed how positive the parents felt about the computer group use. The respondents in this study were well-educated people who had access to a computer. The extent to which the results can be generalized to other parents of children with cancer requires further investigation. There is often a low response rate to online surveys. For example, Murray[38] posted research questions to the Nursenet discussion list, which had more than a thousand subscribers, and completed e-mail interviews with only five subscribers. Of the more than 600 users, this study included only 73 parents (12.2%). As Lakeman[39] suggested, a request for participation that is more friendly and appealing to readers may need to be prepared. The calls for subjects may also need to be posted over a longer period of time to increase response rate.

430 Future generations of caregivers are being exposed to computers as a regular part of school curricula and thus represent a growing base of potential users.[34] For caregivers who are unable or unwilling to access other support services, computer-mediated support groups may indeed represent an attractive alternative. System-

435 atic evaluation of computer-mediated support groups is necessary. Future research should investigate users, helping mechanisms, advantages, and potential disadvantages and risks related to computer-mediated support groups. The results of this study provide direction for further research in this area.

### References

1. Murphy SL. *Deaths: Final data for 1998.* National vital statistics reports; Vol. 48 No. 11. Hyattsville, MD: National Center for Health Statistics; 2000.
2. Moore JB, Mosher RB. Adjustment responses of children and their mothers to cancer: Self-care and anxiety. *Oncol Nurs Forum.* 1997;24(3):519–525.
3. Pelcovitz D, Goldenberg B, Kaplan S, et al. Posttraumatic stress disorder in mothers of pediatric cancer survivors. *Psychosomatics.* 1996;37:116–126.
4. Roberts CS, Piper L, Denny J, Cuddeback G. A support group intervention to facilitate young adults' adjustment to cancer. *Health Soc Work.* 1997;22(2):133–141.
5. Sawyer M, Antoniou G, Toogood I, Rice M. Childhood cancer: A two-year prospective study of the psychological adjustment of children and parents. *J Am Acad Children Adolesc Psychiatry.* 1997;36(12):1736–1743.
6. Sawyer MG, Streiner DL, Antoniou G, Toogood I, Rice M. Influence of parental and family adjustment on the later psychological adjustment of children treated for cancer. *J Am Acad Children Adolesc Psychiatry.* 1998;37(8):815–822.
7. Stuber ML, Christakis DA, Houskamp B, Kazak AE. Posttrauma symptoms in childhood leukemia survivors and their parents. *Psychosomatics.* 1996;37:254–261.
8. Stuber ML, Kazak AE, Meeske K, et al. Predictors of posttraumatic stress symptoms in childhood cancer survivors. *Pediatrics.* 1997;100:958–964.
9. Suris JC, Parera N, Puig C. Chronic illness and emotional distress in adolescence. *J Adolesc Health.* 1996;19(2):153–156.
10. de Bocanegra HT. Cancer patients' interest in group support programs. *Cancer Nurs.* 1992;15(5):347–352.
11. Ray LD, Ritchie JA. Caring for chronically ill children at home: Factors that influence parents' coping. *J Pediatr Nurs.* 1993;8(4):217–225.
12. Carlson-Green B, Morris RD, Krawiecki N. Family and illness predictors of outcome in pediatric brain tumors. *J Pediatr Psychol.* 1995;20(6):769–784.
13. Kupst MJ, Natta MB, Richardson CC, Schulman JL, Lavigne JV, Das L. Family coping with pediatric leukemia: Ten years after treatment. *J Pediatr Psychol.* 1995;20(5):601–617.
14. Mulhern RK, Fairclough DL, Smith B, Douglas SM. Maternal depression, assessment methods, and physical symptoms affect estimates of depressive symptomatology among children with cancer. *J Pediatr Psychol.* 1992;17(3):313–326.
15. Bloom BL. Computer-assisted psychological intervention: a review and commentary. *Clin Psychol Rev.* 1992;12:169–197.
16. Grabowski VM, Jens GP. The collaborative role of the CNS in support groups. *Clin Nurse Spec.* 1993;7(2):99–101.
17. Shapiro J, Simonsen D. Educational/support group for Latino families of children with Down syndrome. *Ment Retard.* 1994;32(6):403–415.
18. Reele BL. Effect of counseling on quality of life for individuals with cancer and their families. *Cancer Nurs.* 1994;17(2):101–112.
19. Rosenberg PP. Support groups: A special therapeutic entry. *Small Group Behavior.* 1984;15:173–186.
20. Yalom ID. *The theory and practice of group psychotherapy,* 4th ed. New York: Basic Books; 1995.
21. Thoits PA. Social support as coping assistance. *J Consult Clin Psychol.* 1986;54:416–423.
22. McGee SJ, Burkett KW. Building a support group for parents of children with brain tumors. *J Neurosci Nurs.* 1998;30(6):345–349.
23. Ainbinder JG, Blanchard LW, Singer GH, et al. A qualitative study of parent-to-parent support for parents of children with special needs. *J Pediatr Psychol.* 1998;23(2):99–109.
24. Feldman JS. An alternative group approach: Using multidisciplinary expertise to support patients with prostate cancer and their families. *J Psychosoc Oncol.* 1993;11(2):83–93.
25. Eaglesham SL. *On-line support groups: Extending communities of concern* [dissertation]. Blacksburg, VA: Virginia Polytechnic Institute and State University; 1996.
26. Weinberg N, Schmale J, Uken J, Wessel K. On-line help: Cancer patients participate in a computer-mediated support group. *Health Soc Work.* 1996;21(1):24–29.
27. Brennan PF, Moore SM, Smyth KA. Alzheimer's disease caregivers' uses of a computer network. *West J Nurs Res.* 1992;14(5):662–673.
28. Klemm P, Hurst M, Dearholt SL, Trone SR. Cyber solace: Gender differences on Internet cancer support groups. *Comput Nurs.* 1999;17(2):65–72.
29. Klemm P, Reppert K, Visich L. A nontraditional cancer support group: The Internet. *Comput Nurs.* 1998;16(1):31–36.
30. Finn J. Computer-based self-help groups: On-line recovery for addictions. *Comput Human Services.* 1996;13(1):21–41.
31. Lamberg L. On-line support group helps patients live with, learn more about the rare skin cancer CTCL-MF. *JAMA.* 1997;277(18):1422–1423.
32. L-Soft. Electronic mailing lists provide support for cancer community worldwide [press release]. Washington, DC: L-Soft; 1998. Available at: http://www.lsoft.com/ACOR-press.html
33. Association of Cancer On-line Resources, Inc. List archives at LISTSERV.ACOR.ORG [On-line], 1999. Available at: http://listserv.acor.org/archives/index.html/Accessed: February 22, 1999.
34. Smyth KA, Harris PB. Using telecomputing to provide information and support to caregivers of persons with dementia. *Gerontologist.* 1993;33(1):123–127.
35. Sharf BF. Communicating breast cancer on-line: Support and empowerment on the Internet. *Women Health.* 1997;26(1):65–84.
36. Noer M, Wandycz K. Senior cybernauts. *Forbes.* 1995;156(7):240–241.
37. Smith J. "Internet patients" turn to support groups to guide medical decisions. *J Natl Cancer Inst.* 1998;90(22):1695–1697.
38. Murray PJ. Nurses' computer-mediated communications on Nursenet: A case study. *Comput Nurs.* 1996;14(4):227–234.
39. Lakeman R. Using the Internet for data collection in nursing research. *Comput Nurs.* 1997;15(5):269–275.

**Address correspondence to:** Hae-Ra Han, PhD, RN, Postdoctoral Fellow, Johns Hopkins University, School of Nursing, 525 North Wolfe Street, Baltimore, MD 21205.

# Exercise for Article 33

## Factual Questions

1. The researchers' review of the literature led them to the conclusion that no prior study had examined the advantages and disadvantages of computer use from whose perspective?

2. What was the mean age of the participants in this study?

3. As each questionnaire was received, what was done as a means of maintaining anonymity and protecting confidentiality?

4. The researchers asked the participants how they learned about the computer groups. For what percentage was this information "unknown"?

5. How many of the participants cited lack of physical contact as a perceived disadvantage of the computer use group?

6. According to the researchers, "noise" refers to what types of posts?

7. Of the more than 600 users of the computer groups, what percentage was included in this study?

## Questions for Discussion

8. What is your understanding of the meaning of the term "convenience sample"? (See lines 118–119.)

9. The researchers determined the interrater reliability of the categorization of the responses of the parents. In your opinion, how important is it to determine interrater reliability when open-ended questions are used? Explain. (See lines 165–172.)

10. The researchers present quantitative results (i.e., numbers of cases, percentages, means, and standard deviations). They also present qualitative results (i.e., discussion of findings using the participants' own words to support interpretations). In your opinion, are both types of equal importance? Explain.

11. The researchers note that collecting data using e-mail "lacks the interaction of face-to-face interviews and nonverbal cues." In your opinion, is this important? Is it offset by the cost savings? Explain. (See lines 401–410.)

12. At the end of the article, the researchers discuss possibilities for future research. Do you agree with their suggestions? Do you have additional suggestions? Explain. (See lines 434–438.)

## Quality Ratings

Directions: Indicate your level of agreement with each of the following statements by circling a number from 5 for strongly agree (SA) to 1 for strongly disagree (SD). If you believe an item is not applicable to this research article, leave it blank. Be prepared to explain your ratings. When responding to criteria A and B, keep in mind that brief titles and abstracts are conventional in published research.

A. The title of the article is appropriate.
   SA   5   4   3   2   1   SD

B. The abstract provides an effective overview of the research article.
   SA   5   4   3   2   1   SD

C. The introduction establishes the importance of the study.
   SA   5   4   3   2   1   SD

D. The literature review establishes the context for the study.
   SA   5   4   3   2   1   SD

E. The research purpose, question, or hypothesis is clearly stated.
   SA   5   4   3   2   1   SD

F. The method of sampling is sound.
   SA   5   4   3   2   1   SD

G. Relevant demographics (for example, age, gender, and ethnicity) are described.
   SA   5   4   3   2   1   SD

H. Measurement procedures are adequate.
   SA   5   4   3   2   1   SD

I. All procedures have been described in sufficient detail to permit a replication of the study.
   SA   5   4   3   2   1   SD

J. The participants have been adequately protected from potential harm.
   SA   5   4   3   2   1   SD

K. The results are clearly described.
   SA   5   4   3   2   1   SD

L. The discussion/conclusion is appropriate.
   SA   5   4   3   2   1   SD

M. Despite any flaws, the report is worthy of publication.
   SA   5   4   3   2   1   SD

# Article 34

# Spiritual Perspectives of Nurses in the United States Relevant for Education and Practice

**Roberta Cavendish**, PhD, RN, CPN, **Barbara Kraynyak Luise**, EdD, RN,
**Donna Russo**, MA, RN, NP-P, **Claudia Mitzeliotis**, MS, RNCS, CASAC,
**Maria Bauer**, RN, MS, **Mary Ann McPartlan Bajo**, RN, **Carmen Calvino**, BS, RN,
**Karen Horne**, MS, RN, **Judith Medefindt**, BS, RN, CIC[*]

ABSTRACT. The purpose of the current study was to describe nurses' spiritual perspectives as they relate to education and practice. A multiple triangulation research design encompassing a questionnaire and a descriptive qualitative content analysis were used with the purpose of capturing a more complete, holistic, and contextual description of nurses' spiritual perspectives. Multiple triangulation included two data sources, two methodological approaches, and nine investigators. Using survey methods, Reed's Spiritual Perspective Scale (SPS) was sent to 1,000 members of Sigma Theta Tau International Nursing Honor Society (STTI). Results support Reed's premise that spirituality permeates one's life. Regardless of gender, participants with a religious affiliation had significantly higher SPS scores than those without one. Nurses having a spiritual base use it in practice. Six themes emerged from the qualitative analysis: Nurses perceive spirituality as strength, guidance, connectedness, a belief system, as promoting health, and supporting practice. The integration of spirituality in nursing curriculums can facilitate spiritual care.

From *Western Journal of Nursing Research, 26*, 196–212. Copyright © 2004 by Sage Publications. Reprinted with permission.

The unmet spiritual needs of patients and families are a cause of angst in health care settings in the United States where a majority of citizens consider themselves religious or spiritual (Gallup, 1996; Gallup & Castelli,
5 1989). Because of 20th-century medical advances, the focus of nursing care is more scientific and technology based. Concurrent with changing models of care is that the spiritual needs of patients are not consistently being assessed by nurses; instead, they are being delegated to
10 the chaplain or others (Mayer, 1992; Narayanasamy, 1999b). Providing spiritual care is inherent in nursing (Chadwick, 1973; Macrae, 1995; Simson, 1986). Nursing's commitment to spiritual care, imbued in the theoretical construct of holistic care, is long standing and
15 universal (Carson, 1989; Shelly & Fish, 1988). In clinical practice, the individual is viewed as a whole, and that which affects one dimension affects all others. Nursing scholars concur with the premise that human beings function as integrated biopsychosocial and spiri-
20 tual beings, greater than the sum of their parts (Banks, 1980; Carson, 1989). With the spiritual dimension considered core (Banks, 1980), spiritual assessments are integral to nursing care plans (Shelly & Fish, 1988). Education for nurses' spiritual development, and to
25 meet human responses in the spiritual domain, varies widely in nursing curriculums (Narayanasamy, 1999b; Van Dover & Bacon, 2001). How to provide spiritual care should be inherent in the nursing curriculum as it was in Nightingale's model for nursing education
30 (Macrae, 1995; Nightingale, 1860/1996; O'Brien, 1999). The ability to provide spiritual care can be learned (Piles, 1990). Nurses perceive that they are ill-prepared to provide spiritual care (Cavendish et al., 2000; Dorff, 1993; Highfield, Taylor, & Amenta,
35 2000). Nurses' perceptions regarding spiritual care need further investigation, or the unmet spiritual needs of patients and families will continue to be a cause of angst in health care settings.

[*] *Roberta Cavendish* is a parent-child health expert, a clinical researcher, and an associate professor in the Department of Nursing at the College of Staten Island City University of New York. *Barbara Kraynyak Luise* is a specialist in community health nursing and an associate professor in the Department of Nursing at the College of Staten Island City University of New York. *Donna Russo* is the clinical educator for behavioral health at St. Vincent Catholic Medical Centers. *Claudia Mitzeliotis* is a psychiatric clinical nurse specialist at the Veterans Administration New York Harbor Healthcare System. *Maria Bauer* is a psychiatric mental health clinical nurse specialist and an adjunct lecturer in the Department of Nursing at the College of Staten Island City University of New York. *Mary Ann McPartlan Bajo* is a staff nurse on the Neurology Unit at Staten Island University Hospital North, Staten Island, New York. *Carmen Calvino* is a patient care coordinator, Staten Island University Hospital, Staten Island, New York. *Karen Horne* is the director of Health/Mental Health Services at the Edwin Gould Services for Children and Families in New York City. *Judith Medefindt* is nurse epidemiologist at Lutheran Medical Center (LMC) in Brooklyn, New York.

## The Foundation of Spiritual Perspectives

40 Society's sustained interest in spirituality correlates with the numbers of individuals and families who expect that their spiritual needs will be met in health care settings (Narayanasamy, 1999b). The ability to meet human responses in the spiritual domain has re-
45 emerged as a critical concern for nursing (Barnum, 1996). Registered nurses who conduct patient assessments and hold primary responsibility for developing plans of care infrequently conduct spiritual assessments or identify spiritual needs (Narayanasamy, 1999b; Tay-
50 lor, 2002). To provide spiritual care, nurses must have spiritual self-awareness and a personal spiritual perspective (Danvers, 1998; Dossey & Keegan, 2000).

According to Clemen-Stone, Eigsti, and McGuire (1995), "Nursing began when humanity began" (p. 2),
55 and the care by a specialized group of people who are ill has existed throughout time. The importance of the spiritual dimension cannot be underestimated. This component is essential for integrating life's demands as well as transcending pain and despair. It allows patients
60 to confront, wrestle with, and reconcile crises. The way suffering is perceived then becomes essential for healing, wellness, and celebration. Nursing clearly identifies the spiritual dimension as part of holistic care, yet the intent to provide that care is often not put into prac-
65 tice. Opportunities that have the potential to enhance spirituality for the patient and the nurse are missed (Cavendish et al., 2000, 2001). Some nurses practice with an infrequent or nonexistent spiritual base (Oldnall, 1996). Nurses are often unable to differentiate
70 spiritual needs from religious needs. Patients' spiritual needs are seen as religious rituals, and spiritual care is often delegated to others (Narayanasamy, 1999a).

*Clarification of the Concepts of Spirituality
and Religion*

A nurse might legitimately question, "In assessing this patient's holistic needs, am I identifying a 'reli-
75 gious need' or a 'spiritual need'?" The answer depends on how the community/nurses/institution use the terms. When essential care-related words are ill-defined, they can confuse caregivers (Dyson, Cobb, & Forman, 1997). When nurses have different meanings for spiri-
80 tual care, they cannot communicate clearly with each other about related care needs. For some nurses, spiritual care means helping patients with maintaining their religious practices and worship. For others, it means helping patients identify what holds the most meaning
85 in their life and then helping them to transcend the pain and suffering that usually accompanies illness. When the nurse defines spiritual needs as only religious needs (including worship and practice aspects), they may omit care for patients' transcendent and relational
90 needs. Omission of spiritual care may occur not because a nurse lacks interest but rather because the nurse defines spiritual care narrowly.

Nurses and others on the health care team must define key terms, distinguish between spirituality and
95 religion, and use them consistently in practice, research, and education. Religion and spirituality have some overlapping areas and similarities. Spirituality and religion focus on the sacred or the divine, both focus on beliefs about the sacred, and both focus on the
100 effects of those beliefs, with practices used to attain or enhance a sense of the sacred. With this knowledge, differences can be clarified.

*Spirituality defined.* Nursing literature defines spirituality as the essence or life principle of a person (Col-
105 liton, 1981), as a sacred journey (Mische, 1982), as the experience of the radical truth of things (Legere, 1984), as giving meaning and purpose in life (Burnard, 1990; Legere, 1984), as a life relationship or sense of connectedness with mystery, a higher power, God, or uni-
110 verse (Bradshaw, 1994; Granstrom, 1985), as a belief that relates a person to the world (Soeken & Carson, 1987), as a unique human capacity for self-transcendence that creates a fulfilling relatedness within oneself, with others, and to the unseen, God, or
115 power greater than the self, and as a unifying and healing force that centers on relationships, development, wholeness, integration, and individual empowerment (Reed, 1992). Spirituality is defined as a universal human phenomenon that recognizes the wholeness of
120 individuals and their connectedness to a higher being; it is the integrating factor in the quest for meaning and purpose in life (Cavendish et al., 2000, 2001). Savett (1997) stated, "Spirituality is humanism and then some. In the clinical setting, it is finding meaning in illness
125 and then exploring that meaning. That process can be therapeutic and healing for the patient and for the healer" (p. 17). One interesting analogy is that spirituality is a force that can be equated with no other and is as mystifying as the wind in that it cannot be seen but
130 is always felt in a spectrum of intensity from still to tranquil or intense. Spirituality is different for each of us. Spirituality includes prayers, meditation, and the use of positive affirmations to obtain a release from fears and worries, finding a purpose and meaning in
135 life, and refocusing on the small joys of everyday life (Benson, 1997). Spirituality is broad and nondogmatic and involves learning and changing. Its energy flows from inward out in a process of subjective growth and connection.

140 *Religion defined.* Religion comes from the Latin word, *religare:* to tie together one of the organized systems of beliefs, practices, and worship of a person, group, or community (O'Conner, 2001). Its energy moves from outward in. This direction is presented
145 through a religion's belief system (e.g., in myths, doctrines, stories, dogma) and is acknowledged when one participates in other practices and observances. Religion can also offer guidance about how to live harmoniously with self, others, nature, and their perceived
150 god(s). Religion, seen "as a system of transcending

ideas" (Reed, 1992, p. 35), is complementary to spirituality. Religion provides the methods for the expression of one's spirituality (Engerbretson, 1996; Labun,
1988; Mayer, 1992; Oldnall, 1996; Reed, 1992). Relig-
155 ion can be seen as a bridge to spirituality in that it encourages ways of thinking, feeling, and behaving that
help people to experience this sense of meaningfulness.
Religious practice is also a way for individuals, often
in the context of sharing a similar orientation with oth-
160 ers, to express their spirituality. Religion includes spirituality; however, a person can be spiritual and not es-
pouse any particular religion or formal practice of religion. From these definitions, religion is a narrower
concept than spirituality.

*Spirituality in Education and Practice*

165   Research-based findings consistently suggest that
nurses' knowledge and skills related to spiritual care is
not adequate because of poor role preparation. A positive correlation exists between the ability of nurses
who have received spirituality education and their abil-
170 ity to provide spiritual care (Clifford & Gruca, 1987;
Harrison & Burnard, 1993; Narayanasamy, 1999b;
Piles, 1990). Clifford and Gruca (1987) stressed the
need for nurses to increase their spiritual awareness,
indicating that nurses need to start with self-reflection
175 of their own spiritual values and attitudes if they are to
help others.

Praill (1995) found that nurses who are present during times of patient distress are more likely to become
involved in a patient's spiritual care, and that nurses
180 offered spiritual care out of the center of their own
spiritual experience, suggesting that they must cultivate
personal spiritual development to provide spiritual
care.

Ross (1994) studied 685 nurses in an attempt to
185 identify factors associated with giving spiritual care.
She discovered that spiritual care could be given at
various levels of involvement with patients. Nurses
who responded at the deepest levels were aware of
their own spirituality, had experienced crises in life,
190 and were sensitive people willing to get involved at a
personal level with their patients. In addition, nurses
who belonged to a religious denomination identified
patients' spiritual needs better than nurses who had no
religious affiliation.

195   Research results indicate that the nurse's perceptions of his or her own spirituality influences the degree to which patients' spiritual needs are identified
and interventions are planned and implemented. Hall
and Lanig (1993) discovered a positive correlation be-
200 tween nurses' self-perception of Christian values and
beliefs and their degree of comfort in providing spiritual care. Chadwick (1973) found that many nurses
were aware of the presence of spiritual needs in some
of their patients but expressed that they would like fur-
205 ther education in this area. Simson (1986) concurred
with these findings and acknowledged that limited

practical guidance is available for nurses who wish to
understand a patient's spiritual needs and practices.

*Contemporary Practice Guidelines for Spiritual Care
in the United States*

The current emphasis on spirituality in society has
210 fueled the demand for nursing sensitivity regarding the
spiritual needs of individuals and families (Narayanasamy, 1999b). The inconsistency with which nurses
provide spiritual care is not congruent with the emphasis placed on spiritual care by nursing codes of conduct
215 and accreditation institutions' guides for practice. Now
that expectation for spiritual care has reached global
proportions (Taylor, 2002), the World Health Organization (WHO, 1998) redefined health. The definition
was revised to include spirituality. The four domains of
220 well-being are physical, mental, social, and spiritual.

In the United States, the Joint Commission on The
Accreditation of Healthcare Organizations (JCAHO)
must accredit all institutions seeking reimbursement for
care rendered for health care organizations. Institution
225 viability is dependent on satisfactory compliance with
JCAHO standards. The increasing demand for spiritual
and religious care prompted the addition of a spiritual
care criterion in accreditation criteria (JCAHO, 2000;
Wright, 1998). This criterion states that (a) institutions
230 must establish guidelines for the documentation of assessments of patients' spiritual beliefs and practices,
(b) pastoral care must be available for patients who
request it, and (c) hospitals must meet the spiritual
needs of dying patients and their families. The goal is
235 for the health care provider to assess the importance of
spirituality as it relates to wellness and healing.
JCAHO offers sample questions to assist nurses in their
endeavor to gather necessary information: "How does
the patient express spirituality?" "What are the pa-
240 tient's spiritual goals?" and "How would the patient
describe his or her philosophy of life?"

The International Council of Nurses (2000), a federation of national nurses' associations (NNAs), represents nurses in more than 120 countries. The ICN Code
245 for Nurses serves as the foundation for ethical nursing
practice throughout the world. The American Nurses
Association (2002) *Code for Nurses* is a guide for
nurses' ethical conduct in the United States. Both codes
contain congruent statements regarding the nurse's role
250 in promoting an environment of respect for a patient's
spirituality or religiosity during the delivery of care.
Patients have named nurses as potential spiritual resource persons (Highfield, 1992; Sodestrom &
Martinson, 1987). In the United States, the American
255 Association of Colleges of Nursing (AACN, 2002)
supports the nursing codes through association mandates to nurse educators. The "how to" of spiritual assessments, use of spiritual assessment tools, nursing
diagnoses, interventions, and outcomes are suggested
260 for inclusion in nursing curriculums. When the dialogue begins in educational programs, confidence will

250

be gained for articulating patients' spiritual needs thereby raising the nurses' comfort level for transferring this theory to practice settings (Altman, 1990).

*A Theoretical Guide for Nursing Practice*

Parse's (1981) model, which is a synthesis of Rogers's (1970, 1980) science of unitary human beings with concepts from existential-phenomenological thought, facilitates the explication of lived experiences and the significance of these experiences to those involved. Parse's model is congruent with triangulation methods. Parse's "man–environment interrelationships" facilitates the explication of emerging patterns of nurses' spiritual perspectives and participative experiences relating to spirituality in education and practice. According to Parse, while providing spiritual care, the meaning of a given health situation is guided by the nurse. Appropriate spiritual interventions to meet human responses in the spiritual domain facilitate the patient's process of transcendence. To remain a facilitator of the patient's spiritual health experience, nurses must be aware of their own personal beliefs.

Parse (1993) acknowledged the importance of the nurse's being present in the moment. The interaction between patient, family, and nurse can be a powerful experience. The goal of spiritual intervention is to enhance quality of life. One must keep in mind that only the patients can define what quality is for them: "Through true presence in living Parse's practice methodology, person and family in the presence of the nurse illuminate meaning, synchronize rhythms, and mobilize transcendence" (p. 18). As the nurse facilitates the therapeutic process, an ever-changing rhythm will develop. Through this experience, the patients will be able to share hopes and dreams as well as their personal belief system.

## Purpose

This research study describes nurses' spiritual perspectives as they relate to education and practice. The study objectives were to describe the spiritual perspectives of nurses, identify the educational needs of nurses related to the spiritual domain, and discuss spiritual care practices.

## Method

*Design*

A multiple triangulation research design encompassing a questionnaire and a descriptive qualitative content analysis were used with the purpose of capturing a more complete, holistic, and contextual description of nurses' spiritual perspectives (Knafl & Breitmayer, 1989; Thurmond, 2001). Multiple triangulation, more than one data source, methodologies, and nine investigators served to strengthen the research findings and reduce bias in all phases of the study (Polit & Hungler, 1995; Thurmond, 2001; Woods & Catanzaro, 1988). Complementary skills support the data source triangulation methodology. Survey methods (Babbie,

1990; Dillman, 1978) were used for data collection. The nurses' responses to the question, "Do you have any views about the importance or meaning of spirituality in your life that have not been addressed by the previous questions?" constituted the qualitative data.

*Sample*

Permission was obtained from Sigma Theta Tau International (STTI) Nursing Honor Society for a national random sample of 1,000 members. A cover letter, questionnaire, demographic form, and stamped return envelope were sent by first-class mail. Data were coded, aggregated, and analyzed as group data to maintain confidentiality. Institutional Review Board (IRB) approval was obtained.

With the $N$ of 545, 55%, the descriptive statistics were run on the demographic variables. Data analysis indicated that age of participants ranged from 21 to 61 years. The majority of participants were women (women: $n = 533$, 97.8%; men: $n = 11$, 2%) and had completed a BS degree ($n = 442$, 81%), followed by more than a BS degree ($n = 103$, 19%). Participants reported a religious affiliation ($n = 541$, 99%) that constituted agnostic ($n = 14$, 2.6%), Buddhist ($n = 6$, 1.1%), Catholic ($n = 201$, 37%), Jewish ($n = 4$, 0.7%), Protestant ($n = 222$, 40%), and individuals who were self-described as other ($n = 94$, 17.2%). The majority of the participants were White ($n = 497$, 91%), then African American ($n = 18$, 3.3%), Asian/Pacific Islander ($n = 115$, 2.8%), Native American/Alaskan ($n = 6$, 1.1%), Hispanic ($n = 4$, 0.7%), and other ($n = 4$, 0.7%). Marital status reported married ($n = 396$, 73%), single ($n = 96$, 17.6%), living with significant other ($n = 12$, 2.2%), and ($n = 346$, 63.6%) had children. Good health status was reported by almost all ($n = 542$, 99.4%).

## Data Collection

Reed's (1986) Spiritual Perspective Scale (SPS) was used. The SPS is a 10-item questionnaire that uses a 6-point Likert-type scale to measure one's spiritual perspective. The SPS tool measures an individual's spiritual perspective to the degree that spirituality permeates one's life and how one engages in spiritually related interactions, reporting a reliability of Cronbach's alpha coefficient of .90. Computing an arithmetic mean of the responses scores the SPS. Scores range from 1 (*low spiritual perspective*) to 6 (*high spiritual perspective*).

The nurses' responses to the question, "Do you have any views about the importance or meaning of spirituality in your life that have not been addressed by the previous questions?" constituted the qualitative data.

## Data Analysis

A Windows 2000 computer program was used for quantitative data entry. Data were entered as an ASCII file, data cleaning was done, and data were transformed

Table 1
*Qualitative Findings*

| Themes and participants' direct quotes |
| --- |

**Spirituality is strength for acceptance**

"I have been through several incidents in my life where I should have died, so I believe I am here for a reason. I believe that things happen the way they are supposed to according to God's plan."

"When a new life arrives, one knows, there must be a God! However, at times of death, disease, pain, makes me question why, usually with no answer."

**Spirituality is a belief system**

"To me, it's a philosophy about living and enters into my decisions and outlook on life."

"Spirituality can be very personal as well as very important and does not require a group."

**Spirituality is guidance**

"Spirituality is what helps me get through the difficult times in my life. It gives me hope."

"If it were not for prayer and my faith, I wouldn't have been able to cope with some of my personal challenges in life. Christ is peace."

**Spirituality is connectedness**

"The meaning of spirituality in my life has had a serious impact on all of my relationships."

"My spiritual connection is my personal relationship with Jesus Christ."

**Spirituality promotes health**

"I feel very strong about the relationship between health and spirituality. They are related."

"Spirituality provides balance and enriches my life."

**Spirituality supports practice**

"My spirituality affects the focus of my care."

"Spirituality is an important part of my practice and a part of my inner strength."

as indicated. The data were analyzed using the SPSS (Version 10.0 for Windows). Parametric and nonparametric statistics were conducted for data analysis. De-
370 scriptive statistics were tabulated noting frequencies, percentages, independent sample $t$ tests, and one-way ANOVAs on demographic data. All statistical analyses were judged based on the predetermined .05 level of significance.

375    The qualitative data were derived from the nurses' response to the question, "Do you have any views about the importance or meaning of spirituality in your life that have not been addressed by the previous questions?" Qualitative data analysis methods included
380 constant comparison of the conceptual linkages, theme identification, theme reduction, and theme validation (Munhall & Oiler-Boyd, 1993). Data were coded by extracting verbatim phrases used to describe spiritual perspectives, spirituality education, and spiritual prac-
385 tices. Data were analyzed for pattern recognition of concepts. Each researcher presented written documentation to the research committee. Themes emerged from the data as commonalities among the codes developed. Two rounds of analysis were conducted for
390 data reduction and theme validation by nine nurse researchers who were experienced in the research method and experts on spirituality.

## Results

There was no significant difference in SPS score by gender, $t(10.2) = .571$, $p = .580$, or by age, looking at
395 age 40 as a divider $t(543) = 1.551$, $p = 122$, or as age 30 as a divider $t(543) = .860$, $p = .390$. In the variable

ethnicity, there was no significance in SPS score $F(5.538) = .595$, $p = .704$. Looking at White vs. non-White, there was no significant difference $t(52.6) =$
400 .288, $p = .775$. When looking at the variable health in the questionnaire, there was a significant difference $t(2.996) = 8.419$, $p = .004$. By combining the unhealthy categories, as there are only three total participants between the two unhealthy categories, there was a sig-
405 nificant difference in the SPS scores of healthy and unhealthy nurses, such that the healthy nurses are less spiritual $t(2.996) = 8.419$, $p = .027$. Marital status was significant. Married persons show a higher SPS score $F(5.539) = 2.558$, $p = .027$, than a single person or a
410 person living with a significant other (the mean difference of SPS score is .8219, $p = .042$). Young (younger than 40 years) and older (older than 41 years) nurses with a religious affiliation had a higher SPS score than their counterparts without a religious affiliation,
415 $F(5.535) = 17.689$, $p = .001$. A Tukey's post hoc comparison was conducted: The findings indicate that agnostics are significantly lower in spirituality than every other group in the questionnaire.

Older nurses are not more likely to have a religious
420 affiliation (approximately 98% of the participants in the younger and the older categories had a religious affiliation). The existence of a religious affiliation was more influential on the SPS score than age for younger (40 years or younger) $t(308) = 5.792$, $p = .001$; and for
425 older (41 years or older) $t(229) = 6.813$, $p = .001$. Men and women with a religious affiliation have a significantly higher SPS score than their same gender coun-

252

terparts without a religious affiliation. Religious affiliation was more important for women $t(5.28) = 8.102$, $p = .001$ than for men $t(8) = 4.641$, $p = .002$. There is no significant difference in the SPS score in the variables nursing degree completed, degree type, length of STTI membership, or years of experience. Findings support Reed's work that spirituality permeates one's life. The arithmetic mean score for participants was (4.9164); standard deviation (.9911); range (1 to 6); and Cronbach's alpha coefficient (.9459).

Qualitative methods used to analyze the written responses included constant comparison of conceptual linkages, theme identification, theme reduction, and theme validation. The research question asked, "Do you have any views about the importance or meaning of spirituality in your life that have not been addressed by the previous questions?" A total of $n = 165$, 30.2%, provided responses to the aforementioned question. Six themes relating to nurses' spiritual perspectives emerged: Spirituality is strength for acceptance; spirituality is a belief system; spirituality is guidance; spirituality is connectedness; spirituality promotes health; spirituality supports practice. (See Table 1.)

The scientific rigor of qualitative research methods is determined not in terms of reliability and validity but in terms of creditability, confirmability, auditability, and fittingness. Creditability is dependent on the researcher's ability to bracket his or her own perspective and on the credibility of the informants (Bogdan & Bilken, 1982). Research meeting minutes were taken to log changes and decisions that were made during the analysis process. Transcriptions of participants' comments were reviewed for accuracy. The criteria for confirmability and creditability were met because the nine expert nurse researchers analyzed the participants' statements and comments. The criterion for auditability was met because the participants' own words have been explicated from the transcripts to validate the themes.

Trustworthiness was enhanced by nurse researchers' consensus for data reduction and theme development (Guba & Lincoln, 1981). Secondary data analysis substantiated the results found on the original analysis. The audit trail was established that consisted of the typed and coded transcripts, research meeting minutes, the data reduction, and data analysis notes including the codes and themes.

## Discussion

The current study demonstrated congruence between nurses who reported having a religious affiliation and their ability to meet patients' spiritual needs. These nurses had higher SPS scores supporting Reed's (1986) work that spirituality becomes intrinsic to one's life. The nurse participants who acknowledged having a spiritual base used it in practice. Because spiritual care has re-emerged as a critical concern for nursing (O'Neill & Kenny, 1998), the knowledge of nurses'

spiritual perspectives can provide a base to (a) develop and support spirituality educational initiatives in the nursing curriculum and (b) strengthen a nurse's ability to use information related to this phenomenon within the nursing process. As facilitator of the patient's nursing care plan, nurses are expected to provide spiritual care. In the United States, nurses must demonstrate compliance with the JCAHO standards for spiritual care evaluation and provide evidence via documentation in patient records. Ethical codes for nursing conduct mandate an environment that respects diverse beliefs and practices.

The current study supports the integration of an educational component on spirituality in the nursing curriculum. Educators cannot assume that nurses have a spiritual foundation for practice that is effective to meet the spiritual needs of patients. Patients and families report that spiritual needs are poorly met in health care settings (Carson, 1989; Narayanasamy, 1999b). The majority of participants stated that they do not feel comfortable dealing with spiritual aspects of care (Granstrom, 1985; Piles, 1990). They are reluctant to provide spiritual care even though patients may expect spiritual interventions, and such interventions may affect the healing process (Dossey & Keegan, 2000). The nurse's scope of practice supports spiritual care (Carson, 1989; Oldnall, 1996).

The strength of the current study is the support for Parse's (1993) theory as relevant to guide spiritual care. One of Parse's assumptions is that a person who agrees to participate in a study about a particular experience can share a description of that experience with the researcher. The nurse participants were able to describe living the experience. Parse's theory facilitates spiritual care through the use of "presence" meaning "to be with" (Emblen & Halstead, 1993). Presence is a form of spiritual care as it provides the nurse with a window of opportunity to enter the world of the patient to give care in the form of empathy and compassion (Gardner, 1992). There are times during nurse-patient interactions when presence is the only therapeutic form of intervention that the nurse can provide (Osterman & Schwartz-Bancrott, 1996). Presence is a purposeful, intended act. The intent to provide spiritual care was evident in the nurses who were aware of their spiritual beliefs.

Conclusions from this research reveal that nurses with religious affiliations have higher SPS scores. Nurses having a spiritual base are more likely to use it in practice. This supports Reed's (1986) work that spirituality permeates one's life. One cannot assume nurses have a foundation to provide spiritual care. The addition of an educational component to the nursing curriculum can facilitate spiritual care for patients and families. Teaching spiritual care concepts to practicing nurses is key to this process. Nurses in the United States perceive spirituality as strength, guidance, connectedness, a belief system, as promoting health, and as supporting practice. The perspectives identified in the current study can be a catalyst for opportunities to enhance spirituality in practice settings.

## References

Altman, H. B. (1990). Syllabus share: "What the teacher wants." In R. A. Neff & M. Weimer (Eds.), *Teaching college: Collected reading for the new instructor* (pp. 45–46). Madison, WI: Magna.

American Association of Colleges of Nursing. (2002). *Hallmarks of the professional nursing practice environment.* Washington, DC: Author.

American Nurses Association. (2002). *Code for nurses.* Kansas City, MO: American Nurses Publishing.

Babbie, E. (1990). *Survey research methods* (2nd ed.). Belmont, CA: Wadsworth.

Banks, R. (1980). Health and the spiritual dimension: Relationships and implications for professional preparation programs. *Journal of School Health, 50,* 195–202.

Barnum, B. S. (1996). *Spirituality in nursing: From traditional to new age.* New York: Springer.

Benson, H. (1997). *Timeless healing: The power and biology of belief.* New York: Scribner.

Bogdan, R., & Bilken, S. (1982). *Qualitative research for education: An introduction to theory and methods.* Boston: Allyn & Bacon.

Bradshaw, A. (1994). *Lighting the lamp: The spiritual dimension of nursing care.* London: Scutari.

Burnard, P. (1990). *Learning human skills: An experimental guide for nurses* (2nd ed.). Oxford, UK: Heinemann.

Carson, V. (1989). *Spiritual dimensions of nursing practice.* Philadelphia: W. B. Saunders.

Cavendish, R., Kraynyak Luise, B., Horne, K., Bauer, M., Gallo, M. A., Medefindt, J., et al. (2000). Opportunities for enhanced spirituality relevant to well adults. *Nursing Diagnosis: International Journal of Nursing Language and Classification, 11,* 151–162.

Cavendish, R., Kraynyak Luise, B., Horne, K., Bauer, M., Medefindt, J., & Russo, D., et al. (2001). Recognizing opportunities for spiritual enhancement in young adults. *Nursing Diagnosis: International Journal of Nursing Language and Classification, 12,* 77–91.

Chadwick, R. (1973). Awareness and preparedness of nurses to meet patients' spiritual needs. In J. A. Shelly & S. Fish (Eds.), *Spiritual care: The nurses' role* (pp. 177–178). Downers Grove, IL: InterVarsity Press.

Clemen-Stone, S., Eigsti, D., & McGuire, S. (1995). *Comprehensive community health nursing* (5th ed.). St. Louis, MO: Mosby Year Book.

Clifford, B., & Gruca, J. (1987). Facilitating spiritual care in rehabilitation. *Rehabilitation Nursing, 12,* 331–333.

Colliton, M. (1981). The spiritual dimensions of nursing. In E. Belland & J. Passos (Eds.), *Clinical nursing* (pp. 901–1012). New York: Macmillan.

Danvers, M. (1998). Keeping in good spirits. *Nursing Management, 5,* 35–37.

Dillman, D. (1978). *Mail and telephone surveys: The total design method.* New York: John Wiley.

Dorff, E. N. (1993). Religion at a time of crisis. *Quality of Life: A Nursing Challenge Monographs, 2,* 56–59.

Dossey, B., & Keegan, L. (2000). Self-assessment: Facilitating healing in self and others. In B. M. Dossey, L. Keegan, & C. Guzzetta (Eds.), *Holistic nursing: A handbook for practice* (3rd ed., pp. 361–374). Rockville, MD: Aspen.

Dyson, J., Cobb, M., & Forman, D. (1997). The meaning of spirituality: A literature review. *Journal of Advanced Nursing, 26,* 1183–1188.

Emblen, J., & Halstead, L. (1993). Spiritual needs and interventions: Comparing the views of patients, nurses, and chaplains. *Clinical Nurse Specialist, 1,* 175–182.

Engerbretson, J. (1996). Considerations in diagnosing in the spiritual domain. *Nursing Diagnosis: The International Journal of Nursing Language and Classification, 7,* 100–107.

Gallup, G. H. (1996). *Religion in America.* Princeton, NJ: Princeton Religious Research Center.

Gallup, G. H., & Castelli, J. (1989). *The people's religion: American faith in the 90s.* New York: Macmillan.

Gardner, D. (1992). Presence. In G. Bulchek & J. McCloskey (Eds.), *Nursing interventions: Treatments for nursing diagnoses* (2nd ed., pp. 316–324). Philadelphia: W. B. Saunders.

Granstrom, S. (1985). Spiritual nursing care for oncology patients. *Topics in Clinical Nursing, 7,* 39–45.

Guba, E., & Lincoln, Y. (1981). *Effective evaluation.* San Francisco: Jossey-Bass.

Hall, C., & Lanig, H. (1993). Spiritual care behaviors as reported by Christian nurses. *Western Journal of Nursing Research, 15,* 730–741.

Harrison, J., & Burnard, P. (1993). *Spirituality and nursing practice.* Aldershot, UK: Averbury.

Highfield, M. (1992). Spiritual health of oncology patients: Nurses and patient perspectives. *Cancer Nursing, 15,* 1–8.

Highfield, M., Taylor, E., & Amenta, M. (2000). Preparation to care: The spiritual care education of oncology and hospice nurses. *Journal of Palliative Nursing, 2,* 53–63.

International Council of Nurses. (2000). The ICN code of ethics for nurses. Retrieved October 19, 2003, from www.icn.ch/icncode.pdf

Joint Commission on the Accreditation of Healthcare Organizations. (2000). *Automated comprehensive accreditation manual for hospitals: The official handbook* [CD-ROM]. Available from www.JCAHO.com

Knafl, K., & Breitmayer, B. (1989). Triangulation in qualitative research: Issue of concept clarity and purpose. In J. M. Morse (Ed.), *Quantitative nursing research: A contemporary dialogue* (pp. 41–47). Rockville, MD: Aspen.

Labun, E. (1988). Spiritual care: An element in nursing care planning. *Journal of Advanced Nursing, 13,* 314–320.

Legere, T. (1984). A spirituality for today. *Studies in Formative Spirituality, 5,* 375–385.

Macrae, J. (1995). Nightingale's spiritual philosophy and its significance for modern nursing. *Image: Journal of Nursing Scholarship, 27,* 8–10.

Mayer, J. (1992). Wholly responsible for a part, or partly responsible for a whole? The concept of spiritual care in nursing. *Second Opinion, 17,* 26–55.

Mische, P. (1982). Toward a global spirituality. In P. Mische (Ed.), *Whole earth papers* (pp. 76–83). East Grange, NJ: Global Education Association.

Munhall, P., & Oiler-Boyd, C. (1993). *Nursing research: A qualitative perspective* (2nd ed.). New York: NLN.

Narayanasamy, A. (1999a). ASSET: A model for actioning spirituality and spiritual care education and training in nursing. *Nurse Education Today, 19,* 274–285.

Narayanasamy, A. (1999b). Learning spiritual dimensions of care from a historical perspective. *Nurse Education Today, 19,* 386–395.

Nightingale, F. (1996). *Notes on nursing.* New York: Dover. (Original work published 1860).

O'Brien, M. (1999). *Spirituality in nursing: Standing on holy ground.* Sudbury, MA: Jones and Bartlett.

O'Conner, S. (2001). Characteristics of spirituality, assessment, and prayer in holistic nursing. *Nursing Clinics of North America, 36,* 33–46.

Oldnall, A. (1996). A critical analysis of nursing: Meeting the spiritual needs of patients. *Journal of Advanced Nursing, 23,* 138–144.

O'Neill, D., & Kenny, E. (1998). Spirituality and chronic illness. *Image: Journal of Nursing Scholarship, 30,* 275–279.

Osterman, P., & Schwartz-Bancrott, D. (1996). Presence: Four ways of being there. *Nursing Forum, 31,* 23–30.

Parse, R. (1981). *Man-living-health: A theory of nursing.* New York: John Wiley.

Parse, R. (1993). Quality of life: Sciencing and living the art of human becoming. *Nursing Science Quarterly, 7,* 16–20.

Piles, C. (1990). Providing spiritual care. *Nurse Educator, 15,* 36–41.

Polit, D. E., & Hungler, B. P. (1995). *Nursing research: Principles and methods* (6th ed.). Philadelphia: J. B. Lippincott.

Praill, D. (1995). Approaches to spiritual care. *Nursing Times, 91,* 55–57.

Reed, P. (1986). Religiousness among terminally ill and healthy adults. *Research in Nursing and Health, 9,* 35–41.

Reed, P. (1992). An emerging paradigm for the investigation of spirituality in nursing. *Research in Nursing and Health, 15,* 349–357.

Rogers, M. (1970). *An introduction to the theoretical base of nursing.* Philadelphia: F. A. Davis.

Rogers, M. (1980). Nursing: A science of unitary man. In J. P. Riehl & C. Roy (Eds.), *Conceptual models for nursing practice* (2nd ed., pp. 329–337). New York: Appleton-Century-Crofts.

Ross, L. (1994). Spiritual care: The nurse's role. *Nursing Standard, 8,* 33–37.

Savett, L. (1997). Spirituality and practice: Stories, barriers and opportunities. *Creative Nursing, 4,* 17.

Shelly, J. A., & Fish, S. (1988). *Spiritual care: The nurses' role.* Downers Grove, IL: InterVarsity Press.

Simson, B. (1986). The spiritual dimension. *Nursing Times, 26,* 41–42.

Sodestrom, K., & Martinson, I. (1987). Patients' spiritual coping strategies: A study of nurse and patient perspectives. *Oncology Nursing Forum, 14,* 41–46.

Soeken, K., & Carson, V. (1987). Responding to the spiritual needs of the chronically ill. *Nursing Clinics of North America, 22,* 603–611.

Taylor, E. J. (2002). *Spiritual care.* Englewood Cliffs, NJ: Prentice Hall.

Thurmond, V. (2001). The point of triangulation. *Journal of Nursing Scholarship, 33,* 253–258.

Van Dover, L., & Bacon, J. (2001). Spiritual care in nursing practice: A close-up view. *Nursing Forum, 36,* 18–30.

Woods, N. F., & Catanzaro, M. (1988). *Nursing research: Theory and practice.* St. Louis MO: Mosby.

World Health Organization. (1998, January). Executive board meeting (Document 101). Geneva, Switzerland: Author.

Wright, K. (1998). Professional, ethical, and legal implications for spiritual care in nursing. *Image: Journal of Nursing Scholarship, 30,* 81–83.

**Acknowledgments**: The members of the Sigma Theta Tau Mu Upsilon Research Committee would like to express their appreciation to the following: the College of Staten Island Department of Nursing and the City University of New York for partial funding from a grant provided by the Professional Staff Congress.

**Address correspondence to:** Roberta Cavendish, Department of Nursing, College of Staten Island CUNY, 2800 Victory Boulevard, Staten Island, NY 10314.

# Exercise for Article 34

## Factual Questions

1. According to Cavendish et al. (2000, 2001), spirituality is defined as a universal human phenomenon that recognizes what?

2. The nurses' responses to what question constituted the qualitative data for this study?

3. A cover letter, questionnaire, demographic form, and stamped return envelope were sent by first-class mail to whom?

4. Reed's (1986) Spiritual Perspective Scale (SPS) was used to measure what?

5. Was the difference between married persons and single persons (including persons living with a significant other) statistically significant? If yes, at what probability level was it significant?

6. What are the values of the arithmetic mean and standard deviation on the Spiritual Perspective Scale?

## Questions for Discussion

7. The introduction, including the literature review, in lines 1 through 295 is somewhat longer than the other introductions to the research reported in this book. In your opinion, are long introductions useful? Explain.

8. In your opinion, is the response rate of 55% adequate for this type of research? (See line 327.)

9. The Spiritual Perspective Scale is described in lines 348–358. Information is provided on internal consistency reliability (i.e., Cronbach's alpha coefficient of .90). Is the omission of validity information in this description important? Explain.

10. The data analysis methods for the qualitative data are described in lines 364–392. In your opinion, is the description sufficiently detailed? Explain.

11. To what extent do the participants' direct quotations in Table 1 help you understand the results? Do you consider them an essential part of the Results section of this research report?

12. Would this research be as informative if the researchers used only the Spiritual Perspective Scale, on which the quantitative results are based, and omitted the qualitative question? Explain.

## Quality Ratings

Directions: Indicate your level of agreement with each of the following statements by circling a number from 5 for strongly agree (SA) to 1 for strongly disagree (SD). If you believe an item is not applicable to this research article, leave it blank. Be prepared to explain your ratings. When responding to criteria A and B, keep in mind that brief titles and abstracts are conventional in published research.

A. The title of the article is appropriate.

SA   5   4   3   2   1   SD

B. The abstract provides an effective overview of the research article.

SA   5   4   3   2   1   SD

C. The introduction establishes the importance of the study.

SA   5   4   3   2   1   SD

D. The literature review establishes the context for the study.

SA   5   4   3   2   1   SD

E. The research purpose, question, or hypothesis is clearly stated.

SA   5   4   3   2   1   SD

F. The method of sampling is sound.

SA   5   4   3   2   1   SD

G. Relevant demographics (for example, age, gender, and ethnicity) are described.

SA   5   4   3   2   1   SD

H. Measurement procedures are adequate.

SA   5   4   3   2   1   SD

I. All procedures have been described in sufficient detail to permit a replication of the study.

SA   5   4   3   2   1   SD

J. The participants have been adequately protected from potential harm.

SA   5   4   3   2   1   SD

K. The results are clearly described.

SA   5   4   3   2   1   SD

L.  The discussion/conclusion is appropriate.

       SA   5   4   3   2   1   SD

M.  Despite any flaws, the report is worthy of publication.

       SA   5   4   3   2   1   SD

# Article 35

## Developing a Residential Care Facility Version of the Observable Indicators of Nursing Home Care Quality Instrument

**Myra A. Aud**, PhD, RN, **Marilyn J. Rantz**, PhD, RN, NHA, FAAN,
**Mary Zwygart-Stauffacher**, PhD, RN,BC–GNP/GCNS, FAAN, **Pam Manion**, MS, RN, CS, GCNS[*]

ABSTRACT. The last decade has seen a substantial growth in the development of residential care facilities (assisted living facilities). Evaluation of the quality of care in this service delivery sector has been hampered by the lack of a consensus definition of quality and the lack of reliable instruments to measure quality. Founded on extensive research on nursing home care quality, a field test of the Residential Care Facility Version of the Observable Indicators of Nursing Home Care Quality Instrument was conducted in 35 residential care facilities in Missouri. Content validity of the 34 items was rated by 4 expert raters as 3.4 on a 4-point scale of relevance. Test-retest was 0.94, interrater reliability was 0.73, and internal consistency was 0.90 for the total scale, indicating excellent results for initial field testing. A focus group confirmed the 5 dimensions of quality of care measured by the instrument as important in residential care settings.

From *Journal of Nursing Care Quality*, 19, 48–57. Copyright © 2004 by Lippincott Williams & Wilkins. Reprinted with permission.

The rapid growth of residential care facilities, also called assisted living facilities or personal care homes, has raised quality concerns for these facilities that parallel concerns for nursing home quality. There are between 30,000 and 40,000 assisted living facilities in the United States caring for an estimated 1 million residents.[1] Driven in part by the increasing number of older adults, consumer demand for alternatives in long-term care, and concerns about nursing home quality, the number of assisted living facilities increased rapidly in the 1990s. Because of that rapid growth, one-third of assisted living facilities have been in operation 5 years or less, and 60% of assisted living facilities have been in operation 10 years or less.[2]

Unlike the nursing home industry, there is no national regulatory standard for assisted living facilities; each state establishes its own definition of "assisted living facility" and its own set of regulations. Assisted living facilities vary in size, services provided, admission policies, resident characteristics, and staff characteristics.[3-5] Evaluation of assisted living facilities is difficult for consumers and health care providers in the face of this variability among facilities and lack of a single definition and regulatory standard. Consumers and health care providers would benefit from a tool to measure assisted living facility care quality. While the literature on quality in long-term care facilities has addressed nursing home care quality, residential care/assisted living facilities have received little attention. Little systematic investigation of assisted living facilities and the quality of care provided has been undertaken.[6]

To explore the feasibility of using a tool designed for measurement of nursing home care quality to measure residential care facility quality, we conducted a pilot test of the Observable Indicators of Nursing Home Care Quality Instrument[7-9] in several residential care facilities in Missouri. The pilot revealed that revision of the nursing home version was necessary to account for differences in care, environment, and residents before it was appropriate for use in residential care facilities. This report describes the revision and subsequent validity and reliability testing of the residential care version. Further development of the residential care version is also described.

The Observable Indicators of Nursing Home Care Quality Instrument (Observable Indicators) was designed to measure the multidimensional concept of nursing home care quality.[10, 11] The creators of the Observable Indicators anticipated its use as a quality improvement tool for nursing homes and as a heuristic guide for consumers, including older adults and their family members, evaluating a facility prospectively when considering a facility for a friend or relative.[12]

The current version of Observable Indicators (6.0, revised July 2002) consists of 42 items. There are 5

[*]*Myra A. Aud*, Sinclair School of Nursing, University of Missouri at Columbia. *Marilyn J. Rantz*, Sinclair School of Nursing, University of Missouri at Columbia. *Mary Zwygart-Stauffacher*, Department of Nursing Systems, University of Wisconsin at Eau Claire. *Pam Manion*, Sinclair School of Nursing, University of Missouri at Columbia.

subscales: communication (5 items), care (9 items), staff (6 items), environment (16 items), and home/family involvement (6 items). The 16 items of the environment subscale are further divided into 3 subscales: space (5 items), odor/cleanliness/condition (5 items), and lighting/noise/atmosphere (6 items). Responses to all items are selected from a 5-point Likert-type scale, with 5 as the response indicating the highest quality and 1 as the response indicating the lowest quality.

The Observable Indicators was designed to be used by health care professionals, nursing home staff, lay people (such as the friends and families of residents), and nursing home residents. A study funded by the National Institutes of Health/National Institute of Nursing Research is in progress for further reliability and validity testing and to determine potential use by regulators. Assessment of the quality of care with the Observable Indicators begins as the observer walks through the facility, its general living spaces, hallways, and other areas commonly available to the public. The walk-through takes approximately 20–30 minutes, depending on the size of the facility. Visiting the facility during usual visiting hours and, if possible, close to a mealtime provides opportunities to note the features included in most of the items. Asking the staff for additional information is appropriate for some items.

**Need for a Residential Care Facility Version**

Quality improvement nurses from the Quality Improvement Project for Missouri (QIPMO) used the Observable Indicators as a part of their consultation site visits to nursing homes. As the QIPMO project expanded to include residential care facilities, the quality improvement nurses in the St. Louis area began to use the Observable Indicators to assess the quality of care in each facility. However, it was immediately apparent that some items in the tool were not appropriate for use in the residential care facility setting. The problems reflected the differences between nursing homes and residential care facilities, particularly differences in resident acuity levels, staffing, special services for confused residents, and rehabilitative therapy services.

*Acuity Levels and Staffing*

Nursing home residents are more frail and more dependent on staff for assistance than the residents of residential care facilities.[13] Direct care staffing numbers are higher in nursing homes so that personal and skilled care needs can be met. Registered nurses have a greater presence in nursing homes because health care needs of residents are greater. In the nursing home version, one item refers to the more active role of direct care staff and another item asks about assistance with eating and drinking, common tasks in nursing homes. However, most residential care facility residents are independent in these tasks. Similarly, the nursing home version has a question about assistance with mobility, another area where most residential care facility residents are independent, even if they use assistive devices. Two other items of the nursing home version specifically address the presence of registered nurses. Registered nurses are scarce in residential care facilities, where the supervisory role is frequently filled by a licensed practical nurse.

*Special Services for Confused Residents in Nursing Homes*

While some residents in residential care facilities may be confused at times or may have mild cognitive impairment, it is more likely that nursing home residents will have special care needs because of moderate to severe cognitive impairment.[13] Three items in the nursing home version are more appropriate to the special environments created in nursing homes for confused residents and especially for those who wander.

*Special Therapy Needs in Nursing Homes*

The Observable Indicators has an item: "Were therapy staff actively working with residents to improve or restore function?" This question, while appropriate for the skilled nursing facility that frequently has an in-house therapy team with services provided at least 5 days per week, is less appropriate in residential care facilities where a physical, occupational, or speech therapist may visit an individual resident as an outpatient in the same way as a therapist would visit a private home. On any given day, there may be no residential care facility residents scheduled to receive therapy services. Additionally, the question, "Were staff helping some residents walk or move about the facility without assistive devices such as canes, walkers, wheelchairs?" is a poor fit for some states' residential care facility regulatory requirements that residents be sufficiently independent in mobility in order to exit the facility without assistance during emergencies.

**Revising the Observable Indicators Instrument**

After an informal test of the Observable Indicators in several residential care facilities, the instrument was revised by the authors. The outcome of that revision is the Observable Indicators of Nursing Home Care Quality: Residential Care Facility Version. The revised instrument has 34 items and retained the 5-point Likert-type response format of the original 42-item nursing home version.

Revision of the nursing home version took 3 forms: deletion of items, rewording of items, and rewording of responses. Two items were reworded; 8 items were deleted; and 2 items were combined into one item. One new item was added to the Residential Care Facility Version: "Were exit doors equipped with monitoring systems?" There also were minor revisions of the wording of the stem and responses of 5 items, but the revisions did not alter the content of the items.

*Validity*

After the initial revision, four experts were asked to review the new Residential Care Facility Version and assess for content validity. Each of the experts was a nursing home administrator licensed to practice in Missouri who had experience with Missouri residential care facilities. Two of the experts were registered nurses and 2 had backgrounds in social work. They were evenly split from urban and nonurban areas of the state of Missouri.

Working independently, the experts were given copies of the revised instrument and a rating form with instructions to rate the relevance of each item on a 4-point rating scale. The choices on the 4-point rating scale were (1) not relevant, (2) somewhat relevant, (3) quite relevant, and (4) very relevant, following content validity measurement outlined by Waltz, Strickland, and Lenz.[14] Although it was not requested in the instructions, all of the experts wrote comments on the rating forms.

*Content validity.* The index of content validity for the total scale was 3.426. For the individual items, when the ratings assigned to each item by the 4 experts were averaged, only 5 of the 34 items had average ratings less than 3.00. The average ratings for those 5 items and the individual ratings by each expert are displayed in Table 1. No items had average ratings less than 2.0.

Table 1
*Summary of the Experts' Average Ratings Less Than 3.0.*

| Item | Mean rating |
| --- | --- |
| Were residents out of their rooms? | 2.00 |
| Were exit doors equipped with monitoring systems? | 2.00 |
| Were residents' rooms personalized with furniture, pictures, and other things from their past? | 2.25 |
| Were homelike things, such as plants and pets, in the residents' rooms? | 2.75 |
| Were visitors visible in the facility? | 2.75 |

All 4 experts wrote comments for the "Were residents out of their rooms?" item on the rating forms. Three of the comments refer to resident preferences. The comments were as follows:

1. Not sure that I understand this one. Out of room is equated to care?
2. Many have private rooms, consider them as apartments. Some choose to stay in and only come out for meals or activities of choice.
3. They have their apartments and it's their choice when to participate.
4. Some residents like to stay in their rooms.

While nursing home quality has been associated with seeing the residents out of their rooms, the emphasis in residential care facilities is on resident autonomy and independence, as well as on social interaction. When residential care facility residents stay in their rooms, this may reflect an institutional philosophy that

supports choice. If the residents choose to remain "at home" in their rooms, this might also attest to the quality of the arrangements of those rooms rather than absence of care or poor facility quality. However, remaining in one's room may also be a reaction to a lack of appealing recreational activities or to the failure of the staff to encourage participation.

Two of the experts wrote comments for the item about exit doors having monitoring systems. One expert explained that state regulations (Missouri) do not require monitoring systems on exit doors "unless resident's condition warrants this." The other expert wrote, "A lot of assisted living facilities do not have alarmed doors. We don't. Residents are free to come and go." Two key points emerge from their comments: (a) decisions about monitoring systems depend on assessment of resident condition, and (b) consideration of resident autonomy influences the use of monitoring systems.

The experts, as inferred from their comments, considered that the 2 items about resident rooms being personalized and the presence of plants and pets actually evaluated resident and family choices rather than the residential care facility and its quality. Comments included "This is a resident choice," and "This is not a facility function." Their ratings and choices again emphasize differences between nursing homes and residential care facilities. Nursing homes exert greater control over the environment of the residents' rooms. Residential care facilities tend to offer more choices to residents. Although individual nursing homes and residential care facilities may depart from these stereotypes of control and choice, nursing homes, in general, offer residents less scope for personalization of living spaces.[15]

The last item addressed the presence of visitors in the facility. One of the experts felt that responses to this item were dependent on time of day or day of week. Another expert asked, "How can someone unfamiliar with the resident or facility know who was present?" That expert also pointed out that visitors could be present but out of sight in the private room of a host-resident. Two experts questioned the usefulness of this item as a measure of the quality of the facility.

In comments related to other items, the experts drew attention to the variations among residential care facilities and to the independence of the residents as compared with nursing home residents as potential influences on responses. For example, comments on the items related to personal hygiene and grooming were: "If they care for their personal needs, we'll allow them to [do it their way]. We want them to stay as independent as possible" and "Some residents do their own personal care." The experts' comments for the items on staff visibility and the presence of a nurse in the facility also pointed out the differences among facilities and residents, and the impact of those differences on the number and type of staff present.

Table 2
*Sample Items from the Observable Indicators of Nursing Home Care Quality: Residential Care Facility Version*

| Were conversations between staff and residents friendly? (Communication) | | | | |
|---|---|---|---|---|
| 1 | 2 | 3 | 4 | 5 |
| Most were not | A few were | Some were | Many were | Most were |

| How often is a nurse present in the facility? (Staff) | | | | |
|---|---|---|---|---|
| 1 | 2 | 3 | 4 | 5 |
| Monthly | Bi-weekly | Weekly | Twice a week | Daily |

| Were odors of urine or feces noticeable in the facility? (Environment) | | | | |
|---|---|---|---|---|
| 1 | 2 | 3 | 4 | 5 |
| Pervasive throughout | Most of the time | Often | Occasionally | Hardly at all |

| Were a variety of activities available for residents? (look for posted schedule, calendars, group meetings, etc.) (Care) | | | | |
|---|---|---|---|---|
| 1 | 2 | 3 | 4 | 5 |
| Rarely seen | A few were | Some were | Many were | Lots were |

*Validity of subscales.* After reviewing the validity of each item, we also reviewed the validity of the subscales. As previously explained, the instrument has 5 major subscales: communication, care, staff, environment, and home/family involvement. The environment subscale is further divided into subscales for (a) odor, cleanliness, condition and (b) lighting, noise, atmosphere. The subscales had excellent validity as evidenced by the average rating for the relevance of all of the items in the subscales: communication, 3.90; care, 3.17; staff, 3.31; environment-a, 3.75; environment-b, 3.46; and home/family involvement, 3.00.

A decision was made to retain both items with a mean rating of 2.00. For the item in the care subscale, "Were residents out of their rooms?" we agreed with one expert comment that an item about residents being out of their rooms was to be equated with better care. We recognized that residents have a right to remain in their rooms, but we believe staff should facilitate engaging residents and their friends in activities and socialization with others. For the "Were exit doors equipped with monitoring systems?" item in the environment-b subscale, we agreed with an expert's comment that it appears that the use of monitoring systems on exit doors is related to specific facility choices based on resident condition or regulatory requirements. The item was retained because of the great variation among residential care facilities, and because recent regulatory changes in Missouri have required monitoring systems on exit doors for some categories of residential care facilities.

We also evaluated the remaining 3 items with ratings of less than 3.0 (see Table 1) that were in the home/family involvement subscale. The items rate the residents' rooms and the use of furnishings to create homelike dwelling places that are connected with the residents' pasts. Environmental design recommendations for residential care facilities emphasize the homelike nature of residential care as opposed to the nursing home environment with its historical links to hospital design.[16] Most residential care facilities encourage the residents and their families to bring in personal belongings to promote a homelike ambiance in resident rooms.

The last item in the home/family involvement subscale rates the visible presence of visitors. As the experts pointed out in their comments, the presence of visitors varies greatly across time of day and day of week. Furthermore, there may be unseen visitors in the residents' private rooms. Unlike the nursing home setting, where visitors are often found in lounge areas and where visitors and residents may be distinguished by cues such as clothing or functional independence, visitors and residents in residential care settings may be indistinguishable. However, we believe the presence of visitors is an indication of family and community involvement that is viewed by consumers as important to quality.[11]

After reviewing the average ratings for each subscale, each item, the distribution of individual expert ratings for the 5 items with mean ratings less than 3.0, and the comments of the experts for the 5 items with mean ratings less than 3.0, we decided to retain all 34 items for the field test of the instrument. The experts together rated no items as "not relevant" (i.e., no items had means of less than 2.0). Although there was a suspicion that these items, and possibly others in the instrument, may be highly site-specific, the instrument, in its first version, was accepted as possessing high content validity and plans were made to assess its reliability. Table 2 displays sample items from the Observable Indicators of Nursing Home Quality: Residential Care Facility Version. The complete instrument is available from the authors.

*Reliability*

Interrater reliability and test-retest reliability were measured for the Residential Care Facility Version of the Observable Indicators of Nursing Home Care Quality Instrument. Content validity assessment answers the question "Does the instrument measure what we want it to measure?" Interrater reliability and test-retest

Table 3
*Summary of Reliability of Results*

| Dimension | Number of items per subscale | Test-retest correlation[*] | Interrater correlation[†] | Cronbach's alpha[‡] |
|---|---|---|---|---|
| Communication | 5 | .81 | .76 | .96 |
| Care | 6 | .88 | .52 | .71 |
| Staff | 4 | .66 | .57 | .38 |
| Environment | 13 | .94 | .79 | .81 |
| Env-OCC[§] | 6 | .86 | .81 | .81 |
| Env-LNA[‖] | 7 | .93 | .66 | .60 |
| Home/family | 6 | .86 | .51 | .76 |
| *Full scale* | *34* | *.94* | *.73* | *.90* |

[*] *N* equal to 140 is the total number of instruments completed.
[†] Spearman's *rho*. Significant at < .0001.
[‡] Cronbach's alpha. Raw alpha values rather than the standardized values are cited because all items are on the same 1–5 point scale.
[§] Env-OCC: odor/cleanliness/condition.
[‖] Env-LNA: lighting/noise/atmosphere.

reliability answer the questions "Do different assessors using the instrument at the same site and at the same time achieve similar results?" and "Does the instrument yield similar results when used again at same sites after a specified time interval?"

The Residential Care Facility Version was tested in 35 licensed residential care facilities in Missouri. A convenience sample of facilities was selected from three geographic regions in the state. Each of the 3 regional teams of quality improvement nurses from the QIPMO project recruited 10 residential care facilities in their respective regions for the reliability field test. The centers of the regions were St. Louis, Columbia, and Kansas City. Initially, 10 facilities were selected in each of the 3 regions. Later, 5 additional facilities in the southeastern quadrant of the state were added to increase the geographic diversity of the sample. The quality improvement nurses were asked to stratify the convenience sample according to facility size with 30% of the facilities licensed for 1–30 residents, 40% of the facilities licensed for 31–60 residents, and 30% of the facilities licensed for more than 61 residents. The quality improvement nurses recruited the facilities to participate in this voluntary evaluation of the instrument.

With the permission of the administrators of the facilities, pairs of QIPMO quality improvement nurses visited each facility twice during the summer and autumn of 2001. There was an interval of 7–10 days between visits. On each visit, the quality improvement nurses walked together through the facility making observations and then independently completed the instrument. Visits to the facilities were made between 8:00 A.M. and 5:00 P.M. from Monday through Friday. No visits were made in evenings or on weekends. Completed assessment tools (*n* = 140) were sent by the nurses to the QIPMO project office.

The statistical analysis included the calculation of Cronbach's alpha for the full scale and subscales and interrater and test-retest item correlations. To quantify the strength of agreement between raters, weighted Kappa coefficients were also calculated for each item.

Table 3 displays the reliability analyses for each subscale and the full scale. The total scale has excellent test-retest reliability, good interrater reliability, and excellent internal consistency. Additionally, most subscales also have excellent and good results. Therefore, preliminary psychometric studies show great promise that the instrument measures quality of residential care facilities, though further testing is needed.

### Revisions of First Version of Tool

After the field test in the 35 residential care facilities, we carefully reviewed the results of the validity and reliability studies for possible revisions to items to improve item and subscale performance. As indicated earlier, the tool we tested had 34 items, some of which the content validity experts questioned. The item "Were residents out of their rooms?" that was questioned by the experts considering validity was deleted. This item had acceptable interrater reliability, but a nonsignificant test-retest correlation suggested a lack of stability over time. We also combined 2 items that addressed the presence and condition of plants and pets in the facility into one item "Were their pets and/or live plants in good condition?" After these changes, the subscale structure was: communication (5 items), care (5 items), staff (4 items), environment (12 items), and home/family (6 items) with the environment subscale further divided into odor/cleanliness/condition (6 items) and lighting/noise/atmosphere (6 items). The total scale was 32 items.

The statistician expressed concern that responses to several items were clustered at one end of the 5-point scale rather than distributed among the range of responses. Therefore, the anchors of these items were revised. The choice "Not Applicable" was added to 2 items.

### Focus Group

Before proceeding with revisions and further testing, we decided we needed to explore additional dimensions of residential care quality and issues raised by the content experts in the comments written on their content validity forms. We recruited five additional experienced residential care administrators to participate in a focus group to discuss their perceptions of quality of residential care. Similar to the four original content experts, these participants had many years of experience as administrators or other direct care staff members in both urban and rural facilities in Missouri and surrounding states.

Using a discussion guide that was similar to the one successfully used to examine nursing home care quality,[10, 11] the focus group participants, after informed consent, were asked to recall particular facilities they had observed in the past that they thought were "excellent places, really doing a good job providing excellent resident care to their residents." Participants were debriefed on what they saw, felt, smelled, heard, and touched in those facilities. We discussed key features they thought were important for quality of care. Descriptions of facilities where they had observed poor quality care were also discussed to better understand care quality in residential care facilities.

The discussion tapes were analyzed to identify additional quality dimensions or additional items to be added to the Residential Care Facility Version. The results of the focus group interview confirmed the appropriateness of 5 dimensions of care quality as discovered in the nursing home research.[10, 11] The results also pointed out the need to add items on the topics of food choices and snack availability, access to telephone and e-mail or other computer-based communication. We added those items to the current Version 7 that is being used in a larger field test that is currently underway in 3 states.

## Discussion

Measuring quality of care in residential care facilities is extremely important, given the dramatic increase in the number of these facilities nationwide. The results of this small-scale field study and follow-up focus group indicate that care quality is an important issue for facility providers, their residents, and the families and friends who visit. It is interesting that while there are many differences between residential care settings and nursing homes, the quality of care dimensions are the same. The major dimensions of communication, care, staff, environment, home, and family involvement that were discovered and confirmed in earlier work in nursing homes[7, 8, 10, 11] appear to be on-target theoretically in residential care settings. However, there are many differences that must be accounted for in the actual items measuring these dimensions.

The emphasis on autonomy and resident choice in residential care facilities is one of these differences. While nursing home staff and regulators have attempted to promote autonomy and choice, the nursing home setting is continually plagued by their reputation of regimes with which residents must comply.[16, 17] Consumers who live in residential care voice their fears

of being forced from their homelike apartments to traditional institutional nursing homes.[18]

The findings of this study are limited because the relatively small sample was selected among facilities in only one state and was not randomly selected. We are currently conducting a larger scale study in which the instrument is being used in 3 states with a larger sample. With further development, we anticipate that the residential care version will be of interest to several constituencies.

An instrument to quickly evaluate quality of care in residential care is of interest to consumers. Families who are attempting to locate care for a loved one need help in judging quality of care. Decisions about moving into a residential care facility cannot be driven by only proximity, which is often the case. Given the range of quality in services that are available, consumers when making a choice need to be knowledgeable about key elements to observe in facilities. We believe that making a good choice based on quality of care is a better choice in the long run. Our research team has information posted on our Web site www.nursinghomehelp.org to help consumers as they are faced with long-term care decisions.

Regulators of residential care facilities will also benefit from having an instrument to measure residential care quality. Typically, regulators focus on compliance with established rules and regulations. The premise of the regulations is that if those minimum standards are met, then there is at least adequate quality of care. Having other ways to quickly evaluate quality of care can be of assistance to regulators who are often stretched across large numbers of facilities in varying geographic regions.

Operators of residential care facilities can also make use of an instrument to measure quality. With the current emphasis on quality improvement programs in all of long-term care,[19] quality improvement teams within facilities can objectively examine their facility and care delivery and design quality improvement projects in areas where they find that they could use improvement.

Obviously, from our point of view as researchers, other researchers interested in understanding and conducting studies in residential care settings can benefit from an instrument measuring residential care quality. Given the results of this field study, we think the Residential Care Version of the Observable Indicators holds much promise for researchers. The initial validity and reliability studies indicate that it has reasonably sound reliability and excellent validity. We anticipate that the revisions made on the basis of this field study will improve the performance of individual items, subscales, and total scale. We are confident that the dimensions of quality of care (communication, care, staffing, environment, and home/family involvement) are theoretically sound and appropriate for this setting. We encourage other researchers to contact us for the most recent version of the Observable Indicators of Nursing Home Care Quality: Residential Care Facility Version Instrument.

### References

1. PriceWaterhouseCoopers. *An Overview of the Assisted Living Industry, 1998.* Fairfax, VA: Assisted Living Federation of America; 1998.
2. Hawes C, Rose M, Phillips CD. *A National Study of Assisted Living for the Frail Elderly: Results of a National Survey of Facilities.* Beachwood, OH: Meyers Research Institute; 1999.
3. Zimmerman S, Eckert JK, Wildfire JB. The process of care. In: Zimmerman S, Sloane PO, Eckert JK, eds. *Assisted Living: Needs, Practices, and Policies in Residential Care for the Elderly.* Baltimore, MD: Johns Hopkins University Press; 2001:198–223.
4. Morgan LA, Gruber-Baldini AL, Magaziner J. Resident characteristics. In: Zimmerman S, Sloane PO, Eden JK, eds. *Assisted Living: Needs, Practices, and Policies in Residential Care for the Elderly.* Baltimore, MD: Johns Hopkins University Press; 2001:144–172.
5. Hodlewsky RT. Staffing problems and strategies in assisted living. In: Zimmerman S, Sloane PO, Eckert JK, eds. *Assisted Living: Needs, Practices, and Policies in Residential Care for the Elderly.* Baltimore, MD: Johns Hopkins University Press; 2001:78–91.
6. Hawes C. Introduction. In: Zimmerman S, Sloane PO, Eckert JK, eds. *Assisted Living: Needs, Practices, and Policies in Residential Care for the Elderly.* Baltimore, MD: Johns Hopkins University Press; 2001:1–6.
7. Rantz MJ, Mehr DR, Petroski GF, et al. Initial field-testing of an instrument to measure: Observable indicators of nursing home quality. *J Nurs Care Qual.* 2000;14(3):1–12.
8. Rantz MJ, Mehr DR. A quest to understand and measure nursing home quality of care. *Long-Term Care Interface.* 2001;2(7):34–38.
9. Rantz M, Jensdottir AB, Hjaltadottir I, et al. International field test results of the observable indicators of nursing home care quality instrument. *Int Nurs Rev.* 2002;49(4):234–242.
10. Rantz MJ, Mehr D, Popejoy L, et al. Nursing home care quality: A multidimensional theoretical model. *J Nurs Care Qual.* 1998;12(3):30–46.
11. Rantz MJ, Zwygart-Stauffacher M, Popejoy L, et al. Nursing home care quality: A multidimensional theoretical model integrating the views of consumers and providers. *J Nurs Care Qual.* 1999;14(1):16–37.
12. Rantz M, Popejoy L, Zwygart-Stauffacher M. *The New Nursing Homes: A 20-Minute Way to Find Great Long-Term Care.* Minneapolis, MN: Fairview Press; 2001.
13. Kane RA, Kane RL, Ladd RC. *The Heart of Long-Term Care.* New York: Oxford University Press; 1998.
14. Waltz CF, Strickland OL, Lenz ER. *Measurement in Nursing Research.* Philadelphia: FA Davis; 1984.
15. Schwarz B. Assisted living: An evolving place type. In: Schwarz B, Brent R, eds. *Aging, Autonomy, and Architecture: Advances in Assisted Living.* Baltimore, MD: Johns Hopkins University Press; 1999: 185–206.
16. Regnier VA, Scott AC. Creating a therapeutic environment: Lessons from Northern European models. In: Zimmerman S, Sloane PO, Eckert JK, eds. *Assisted Living: Needs, Practices, and Policies in Residential Care for the Elderly.* Baltimore, MD: Johns Hopkins University Press; 2001:53–77.
17. Regnier VA. The definition and evolution of assisted living within a changing system of long-term care. In: Schwarz B, Brent R, eds. *Aging, Autonomy, and Architecture: Advances in Assisted Living.* Baltimore, MD: Johns Hopkins University Press; 1999:3–19.
18. Frank J. How can I stay?: The dilemma of aging in place in assisted living. In: Schwarz B, ed. *Assisted Living: Sobering Realities.* New York: Haworth Press; 2001:15–30.
19. Kane RA. Long-term care and a good quality of life: bringing them closer together. *Gerontologist.* 2001;41(3):293–304.

**Acknowledgments**: The authors wish to acknowledge the contributions of the other quality improvement nurses who participated in this field study: Carol Siem, Katy Nguyen, Elizabeth Sutherland, De Minner, Amy Vogelsmeier, Clara Boland, and Dale Potter. We also wish to thank Greg Petroski for statistical support and Steve Miller for data support.

**Address correspondence to:** Myra A. Aud, PhD, RN, Sinclair School of Nursing (S 422), University of Missouri at Columbia, Columbia, MO 65211. E-mail: audm@health.missouri.edu

# Exercise for Article 35

## Factual Questions

1. Responses to all items on the Observable Indicators of Nursing Home Care Quality: Residential Care Facility Version Instrument are selected from a 5-point Likert-type scale. What does a response of 5 indicate?

2. Although it was not requested in the instructions, how many of the experts wrote comments on the rating forms?

3. How many of the 34 items had average ratings by the experts of less than 3.00?

4. The researchers point out that interrater reliability answers this question: "Do different assessors using the instrument at the same site and at the same time achieve similar results?" According to the researchers, what question does test-retest reliability answer?

5. Which "dimension" has the lowest test-retest reliability?

6. How many additional experienced residential care administrators participated in the focus group to discuss their perceptions of quality of residential care?

## Questions for Discussion

7. The experts who examined the instrument for content validity worked independently. In your opinion, is it desirable to have them work independently *or* would it have been better if they worked in consultation with each other? (See lines 170–173.)

8. What is your opinion on the researchers' decision to retain the two items with expert ratings of 2.00? (See Table 1 and lines 275–293.)

9. Keeping in mind that the complete instrument is available from the authors (see lines 335–336 and 534–538), are the sample items in Table 2 sufficient for a research report of this type? To what extent do the items help you understand what the instrument measures?

10. The researchers discuss the content validity of the instrument in lines 180–336. Based on this information, are you convinced that the instrument has a high level of content validity? Explain.

11. The researchers state that the total scale (i.e., full scale) has "excellent" test-retest reliability. Do you agree? Explain. (See lines 385–387 and Table 3.)

12. To what extent, if any, did the focus group part of this research convince you that the instrument is valid? (See lines 418–454.)

## Quality Ratings

Directions: Indicate your level of agreement with each of the following statements by circling a number from 5 for strongly agree (SA) to 1 for strongly disagree (SD). If you believe an item is not applicable to this research article, leave it blank. Be prepared to explain your ratings. When responding to criteria A and B, keep in mind that brief titles and abstracts are conventional in published research.

A. The title of the article is appropriate.

    SA   5   4   3   2   1   SD

B. The abstract provides an effective overview of the research article.

    SA   5   4   3   2   1   SD

C. The introduction establishes the importance of the study.

    SA   5   4   3   2   1   SD

D. The literature review establishes the context for the study.

    SA   5   4   3   2   1   SD

E. The research purpose, question, or hypothesis is clearly stated.

    SA   5   4   3   2   1   SD

F. The method of sampling is sound.

    SA   5   4   3   2   1   SD

G. Relevant demographics (for example, age, gender, and ethnicity) are described.

    SA   5   4   3   2   1   SD

H. Measurement procedures are adequate.

    SA   5   4   3   2   1   SD

I. All procedures have been described in sufficient detail to permit a replication of the study.

    SA   5   4   3   2   1   SD

J. The participants have been adequately protected from potential harm.

    SA   5   4   3   2   1   SD

K. The results are clearly described.

    SA   5   4   3   2   1   SD

L. The discussion/conclusion is appropriate.

    SA   5   4   3   2   1   SD

M. Despite any flaws, the report is worthy of publication.

    SA   5   4   3   2   1   SD

# Article 36

## Preverbal, Early Verbal Pediatric Pain Scale (PEPPS): Development and Early Psychometric Testing

**Alyce A. Schultz**, RN, PhD, **Ellen Murphy**, RN, MSN, **Jennifer Morton**, RN, BSN,
**Audrey Stempel**, RN, MSEd, **Carole Messenger-Rioux**, RN, NNP, **Kathleen Bennett**, RN[*]

ABSTRACT. The Preverbal, Early Verbal Pediatric Pain Scale (PEPPS) is conceptualized to measure the established pain response in toddlers, a pediatric group void of pain assessment scales. It consists of seven categories, each with weighted indicators. Scores can range from 0 to 26. Using a blinded, cross-sectional design, 40 children, aged 12 to 24 months, were videotaped throughout their postoperative stay in the postanesthesia care unit. Vignettes were randomly selected and viewed by four experienced pediatric nurses. Results indicated that the PEPPS was easy to use and demonstrated acceptable interrater and intrarater reliability. Early evidence of construct validity was established by statistically significant differences in premedication and postmedication pain scores.

From *Journal of Pediatric Nursing*, 14, 19–27. Copyright © 1999 by the W.B. Saunders Company. Reprinted with permission.

Before the late 1970s, clinical and empirical work on pain and pain management focused entirely on adults. It was not until 1977 that the term "pain" even appeared in medical and nursing pediatric textbooks.
5 Twenty years later, the assessment and management of pain in children continue to challenge health professionals, with the assessment and management of pain in the nonverbal child being particularly difficult (Anand & Craig, 1996).
10 Children who have similar diagnoses and procedures receive far less pain management than their adult counterparts (Schechter, 1989; Truog & Anand, 1989). Yet, empirical evidence supports that the experience of pain impedes healing and recovery in very young chil-
15 dren just as it does in adults and older children (Eland & Coy, 1990; Fitzgerald & Anand, 1993; Marchette, Main, & Redick, 1989; Stevens & Franck, 1995). The ethical justification for this undertreatment of pain in the young has been questioned (Walco, Cassidy, &
20 Schechter, 1994).

Research-based protocols for the assessment and management of pain have been developed for adults and children who are old enough to self-report their

pain (AHCPR, 1992; Schmidt, Holiday, Kleiber, Peter-
25 sen, & Phearman, 1994). It is now generally accepted that children older than 4 years of age are able to accurately self-report painful experiences. Although there is still debate, children as young as 3 years of age have been reported as reliable if they are able to count to 10
30 and understand the scales (Keck, Gerkensmeyer, Joyce, & Schade, 1996; Knott et al., 1994; Wong & Baker, 1988). Development of assessment scales for preverbal, early verbal children remains a priority (NINR, 1994).
35 Recent work has contributed assessment scales for infants (Barrier, Attia, Mayer, Amiel-Tison, & Shnider, 1989; Krechel & Bildner, 1995; Lawrence et al., 1993; Stevens, Johnston, Petryshen, & Taddio, 1996; Taddio, Nulman, Koren, Stevens, & Koren, 1995). The toddler,
40 however, continues to be included with older children who are capable of self-report (McGrath et al., 1985; Merkel, Voepel-Lewis, Shayevitz, & Malviya, 1997; Robieux, Kumar, Radhakrishman, & Koren, 1991). The purpose of this research was to develop and vali-
45 date psychometric properties of the Preverbal, Early Verbal Pediatric Pain Scale (PEPPS), designed specifically for the toddler population.

### Background

This selected review of the literature addresses work in the assessment of pain in preverbal, early ver-
50 bal children, defined as less than 3 years of age. No studies were found that specifically addressed behaviors in the toddler population.

### Behavioral Categories

A number of studies have been conducted to evaluate specific behavioral responses by infants and tod-
55 dlers to painful stimuli (i.e., cry, facial expressions, and body movements) (Table 1). Supporting the work of earlier research, investigators reported that although the cry response may differ across the developmental stages, from preterm to toddler, experienced practitio-
60 ners were able to recognize and differentiate among

---

[*]All authors are at the Maine Medical Center, Portland, Maine.

cries suggestive of fussiness, hunger, and pain. They further concluded that the cry response alone is not adequate to measure the immediate pain response, particularly in preterm infants who do not always use cry in response to painful stimuli (Grunau & Craig, 1987; Grunau, Johnston, & Craig, 1990; Fuller, Horii, & Conner, 1989; Porter, Miller, & Marshall, 1986).

Table 1
*Pain Behaviors*

| Category | Descriptors | Authors |
| --- | --- | --- |
| Cry/vocaliza-tion | Latency to cry, duration of cry cycle, frequency, melody, and dys-phonia | Owens & Todt, 1984; Porter, Miller, & Marshall, 1986; Fuller, Horii, & Conner, 1989; Grunau, Johnston, & Craig, 1990; Ste-vens, Johnston, & Grunau, 1995 |
| Facial expres-sions | Brow activity, nasal root, eyes, mouth, chin, and tongue | Izard, 1982; Izard, Hembree, & Hueb-ner, 1987; Grunau & Craig, 1987; Craig, Grunau, & Aquon-Assee, 1988; Grunau et al., 1990; Fuller & Conner, 1995 |
| Body movement | Limb movements, thrashing, jerk-ing, wiggling, withdrawing, kicking, and torso rigidity | Craig, McMahon, Morison, & Zaskow, 1984; Dole, 1986; Johnston & Strada, 1986; Mills, 1989; Bozzette, 1993 |

Facial expressions have also been found to differ in response to varying painful stimuli according to age (Attia, Amiel-Tison, Mayer, Shnider, & Barrier, 1987; Grunau & Craig, 1987; Grunau et al., 1990; McGrath et al., 1985). Composite scores, based on 10 facial actions, were found to differ with different stimuli and to differ from the cry response (Grunau & Craig, 1987; Grunau et al., 1990). Body movements that also differ developmentally have been linked with the pain response. Specific movements of the body have been studied individually for their correlation with painful stimuli (Craig, McMahon, Morison, & Zaskow, 1984; Attia et al., 1987; Barrier et al., 1989; McGrath et al., 1985; Gauvain-Piquard, Rodary, Rezvani, & Lemerle, 1987).

Sociability, consolability, and readiness to feed or suck have not been consistently included in behavioral work assessing pain in very young children. Yet, early work on the management of pain in very young children suggests that the postoperative engagement of parents with their child is consoling to the child. Further research correlating the response of children to these interventions and the subsequent reduction of pain is needed.

*Assessment Scales*

A recent publication by the National Institute of Nursing Research (1994) devoted an entire chapter to the measurement of pain in the preverbal child. It was noted that although valid pain assessment scales have been developed for older children and adults, no valid and reliable scales exist for the very young.

Health care providers are somewhat reticent to accept the use of behavioral characteristics as adequate in the management of painful responses in very young children. Although physiological measures are viewed as more objective, they are inconclusive in determining the presence of pain (Brown, 1987; Maxwell, Yaster, Wetzel, & Niebyl, 1987; Taddio et al., 1995; Tarbell, Cohen, & March, 1992). Most of the physiological indicators (e.g., taking nonmonitored heart rate or blood pressure) produce stressful stimuli in the process of their measurement, thereby negating their reliability and validity as representative of pain. Hence, emphasis has focused on the observation of changes in behavior when developing scales for very young children.

Published scales for preverbal, early verbal children were reviewed for inclusion of varying behavioral categories and reported psychometric testing (Table 2). The review indicated that several tools are available specifically for the infant population, from premature infants through 1 year of age. Other scales used to measure pain in early verbal children, however, also included older, verbal children. All the scales included indicators for facial expression, cry, and body posture. A variety of descriptors were used within each category. In several scales, the various movements of the legs, torsos, and even arms were measured separately (Barrier et al., 1989; Lawrence et al., 1993; McGrath et al., 1985; Merkel et al., 1997). This division of body responses resulted in heavier scale weights for body movements than for cry and facial expressions. No theoretical explanations were given for these decisions. The Postoperative Pain Scale (POPS), developed for use with infants, included all the behavioral categories (Barrier et al., 1989) as compared with the Premature Infant Pain Profile (PIPP), which focused primarily on facial movements (Stevens et al., 1996).

All the scales reported some estimation of reliability and validity (Table 2). Construct validity was addressed primarily using the known groups technique whereby premedication and postmedication pain scale scores were compared for significant differences. Convergent validity, another approach to measuring construct validity, was examined most frequently by comparing the scale under study with the visual analogue scale as determined by nursing staff (Lawrence et al., 1993; McGrath et al., 1985; Robieux et al., 1991; Taddio et al., 1995; Tarbell et al., 1992); other investigators reported validity testing of their new scales with other published but nonvalidated scales (Krechel & Bildner, 1995; Merkel et al., 1997). Only one study reported that the raters or scale evaluators were blinded to the pain medication or painful procedure (Robieux et al., 1991). Interestingly, the child must be awake to use

Table 2
*Behavioral Categories*

| Scales | Age range | Facial | Cry | Consolability & sociability | Body posture | Sucking/ feeding | Reliability & validity | Authors |
|--------|-----------|--------|-----|------------------------------|--------------|------------------|-------------------------|---------|
| PIPP | Premature infants | ✓ | | | | | IRR, Construct | Stevens et al., 1996 |
| CRIES | Neonates | ✓ | ✓ | | | | IRR, Construct | Krechel & Bildner, 1995 |
| POPS | 1–7 months | ✓ | ✓ | ✓ | ✓ | | Construct | Barrier et al., 1989 |
| NIPS | 2–6 months | ✓ | ✓ | | ✓ | ✓ | IRR, Int. Consistency Construct | Lawrence et al., 1993 |
| MBPS | 4–6 months | ✓ | ✓ | | ✓ | | IRR Intrarater Int. Consistency, Construct | Taddio et al., 1995 |
| BPS | Infant/ toddler | ✓ | ✓ | | ✓ | | Construct | Robieux et al., 1991 |
| FLACC | 2 months–7 years | ✓ | ✓ | ✓ | ✓ | | IRR, Construct | Merkel et al., 1997 |
| TPPPS | 1–5 years | ✓ | ✓ | | | | IRR, Construct | Tarbell et al., 1992 |
| CHEOPS | 1–7 years | ✓ | ✓ | | ✓ | | IRR, Construct | McGrath et al., 1985 |

Abbreviations: PIPP, Premature Infant Pain Profile; CRIES, Crying, Requires oxygen, Increased vital signs, Expression, Sleeplessness; POPS, Postoperative Pain Scale; NIPS, Neonatal Infant Pain Scale; MBPS, Modified Behavioral Pain Scale; BPS, Behavioral Pain Scale; FLACC, Facial expression, Leg movement, Activity, Cry, Consolability; TPPPS, Toddler Preschooler Postoperative Pain Scale; CHEOPS, Children's Hospital of Eastern Ontario Pain Scale.

the Toddler Preschooler Postoperative Pain Scale (TPPPS) (Tarbell et al., 1992). All the scales were evaluated during needle-stick procedures or during the immediate postoperative period. The Children's Hospi-
155 tal of Eastern Ontario Pain Scale (CHEOPS) was later tested with children, aged 4 to 7 years, outside the recovery room with less than satisfactory correlations to self-reported pain (Beyer, McGrath, & Berde, 1990).

No scale specifically measured postoperative pain
160 in the toddler. Thus, the first phase of this project was to develop an assessment scale that would measure "the established pain response" or the pain stimulated by surgery in preverbal, early verbal children. This "pain response" was envisioned as a composite picture
165 characterized by physiological changes in heart rate and behavioral changes in facial expression, cry, body posture, sociability, consolability/state of restfulness, and sucking/feeding.

### Development of the PEPPS

Seven pediatric nurses, each with 7 to 18 years of
170 pediatric experience, established a Pediatric Pain Committee to address the issues of pain assessment and management in preverbal, early verbal children, from premature infants to toddlers, of approximately 36 months. They were particularly concerned with pain
175 assessment of children who were unable to self-report the location and severity of their pain. In developing domains for the scale, they followed the stages suggested by Green and Lewis (1986) for establishing content validity: (1) review of relevant literature, (2) per-
180 sonal reflection of the developer's ideas about the con-

cept under study, (3) identification of components of the concept, (4) generation of multiple items that demonstrate the concept, and (5) empirical examination of the interrelationship of items and how they cluster
185 around the components of the concept.

The investigators closely observed and recorded postoperative behaviors of young children. They simultaneously completed an extensive review of the literature on pain in preverbal children. Based on consensus,
190 items that reflected the multifaceted construct of pain were generated in physiological and behavioral categories. A preliminary version of the pain assessment scale was shared with pediatric physicians, anesthesiologists, and staff nurses within the various settings where very
195 young children were provided postoperative care. Feedback from these health care providers was incorporated into the scale.

The investigators then used the scale postoperatively with a variety of preverbal, early verbal children
200 to establish face validity and utility. In preparation for further psychometric testing of the instrument, a pilot study was conducted by the investigators within their practice settings. Four investigators established interrater reliability among themselves and then with an-
205 other nurse in their same practice setting by simultaneously observing children during their postoperative period. All nurses using the scale reported that the scale was easy to use and intuitively captured the pain behaviors in this age group. Twenty-six observations
210 on 10 children were completed. Pearson's correlation revealed significantly high agreement ($r = .97$, $p \le$

267

.000) among the nurses who used the scale. The results of this pilot study were reported at an international pain conference in 1994 (Murphy et al., 1994).

The strongest recommendations from the conference suggested that the scale should be targeted specifically at the toddler population, as these children are developmentally different from the infant population, but cannot use the self-report scales. The investigators returned to the bedside to focus on toddler behaviors exhibiting pain. The current version of the PEPPS contains seven categories, each containing two to four indicators of varying levels of responses to painful stimuli. Descriptors were identified that reflected behaviors ranging from the subtleties of mild pain to the demonstrative nature of severe pain (Table 3). Categorical scores can range from 0 to 4 in all categories except for the sucking/feeding category where scores range from 0 to 2. The desire to eat or suck after surgery may be more closely correlated with the feeling of nausea than pain. Total scores are determined by summing the categorical scores and can range from 0 to 26.

## Methodology

The purpose of this study was to empirically examine the psychometric properties of the PEPPS. Psychometric evaluation is designed to examine the degree to which an instrument measures the same concept time after time and the extent to which it measures what it is intended to measure (Burns & Grove, 1993; Carmines & Zeller, 1979). This evaluation included examination of reliability and validity. The blinded, cross-sectional study was approved by the hospital's Institutional Review Board and conducted in the postanesthesia care unit (PACU) of a 606-bed tertiary care hospital in northern New England.

### Sample

Subjects were a convenience sample of children between the ages of 12 and 24 months scheduled for urologic or general abdominal surgery. Children with known developmental delays were excluded from the study.

### Procedure

Parents of children who met the study criteria were approached by the primary investigator or study coordinator for informed consent in the waiting area the morning of surgery. The study was carefully described, with particular emphasis on the option of participating and the certainty that postoperative care would not be altered by the study. Parents were assured confidentiality and the right to withdraw at any time with no adverse effects on their child's postoperative care. Parents were given a copy of the signed informed consent and an additional flyer that described the study and provided names and phone numbers of the primary investigator and study coordinator. After surgery, the children were admitted to a private treatment room within PACU. A PACU nurse was assigned to provide individual care to each child. Standard perioperative care was not altered. Parents were present in the PACU and held the children as soon as they emerged from anesthesia. The children were videotaped throughout their PACU experience, using a Panasonic AG-450 S-VHS camcorder with an Audio-Technica AT815a shotgun microphone and Maxell ST-126 BQ S-VHS videotape. The study coordinator collected demographic data, baseline pulse, and preoperative and intraoperative medication information from the chart. Heart rate and pulse oximetry were recorded every 5 minutes during the PACU period, as were the time and dose of postoperative pain medications.

Table 3 *how they scored*
*Preverbal, Early Verbal Pediatric Pain Scale (PEPPS)©*

| Heart Rate | Body Posture |
|---|---|
| 4—40 beats/min above baseline | 4—Sustained arching, flailing, thrashing and/or kicking |
| 3—31–40 beats above baseline | 3—Intermittent or sustained movement with or without periods of rigidity |
| 2—21–30 beats above baseline | |
| 1—10–20 beats above baseline | 2—Localization with extension or flexion or stiff and nonmoving |
| 0—baseline range | |
| **Facial** | 1—Clenched fists, curled toes and/or reaching for, touching wound or area |
| 4—Severe grimace; brows lowered, tightly drawn together; eyes tightly closed | 0—Body at rest, relaxed positioning |
| 2—Grimace; brows drawn together; eyes partially closed, squinting | **Sociability** |
| 0—Relaxed facial expression | 4—Absent eye contact, response to voice and/or touch |
| **Cry (Audible/Visible)** | 2—With effort, responds to voice and/or touch, makes eye contact, difficult to obtain and maintain |
| 4—Screaming | |
| 3—Sustained crying | |
| 2—Intermittent crying | |
| 1—Whimpering, groaning, fussiness | 0—Responds to voice and/or touch, makes eye contact and/or smiles, easy to obtain and maintain; sleeping |
| 0—No cry | |
| **Consolability/State of Restfulness** | |
| 4—Unable to console, restlessness, sustained movement | **Sucking/Feeding** |
| 2—Able to console, distract with difficulty, intermittent restlessness, irritability | 2—Lack of sucking, refusing food, fluids |
| | 1—Disorganized sucking, attempting to eat or drink but discontinues |
| 1—Distractible, easy to console, intermittent fussiness | 0—Sucking, drinking and/or eating well |
| 0—Pleasant, well integrated | 0—N/A; NPO and/or does not use oral stimuli |

Total score: _____

*face validity* ✓

*convenience sample — people that were available*

Two to four vignettes 2 to 3 minutes long were selected for each study child for a total of 120 vignettes. Vignettes were selected to include behaviors exhibited before and after pain medication. Premedication time was defined as 10 minutes before receiving medication. Postmedication time was defined as 5 to 7 minutes after receipt of fentanyl, 7 to 10 minutes after morphine, and 20 minutes after Tylenol or B&O suppository (McEvoy, 1996). These times represent the peak periods of expected analgesic effect for each medication. Other vignettes were randomly selected from time periods that did not fit into either the premedication or the postmedication definition; these were labeled *nonmedication* vignettes. Thus, nonmedication vignettes were those time periods at least 10 minutes before any administration of pain medication or after the time of expected peak action. All vignettes were carefully selected so that no evidence of medication administration was visible. The vignettes were then randomly ordered into seven viewing tapes, each containing 15 to 20 vignettes.

Four pediatric nurses, blinded to the administration of pain medications, individually viewed each tape and scored each vignette using the PEPPS. Each viewer followed a protocol for viewing the vignettes (Table 4). Each vignette had its own scoring form. The scoring sessions were scheduled approximately 4 weeks apart. The pediatric nurses who scored the vignettes were part of the research team that developed the scale but were not involved in caring for these children preoperatively or postoperatively or in preparing the vignettes.

Table 4
*Guidelines for Reviewing PEPPS Tapes*

Each of you will receive a copy of the tape for review. A Master Copy of all tapes will be retained in the audiovisual department.

1. Carefully fill out the information in the upper right hand corner of the assessment form.
2. Select an area for viewing that is free from distractions.
3. View the complete vignette WITHOUT PAUSING. DO NOT REWIND THE TAPE AT ANY TIME DURING THE VIEWING. Instant replay is not allowed. YOU CAN AND PROBABLY SHOULD STOP the tape between vignettes so you can complete each scoring.
4. Record a PEPPS score for each vignette (approximately 2 to 3 minutes). If you have any additional comments, please put them on the forms.
5. When you are finished with the viewing, return the tape and all copies of the PEPPS to either Alyce Schultz or Ellen Murphy.

*Reliability Measurement*

Three approaches were used to examine reliability: interrater reliability, intrarater reliability, and internal consistency. Pearson's correlation was used to determine interrater and intrarater reliability. To determine interrater reliability, the four raters independently viewed and scored the behaviors captured on the 120 vignettes. To determine intrarater reliability, the raters viewed 14 vignettes a second time 2 months after the

first viewing. Internal consistency of the scale was measured using Cronbach's alpha.

*Validity Measurement*

Empirical analysis of the content validity, as described by Green and Lewis (1986), was addressed by examining variations in the categorical scores and in the total pain scores. Representativeness of the indicators within each category was further probed by the primary investigator and study coordinator who were not involved in scoring the vignettes. All indicators within each category were examined for their frequency in scoring the varying intensities of pain response behaviors.

Construct validity was examined by testing the theoretical assumption that pain can be expected to decrease after the administration of appropriate doses of analgesic medications. Using the known groups approach, sometimes referred to as contrasting groups, premedication scores were compared with postmedication scores (Woods & Catanzaro, 1988).

## Findings

*Demographics*

A total of 40 children, 35 boys and 5 girls, participated in the study. The children ranged in age from 12 to 24 months, with a mean age of 16.2 months. Seven children had inguinal hernia repairs, nine had hypospadius repairs, eight had an orchipexy, three had ureteral reimplantations; the other 13 children had a variety of urologic or abdominal procedures. Thirty-nine children received intraoperative pain medications.

*Reliability Data*

Interrater correlations ranged from .90 to .96. Intrarater correlations ranged from .96 to .98. Cronbach's coefficient alpha for the total scale was .89. Interitem correlations ranged from .15 for Sucking/Feeding and Heart Rate to .88 for Consolability and Cry (Table 5). Similarly, item to total scale correlations for Sucking/Feeding and Heart Rate were .37 and .38, respectively. Eliminating these items would only slightly improve the internal consistency.

Table 5
*Item-to-Item Correlations*

| | Heart rate | Facial | Cry | Body posture | Sociability | Consolability | Sucking/feeding |
|---|---|---|---|---|---|---|---|
| Heart Rate | – | | | | | | |
| Facial | .2813 | – | | | | | |
| Cry | .3803 | .7789 | – | | | | |
| Body Posture | .2874 | .6564 | .7388 | – | | | |
| Sociability | .3722 | .6455 | .7667 | .7149 | | | |
| Consolability | .4056 | .7433 | .8768 | .7869 | .8497 | – | |
| Sucking/Feeding | .1536 | .2920 | .3296 | .3233 | .3405 | .3990 | – |

*Validity Data*

Content validity was addressed during the development of the scale and by examining the utilization of items in scoring the pain response behaviors. Total pain scores covered the entire possible range of 0 to 26, with a mean score of 8.4 (*SD*, 6.57). Fifty-seven percent of the vignettes depicted pain scores of 8 or less. Only 15% of the scores were higher than 16. All items were used to score pain, with items reflecting severe pain used less frequently.

Construct validity was assessed, using the known-group method, by comparing premedication and postmedication pain scores. Twenty children received medication in PACU, with six children receiving medication twice for a total of 26 premedication vignettes. Twenty-five corresponding postmedication vignettes were available. One child was discharged from the PACU before the established time for peak performance of the analgesic (i.e., Tylenol). Using paired *t* test, there was a statistically significant difference in the premedication and postmedication scores for the 25 pairs, *t* = 14.58, *p* = .0000. There was a statistically significant difference among the pain scores for premedication, postmedication, and nonmedication behaviors, $F(2,477) = 145.29$, $p < .001$ (Fig. 1). Using Scheffe as the post hoc test of comparison, pain scores for postmedication-related behaviors were significantly lower than scores for nonmedication and premedication behaviors ($p < .05$), and pain scores for nonmedication-related behaviors were significantly lower than scores for premedication behaviors ($p < .05$).

### Discussion

This phase of psychometric testing supports early evidence that the PEPPS is a valid and reliable scale for measuring immediate postoperative pain in the toddler, an age group void of published pain assessment scales. Two- to three-minute vignettes of the postoperative behaviors of children provided sufficient time for the viewers to assess behaviors exhibiting pain, as compared with those behaviors that exhibited a non-painful or less painful state. It is hypothesized that nurses who are taking care of the children could complete the scale in even less time because the behaviors in the PEPPS are the same behaviors reportedly used in the systematic assessment of the experienced pain response.

The sample for the study was selected from toddlers between the ages of 12 and 24 months who were scheduled for urologic or general abdominal surgery. This selection process resulted in an overrepresentation of males in the sample. However, the sample is representative of the children in this age group who are undergoing these types of surgical procedures. Future studies should address this limitation by following children after other types of surgery and equalizing representation of females. Expanding the study to include toddlers up to the age of 36 months may also

help address this gender bias. The sample in this study was Caucasian, representative of the population within the state. Future studies should be conducted in facilities where possible ethnic differences can be assessed.

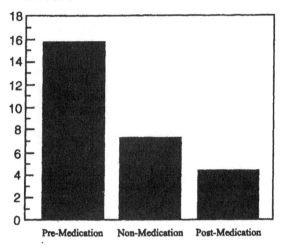

Scale Score

*Figure 1.* Comparison of mean pain scores for pre-medication, post-medication, and non-medication responses.

High interrater and intrarater reliability were evident. Generalization of these findings is limited because the raters were also members of the team that developed the scale. In the pilot study, four nurses who developed the scale and five nurses not involved in the development of the scale were able to achieve high interrater reliability ($r = .97$). The "uninvolved" nurses reported the scale as easy to use and indicative of pain response behaviors in the toddler. It will be important in future studies to use health care providers who were not intimately involved in the development of the scale to provide further estimates of reliability and utility.

Internal consistency among the categories was supported. The high item-to-total score correlations suggest that varying categories are measuring facets of the same construct, supporting the gestalt of the construct. The overall alpha of .89 suggests that the scale reflects subtle discriminations in levels of the construct (Burns & Grove, 1993). It is important to note, however, that the item-to-item correlations for the five behavioral categories (i.e., facial, cry, body posture, sociability, and consolability) ranged from .66 to .88, somewhat higher than the interitem correlations of .30 to .70 recommended by Nunnally (1978). Internal consistency should continue to be assessed in future studies. Although the categories of Heart Rate and Sucking/Feeding could be eliminated without adversely affecting internal consistency, it is too premature in the use of the instrument to support their elimination. Heart Rate as a poor indicator of pain has been reported by other investigators (Taddio et al., 1995; Tarbell et al.,

270

1992). Many children who are emerging from anesthesia are not yet ready to take fluids orally due to an upset stomach rather than pain. Close attention to the Sucking/Feeding category should be emphasized as the scale is tested further away from the PACU setting.

Early evidence of construct validity is supported by the significant differences in pain scores for children before receipt of pain medications as compared with their scores after analgesic administration. This analysis provided power of 1.00, with an alpha of .01, for the differences found in the premedication and postmedication scores (Borenstein & Cohen, 1988).

Almost all the children (39/40) were given pain medication intraoperatively. This anticipatory pain management appeared to work for half the children who, based on the intuitive assessment of pain by the PACU nurse caregiver, were not given pain medication during their PACU stay. From this experience, one could also extrapolate support for scores of the non-medication vignettes falling somewhere between the higher scores, when the PACU nurse determined the child needed medication, and the lowest scores, representing relief from pain after administration of an analgesic. Future examination of construct validity may provide further explanation for these findings.

The analysis provided additional validity for the domains of the scale. All the indicators within each category were used with varying frequency to capture descriptors of pain behaviors. The items suggesting greater pain were not used as often as those representing mild or moderate pain. This finding may be strongly related to the fact that all but one child received intraoperative pain medication. Further, the children in this study all had pain medication orders for their PACU stay. The children were not allowed to experience severe pain for the benefit of the study. Pain medication orders do not necessarily continue for those children after their immediate recovery period. The broad use of all the indicators should be reviewed in future studies, particularly as the scale is used by health care providers in an inpatient setting.

Using a pain assessment scale that is not specifically developed to represent the developmental stage of the toddler may leave these young children at a disadvantage for appropriate and adequate postoperative pain management. Early evidence for construct validity, reliability, and utility of the PEPPS for use in the immediate postoperative recovery period is supported by this study. Its usefulness outside this setting cannot be generalized until the scale is tested during extended postoperative experiences. Psychometric testing of newly developed scales is a continuous process and must be addressed with each study.

## References

Anand, K.J.S., & Craig, K.D. (1996). Editorial. New perspectives on the definition of pain. *Pain, 67*, 3–6.

Attia, J., Amiel-Tison, A., Mayer, M.N., Shnider, S.M., & Barrier, G. (1987). Measurement of postoperative pain and narcotic administration in infants using a new clinical scoring system. *Anesthesiology, 67*(3A), 66.

Barrier, G., Attia, J., Mayer, M.N., Amiel-Tison, C., & Shnider, S.M. (1989). Measurement of post-operative pain and narcotic administration in infants using a new clinical scoring system. *Intensive Care Medicine, 15*(Suppl 1), S37–S39.

Beyer, J.E., McGrath, P.J., & Berde, C.B. (1990). Discordance between self-report and behavioral measures in 3–7-year-old children following surgery. *Journal of Pain and Symptom Management, 5*, 350–356.

Borenstein, M., & Cohen, J. (1988). *Statistical power analysis: A computer program*. Hillsdale, JH: Lawence Erlbaum Associates, Inc.

Bozzette, M. (1993). Observation of pain behavior in the NICU: An exploratory study. *Journal of Perinatology Neonatology Nursing, 7*, 76–87.

Brown, L. (1987). Physiological responses to cutaneous pain in neonates. *Neonatal Network, 6*(3), 18–22.

Burns, N., & Grove, S.K. (1993). *The practice of nursing research: Conduct, critique, & utilization*. Philadelphia: W.B. Saunders Company.

Carmines, E.G., & Zeller, R.A. (1979). *Reliability and validity assessment*. Newbury Park, CA: Sage University Paper.

Craig, K.D., Grunau, R.V.E., & Aquon-Assee, J.C. (1988). Judgement of pain in newborns: Facial activity and cry as determinants. *Canadian Journal of Behavioral Science, 20*, 442–451.

Craig, K.D., McMahon, R.J., Morison, J.D., & Zaskow, C. (1984). Development changes in infant pain expression during immunization injections. *Social Science in Medicine, 19*, 1331–1337.

Dole, J.C. (1986). A multidimensional study of infants' responses to painful stimuli. *Pediatric Nursing, 12*, 27–31.

Eland, J., & Coy, J. (1990). Assessing pain in the critically ill child. *Focus on Critical Care, 17*, 469–475.

Fitzgerald, M., & Anand, K.J.S. (1993). Developmental neuroanatomy and neurophysiology of pain. In N.L. Schechter, C.B. Berde, & M. Yaster (Eds.), *Pain in infants and children* (pp. 11–31). Philadelphia: Williams and Wilkins.

Fuller, B.F., & Conner, D.A. (1995). The effect of pain on infant behaviors. *Clinical Nursing Research, 4*, 253–273.

Fuller, B.F., Horii, Y., & Conner, D. (1989). Vocal measures of infant pain. In S.G. Funk, E.M. Tornquist, L.A. Copp, M.T. Champagne, & R.A. Weise (Eds.), *Key aspects of comfort: Management of pain, fatigue, and nausea* (pp. 46–51). New York: Springer Publishing Co.

Gauvain-Piquard, A., Rodary, C., Rezvani, A., & Lemerle, J. (1987). Pain in children aged 2–6 years: A new observational rating scale elaborated in a pediatric oncology unit—preliminary report. *Pain, 31*, 177–188.

Green, L., & Lewis, F. (1986). *Measurement evaluation in health education and health promotion*. Palo Alto, CA: Mayfield.

Grunau, R.V.E., & Craig, K.D. (1987). Pain expression in neonates: Facial action and cry. *Pain, 28*, 395–410.

Grunau, R.V.E., Johnston, C.C., & Craig, K.D. (1990). Neonatal facial and cry responses to invasive and non-invasive procedures. *Pain, 42*, 295–305.

Izard, C.E. (1982). *Measuring emotions in infants and children*. New York: Cambridge University Press.

Izard, C.E., Hembree, E.A., & Huebner, R.R. (1987). Infant's emotional expressions to acute pain: Developmental change and stability of individual differences. *Developmental Psychology, 23*, 105–113.

Johnston, C.C., & Strada, M.E. (1986). Acute pain response in infants: A multidimensional description. *Pain, 24*, 373–382.

Keck, J.F., Gerkensmeyer, J.E., Joyce, B.A., & Schade. J.G. (1996). Reliability and validity of the FACES and word descriptor scales to measure procedural pain. *Journal of Pediatric Nursing, 11*, 368–374.

Knott, C., Beyer, J., Villarruel, A., Denyes, M., Erickson, V., & Willard, G. (1994). Using the oucher: Developmental approach to pain assessment in children. *MCN, 19*, 314–320.

Krechel, S., & Bildner, J. (1995). Cries: A new neonatal post-op pain assessment score. Initial testing of validity and reliability. *Paediatric Anaesthesia, 5*, 53–61.

Lawrence, J., Alcock, D., McGrath, P., Kay, J., MacMurray, S., & Dulberg, C. (1993). The development of a tool to assess neonatal pain. *Neonatal Network, 12*, 59–67.

Marchette, L., Main, R., & Redick, E. (1989). Pain reduction during neonatal circumcision. *Pediatric Nursing, 15*, 207–210.

Maxwell, L.G., Yaster, M., Wetzel, R.C., & Niebyl, J.R. (1987). Penile nerve block for newborn circumcision. *Obstetrics and Gynecology, 70*, 415–419.

McEvoy, G.K. (1996). American Hospital Formulary Service Drug Information. Bethesda, MD: American Society of Health System Pharmacists, Inc.

McGrath, P.J., Johnson, G., Goodman, J.T., Schillinger, J., Dunn, J., & Chapman, J.A. (1985). CHEOPS: A behavioral scale for rating postoperative pain in children. In H.L. Fields (Ed.), *Advances in pain research and therapy* (Vol. 9, pp. 395–402). New York: Raven Press.

Merkel, S.I., Voepel-Lewis, T., Shayevitz, J.R., & Malviya, S. (1997). The FLACC: A behavioral scale for scoring postoperative pain in young children. *Pediatric Nursing, 23*, 293–297.

Mills, N.M. (1989). Pain behavior in infants and toddlers. *Journal of Pain and Symptom Management, 4*, 184–190.

Murphy, E., Bennett, K., Ent, S., Messenger-Rioux, C., Morton, J., Stempel, A., & Thompson, B. (1994, June). Development of a pain assessment scale for the preverbal, early-verbal child (Abstract No. 160). Presented at The

Third International Symposium on Pediatric Pain. Children and Pain: Integrating Science and Care. Philadelphia, PA.

National Institute of Nursing Research. (1994). National Nursing Research Agenda: Volume 6. *Symptom management: Acute pain.* Bethesda, MD: National Institutes of Health, U.S. Department of Health and Human Services.

Nunnally, J.C. (1978). *Psychometric theory.* New York: McGraw Hill Book Company.

Owens, M.E., & Todt, E.H. (1984). Pain in infancy: Neonatal reaction to a heel lance. *Pain, 20,* 77–86.

Porter, F.L., Miller, R.H., & Marshall, R.E. (1986). Neonatal pain cries: Effect of circumcision on acoustic features and perceived urgency. *Child Development, 57,* 790–802.

Robieux, I., Kumar, R., Radhakrishnan, S., & Koren, G. (1991). Assessing pain and analgesia with a lodocaine-prilocaine emulsion in infants and toddlers during venipuncture. *Journal of Pediatrics, 118,* 971–973.

Schechter, N.L. (1989). The undertreatment of pain in children: An overview. *Pediatric Clinics of North America, 36,* 781–794.

Schmidt, K., Holiday, D., Kleiber, C., Petersen, M., & Phearman, L. (1994). Implementation of the AHCPR pain guidelines for children. *Journal of Nursing Care Quality, 8*(3), 68–74.

Stevens, B.J., & Franck, L. (1995). Special needs of preterm infants in the management of pain and discomfort. *JOGNN, 24,* 856–862.

Stevens, B.J., Johnston, C.C., & Grunau, R.V.E. (1995). Issues of assessment of pain and discomfort in neonates. *JOGNN, 24,* 849–855.

Stevens, B., Johnston, C., Petryshen, P., & Taddio, A. (1996). Premature Infant Pain Profile: Development and initial validation. *Clinical Journal of Pain, 12,* 13–22.

Taddio, A., Nulman, I., Koren, B.S., Stevens, B., & Koren, G. (1995). A revised measure of acute pain in infants. *Journal of Pain and Symptom Management, 10,* 456–463.

Tarbell, S.E., Cohen, T., & March, J.L. (1992). The toddler–preschooler postoperative pain scale: An observational scale for measuring postoperative pain in children aged 1–5. Preliminary report. *Pain, 50,* 273–280.

Truog, R., & Anand, K.J.S. (1989). Management of pain in the postoperative neonate. *Clinics in Perinatology, 16*(1), 61–78.

U.S. Department of Health and Human Services, Public Health Service, Agency for Health Care Policy and Research. (1992). *Acute pain management: Operative or medical procedures and trauma. Clinical practice guideline.* DHHS Pub. No. (AHCPR) 92-0032. Silver Spring, MD: AHCPR Clearinghouse.

Walco, G.A., Cassidy, R.C., & Schechter, N.L. (1994). Pain, hurt, and harm: The ethics of pain control in infants and children. *The New England Journal of Medicine, 331,* 541–544.

Wong, D., & Baker, C. (1988). Pain in children: Comparison of assessment scales. *Pediatric Nursing, 14,* 9–17.

Woods, N.F., & Catanzaro, M. (1988). *Nursing research. Theory and practice.* St. Louis: C.V. Mosby Company.

**Note:** This work was supported, in part, by a grant from the Maine Medical Center Medical Research Committee.

**Address reprint requests to:** Alyce A. Schultz, RN, PhD, Maine Medical Center, 22 Bramhall Street, Portland, ME 04102.

# Exercise for Article 36

## Factual Questions

1. "Preverbal, early verbal" children are defined as being less than how many years of age?

2. Physiological indicators (e.g., taking blood pressure) negate what?

3. In 1986, Green and Lewis suggested how many stages for establishing content validity?

4. "Premedication time" was defined as how many minutes before receiving medication?

5. In Table 5, which correlation coefficient represents the strongest relationship?

6. In this study, what percentage of the scores on the PEPPS was higher than 16?

7. Was there a statistically significant difference among the pain scores for premedication, postmedication, and nonmedication?

## Questions for Discussion

8. The researchers state that they used a "convenience sample." In your opinion, is this an important issue? Explain. (See lines 245–247.)

9. This study used children undergoing surgery. In your opinion, is it safe to generalize the results to children who are not undergoing surgery? Explain.

10. The researchers state that the four pediatric nurses were "blinded to the administration of pain medications." What do you think this means? Is it important? Explain. (See lines 299–301.)

11. Do you agree with the first sentence under the heading "Discussion"? (See lines 383–387.)

12. If you were to conduct another study on the same topic, what changes in the research methodology, if any, would you make?

## Quality Ratings

Directions: Indicate your level of agreement with each of the following statements by circling a number from 5 for strongly agree (SA) to 1 for strongly disagree (SD). If you believe an item is not applicable to this research article, leave it blank. Be prepared to explain your ratings. When responding to criteria A and B, keep in mind that brief titles and abstracts are conventional in published research.

A. The title of the article is appropriate.

   SA   5   4   3   2   1   SD

B. The abstract provides an effective overview of the research article.

   SA   5   4   3   2   1   SD

C. The introduction establishes the importance of the study.

   SA   5   4   3   2   1   SD

D. The literature review establishes the context for the study.

   SA   5   4   3   2   1   SD

E. The research purpose, question, or hypothesis is clearly stated.

   SA   5   4   3   2   1   SD

F.  The method of sampling is sound.

    SA   5   4   3   2   1   SD

G.  Relevant demographics (for example, age, gender, and ethnicity) are described.

    SA   5   4   3   2   1   SD

H.  Measurement procedures are adequate.

    SA   5   4   3   2   1   SD

I.  All procedures have been described in sufficient detail to permit a replication of the study.

    SA   5   4   3   2   1   SD

J.  The participants have been adequately protected from potential harm.

    SA   5   4   3   2   1   SD

K.  The results are clearly described.

    SA   5   4   3   2   1   SD

L.  The discussion/conclusion is appropriate.

    SA   5   4   3   2   1   SD

M.  Despite any flaws, the report is worthy of publication.

    SA   5   4   3   2   1   SD

# Article 37

# Revised Susceptibility, Benefits, and Barriers Scale for Mammography Screening

Victoria L. Champion[*]

ABSTRACT. The purpose of this research was to revise scales measuring perceived susceptibility to breast cancer and perceived benefits and barriers to mammography utilization. A total of 618 women age 50 and over who were enrolled in a large intervention study participated in data collection. Scales were revised beginning with focus group input. Analyses included internal consistency reliability, test-retest reliability, factor analysis, confirmatory analysis, and known group techniques to test construct validity. Internal consistency ranged from .75 to .88, and test reliabilities from .59 to .72. Construct validity was confirmed with exploratory and confirmatory factor analyses, as well as known group techniques. Overall, these scales represent an improvement in those previously reported.

From *Research in Nursing & Health*, *22*, 341–348. Copyright © 1999 by John Wiley & Sons, Inc. Reprinted with permission.

Breast cancer mortality is beginning to decrease in white women across all age groups, with deaths decreasing by approximately 6% from 1989 to 1992 (Chevarley & White, 1997). This mortality decline is thought to be due mainly to mammography screening. Although this trend is encouraging, statistics for overall mortality are still problematic. It is estimated that in 1999 approximately 43,300 women will die of breast cancer (Landis, Murray, Bolden, & Wingo, 1999). Because mammography has been shown to decrease breast cancer mortality by 25%–35% in women age 50 and over when consistently used, it is extremely important to maintain screening in this age group (Andersson et al., 1988; Roberts et al., 1990; Shapiro, 1989; Shapiro, Venet, Strax, Venet, & Roeser, 1982; Tabar & Dean, 1987).

Most current estimates are that between 20% and 50% of women 40 and over have the recommended yearly mammograms (Chevarley & White, 1997). Interventions based upon the Health Belief Model (HBM) variables of perceived susceptibility, benefits, and barriers (Becker, 1974) have been shown to increase breast cancer screening significantly (Champion & Huster, 1995). Previous development of susceptibility, benefits, and barriers scales related to mammography has been useful in both descriptive and intervention work in general populations (Champion, 1993; 1995). The current work extends instrument development to a Health Maintenance Organization (HMO) population. The purpose of the current research was to test revised scales measuring susceptibility to breast cancer and benefits and barriers related to mammography screening for validity and reliability in an HMO and general medicine clinic population.

Perceived susceptibility and perceived severity were together identified as a threat and initially combined in the HBM as a predictor of preventive behaviors (Becker, 1974). Theoretically, before health-promoting behaviors will occur, a threat must be recognized. In the case of mammography, a woman must perceive both that breast cancer is serious and that there is a possibility that she is personally at risk for breast cancer. Because little variance usually is found in breast cancer severity, perceived susceptibility alone is used as the threat variable. An increase in perceived susceptibility has been linked to an increase in breast cancer screening (Stein, Fox, Murata, & Morisky, 1992; Zapka, Hosmer, Constanza, Harris, & Stoddard, 1992).

In addition to perceived susceptibility, perceived benefits to taking action and perceived barriers to action are central constructs of the HBM. Perceived benefits refer to the perception of positive outcomes thought to accrue from a behavior. In the case of mammography screening, benefits relate to the potential to discover breast cancer early, thereby avoiding death. Perceived barriers refer to negative attributes related to the health action. For mammography screening, barriers might include fear of cancer, pain, cost, time, or fear of radiation. Theoretically, a perception of more benefits to screening combined with perception of few barriers will be associated with breast cancer screening. Many investigators have verified the usefulness of perceived benefits and barriers in predicting mammography behavior. They have demonstrated that increased benefits and decreased barriers are linked to increased screening (Champion, 1992; Rakowski et al., 1992; Rakowski, Rimer, & Bryant, 1993; Slenker & Grant, 1989; Tho-

---

[*]*Victoria L. Champion*, Mary Margaret Walther professor of nursing and associate dean for research, Indiana University School of Nursing.

mas, Fox, Leake, & Roetzheim, 1996). In addition, in several intervention studies investigators have demonstrated the usefulness of including these constructs in communication messages designed to increase screening (Champion & Huster, 1995; King et al., 1993; Rimer et al., 1992). Beliefs about susceptibility, benefits, and barriers have been found to differentiate women in various stages related to mammography compliance (Champion & Skinner, 1999; Skinner, Champion, Gonin, & Hanna, 1997). In order to test theoretical relationships between revised scale scores and stages of compliance with screening recommendations, the Transtheoretical Model was used in this study (Rakowski et al., 1993). The conceptual definitions in this study, which also were used for previous instrument development, are shown in Table 1.

The stages of precontemplation, contemplation, action, relapse precontemplation, and relapse contemplation were used. In the Transtheoretical Model, any behavior change or adoption is conceptualized as a continuum. Action is defined as current compliance. Women may also relapse or become noncompliant after initial screening. They are then staged as relapse precontemplation or relapse contemplation.

The ability to identify the relationships between susceptibility, benefits and barriers, and compliance with mammography recommendations has been critical in determining their influence on screening behavior. The perceived susceptibility to breast cancer scale was developed and reported initially in 1984 (Champion, 1984) and underwent subsequent revision (Champion, 1993). Benefits and barriers scales for mammography were developed later and reported by Champion (1995). Initial development of the perceived susceptibility scale as reported by Champion (1984) started with extensive review of the theoretical and empirical literature. Initially, 20–24 items were written to measure susceptibility. Content validity was established through a panel of eight judges who were familiar with the HBM. Items were retained if there was a 75% agreement among judges. Approximately half of the original items reached the 75% agreement criterion. All items were anchored with a five-point Likert scale with response options from "strongly agree" to "strongly disagree." Data were collected with a general population.

The susceptibility scale as initially developed retained six items after factor analysis and item deletion (Champion, 1984). The initial testing of the susceptibility scale demonstrated beginning validity and reliability. The susceptibility scale was revised again using a random sample of 581 women (Champion, 1993). Content validity was judged by an expert panel consisting of nationally known researchers and theoreticians. A consensus of three experts was necessary for item retention. Five items were retained in this analysis for susceptibility. Exploratory factor analysis was completed and all items loaded at .84 or above on the sus-

ceptibility factor. A Cronbach alpha of .93 was realized with a test-retest reliability of .70. Predictive validity was demonstrated when susceptibility was significantly correlated with breast cancer screening behavior.

Table 1
*Conceptual Definitions of Major Study Variables*

| | |
|---|---|
| Perceived susceptibility | Perceived beliefs of personal threat or harm related to breast cancer |
| Perceived benefits (mammography) | Perceived positive outcomes of obtaining a mammogram |
| Perceived barriers | Perceived emotional, physical, or structural concerns related to mammography behaviors |
| Precontemplation | Never had a mammogram and not thinking about having one in the next 6 months |
| Contemplation | Never had a mammogram but thinking about having one in the next 6 months |
| Action | Had a mammogram within the last 15 months |
| Relapse precontemplation | Last mammogram 15 months ago or more and not thinking about having one in the next 6 months |
| Relapse contemplation | Last mammogram 15 months ago or more and thinking about having one in the next 6 months |

The initial benefits and barriers scales were developed in relation to the behavior of breast self-examination and reported by Champion (1984). They included a total of five benefits items and eight barriers items. The two scales were found to have Cronbach's alpha of .61 and .76, respectively. This scale was revised in 1995 (Champion, 1995) to reflect benefits and barriers to mammography. Because benefits and barriers for mammography may be different from those for Breast Self-Examination (BSE), a thorough examination of the literature and theory was completed again prior to the revision. Items were developed on the basis of literature and theoretical definitions. Eight items initially were developed for each scale and sent to a panel of experts for content validity. The benefits and barriers to mammography scales were tested at the same time the second testing for the susceptibility scale was done. A total of 581 women participated. Confirmatory factor analysis supported construct validity. Confirmatory factor analysis revealed factor loadings of .44 or above for each of six benefits items and five barriers items. Correlational analysis confirmed theoretical relationships, further supporting validity. The Cronbach alpha was .79 for the benefit scale and .73 for the barrier scale. Test-retest correlations were somewhat lower, as reported in the summary by Champion (1995). This was thought to reflect actual changes in attitudes rather than inconsistency across measurements. The current work required scales that were valid and reliable for an HMO population. Validity and reliability are sample specific; therefore, further testing was required.

## Method

### Participants

Revision of the HBM scales took place within a large intervention study to increase breast cancer screening in women age 50 and over ($N = 804$) who were members of an HMO and general medicine clinic.

The mean age of participants was 61.15 ($SD = 9.66$). Mean educational level was 12.5 years ($SD = 2.70$). Forty-six percent were married, 25% widowed, and 21% divorced. The remaining participants were never married, living with a partner, or separated. Sixty-eight percent were Caucasian and 30% African American, with the remainder being of Asian, Native American, or Hispanic descent. Eligibility criteria included being age 50 or over, not having had a mammogram in the last 15 months, not having had breast cancer, and being able to read and write English. There was a response rate of 39% from eligible women. Reasons for declining were related to hesitancy to commit to a longitudinal intervention study.

### Instrument

The work of refinement began with a review of susceptibility, benefits, and barriers items from past work by the principal investigator and an advisory panel. In addition, items were presented to two focus groups of women age 50 and over to assess clarity of meaning. Women also were asked for additional items not included. Focus group comments did not contain any information suggesting needed changes in items. Prior results for the susceptibility scale indicated that all items were highly correlated; thus, two redundant items were deleted prior to testing. Three items were retained and related to perceived risk of developing breast cancer at different times in a woman's life.

Five items were retained for the benefit scale. The original item, "When I get a recommended mammogram, I feel good about myself" was deleted because it had the lowest factor loading in previous work. Other changes in benefits items were made after clarifications from a focus group. For example, a previous item, "Having a mammogram or x-ray of the breast will decrease my chances of requiring radical or disfiguring surgery for breast cancer," was changed to, "If I find a lump through a mammogram, my treatment for breast cancer may not be as bad." The items relating to decreased worry, finding breast lumps early, treatment not being as bad, best way of finding a very small lump, and decreasing chances of dying were retained.

The barriers scale also was revised. Initially, there were five items that respectively addressed worry about breast cancer, embarrassment, time, pain, and money. Items were added that related to understanding what will be done, knowing how to go about getting a mammogram, rudeness of personnel, radiation, remembering to schedule a mammogram, being too old

to have a mammogram, and having other problems that are more important. The additional items were recommended as a result of the two focus group discussions. The original cost item was dropped because the current population had cost completely covered. The additional barriers are reflected in the new items. A total of 11 items were included on the revised scale. Items comprising the barrier scales do potentially represent different dimensions, raising the question of a homogeneous set of items. Past analysis has demonstrated unidimensionality of items; unidimensionality was reexamined as part of the work of revision.

### Procedures

Eligible women from the HMO were identified by computer and sent an introductory letter signed by the medical director of the HMO. This letter was followed by a telephone call from a research assistant, who further described the study and asked each woman if she would be willing to participate. If agreement was obtained, the participant was sent an informed consent statement and a questionnaire that included the scales for susceptibility, benefits, and barriers. Upon return of the completed questionnaire, women were assigned to a control or intervention group. Following intervention, a second data collection occurred, via a mailed questionnaire. In this report, the second data set was used for test-retest calculations. Because the intervention may have changed actual beliefs, only control group women were used for test-retest computations.

Eligibility criteria were the same for the general medicine clinic, but the procedure was slightly different at this site. Again, a computer-generated list of eligible women was developed. These women then were approached by a research assistant when they came to the clinic for an appointment. If they agreed to be in the study, informed consent was completed, and the questionnaire data were collected at this time. After entry into the study, the same procedure was used for randomization of the intervention delivery and follow-up data collection.

## Results

### Construct Validity

The construct validity of the revised 19 items was examined using two types of factor analysis. First, an exploratory factor analysis using principal components extraction with a varimax rotation was completed. Varimax rotation was selected because the items were expected to factor into three independent scales. A varimax rotation provides a solution that is often more conceptually clear than oblique rotation (Kim & Mueller, 1978). Three factors were selected and accounted for 54% of the variance. The three factors also represented eigenvalues that were greater than 1. The rotated factor matrix using all 19 items with a forced three-factor solution is presented in Table 2. Factor extraction was guided by theory and eigenvalues, as well as the criterion that items greater than .4 would be re-

tained, as suggested by Nunnally (1978). As can be
270 seen in Table 2, all items loaded on their respective
factors at .4 or above. Susceptibility items loaded on
Factor 3 and all had high loadings with Factor 3 (.87 or
above). Benefit items loaded on Factor 2 and again
were correlated strongly, yielding loadings between .55
275 and .75. Barrier items loaded on Factor 1 with loadings
between .48 to .79. Items did not overlap scales. That
is, after loading on a primary scale, the same item did
not load at above .3 on any other scale.

Table 2
*Exploratory Factor Analyses for Scale Items*

|        | Factor 1 | Factor 2 | Factor 3 |
|--------|----------|----------|----------|
| SUS 1  |          |          | .91      |
| SUS 2  |          |          | .89      |
| SUS 3  |          |          | .87      |
| BEN 1  |          | .55      |          |
| BEN 2  |          | .71      |          |
| BEN 3  |          | .73      |          |
| BEN 4  |          | .75      |          |
| BEN 5  |          | .75      |          |
| BAR 1  | .64      |          |          |
| BAR 2  | .72      |          |          |
| BAR 3  | .68      |          |          |
| BAR 4  | .79      |          |          |
| BAR 5  | .75      |          |          |
| BAR 6  | .64      |          |          |
| BAR 7  | .66      |          |          |
| BAR 8  | .64      |          |          |
| BAR 9  | .48      |          |          |
| BAR 10 | .67      |          |          |
| BAR 11 | .70      |          |          |

*Note.* SUS = susceptibility; BEN = benefits; BAR = barriers.

Items also were subjected to confirmatory factor
280 analysis using LISREL (Joreskog & Sorbom, 1989).
Exploratory factor analysis is limited in that possible
relationships are not reconfirmed and data to establish
a relationship are not based on theory. The measurement model of LISREL allowed exploration of how
285 well the latent variables (susceptibility, benefits, and
barriers) were measured by the items. Confirmatory
factor analysis has advantages over an exploratory approach in that relationships are hypothesized between
the observed variables and latent variables; thus, it tests
290 how well items fit with theoretical concepts. A covari-
ance matrix of the 19 items was used as input in testing
the model. Fit of the model to the data was tested by
the Goodness of Fit Index, which is a measure of similarity between the correlation matrix analyzed and that
295 predicted by the estimated model. Boyd, Frye, and
Aaronson (1988) suggest that a value of close to .9 is a
good fit. The Goodness of Fit ratio for these data was
.87 and *t* values for each item were tested for fit with
each latent construct. All *t* values, shown in Table 3,
300 were significant for each item and for the identified
latent variable. Lambda values, which are interpreted
like factor loadings, ranged from .68 to .90 for the sus-

ceptibility scale, .40 to .83 for the benefit scale, and .44
to .69 for the barrier scale.

*Reliability*

305     Item analysis was completed using two criteria established by Nunnally (1978). In order to identify
poorly functioning items, an increase of more than .10
in the total scale reliability when that item was deleted
or correlation of less than .30 between an item and the
310 total subscale score was identified. All items on the
susceptibility score met the criteria for inclusion, and a
standardized item alpha of .87 was obtained for the
final scale. The three items each correlated with the
scale at .72 or above. For the benefit scale, corrected
315 item-total correlations revealed all items to be between
.37 and .57. Deleting items did not increase the alpha.
A final standardized item alpha of .75 was obtained.
The barrier scale had 11 items, all of which correlated
at .41 or above on the corrected item-total scale. Delet-
320 ing any item would not have increased the standardized
item alpha significantly; therefore, all items were retained. A final standardized alpha of .88 was obtained.

For women in the control group, Time 2 data collection followed Time 1 by about 6 weeks. All test-
325 retest correlations for control group women were significant at the .01 level: perceived susceptibility ($r =$
.62), perceived benefits ($r = .61$), and perceived barriers ($r = .71$).

*Predictive Validity*

Theoretically, scale scores should be different for
330 groups of women in different stages of mammography
action. Questions were asked about mammography
history, date of last mammogram, and whether the
women intended to have one in the next 6 months at
both Time 1 and Time 2. Answers to these questions
335 were combined in computer-defined statements that
characterized women as in a precontemplation, contemplation, action, relapse precontemplation, or relapse
contemplation stage. To test theoretical relationships
between scale scores and stage of mammography com-
340 pliance, one-way analysis of variance was computed
followed by Tukey's post hoc tests. Results are displayed in Table 4. Because some women became compliant 6 weeks following intervention, the action stage
was relevant for women who had obtained mammo-
345 grams. Both benefits and barriers had extremely significant overall *F* values, while susceptibility had a
lower but significant overall *F* value. For the overall
benefit score, precontemplators were significantly different from contemplators, relapse contemplators, or
350 those in action, indicating that those who had never had
a mammogram and did not intend to have one did not
perceive as many benefits to the procedure as did those
who had either had a mammogram in the past or were
currently compliant. Relapse precontemplators were
355 different from relapse contemplators or those in action,

Table 3
*Confirmatory Factor Loadings for Scale Items*

| | Lambda | *t* Value |
|---|---|---|
| **Susceptibility** | | |
| 1. It is likely that I will get breast cancer. | .68 | 20.59 |
| 2. My chances of getting breast cancer in the next few years are great. | .90 | 25.92 |
| 3. I feel I will get breast cancer sometime during my life. | .77 | 20.93 |
| **Benefits** | | |
| 1. If I get a mammogram and nothing is found, I do not worry as much about breast cancer. | .40 | 9.08 |
| 2. Having a mammogram will help me find breast lumps early. | .51 | |
| 3. If I find a lump through a mammogram, my treatment for breast cancer may not be as bad. | .60 | 15.20 |
| 4. Having a mammogram is the best way for me to find a very small lump. | .73 | 15.36 |
| 5. Having a mammogram will decrease my chances of dying from breast cancer. | .83 | 18.73 |
| **Barriers** | | |
| 1. I am afraid to have a mammogram because I might find out something is wrong. | .56 | 14.99 |
| 2. I am afraid to have a mammogram because I don't understand what will be done. | .51 | 17.75 |
| 3. I don't know how to go about getting a mammogram. | .44 | 16.18 |
| 4. Having a mammogram is too embarrassing. | .69 | 21.22 |
| 5. Having a mammogram takes too much time. | .60 | 19.15 |
| 6. Having a mammogram is too painful. | .68 | 13.99 |
| 7. People doing mammograms are rude to women. | .56 | 15.78 |
| 8. Having a mammogram exposes me to unnecessary radiation. | .57 | 16.01 |
| 9. I cannot remember to schedule a mammogram. | .47 | 11.06 |
| 10. I have other problems more important than getting a mammogram. | .58 | 15.92 |
| 11. I am too old to need a routine mammogram. | .53 | 16.45 |

indicating that those who had not thought about mammograms perceived fewer benefits than those who had one in the past and were thinking about getting one or those currently compliant. Perceived barriers demonstrated even greater differences. Those who had never had a mammogram had significantly higher barrier scores than those who had either had one and relapsed or were currently in action. All other groups had significantly higher barrier scores than those currently in action.

Women were divided into compliant and noncompliant groups 6 weeks post intervention. Three independent *t* tests were computed using the dependent variables of susceptibility, benefits, and barriers respectively. For susceptibility, a significant difference between groups did not emerge. For benefits, the difference was significant ($t(2,676) = 2.88$, $p = .004$), with those who became compliant perceiving more benefits. For the barrier scale, a more significant difference emerged ($t(2,665) = 7.28$, $p \leq .001$), with compliant women having the fewest perceived barriers.

### Discussion

Findings reported in this manuscript reflect the continued revision of susceptibility, benefits, and barriers scales for mammography utilization. Overall, both validity and reliability were confirmed with the revised scales.

Content validity was improved by having both expert and focus groups of women react to items. On the basis of these results, changes were made, including deleting some susceptibility items and adding some barrier items. Construct validity was tested using both exploratory and confirmatory factor analysis because they represent different conceptual processes in establishing validity. Unidimensionality of all three scales was supported by both exploratory factor analyses and confirmatory factor analyses. Even with three items, the susceptibility scale retained very high correlations among individual items, as identified both by the exploratory and confirmatory factor analyses. This was consistent with the past work on the version of the susceptibility scale that included five items (Champion, 1993).

The benefits and barriers scales also demonstrated strong construct validity, with high correlations between items and the respective scales for both exploratory and confirmatory analysis. Overall, correlations were stronger for these revised items than for previously reported scales (Champion, 1995). Correlations of benefits items with the respective scale revealed all items above .57 on factor analyses, higher than what was reported previously (Champion, 1993). In addition, using factor analysis, most of the barrier items also evidenced higher correlations than reported previously (Champion, 1995), again providing evidence of improved construct validity.

Theoretically, these scales also should be related to stage of mammography compliance. Using data from 6 weeks post intervention, all three scales did differentiate between women who were at different stages of mammography compliance. Skinner et al. (1997) demonstrated similar results for both benefits and barriers. Thus, given the short timeframe for follow-up, the scales were consistent and theoretical relationships were upheld. It is probable that these results do not reflect the full potential of these scales to predict compliance. More women might have become compliant if

Table 4
*Scale Differences by Mammography Stage*

| | Precontemplation (a) | | Contemplation (b) | | Relapse precontemplation (c) | | Relapse contemplation (d) | | Action (e) | |
|---|---|---|---|---|---|---|---|---|---|---|
| | M | SD | M | SD | M | SD | M | SD | M | SD |
| **Susceptibility** | | | | | | | | | | |
| | 6.51 | 5.33 | 7.38 | 2.44 | 6.93 | 2.50 | 7.40 | 2.43 | 7.47 | 2.54 |
| $F(4,654) = 2.46, p = .04$ | | | | | | | | | | |
| **Benefits** | | | | | | | | | | |
| | 17.98 | 4.33 | 20.26 | 2.30 | 19.01 | 3.55 | 20.23 | 2.96 | 20.55 | 3.09 |
| $F(4,673) = 9.26, p = .001$; a diff b, d, e; c diff d, e | | | | | | | | | | |
| **Barriers** | | | | | | | | | | |
| | 26.12 | 6.63 | 26.37 | 4.84 | 22.65 | 6.35 | 20.12 | 6.55 | 17.92 | 5.30 |
| $F(4,662) = 26.49, p = .001$; a, b diff c, d, e; c diff d, e | | | | | | | | | | |

measurements had been taken 2–3 months post intervention, as it often takes 1 or 2 months to obtain a mammography appointment.

425     Overall, items reflected strong internal consistency reliability and test-retest reliability. The susceptibility scale showed a slight decrease in internal consistency reliability with only three items: .87 for the current data as compared to .93 reported previously (Champion, 430 1993). This decrease in internal consistency reliability is not considered significant. The test-retest reliability for susceptibility was somewhat decreased at .62. Because test-retest reliability may be due to inconsistency within the scale or to actual changes in attitude, however, 435 a correlation of .62 is considered acceptable (Carmines & Zeller, 1990). Both benefits and barriers scales were relatively stable as compared to previous work. Internal consistency reliability for the barriers scale was increased (.88) as compared to .73 in the 440 previous work. Test-retest reliabilities were higher for both benefits and barriers. For the current data, test-retest reliability was .61 for benefits and .71 for barriers as compared to previous findings (Champion, 1995) of .38 for benefits and .60 for barriers. Overall, these 445 differences seemed to reflect changes for the better in both mammography barriers and benefits scales.

    All three scales have potential use for nursing practice and research. The constructs of susceptibility, benefits, and barriers have been shown in past work to 450 be related to mammography behavior (Aiken, West, Woodward, & Reno, 1994; Champion & Huster, 1995; Hyman, Baker, Ephraim, Moadel, & Philip, 1994; Rakowski et al., 1992; Rakowski, Fulton, & Feldman, 1993). Results of this past research, along with current 455 results, indicate that the scales are valid and reliable. The susceptibility scale was refined to include only three items, which maintained good validity and reliability. The benefit scale was clarified, with five items retained. The barrier scale was enlarged somewhat to 460 reflect additional barriers identified by women currently considering mammography utilization. Validity and reliability should be reassessed with each new population. Research interventions to promote change could include modification of risk perceptions, benefits 465 perceptions, or barriers perceptions. For example, if a woman did not believe she was susceptible to breast cancer, she could be counseled on her individual risk profile. The benefits of mammography could be discussed. Finally, individual barriers could be identified 470 and joint solutions to overcome these barriers developed. Because scales have been thoroughly tested, research using these constructs is supported. The scales also are useful in that they may be quickly administered in a clinical situation, and they allow for immedi-475 ate assessments and interventions based upon the results.

    The current study has several limitations. First, there was a short timeframe for assessment of mammography compliance following the intervention, 480 which may not have allowed all women who were so disposed to obtain mammography. Second, mammography behavior was based on self-reports. Finally, although the constructs were related to mammography, the variance accounted for is not complete. Additional 485 predictors need to be identified.

## References

Aiken, L. S., West, S. G., Woodward, C. K., & Reno, R. R. (1994). Health beliefs and compliance with mammography-screening recommendations in asymptomatic women. *Health Psychology, 13*, 122–129.

Andersson, I., Aspegren, K., Janzon, L., Landberg, T., Lindholm, K., Linell, F., Ljunberg, O., Ranstam, J., & Sigfusson, B. (1988). Mammographic screening and mortality from breast cancer: The Malmo Mammographic Screening Trial. *British Journal of Medicine, 297*, 943–948.

Becker, M. H. (Ed.). (1974). The Health Belief Model and personal health behavior. Thorofare, NJ: Charles B. Slack.

Boyd, C. J., Frye, M. A., & Aaronson, L. S. (1988). Structural equation models and nursing research. Part I. *Nursing Research, 37*, 249–252.

Carmines, E., & Zeller, R. (1990). Reliability and validity assessment. Newbury Park, CA: Sage.

Champion, V. L. (1984). Instrument development for Health Belief Model constructs. *ANS: Advances in Nursing Science, 6*, 73–85.

Champion, V. L. (1992). The relationship of age to factors influencing breast self-examination practice. *Health Care for Women International, 13*, 1–9.

Champion, V. L. (1993). Instrument refinement for breast cancer screening behaviors. *Nursing Research, 42*, 139–143.

Champion, V. L. (1995). Development of a benefits and barriers scale for mammography utilization. *Cancer Nursing, 18*, 53–59.

Champion, V. L., & Huster, G. (1995). Effect of interventions on stage of mammography adoption. *Journal of Behavioral Medicine, 18*, 169–187.

Champion, V. L., & Skinner, C. S. (1999). Differences in perceptions of risk, benefits, and barriers by stage of mammography adoption. Manuscript submitted for publication.

Chevarley, F., & White, E. (1997). Recent trends in breast cancer mortality among white and black U.S. women. *American Journal of Public Health, 87*, 775–781.

Hyman, R. B., Baker, S., Ephraim, R., Moadel, A., & Philip, J. (1994). Health belief model variables as predictors of screening mammography utilization. *Journal of Behavioral Medicine, 17,* 391–406.

Joreskog, K. G., & Sorbom, D. (1989). LISREL VII: A guide to the program and applications. (2nd ed). Chicago: Scientific Software, Inc.

Kim, J., & Mueller, C. W. (1978). Factor analyses: Statistical methods and practical solutions. Beverly Hills, CA: Sage.

King, E. S., Resch, N., Rimer, B., Lerman, C., Boyce, A., & McGovern-Gorchov, P. (1993). Breast cancer screening practices among retirement community women. *Preventive Medicine, 22,* 1–19.

Landis, S., Murray, T., Bolden, S., & Wingo, P. (1999). *Cancer statistics. CA: A Cancer Journal for Clinicians, 49,* 8–32.

Nunnally, J. C. Psychometric theory (2nd Ed.). McGraw-Hill Publishing Co.: New York, 1978.

Rakowski, W., Dube, C. E., Marcus, B. H., Prochaska, J. O., Velicer, W., & Abrams, D. B. (1992). Assessing elements of women's decisions about mammography. *Health Psychology, 11,* 111–118.

Rakowski, W., Fulton, J. P., & Feldman, J. (1993). Women's decision making about mammography: A replication of the relationship between stages of adoption and decisional balance. *Health Psychology, 12,* 209–214.

Rakowski, W., Rimer, B. K., & Bryant, S. A. (1993). Integrating behavior and intention regarding mammography by respondents in the 1990 National Health Interview Survey of health promotion and disease prevention. *Public Health Reports, 108,* 605–624.

Rimer, B. K., Resch, N., King, E., Ross, E., Lerman, C., Boyce, A., Kessler, H., & Engstrom, P. F. (1992). Multistrategy health education program to increase mammography use among women ages 65 and older. *Public Health Reports, 107,* 369–380.

Roberts, M. M., Alexander, F. E., Anderson, T. J., Chetty, U., Donnan, P. T., Forrest, P., Hepburn, W., Huggins, A., Kirkpatrick, A. E., Lamb, J., Muir, B. B., & Prescott, R. J. (1990). Edinburgh trial of screening for breast cancer: Mortality at seven years. *The Lancet, 335,* 241–246.

Shapiro, S. (1989). Determining the efficacy of breast cancer screening. *Cancer, 63,* 1873–1880.

Shapiro, S., Venet, W., Strax, P., Venet, L., & Roeser, R. (1982). Prospects for eliminating racial differences in breast cancer survival rates. *American Journal of Public Health, 72,* 1142–1145.

Skinner, C. S., Champion, V. L., Gonin, R., & Hanna, M. (1997). Do perceived barriers and benefits vary by mammography stage? *Psychology, Health and Medicine, 2,* 65–75.

Slenker, S. E., & Grant, M. C. (1989). Attitudes, beliefs, and knowledge about mammography among women over forty years of age. *Journal of Cancer Education, 4,* 61–65.

Stein, J. A., Fox, S. A., Murata, P. J., & Morisky, D. E. (1992). Mammography usage and the Health Belief Model. *Health Education Quarterly, 19,* 447–462.

Tabar, L., & Dean, P. B. (1987). The control of breast cancer through mammography screening. What is the evidence? *Radiologic Clinics of North America, 25,* 993–1005.

Thomas, L., Fox, S., Leake, B., & Roetzheim, R. (1996). The effects of health beliefs on screening mammography utilization among a diverse sample of older women. *Women and Health, 24,* 77–91.

Zapka, J. G., Hosmer, D., Constanza, M. E., Harris, D. R., & Stoddard, A. (1992). Changes in mammography use: Economic, need, and service factors. *American Journal of Public Health, 82,* 1345–1351.

**Note**: Grant sponsor: National Center for Nursing Research (NIH). Grant sponsor: National Cancer Institute (NCI); grant number: R01 CA 58606.

**Address correspondence to**: Victoria L. Champion, Indiana University School of Nursing, 1111 Middle Drive, Indianapolis, IN 46202.

# Exercise for Article 37

## Factual Questions

1. The acronym HBM stands for what words?

2. In the initial development of the perceived susceptibility scale by Champion (1984), how was content validity established?

3. Why were only control group women used for test-retest computations?

4. As a result of the exploratory factor analyses, the researcher states, "Items did not overlap." What does this statement mean?

5. What is the value of *r* for the test-retest reliability of the perceived benefits scale determined using the control group women?

6. According to Table 4, which group had the highest mean benefits score? What was their mean score?

7. According to Table 4, which group had the lowest mean benefits score? What was their mean score?

## Questions for Discussion

8. In lines 160–162, the researcher states, "Validity and reliability are sample specific; therefore, further testing was required." In your own words, explain what you think the researcher means by this statement.

9. In lines 199–204, the researcher describes how the wording of one item was changed. Do you think that the change improved the item? Explain.

10. In lines 227–253, the researcher describes how participants were recruited for the study. However, the researcher does not specify the percentage who declined to participate. Would you be interested in having this information? Why? Why not?

11. The items for the three scales are presented in Table 3. What is your opinion of the items?

12. The researcher states that mammography behavior was based on self-reports, which is a limitation of the study. In your opinion, how important is this limitation? (See lines 481–482.)

13. Has this study convinced you that the three scales are reasonably reliable and valid for the participants who were tested? Explain.

## Quality Ratings

Directions: Indicate your level of agreement with each of the following statements by circling a number from 5 for strongly agree (SA) to 1 for strongly disagree (SD). If you believe an item is not applicable to this research article, leave it blank. Be prepared to explain your ratings. When responding to criteria A and B, keep in mind that brief titles and abstracts are conventional in published research.

A. The title of the article is appropriate.

   SA   5   4   3   2   1   SD

B. The abstract provides an effective overview of the research article.

   SA   5   4   3   2   1   SD

C. The introduction establishes the importance of the study.

   SA   5   4   3   2   1   SD

D. The literature review establishes the context for the study.

   SA   5   4   3   2   1   SD

E. The research purpose, question, or hypothesis is clearly stated.

   SA   5   4   3   2   1   SD

F. The method of sampling is sound.

   SA   5   4   3   2   1   SD

G. Relevant demographics (for example, age, gender, and ethnicity) are described.

   SA   5   4   3   2   1   SD

H. Measurement procedures are adequate.

   SA   5   4   3   2   1   SD

I. All procedures have been described in sufficient detail to permit a replication of the study.

   SA   5   4   3   2   1   SD

J. The participants have been adequately protected from potential harm.

   SA   5   4   3   2   1   SD

K. The results are clearly described.

   SA   5   4   3   2   1   SD

L. The discussion/conclusion is appropriate.

   SA   5   4   3   2   1   SD

M. Despite any flaws, the report is worthy of publication.

   SA   5   4   3   2   1   SD

# Article 38

# Nurse Entrance Test Scores:
# A Predictor of Success

**Sherri Orso Ellis**, MSN, RN[*]

ABSTRACT. A program evaluation was conducted to determine if requiring higher scores on critical thinking components of the Nurse Entrance Test would have a positive effect on the percentage of students that could be retained in a diploma nursing program. The program evaluation revealed that using the Nurse Entrance Test as a tool for admissions screening, specifically portions of the examination that predict critical thinking, was effective in helping to predict success through level 1 nursing courses.

From *Nurse Educator*, 31, 259–263. Copyright © 2006 by Lippincott Williams & Wilkins. Reprinted with permission.

According to the U.S. Department of Health and Human Services,[1] anticipated shortages in numbers of nurses available to meet healthcare needs in the United States will reach 29% by the year 2020 if current trends
5 remain unchanged. A dwindling supply of qualified faculty in nursing schools throughout the country further compounds the problem by limiting the number of applicants who can be accepted into nursing programs. Student attrition becomes a major focus as nursing
10 programs attempt to discover and implement effective interventions aimed at increasing retention rates.[2]

Statistics reported by the National Council of State Boards of Nursing reveal that the number of first time applicants sitting for the NCLEX-RN, the national li-
15 censure examination for registered nurses, decreased by 20% from 1995 to 2003.[2] Additional data from the U.S. Department of Health and Human Services indicate declining numbers of graduates from diploma, associate degree (AD), and baccalaureate programs.
20 Only 4% of graduates in 1999 were from diploma programs compared with 9% in 1992. This is partially due to the fact that over the past few decades, many hospital-based diploma programs have closed.[1] The latest data compiled and reported by the National
25 League for Nursing (NLN) reveal that as of the year 2000, only 78 diploma nursing programs remained in operation.[3] The need exists to make the most efficient use of available resources, faculty, and allocated dol-

lars by implementing measures to effectively lower
30 attrition rates in schools of nursing.[2]

The only diploma program offered in the state of Louisiana is the Baton Rouge General Medical Center School of Nursing (BRGMC SON), located in the capital city of Baton Rouge. The school's mission is to
35 prepare registered nurses for entry-level practice. The program is designed for completion over a 3-year period. Major components include 25 hours of prerequisite college credit in specific core courses, 3 levels of intense coursework, and a substantial number of hours
40 focused on clinical experiences.

## Background

As with most nursing programs, the director and faculty of BRGMC SON were concerned about high attrition rates. Since 1998, the school has used the Nurse Entrance Test (NET) as a tool for the identifica-
45 tion of qualified applicants. Informal trending of NET scores and student performance data compiled by the director of the school of nursing revealed that after admission to the program, approximately one-third of the students were not successfully passing level 1
50 courses. Trended data of NET scores suggested that candidates with lower scores on areas of the test that predicted critical thinking ability were more likely to be unsuccessful. This initial observation prompted the admissions committee to adopt a change in admission
55 criteria.[4]

## Change in Admission Criteria

Prior to 2005, candidates for admission were required to complete 8 specific college credit courses with a grade of "C" or better, maintain a grade point average of at least 2.7, and provide evidence that they
60 had completed a computer literacy course and either a high school or college chemistry course with a grade of "C" or better. Candidates were required to take the NET, achieve a composite percentile of 50 or better, and score an average of 50 or better on the "critical
65 thinking appraisal" section of the test. With the change in admission criteria, applicants accepted into the program in the spring of 2005 were required to meet higher standards for admission with regard to NET

[*]*Sherri Orso Ellis* is instructor, School of Nursing, Baton Rouge General Medical Center, Baton Rouge, LA.

70 scores. The required composite percentile remained 50 or above. However, in addition to this requirement, applicants for 2005 were required to score 50% or better on each component of the critical thinking appraisal portion of the NET. Components in this section include inferential reading, main idea of passage, and predict-
75 ing of outcomes.

### Need for Program Evaluation

To address the impact of this change, a committee was formed to compare retention in the program between before and after the change in admission criteria. To date, those admitted under the new criteria have
80 completed level 1 nursing courses. These courses include pharmacology, fundamentals of nursing, and a course introducing medical-surgical nursing. The medical-surgical course incorporates basic medical-surgical topics, with an increased emphasis on patho-
85 physiology.

A program evaluation project was initiated to determine if increasing the admissions criteria to require higher NET scores on portions of the examination that predict critical thinking ability would result in a higher
90 percentage of students being retained in the program. A secondary purpose of this evaluation was to determine if increased NET scores on the critical thinking analysis portion of the examination significantly increased the proportion of students retained at the end of level 1
95 nursing courses.

### Review of Literature

The NET, developed by Educational Resources, Inc. (ERI), is a diagnostic instrument used by diploma, AD, and baccalaureate nursing programs as part of admissions criteria and as a tool for identifying "at-
100 risk" student populations. The NET provides diagnostic scores for essential skills areas, including math, reading comprehension, reading rate, critical thinking appraisal, test-taking skills, and learning styles. The test also scores certain nonacademic indicators, such as
105 stress level and social interaction in addition to providing composite percentages and percentile scores. All or some of these scores may be used as diagnostic tools or for screening purposes, depending on individual institution needs.[5]
110 Although use of the NET varies, several researchers have published studies on the use of the NET as a predictor of student success. One study conducted by Sayles et al.[6] sought to determine if there was a positive correlation between NET and PreRN scores, suc-
115 cessful completion of an AD program, and subsequent success on NCLEX-RN. Sayles et al. documented that maintaining a higher grade point average (numerical value not assigned) for nursing-related courses, math, reading, and NET composite scores, the PreRN com-
120 posite score, and the grade earned on the highest level nursing course, which teaches concepts related to circulation and oxygenation, were all found to have statistical significance. The results of this study indicated

125 that standardized tests such as the NET could be successfully used as tools to screen applicants for admission, predict success in nursing programs, and to identify at-risk students.

Various studies[6–8] have helped to validate the premise that early identification and intervention for stu-
130 dents categorized as at risk can help improve retention and increase the likelihood of academic success. The NET is often used as a tool to identify at-risk student populations. Students entering the AD nursing program at Texas Woman's University (TWU), many of whom
135 speak English as a second language, are required to take the NET test. Data collected at this institution revealed that students who scored less than 55% on reading comprehension were more likely to be unsuccessful in the program. Based on these data, TWU developed
140 the Student Success Program with the goal of improving retention. Students who fall into this at-risk group are required to enter the Student Success Program. Within this program, they participate in regular nursing courses along with additional courses specially de-
145 signed to help them become expert learners, improve language and communication skills, and overcome cultural barriers. Although it is in its early stages, the program has shown to be successful in helping to retain students throughout the program.[7]
150 Symes et al.[9] reported a follow-up evaluation of the Nursing Success Program established at TWU in the fall of 2000. This program was established to identify at-risk nursing students and to provide early intervention, with the goal of increasing retention rates
155 throughout the program. According to this report, the decision to use reading comprehension as a tool for the identification and advisement of this student population originated from earlier data showing a relationship between low reading comprehension scores on the
160 NET and high attrition rates. Results of this study indicate that reading comprehension scores on the NET test have a significant relationship to retention in the nursing program.

Numerous studies to help validate the use of the
165 NET as a predictor of success in nursing programs have been conducted by ERI. Simmons et al.[8] collected data from nursing programs in 12 states that used the NET as a part of admissions criteria or for screening at-risk student populations. The sample was representa-
170 tive of each of the 3 program types. Overall findings indicated that NET composite scores and reading comprehension scores were most significant in predicting student success. Higher NET scores on inferential reading were correlated with better critical thinking skills.
175 It was determined that early identification of at-risk students may positively affect attrition rates by helping nursing programs to initiate early interventions aimed at retention.

In some instances, use of the NET as a predictor of
180 success has been shown to have no significance. Gallagher et al.[10] studied a random sample of 121 students

from William Rainey Harper College who took both the Registered Nurse Entrance Exam before admission and the NET before entering nursing courses in the fall 1995 term. Both the Registered Nurse Entrance Exam and the NET were examined for their ability to predict success in the first nursing course, and to determine if the NET would be a better predictor of success for use in their nursing program. The study revealed that with the exception of mathematics, NET scores had no significant relationship to success for students who scored a "C" or better compared with those who scored less than a "C" in the first nursing course.

## Conceptual Framework

According to the NET Technical and Developmental Report published by ERI,[5(p32)] "the critical thinking appraisal of the NET has been reported to predict success in certain types of professions or instructional programs in which critical thinking is known to play an important role." The NET evaluates critical thinking ability by the participant's success on three sections of the test that include inferential reading, predicting outcomes, and main idea of passage. Developers of the NET propose that the mental activities required to execute the nursing process are analogous to the mental processes required to critically think and that the two processes are "closely related cognitive skills."[5(p33)]

Although there is an abundance of research that recognizes critical thinking as an essential core component of nursing, the concept can be hard to define. Hynes and Bennett[11(p26)] wrote that critical thinking, as defined by Fowler, is making informed and purposeful decisions by looking beyond the obvious and, as defined by Bittner and Tobin, as "a process influenced by knowledge and experience using strategies such as reflective thinking as a part of learning to identify the issues and opportunities and holistically synthesize the information in nursing practice." In a recent article, Turner[12] documented that critical thinking, although widely discussed and examined, has multiple definitions and lacks clarity. She cites the usage of overlapping terms such as *decision making*, *problem solving*, and *clinical reasoning* in the literature devoted to the concept of critical thinking. No matter how critical thinking is defined, most agree that it is required by nurses to practice in a safe and competent manner, with the ability to make sound judgments that will positively affect patient outcomes.

The Critical Thinking Model for Nursing Judgment, developed by Kataoka-Yahiro and Saylor,[13] provides insight into the process of critical thinking. This model dictates that critical thinking is not simply the nursing process. It is a process affected by five factors: experience, knowledge base, attitude, standards, and competencies. The authors make reference to the fact that the NLN includes criteria specific to critical thinking in its standards for accreditation. With this emphasis on critical thinking as a necessary component of nursing

curriculum, nurse educators are challenged to discover methods of measuring and evaluating students' ability to think critically.[13]

## Methods

### Sample

The population for this program evaluation consisted of students admitted into the nursing program in the spring of 2003, 2004, and 2005. The total sample size included 137 students. For the purpose of analysis, the groups were divided into those students admitted before changes in admission criteria ($n = 82$) and those admitted after changes in admission criteria ($n = 55$).

### Protection of Rights

This evaluation process required no active subject participation. Approval to use data from school records was granted by the director of the school. All data were obtained from records on file with the school. Institutional Review Board approval was obtained from Southeastern Louisiana University prior to data collection.

### Variables

The dependent variables in this evaluation were retention in the program, specifically retention at the end of level 1 nursing courses, and the status at the end of level 1 nursing courses. Independent variables included inferential reading, predicting outcomes, and main idea of passage scores on the NET exam. Other variables considered were age, gender, marital status, NET composite percentile, math and reading comprehension percentages, and semester of enrollment.

### Design and Procedure

Descriptive statistics were examined to summarize the sample characteristics. A percentage was calculated for those students retained in the program at level 1 before and after changes in admissions criteria. A $\chi^2$ analysis was performed to determine if a significant difference existed in the proportion of students retained in the program before and after the admissions criteria changes. Table 1 contains demographic data and represents percentages scored on the NET for the two groups.

## Results

Data were analyzed using the SPSS program. The first group represents students who entered the program in 2003 and 2004, before the requirement of higher NET scores on the critical thinking analysis portion of the exam. According to percentages calculated between the two groups, 89.1% of the students in group 2 were retained at the end of level 1 nursing courses compared with 70.7% in group 1. At the end of level 1 nursing courses, 24 students (29.3%) were no longer in the program. Fifty-eight students (70.7%) were retained. Group 2 consisted of 55 students admitted in the spring of 2005, after the implementation of higher NET scores for admission. At the end of level 1 nursing courses,

Table 1
*Demographic Characteristics of Students in Old and New Criteria*

| Variables | Old criteria ($n = 82$) | | New criteria ($n = 55$) | |
|---|---|---|---|---|
| | $n$ | % | $n$ | % |
| Gender | | | | |
| Male | 13 | 15.9 | 4 | 7.3 |
| Female | 69 | 84.1 | 51 | 92.7 |
| Marital status | | | | |
| Married | 38 | 46.3 | 18 | 32.7 |
| Single | 44 | 53.7 | 37 | 67.3 |
| # of NET attempts | | | | |
| 1 | 61 | 74.4 | 34 | 61.8 |
| > 1 | 21 | 25.6 | 21 | 38.2 |
| NET composite percentile | | | | |
| < 50 | 1 | 1.2 | – | – |
| 50–70 | 22 | 26.8 | 9 | 16.4 |
| 71–80 | 19 | 23.2 | 12 | 21.8 |
| 81–100 | 40 | 48.8 | 34 | 61.8 |
| Math % | | | | |
| < 50 | 1 | 1.2 | – | – |
| 50–70 | 20 | 24.4 | 16 | 29.1 |
| 71–80 | 43 | 52.4 | 20 | 36.4 |
| 81–100 | 18 | 22.0 | 19 | 34.5 |
| Reading % | | | | |
| < 50 | – | – | – | – |
| 26–50 | 2 | 2.4 | – | – |
| 51–75 | 54 | 65.9 | 32 | 58.2 |
| > 75 | 26 | 31.7 | 23 | 41.8 |
| Inferential reading % | | | | |
| < 50 | – | – | – | – |
| 26–50 | 14 | 17.1 | 4 | 7.3 |
| 51–75 | 45 | 54.9 | 31 | 56.4 |
| > 75 | 23 | 28.0 | 20 | 36.4 |
| Main idea of passage % | | | | |
| < 50 | – | – | – | – |
| 26–50 | 3 | 3.7 | – | – |
| 51–75 | 32 | 39.0 | 19 | 34.5 |
| > 75 | 47 | 57.3 | 36 | 65.5 |
| Predicting outcomes % | | | | |
| < 50 | – | – | – | – |
| 26–50 | 13 | 15.9 | 2 | 3.6 |
| 51–75 | 61 | 74.4 | 50 | 90.9 |
| > 75 | 8 | 9.8 | 3 | 5.5 |
| Level 1 status | | | | |
| Out of program | 24 | 29.3 | 6 | 10.9 |
| Retained | 58 | 70.7 | 49 | 89.1 |

6 students (10.9%) were no longer in the program and 49 students (89.1%) were retained.

To determine statistical significance, a $\chi^2$ analysis was performed; $\chi^2$ is a nonparametric statistic that compares the actual number in a group with the expected number. The question answered by a $\chi^2$ is if the expected number and the actual number within the groups that are being compared differ significantly. The $\chi^2$ analysis of the 2 groups showed that a significantly higher proportion of students within group 2 were retained in the program at the end of level 1 nursing courses. With a sample size of 137 and 1 degree of freedom, $\chi^2$ was equal to 6.488 ($\chi^2 = 6.488$, $df = 1$, $N =$ 137). Statistical significance was established at the .05 level ($p = .011$).

## Discussion

The program evaluation was conducted to determine if raising admission requirements to include higher expected scores on critical thinking portions of the NET would have a positive effect on the numbers of students that could be retained in the program. Research related to student success in diploma nursing programs is limited, and there is currently no research available on the use of NET scores as a predictor of success or as a screening tool for admissions in diploma nursing programs. However, the results of this evaluation are consistent with findings from research studies conducted with associate and baccalaureate nursing programs where NET scores were used to predict student success. Math and reading comprehension NET scores have shown to be useful in identifying at-risk students and providing direction when counseling and advising students and have been shown to have a positive correlation with success on NCLEX-RN.[6]

Although there are no research studies specific to diploma programs, research conducted with AD and baccalaureate programs showed that students who scored higher on the math and reading comprehension sections of the test were more likely to be successful in nursing programs.[5,6]

The results of the program evaluation indicate that a significantly higher proportion of students who were required to have higher critical thinking scores on the NET prior to admission were retained in the program through level 1 nursing courses. Although there is currently no research specific to the use of critical thinking portions of the NET as an admissions tool, there is a large segment of literature depicting critical thinking as a necessary component of nursing. A concept analysis conducted by Turner[12] on the subject of critical thinking found over 646 literary sources since 1981. The model of Kataoka-Yahiro and Saylor[13(p351)] was created to promote critical thinking as "an essential part of autonomous, excellent nursing practice." Nurses are routinely called upon to accurately assess the health needs of acutely ill patients and to respond with appropriate interventions. Because we know that knowledge alone is not enough to ensure safe actions and sound clinical judgment, nurse educators are challenged to incorporate the critical thinking component in their programs. The BRGMC SON places emphasis on clinical performance. Students are required to synthesize the knowledge attained in the classroom and demonstrate the ability to apply that knowledge in the clinical setting. This program evaluation indicates that using critical thinking NET scores may prove to be one effective method of identifying prospective students who possess critical thinking skills that can be further developed to foster success in the program.

The process of using higher critical thinking scores on the NET as an admissions tool for the BRGMC SON diploma program will require further evaluation. A follow-up study will be conducted after those students admitted to the spring 2005 class have completed the program and have had an opportunity to take the NCLEX-RN exam. Further analysis of data at that time will help determine if NET critical thinking scores can help predict success beyond level 1 nursing courses. Proportions of students retained throughout the program to graduation and eventual success on the NCLEX-RN examination will be evaluated to determine the effectiveness of critical thinking NET scores as an early predictor of success.

## Limitations

There are several limitations that must be considered when reviewing the results of this program evaluation. First, this evaluation was conducted with data from a diploma nursing program. There are limited numbers of diploma programs still in operation throughout the United States. The results of this evaluation may not be applicable to other types of nursing programs. Second, changes in admissions criteria at this school of nursing became effective in the spring semester of 2005. At the time of this evaluation, students admitted for the year 2005 had completed only level 1 courses. Therefore, a determination of the effect of increased critical thinking NET scores throughout the program cannot yet be determined. Finally, the author recognizes that other extraneous variables, such as age, gender, marital status, and grade point average, exist and could possibly affect success or nonsuccess in the program.

## Implications

Because of the growing shortage of nurses, the need exists for educators to find ways to identify the most qualified applicants and those who will most likely be successful in nursing programs. The results of this program evaluation have helped establish that using the NET critical thinking analysis as a screening tool for admissions may be one way to achieve this goal. A follow-up study is recommended to determine if critical thinking analysis NET scores will affect success beyond level 1 nursing courses.

## Conclusion

Critical thinking is a necessary component of nursing practice. The use of purposeful, goal-directed thinking helps guide nurses as they use their experience, knowledge, and intuitiveness to make decisions that impact patient care.[14] Nursing faculty are being challenged to find ways to identify applicants with critical thinking skills and to foster those skills throughout their nursing programs to produce competent, skilled, novice nurses who have the ability to make sound clinical nursing judgments. Rote memorization and retention of knowledge are not enough.

Nursing faculty are charged with the task of identifying those nursing students with good critical thinking skills and helping to further develop the skills that will be necessary to synthesize information using the critical thinking process. Also, they have a responsibility to identify those students who are weak in the area of critical thinking and to use teaching methods that will help develop the ability to make sound decisions. This program evaluation indicates that using the critical thinking analysis portion of the NET in conjunction with other interventions can be an effective method of screening applicants for admission and helping identify those potential candidates who have a higher probability of success in early nursing courses.

## References

1.  Health Resources and Services Administration. Projected supply, demand, and shortages of registered nurses: 2000–2020. 2002. Available at: http://bhpr.gov/healthworkforce/reports/rnproject/default.htmAmerican. Accessed October 24, 2005.
2.  Association of Colleges of Nursing. Nursing shortage fact sheet. Available at: http://www.aacn.nche.edu/Media/Backgrounders/shortagefacts.htm. October 24, 2005.
3.  National League for Nursing. Table 407. Number of diploma nursing programs, students and graduates, academic years: 1975–76 to 1999–2000. Available at: http://bhpr.hrsa.gov/healthworkforce/reports/factbook02/FB407.htm. Accessed October 24, 2005.
4.  Baton Rouge General School of Nursing. *A Diploma Program in Nursing [Brochure]*. Baton Rouge, LA: Baton Rouge General; 2004.
5.  Educational Resources, Inc. *Nurse Entrance Test: Technical & Developmental Report*. Shawnee Mission, Kan: Educational Resources, Inc; 2004.
6.  Sayles S, Shelton D, Powell H. Predictors of success in nursing education. *Assoc Black Nurs Faculty*. 2003;14(6):116–120.
7.  Symes L, Tart K, Travis L, Toombs MS. Developing and retaining expert learners. *Nurse Educ*. 2002;27(5):227–231.
8.  Simmons LE, Haupt GA, Davis L. *The Usefulness of the Nurse Entrance Test (NET) for Prediction of Successful Completion in a Nursing Program*. Shawnee Mission, Kan: Educational Resources, Inc; 2004.
9.  Symes L, Tart K, Travis L. An evaluation of the Nursing Success Program. *Nurse Educ*. 2005;30(5):217–220.
10. Gallagher PA, Bomba C, Crane LR. Using an admissions exam to predict student success in an ADN program. *Nurse Educ*. 2001;26(3):132–135.
11. Hynes P, Bennett J. About critical thinking. *Can Assoc Crit Care Nurs*. 2004;15(3):26–29.
12. Turner P. Critical thinking in nursing education and practice as defined in the literature. *Nurs Educ Perspect*. 2005;26(5):272–277.
13. Kataoka-Yahiro M, Saylor C. A critical thinking model for nursing judgment. *J Nurs Educ*. 1994;33(8):351–356.
14. L'Eplattenier N. Tracing the development of critical thinking in baccalaureate nursing students. *J N Y State Nurses Assoc*. 2001;32(2);27–32.

**Address correspondence to**: Sherri Orso Ellis, School of Nursing, Baton Rouge General Medical Center, Baton Rouge, LA 70806, USA. E-mail: sherri.ellis@brgeneral.org

# Exercise for Article 38

## Factual Questions

1.  The critical thinking portion of the NET contains what three components?

2.  This study included how many participants who were admitted after changes in admission criteria?

3.  Under the old criteria, what percentage of the participants were retained?

4.  Under the new criteria, what percentage of the participants were retained?

5.  Is the difference between the answers to Questions 3 and 4 statistically significant? If yes, at what probability level?

6.  What percentage of participants under the new criteria had a NET composite percentile of 81 to 100?

## Questions for Discussion

7.  How helpful was the Conceptual Framework in helping you understand this study? (See lines 194–240.)

8.  How important is the issue of protecting participants' rights? (See lines 248–254.)

9.  Is the demographic information on gender and marital status in Table 1 important for understanding this study? Explain. (See Table 1.)

10. Do you think that the planned follow-up is important? Explain. (See lines 358–368 and 393–396.)

11. Do you agree with the second limitation discussed by the researcher? (See lines 376–382.)

12. In the Contents of this book, this article is classified as an example of Test Reliability and Validity Research. In your opinion, would it also be appropriate to classify it as an example of Program Evaluation/Process Evaluation? Explain.

## Quality Ratings

Directions: Indicate your level of agreement with each of the following statements by circling a number from 5 for strongly agree (SA) to 1 for strongly disagree (SD). If you believe an item is not applicable to this research article, leave it blank. Be prepared to explain your ratings. When responding to criteria A and B, keep in mind that brief titles and abstracts are conventional in published research.

A.  The title of the article is appropriate.

    SA   5   4   3   2   1   SD

B.  The abstract provides an effective overview of the research article.

    SA   5   4   3   2   1   SD

C.  The introduction establishes the importance of the study.

    SA   5   4   3   2   1   SD

D.  The literature review establishes the context for the study.

    SA   5   4   3   2   1   SD

E.  The research purpose, question, or hypothesis is clearly stated.

    SA   5   4   3   2   1   SD

F.  The method of sampling is sound.

    SA   5   4   3   2   1   SD

G.  Relevant demographics (for example, age, gender, and ethnicity) are described.

       SA   5   4   3   2   1   SD

H.  Measurement procedures are adequate.

       SA   5   4   3   2   1   SD

I.  All procedures have been described in sufficient detail to permit a replication of the study.

       SA   5   4   3   2   1   SD

J.  The participants have been adequately protected from potential harm.

       SA   5   4   3   2   1   SD

K.  The results are clearly described.

       SA   5   4   3   2   1   SD

L.  The discussion/conclusion is appropriate.

       SA   5   4   3   2   1   SD

M.  Despite any flaws, the report is worthy of publication.

       SA   5   4   3   2   1   SD

# Article 39

# A Meta-Analysis of Interventions to Promote Mammography Among Ethnic Minority Women

**Hae-Ra Han**, PhD, RN, **Jong-Eun Lee**, PhD, RN, **Jiyun Kim**, PhD, RN, **Haley K. Hedlin**, BA, **Heejung Song**, PhD, **Miyong T. Kim**, PhD, RN, FAAN[*]

## ABSTRACT

*Background*: Although many studies have been focused on interventions designed to promote mammography screening among ethnic minority women, few summaries of the effectiveness of the interventions are available.

*Objective*: The aim of this study was to determine the effectiveness of the interventions for improving mammography screening among asymptomatic ethnic minority women.

*Methods*: A meta-analysis was performed on intervention studies designed to promote mammography use in samples of ethnic minority women. Random-effects estimates were calculated for interventions by measuring differences in intervention and control group screening rates postintervention.

*Results*: The overall mean weighted effect size for the 23 studies was 0.078 ($Z = 4.414$, $p < .001$), indicating that the interventions were effective in improving mammography use among ethnic minority women. For mammography intervention types, access-enhancing strategies had the biggest mean weighted effect size of 0.155 ($Z = 4.488$, $p < .001$), followed by 0.099 ($Z = 6.552$, $p < .001$) for individually directed approaches such as individual counseling or education. Tailored, theory-based interventions resulted in a bigger effect size compared with nontailored interventions (effect sizes = 0.101 vs. 0.076, respectively; $p < .05$ for all models). Of cultural strategies, ethnically matched intervention deliveries and offering culturally matched intervention materials had effect sizes of 0.067 ($Z = 2.516$, $p = .012$) and 0.051 ($Z = 2.365$, $p = .018$), respectively.

*Discussion*: Uniform improvement in mammography screening is a goal to address breast cancer disparities in ethnic minority communities in this country. The results of this meta-analysis suggest a need for increased use of a theory-based, tailored approach with enhancement of access.

From *Nursing Research*, 58, 246–254. Copyright © 2009 by Lippincott Williams & Wilkins. Reprinted with permission.

Despite considerable progress in breast cancer control in the United States over the past 20 years, ethnic minority women continue to face an unequal burden of cancer (Chu, Miller, & Springfield, 2007; Lantz et al., 2006). For example, African American and Hispanic women are more likely to be diagnosed at an advanced stage of breast cancer (American Cancer Society, 2008; Lantz et al., 2006) and have worse stage-for-stage survival than do White women (Carey et al., 2006; Shavers, Harlan, & Stevens, 2003). Traditionally, Asian American women have had lower breast cancer incidence rates than White women had (American Cancer Society, 2008). Over the past decade, however, the incidence of breast cancer in Asian women has been increasing at a much higher rate than that of White women (annual increase of 6.3% vs. < 1.5%; Deapen, Liu, Perkins, Bernstein, & Ross, 2002). In addition, similar to Black and Hispanic women, Asian American women are significantly more likely than White women to discover breast cancer at a later stage (Miller, Hankey, & Thomas, 2002).

Researchers have ascribed a large portion of this disparity in the late-stage diagnosis and poor survival of breast cancer to racial and ethnic differences in the utilization of mammography screening, which is a critical strategy in early detection and timely treatment of breast cancer (Smith-Bindman et al., 2006). The U.S. Preventive Services Task Force (2002) recommends that women have a mammogram every 1–2 years beginning at age 40 years. Although differences in mammography rates between White and African American women have narrowed during the past decade (Smigal et al., 2006), ethnic differences in screening do persist in some groups. The American Cancer Society's most recent annual report of cancer statistics revealed that regular use of mammography was especially low among Hispanic and Asian women relative

[*]*Hae-Ra Han*, PhD, RN, is associate professor, School of Nursing; *Jong-Eun Lee*, PhD, RN, is postdoctoral fellow, School of Nursing; *Jiyun Kim*, PhD, RN, is postdoctoral fellow, School of Nursing; *Haley K. Hedlin*, BA, is doctoral student, Bloomberg School of Public Health; *Heejung Song*, PhD, is research associate, Bloomberg School of Public Health; and *Miyong T. Kim*, PhD, RN, FAAN, is professor, School of Nursing, Bloomberg School of Public Health, and School of Medicine, The Johns Hopkins University, Baltimore, Maryland.

to the national level (Cokkinides, Bandi, Siegel, Ward, & Thun, 2007). According to a recent report on national surveys (Town, Wholey, Feldman, & Burns, 2007), ethnic minority women are less likely than their White counterparts to have health insurance (69.7% vs. 87%). Minority women who lack health insurance or have lived in the United States for less than 10 years have been found particularly vulnerable to insufficient mammography screening (Cokkinides et al., 2007; Purc-Stephenson & Gorey, 2008; Rakowski et al., 2006).

Many studies have been focused on promoting mammography screening among ethnic minority women using a variety of intervention strategies. For example, *promotora* (lay health advisor) interventions have been generally well received by ethnic minority women, positively affecting their use of preventive health services, including mammography (Erwin et al., 2003; Mock et al., 2007; Navarro et al., 1998; Taylor et al., 2002). Without a sufficient amount of monitoring, support, and opportunities for advancement, however, the utility of the *promotora* approach is uncertain because the content and frequency of interactions between the *promotora* and the study participant may change by the discretion of the *promotora* (Suarez et al., 1997; Wasserman, Bender, & Lee, 2007). Well-validated theories can be used to guide an intervention effectively by specifying the ingredients and correct implementation of the intervention, making replication of the intervention easier (Sidani & Braden, 1998). Theory-guided tailored interventions (i.e., providing intervention materials adjusted to the characteristics of an individual) have been effective in promoting various forms of health behavior such as healthy diet (Park et al., 2008; Resnicow et al., 2008) and smoking cessation (Schumann et al., 2008). Likewise, recent strategies to promote breast cancer screening include theory-based tailored interventions (Allen & Bazargan-Hejazi, 2005; Champion et al., 2006, 2007; Jibaja-Weiss, Volk, Kingery, Smith, & Holcomb, 2003), although no systematic evaluation of this intervention approach across studies has been done.

The purpose of this meta-analysis was to determine the effects of intervention programs on mammography screening among ethnic minority women. Identification of the determinants of mammography use can facilitate more effective strategies to reduce barriers to breast cancer screening. Meta-analyses of mammography interventions (Denhaerynck et al., 2003; Edwards et al., 2006; Legler et al., 2002; Sohl & Moyer, 2007; Yabroff & Mandelblatt, 1999) found that combined approaches enhancing access—in addition to individual strategies such as reminder letters, telephone calls, or personal contact—can increase mammography use. Specifically, in the Legler et al. (2002) meta-analysis, access-enhancing strategies were the strongest intervention approach, resulting in an increase in mammography use by 18.9% (95% confidence interval [CI] =

10.4–27.4), followed by individually directed interventions in a healthcare setting (17.6%; 95% CI = 11.6–24.0). Yabroff and Mandelblatt (1999) included two studies that used access-enhancing strategies (financial incentives) in their meta-analysis but did not perform meta-analysis with two interventions. They found that patient-targeted behavioral interventions improved mammography utilization by 13.2% (95% CI = 4.7–21.2). Effect sizes of interventions using social networks were revealed to be in the range of 5.8% (Legler et al., 2002) to 12.6% (Yabroff & Mandelblatt, 1999).

However, most previous meta-analyses have not been focused specifically on ethnic minority women, nor have culturally tailored or recent intervention approaches most effective for these groups of women with traditionally lower use of mammography been discussed. The goal of this study was to fill this gap by conducting analyses on more recent studies (published since September 2000, where the review by Legler et al., 2002, left off) that were targeted specifically to ethnic minority women. Specifically, the objective of the meta-analysis was to describe mammography intervention approaches used for ethnic minority (Asian American, African American, and Hispanic) women in the United States.

## Methods

### Study Selection

Literature for this review was identified using electronic searches of databases and hand searches from reference collections. The literature search was limited to articles published in the English language from 2000 onwards. Two authors independently searched Medline, CINAHL, PsycINFO, and Web of Science using combinations of the key word phrases *Asian, African American, Hispanic* or *Latino, breast cancer screening, mammography, experimental studies, interventions,* and *intervention studies.*

The electronic and hand searches generated a combined total of 749 titles and abstracts for assessment. Screening of relevant studies for inclusion was conducted using titles and abstracts based on the following criteria: (a) the study aimed to increase use of mammography screening among asymptomatic women, either exclusively or in addition to other health behaviors; (b) the study included more than 40% of women with ethnic minority background (i.e., Asian American, Black, or Hispanic) in the sample; (c) outcomes were based on a woman's adherence to mammography screening, documented either by self-report or in a clinical database or medical record; (d) an experimental or quasi-experimental design was used in the study; and (e) the study was reported between September 2000 and August 2008. Not included were international studies because the focus was on intervention strategies to improve breast cancer screening among ethnic minority women in the United States.

150   The titles and abstracts of all identified studies were reviewed by two study team members. Of these 749 studies, 607 were excluded. A total of 142 full-text articles were reviewed systematically to confirm eligibility for this study. Of the 142 articles examined, 43
155   did not include more than 40% of ethnic minority women, or ethnicity was unclear; 23 did not have a control group; 2 were only system directed; and 6 did not specify an intervention component clearly. In addition, 13 did not include enough information to calculate
160   an effect size; 18 did not include a woman's adherence to mammography screening as an outcome; and 14 had an international study setting or reported on the same sample as another that was already included. As a result, a total of 23 studies were included in the meta-
165   analysis (Figure 1).

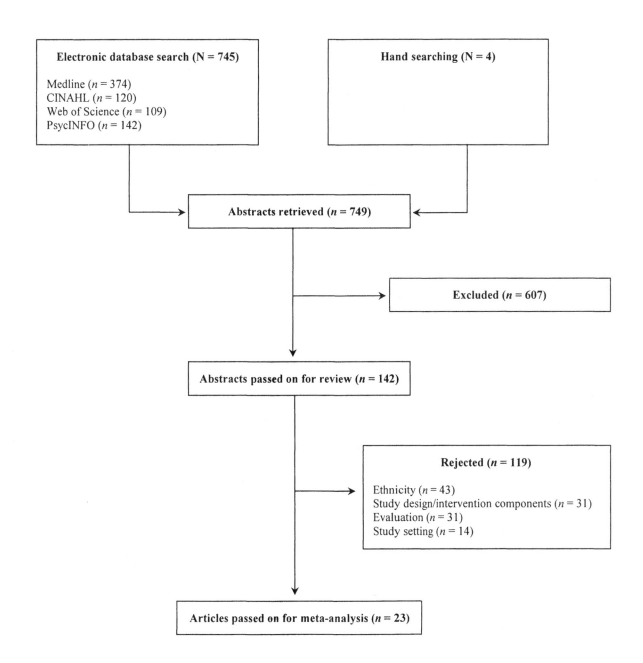

*Figure 1*. Summary of the study selection process.

*Study Coding*

The specific outcome of interest in this analysis was the difference in the proportion of mammography screening in the intervention group versus the control group. A number of variables were selected for inclu-
170 sion in the database of articles. The following were coded: first author, year, study design, setting, sample (percentage of ethnic minority women), unit of assignment, type of intervention, intervention period, time to outcome measure (months), method of outcome
175 ascertainment, number of participants in the study groups, mean age of the study sample, proportion of mammography screening for the treatment and control groups, theory, control group (no intervention, minimal intervention or usual care, or other non-breast-cancer
180 intervention), any cultural strategies used, and study quality. Following the typology used in previous reviews (Legler et al., 2002; Rimer, 1994), interventions were categorized as follows: (a) individual directed (e.g., one-on-one counseling, tailored and nontailored
185 letters and reminders, and telephone counseling), (b) system directed (e.g., provider prompts), (c) access-enhancing (e.g., mobile vans and reduced-cost mammograms), (d) social network (e.g., peer educators and lay health advisors), (e) community education, (f) mass
190 media, and (g) multiple strategies (combinations of the intervention approaches listed above). As in a prior review (Legler et al., 2002), in five studies comparing two or more intervention groups to one control group, the intervention with the most components (i.e., highest
195 dose group) was considered. To rate study quality, four items were used from relevant literature (Jadad et al., 1996; Soeken, Lee, Bausell, Agelli, & Berman, 2002). The range of total quality scores was 0 to 4 (Table 1). For the purpose of this analysis, studies with scores of
200 1–2 were considered to be *low quality* and those with scores of 3–4 were considered to be *high quality*. Using Microsoft Excel, two raters independently coded the variables. Every discrepancy was identified and resolved by discussion among team members. The aver-
205 age $\kappa$ for coding agreement was sufficient, 0.86.

Table 1
*Study Quality Ratings*

| Items | Scores |
|---|---|
| Study design | 0 = Nonrandomized prospective experiment<br>1 = Randomized experiment |
| Outcome measure | 0 = Subjective measure of mammogram receipt (self-reports)<br>1 = Objective measure of mammogram receipt (claims data, chart review) |
| Clarity of outcome definition | 0 = No definition of study outcome (mammogram adherence)<br>1 = Clearly defined mammogram adherence |
| Information on withdrawal | 0 = Not clearly discussed<br>1 = The number and the reasons for withdrawals in each group are stated |

*Analysis*

Stata (StataCorp LP, College Station, TX) was used to conduct the data analysis. An effect size (*d*) was calculated for each study using the difference in the postintervention adherence rates between the interven-
210 tion and control groups ($p_i$ and $p_c$, respectively). An overall mean weighted effect size (MWES) for the 23 studies was computed using the *meta* command in Stata, which weights *d* by the inverse of the estimated study variance in fixed-effects models. For the effect
215 size of $d = p_i - p_c$, the study variance was defined to be $p_i (1 - p_i)/n_i + p_c (1 - p_c)/n_c$, where $n_i$ and $n_c$ are the number of participants in the intervention and control groups, respectively (DerSimonian & Laird, 1986). A test for heterogeneity of the intervention effects was
220 performed using the DerSimonian and Laird (1986) *Q* statistic. When significant, a random-effects model was used to accommodate this heterogeneity (DerSimonian & Laird, 1986). This process was repeated to calculate MWES for various subgroups of the 23 studies. In ad-
225 dition, 95% CIs were estimated for each MWES.

The sensitivity analyses consisted of refitting the meta-analysis for the overall MWES to determine whether the results varied by potentially influential studies (i.e., extreme effect size, large sample size) or
230 study quality. A leave-one-out approach was taken and the overall MWES was reestimated by removing the influential studies one at a time. Also conducted were meta-analyses restricted to high- and low-quality studies to compare to the overall MWES. Finally, addi-
235 tional analyses using funnel plot and fail-safe *N* were performed to examine publication bias. In the absence of publication bias, the plot should be symmetric, resembling an inverted funnel (Light & Pillemer, 1984). Because visual inspection of the funnel plot involves
240 subjective interpretation, Rosenthal's (1984) fail-safe *N* was calculated also. This calculation is an estimate of the number of studies having no effect (i.e., zero effect size) that is needed to reduce the overall effect size in the meta-analysis from significant to nonsignificant. If
245 the estimated fail-safe *N* is greater than a cutoff value (formula = $5k + 10$, where *k* is the number of studies in the meta-analysis; Rosenthal, 1984), it is suggested that there is no evidence of publication bias.

**Results**

*Study Characteristics*

Of the 23 studies, 6 studies included predominantly
250 African Americans; 2 studies, Hispanics; 5 studies, Asians; and 10 studies, combined ethnic samples. Randomized experimental study design (61%), group-level assignment (57%), and community setting (83%) were common features of the studies. Sample sizes varied;
255 smaller studies included < 100 participants in the sample, whereas the biggest study was done on > 5,000 women, totaling 22,849 women. (See Table, Supplemental Digital Content 1, which summarizes the characteristics of studies included in this meta-analysis,

260 http://links.lww.com/A1244.) This table is also included on the Editor's Web site at http://www.nursing-research-editor.com.

The studies used single or multiple intervention strategies, with individually directed print materials being the most frequently used approach, followed by peer or lay health worker education or support and telephone counseling. Access-enhancing strategies such as low- or no-cost mammograms, making appointments, mobile vans, or vouchers were included in 6 studies. For the comparison group, 15 studies (65%) provided no intervention or usual care; 6 studies, minimal intervention; and 2 studies, other active nonbreast intervention (e.g., education on cholesterol or physical activity). Self-report rather than medical records was more frequently used as a method of outcome measurement (74% vs. 26%). The Health Belief Model was the most popular theory and was used in 6 studies alone or in combination with other theories such as Transtheoretical Model of Change and Social Learning theory, although in 9 studies, the theoretical approach was unspecified. These theories offered a basis for targets of individualized tailoring (e.g., providing intervention materials attuned to the characteristics of a person) in 4 studies. Most interventions involved some form of cultural strategies except for 2 (both conducted in a healthcare setting). Culturally matched intervention materials and ethnically matched intervention deliveries were equally common, whereas 5 studies indicated participation of members of the target ethnic community as a way of increasing cultural sensitivity of their intervention. Nine (39%) of the studies received a high quality rating, whereas 14 (61%) were rated as low quality.

*Pooled Results*

The estimated intervention effect and 95% CI for each study are presented in Table 2. As shown in Table 2, the overall MWES for the 23 studies was 0.078 ($Z$ = 4.414, $p < .001$) with a 95% CI of 0.043 to 0.113, indicating that the interventions were effective in improving mammography screening among ethnic minority women. This effect size was computed using a random-effects model to account for significant heterogeneity among interventions as indicated by a significant $Q$ statistic ($Q = 92.95$, $df = 22$, $p < .001$).

Table 2
*Estimated Effect Sizes With 95% Confidence Intervals (CIs)*

| Element | Category | No. of studies | Effect size (95% CI) |
|---|---|---|---|
| Overall | | 23 | 0.078 (0.043 to 0.113) |
| Intervention type[a,b] | Individual-directed | 19 | 0.099 (0.073 to 0.110) |
| | Access-enhancing | 6 | 0.155 (0.087 to 0.223) |
| | Social network | 6 | −0.023 (−0.078 to 0.032) |
| | Community education | 4 | 0.013 (−0.067 to 0.094) |
| | Mass media | 4 | 0.065 (−0.007 to 0.138) |
| Theory | Theory based | 14 | 0.090 (0.042 to 0.137) |
| | Nontheory based | 9 | 0.062 (0.009 to 0.116) |
| Tailored | Yes[c] | 4 | 0.101 (0.057 to 0.145) |
| | No | 19 | 0.076 (0.035 to 0.116) |
| Cultural strategies[b] | Involved target community members | 5 | 0.074 (−0.055 to 0.203) |
| | Culturally matched materials | 15 | 0.051 (0.009 to 0.092) |
| | Matched intervention deliveries | 14 | 0.067 (0.015 to 0.120) |
| Setting | Healthcare[c] | 4 | 0.113 (0.081 to 0.114) |
| | Community | 19 | 0.067 (0.027 to 0.107) |
| Ethnic groups[d] | African American | 9 | 0.098 (0.023 to 0.174) |
| | Asian Pacific Islanders | 5 | 0.094 (0.000 to 0.189) |
| | Hispanic | 5 | 0.036 (−0.034 to 0.106) |
| Quality | High (3 or 4)[c] | 9 | 0.099 (0.076 to 0.122) |
| | Low (1 or 2) | 14 | 0.061 (0.008 to 0.114) |

[a]Type of intervention: individual-directed = counseling (in person, telephone), letters, reminders; access-enhancing = facilitated scheduling, mobile vans, vouchers, reduced-cost or free mammograms; social network = peer leaders or lay health advisors; community education = community workshops, seminars.
[b]Studies may be classified as using more than one type of intervention or cultural strategies.
[c]Fitted with a fixed-effects model ($p$ for $Q$ statistic > .05).
[d]Included studies with samples > 40% of specified ethnic groups.

*Subgroup Analyses*

Also shown in Table 2 is the effectiveness of the different intervention methods. Access-enhancing interventions had the biggest MWES of 0.155 ($n = 6$, $Z = 4.488$, $p < .001$), followed by individually directed interventions ($n = 19$, MWES $= 0.099$, $Z = 6.552$, $p < .001$). Estimated effect sizes for other intervention approaches involving mass media ($n = 4$, MWES $= 0.065$, $Z = 1.759$, $p = .079$), community education ($n = 4$, MWES $= 0.013$, $Z = 0.324$, $p = .746$), or social networks ($n = 6$, MWES $= -0.023$, $Z = -0.817$, $p = .414$) were not statistically significant.

Tailoring an intervention according to the individual's characteristics based on valid behavioral theory was more effective than not doing so, with the MWES being 0.101 ($n = 4$, $Z = 4.476$, $p < .001$) and 0.076 ($n = 19$, $Z = 3.677$, $p < .001$), respectively. Theory-based interventions ($n = 14$) resulted in a bigger effect size compared with nontheory-based interventions ($n = 9$; effect sizes $= 0.090$ vs. $0.062$, respectively; $p < .05$ for all tests). Of cultural strategies, ethnically matched intervention deliveries ($n = 14$, MWES $= 0.067$, $Z = 2.516$, $p = .012$) and culturally matched intervention materials ($n = 15$, MWES $= 0.051$, $Z = 2.365$, $p = .018$) significantly improved mammography screening. Interventions involving members of the target community were a cultural strategy, with the biggest effect size of 0.074 ($n = 5$, $Z = 1.124$, $p = .261$), but the result was not significant. Interventions delivered in healthcare settings ($n = 4$) were associated with a bigger effect size compared with interventions done in community settings ($n = 19$; MWES $= 0.113$ vs. $0.067$; $p < .01$ for all models). When combined intervention effects were examined for each ethnic group (included studies with samples > 40% of specified ethnic groups), the estimated intervention effect was significant for African American women with a MWES of 0.098 ($n = 9$, $Z = 2.550$, $p = .011$). Studies with other ethnic minority women yielded no significant findings with a MWES of 0.094 for Asian and Pacific Islanders ($n = 5$, $Z = 1.955$, $p = .051$) and 0.036 for Hispanic women ($n = 5$, $Z = 1.004$, $p = .315$).

*Sensitivity Analyses*

Sensitivity analyses were conducted using potentially influential studies such as Kim and Sarna (2004), Sauaia et al. (2007), and Welsh, Sauaia, Jacobellis, Min, and Byers (2005) to gauge the impact on the variability of effect sizes. When the Kim and Sarna study was removed, the MWES for remaining studies was 0.069 ($Z = 4.153$, $p < .001$). Removing Sauaia et al. resulted in a MWES of 0.082 ($Z = 4.292$, $p < .001$) for the remaining studies. Without Welsh et al., the MWES for the other 22 studies was 0.085 ($Z = 5.198$, $p < .001$). Also performed were analyses with studies of high- versus low-quality ratings (quality rating 3–4 vs. 1–2). The MWES for the high-quality studies ($n = 9$) was 0.099 ($Z = 8.452$, $p < .001$), whereas the MWES for the low-quality studies ($n = 14$) was 0.061 ($Z = 2.239$, $p = .025$).

*Publication Bias*

The likelihood of publication bias was examined by first plotting the standard error by the natural logarithm of the logged odds ratio for the estimated effect sizes. The funnel plot appeared slightly asymmetrical. The fail-safe $N$, however, indicated that 411 nonsignificant studies would be necessary (cutoff = 125) to show that these interventions used to promote mammography screening among traditionally nonadherent ethnic minority women have no effect on mammography adherence, making the aggregate result from this analysis fairly robust.

## Discussion

The results indicate that there was an average of 7.8% increase in the rate of mammography use for minority women in the treatment groups receiving a variety of interventions. Access-enhancing interventions yielded the biggest increase in mammography use (15.5%), followed by individually directed interventions (9.9%). Even though the result cannot be compared directly with those of other meta-analyses due to different study selection criteria and intervention typology, this finding is similar to that of Legler et al. (2002) and Yabroff and Mandelblatt (1999).

Interventions using social networks such as *promotoras* or lay health advisors were associated with a small and negative effect size (i.e., reduced mammography screening rates after intervention). The finding of the negative effect size associated with *promotora* interventions might have been a result of study design. Specifically, the six *promotora* interventions included in the meta-analysis (Earp et al., 2002; Fernandez-Esquer, Espinoza, Torres, Ramirez, & McAlister, 2003; Nguyen, Vo, McPhee, & Jenkins, 2001; Powell et al., 2005; Sauaia et al., 2007; Welsh et al., 2005) were all nonrandomized, community-based trials with mostly large sample sizes (mean sample size = about 2,299) and low quality ratings; five studies received a quality rating of 2 and one study received a quality rating of 1. Our finding indicates that *promotora* interventions may be better suited for smaller community applications. When a large-scale community-based intervention trial is planned, interventions using *promotoras* may need to be considered as an alternative with well-prepared *promotora* training and a rigorous monitoring plan.

In analyzing effect sizes by the use of theory, the results indicated that theory-based interventions were more effective than nontheory-based interventions. Tailored interventions guided by theory also resulted in a greater effect size than did nontailored interventions. Indeed, tailored interventions included in this meta-analysis used single or multiple theories to structure the content of the intervention messages. Considering the few tailored interventions with larger improvement in mammography screening, more tailored intervention studies based on valid theories are warranted.

Interventions involving target community members as a way to enhance cultural sensitivity yielded a bigger effect size as compared with interventions using other cultural strategies (e.g., providing culturally matched materials or matching intervention deliveries), although the random-effects model for testing of its effect was not statistically significant. We cannot compare the result with those of other meta-analyses because no previous meta-analyses specifically examined cultural strategies as part of intervention typology. The nonsignificance might be attributable to the small number of studies in this category ($n = 5$). Although the finding offers some implications in designing mammography-enhancing interventions for ethnic minority women, future meta-analysis is needed as more empirical evidence becomes available.

Consistent with previous meta-analysis (Legler et al., 2002), it was found that the intervention effect was bigger for studies conducted in a healthcare setting (e.g., health maintenance organizations and community health centers) than for the community-based studies. Healthcare settings naturally offer increased contact with medical providers. It is likely that women in the healthcare setting might have had fewer barriers to screening, with more support for obtaining mammograms through individualized letters or counseling (Champion et al., 2007; Young, Waller, & Smitherman, 2002), scheduling of screening appointments (Beach et al., 2007), or case management (Beach et al., 2007; Dietrich et al., 2006). As Legler et al. (2002) pointed out, additional support or cues are necessary to facilitate mammography use even when access may no longer be a problem.

Effect sizes for studies including more than 40% African American and more than 40% Asian or Pacific Islander women were similar (9.8% and 9.4%, respectively), although the effect size for Asian or Pacific Islander women was marginally significant ($p = .051$); however, the MWES (3.6%) was not statistically significant for comparisons consisting of more than 40% Hispanic women. The estimated effect for intervention groups with more than 40% African American women in the Legler et al. (2002) meta-analysis was 11.6% (95% CI = 6.4–16.7), slightly bigger than that in this study. Although no published analysis of intervention effects for Asian or Pacific Islanders or Hispanic women were found, the nonsignificant result might have been due, in part, to the small number of studies available for these subgroup analyses (five studies each for Asian or Pacific Islander and Hispanic women). A careful examination of the characteristics of each individual study included in the ethnic subgroup analyses also revealed some design issues—particularly for studies involving Hispanic women—that are worth pointing out: three out of five studies with more than 40% Hispanic women (Fernandez-Esquer et al., 2003;

Sauaia et al., 2007; Welsh et al., 2005) used a nonrandomized experimental design with a large sample size ($N > 5,000$ for Sauaia et al., 2007, and Welsh et al., 2005). A large-scale community trial is likely to put researchers in a less controlled situation. Diffusion might occur between groups, or control communities may receive interventions with substantial amounts through other mechanisms (e.g., the Breast and Cervical Cancer Program for free mammograms). A traditional randomized controlled trial could pose ethical and logistical dilemmas in community research because control groups do not benefit from study participation, which is often perceived as *unfair* (Learmonth, 2000). Nevertheless, this analysis suggests that more tightly controlled trials may be necessary to improve mammography screening among minority groups, particularly Hispanic women. Researchers may need to consider and engage more actively in alternative research designs (e.g., waiting list design and attention control design) to ensure that the benefits of the research are made available to all ethnic minority communities (Corbie-Smith et al., 2003).

Several limitations of this meta-analysis should be noted. One limitation is the reliance of this review on published sources in Medline, CINAHL, PsycINFO, and Web of Science databases. This might have led to an overestimation or underestimation of effect sizes by excluding unpublished sources (e.g., dissertations) or government documents that might not be readily available, although researchers have found no differences related to inclusion or exclusion of unpublished literature (Conn, Valentine, Cooper, & Rantz, 2003). Second, due to the focus of interest in ethnic minority women in the United States who face unique cultural and linguistic challenges, this review was limited to articles of samples in the United States; thus, the findings may not be generalizable to studies that have been conducted in other countries. Third, as is common in meta-analyses, the uneven quality and quantity of studies are also limitations. An attempt was made to address this issue by offering estimates for high- versus low-quality studies. Several analyses included only four to six studies with nonsignificant MWES. Findings from the analyses with only a small number of studies should be considered as preliminary evidence and not definitive estimates of the effectiveness of the studies. It will be important to conduct additional analyses when results from more studies become available. Finally, most studies included in this meta-analysis used multiple intervention components. One problem in interventions with multiple components is that it is difficult to tease out the effect of each individual component. Some researchers suggest conducting factorial design studies to address this issue (Legler et al., 2002), although the cost to conduct such studies would likely be higher.

In conclusion, uniform improvement in cancer screening is a national goal to address cancer dispari-

530 ties among ethnic minority communities in the United States. The results of this meta-analysis suggest important directions for the design of future interventions to promote mammography screening among ethnic minority women. Access-enhancing strategies are an important intervention component for minority women
535 who are likely to lack the resources to obtain mammography screening readily. Also highlighted in this analysis is a need for increased use of a theory-based, tailored approach. More active engagement of community partners in the research process should be considered
540 also to improve screening outcomes. Finally, based on the pooled MWES estimated in this meta-analysis, well-controlled studies are needed to improve the effectiveness of mammography intervention programs among ethnic minority women, particularly among
545 Hispanic women. Consistent use of the rate difference of mammography screening as an outcome measure is important for additional meta-analyses and promotion of further knowledge development in this important area.

## References

*Allen, B. Jr., & Bazargan-Hejazi, S. (2005). Evaluating a tailored intervention to increase screening mammography in an urban area. *Journal of the National Medical Association, 97*(10), 1350–1360.

American Cancer Society. (2008). *Cancer facts and figures 2008.* Atlanta, GA: Author.

*Avis, N. E., Smith, K. W., Link, C. L., & Goldman, M. B. (2004). Increasing mammography screening among women over age 50 with a videotape intervention. *Preventive Medicine, 39*(3), 498–506.

*Beach, M. L., Flood, A. B., Robinson, C. M., Cassells, A. N., Tobin, J. N., Greene, M. A., et al. (2007). Can language-concordant prevention care managers improve cancer screening rates? *Cancer Epidemiology, Biomarkers & Prevention, 16*(10), 2058–2064.

Carey, L. A., Perou, C. M., Livasy, C. A., Dressler, L. G., Cowan, D., Conway, K., et al. (2006). Race, breast cancer subtypes, and survival in the Carolina Breast Cancer Study. *JAMA, 295*(21), 2492–2502.

*Champion, V. L., Springston, J. K., Zollinger, T. W., Saywell, R. M. Jr., Monahan, P. O., Zhao, Q., et al. (2006). Comparison of three interventions to increase mammography screening in low income African American women. *Cancer Detection and Prevention, 30*(6), 535–544.

*Champion, V., Skinner, C. S., Hui, S., Monahan, P., Juliar, B., Daggy, J., et al. (2007). The effect of telephone versus print tailoring for mammography adherence. *Patient Education and Counseling, 65*(3), 416–423.

Chu, K. C., Miller, B. A., & Springfield, S. A. (2007). Measures of racial/ethnic health disparities in cancer mortality rates and the influence of socioeconomic status. *Journal of the National Medical Association, 99*(10), 1092–1100, 1102–1104.

Cokkinides, V., Bandi, P., Siegel, R., Ward, E. M., & Thun, M. J. (2007). *Cancer prevention & early detection facts & figures 2008.* Atlanta, GA: American Cancer Society.

Conn, V. S., Valentine, J. C., Cooper, H. M., & Rantz, M. J. (2003). Grey literature in meta-analyses. *Nursing Research, 52*(4), 256–261.

Corbie-Smith, G., Ammerman, A. S., Katz, M. L., St. George, D. M., Blumenthal, C., Washington, C., et al. (2003). Trust, benefit, satisfaction, and burden: A randomized controlled trial to reduce cancer risk through African-American churches. *Journal of General Internal Medicine, 18*(7), 531–541.

*Danigelis, N. L., Worden, J. K., Flynn, B. S., Skelly, J. M., & Vacek, P. M. (2005). Increasing mammography screening among low-income African American women with limited access to health information. *Preventive Medicine, 40*(6), 880–887.

Deapen, D., Liu, L., Perkins, C., Bernstein, L., & Ross, R. K. (2002). Rapidly rising breast cancer incidence rates among Asian-American women. *International Journal of Cancer, 99*(5), 747–750.

Denhaerynck, K., Lesaffre, E., Baele, J., Cortebeeck, K., Van Overstraete, E., & Buntinx, F. (2003). Mammography screening attendance: Meta-analysis of the effect of direct-contact invitation. *American Journal of Preventive Medicine, 25*(3), 195–203.

DerSimonian, R., & Laird, N. (1986). Meta-analysis in clinical trials. *Controlled Clinical Trials, 7*(3), 177–188.

*Dietrich, A. J., Tobin, J. N., Cassells, A., Robinson, C. M., Greene, M. A., Sox, C. H., et al. (2006). Telephone care interventions to improve cancer

screening among low-income women: A randomized, controlled trial. *Annals of Internal Medicine, 144*(8), 563–571.

*Duan, N., Fox, S. A., Derose, K. P., & Carson, S. (2000). Maintaining mammography adherence through telephone counseling in a church-based trial. *American Journal of Public Health, 90*(9), 1468–1471.

*Earp, J. A., Eng, E., O'Malley, M. S., Altpeter, M., Rauscher, G., Mayne, L., et al. (2002). Increasing use of mammography among older, rural African American women: Results from a community trial. *American Journal of Public Health, 92*(4), 646–654.

Edwards, A. G., Evans, R., Dundon, J., Haigh, S., Hood, K., & Elwyn, G. J. (2006). Personalised risk communication for informed decision making about taking screening tests. *Cochrane Database of Systematic Reviews,* (4), CD001865.

Erwin, D. O., Ivory, J., Stayton, C., Willis, M., Jandorf, L., Thompson, H., et al. (2003). Replication and dissemination of a cancer education model for African American women. *Cancer Control, 10*(5 Suppl.), 13–21.

*Fernandez-Esquer, M. E., Espinoza, P., Torres, I., Ramirez, A. G., & McAlister, A. L. (2003). A su salud: A quasi-experimental study among Mexican American women. *American Journal of Health Behavior, 27*(5), 536–545.

*Husaini, B. A., Sherkat, D. E., Levine, R., Bragg, R., Van, C. A., Emerson, J. S., et al. (2002). The effect of a church-based breast cancer screening education program on mammography rates among African-American women. *Journal of the National Medical Association, 94*(2), 100–106.

Jadad, A. R., Moore, R. A., Carroll, D., Jenkinson, C., Reynolds, D. J., Gavaghan, D. J., et al. (1996). Assessing the quality of reports of randomized clinical trials: Is blinding necessary? *Controlled Clinical Trials, 17*(1), 1–12.

*Jibaja-Weiss, M. L., Volk, R. J., Kingery, P., Smith, Q. W., & Holcomb, J. D. (2003). Tailored messages for breast and cervical cancer screening of low-income and minority women using medical records data. *Patient Education and Counseling, 50*(2), 123–132.

*Kim, Y. H., & Sarna, L. (2004). An intervention to increase mammography use by Korean American women. *Oncology Nursing Forum, 31*(1), 105–110.

Lantz, P. M., Mujahid, M., Schwartz, K., Janz, N. K., Fagerlin, A., Salem, B., et al. (2006). The influence of race, ethnicity, and individual socioeconomic factors on breast cancer stage at diagnosis. *American Journal of Public Health, 96*(12), 2173–2178.

Learmonth, A. M. (2000). Utilizing research in practice and generating evidence from practice. *Health Education Research, 15*(6), 743–756.

Legler, J., Meissner, H. L, Coyne, C., Breen, N., Chollette, V., & Rimer, B. K. (2002). The effectiveness of interventions to promote mammography among women with historically lower rates of screening. *Cancer Epidemiology, Biomarkers & Prevention, 11*(1), 59–71.

Light, R. J., & Pillemer, D. B. (1984). *Summing up: The science of reviewing research.* Cambridge, MA: Harvard University Press.

*Maxwell, A. E., Bastani, R., Vida, P., & Warda, U. S. (2003). Results of a randomized trial to increase breast and cervical cancer screening among Filipino American women. *Preventive Medicine, 37*(2), 102–109.

Miller, B. A., Hankey, B. F., & Thomas, T. L. (2002). Impact of sociodemographic factors, hormone receptor status, and tumor grade on ethnic differences in tumor stage and size for breast cancer in US women. *American Journal of Epidemiology, 155*(6), 534–545.

*Mishra, S. I., Bastani, R., Crespi, C. M., Chang, L. C., Luce, P. H., & Baquet, C. R. (2007). Results of a randomized trial to increase mammogram usage among Samoan women. *Cancer Epidemiology, Biomarkers & Prevention, 16*(12), 2594–2604.

Mock, J., McPhee, S. J., Nguyen, T., Wong, C., Doan, H., Lai, K. Q., et al. (2007). Effective lay health worker outreach and media-based education for promoting cervical cancer screening among Vietnamese American women. *American Journal of Public Health, 97*(9), 1693–1700.

*Moskowitz, J. M., Kazinets, G., Wong, J. M., & Tager, I. B. (2007). "Health is strength": A community health education program to improve breast and cervical cancer screening among Korean American women in Alameda County, California. *Cancer Detection and Prevention, 31*(2), 173–183.

Navarro, A. M., Senn, K. L., McNicholas, L. J., Kaplan, R. M., Roppe, B., & Campo, M. C. (1998). Por La Vida model intervention enhances use of cancer screening tests among Latinas. *American Journal of Preventive Medicine, 15*(1), 32–41.

*Nguyen, T., Vo, P. H., McPhee, S. J., & Jenkins, C. N. (2001). Promoting early detection of breast cancer among Vietnamese-American women. Results of a controlled trial. *Cancer, 91*(1 Suppl), 267–273.

Park, A., Nitzke, S., Kritsch, K., Kattelmann, K., White, A., Boeckner, L., et al. (2008). Internet-based interventions have potential to affect short-term mediators and indicators of dietary behavior of young adults. *Journal of Nutrition Education and Behavior, 40*(5), 288–297.

*Powell, M. E., Carter, V., Bonsi, E., Johnson, G., Williams, L., Taylor-Smith, L., et al. (2005). Increasing mammography screening among African American women in rural areas. *Journal of Health Care for the Poor and Underserved, 16*(4 Suppl. A), 11–21.

Purc-Stephenson, R. J., & Gorey, K. M. (2008). Lower adherence to screening mammography guidelines among ethnic minority women in America: A meta-analytic review. *Preventive Medicine, 46*(6), 479–488.

Rakowski, W., Meissner, H., Vernon, S. W., Breen, N., Rimer, B., & Clark, M. A. (2006). Correlates of repeat and recent mammography for women ages 45 to 75 in the 2002 to 2003 Health Information National Trends Survey (HINTS 2003). *Cancer Epidemiology, Biomarkers & Prevention, 15*(11), 2093–2101.

Resnicow, K., Davis, R. E., Zhang, G., Konkel, J., Strecher, V. J., Shaikh, A. R., et al. (2008). Tailoring a fruit and vegetable intervention on novel motivational constructs: Results of a randomized study. *Annals of Behavioral Medicine, 35*(2), 159–169.

*Reuben, D. B., Bassett, L. W., Hirsch, S. H., Jackson, C. A., & Bastani, R. (2002). A randomized clinical trial to assess the benefit of offering on-site mobile mammography in addition to health education for older women. *American Journal of Roentgenology, 179*(6), 1509–1514.

Rimer, B. K. (1994). Mammography use in the U.S.: Trends and the impact of interventions. *Annals of Behavioral Medicine, 16*(4), 317–326.

Rosenthal, R. (1984). *Meta-analysis procedures for social research.* Beverly Hills, CA: Sage.

*Sauaia, A., Min, S. J., Lack, D., Apodaca, C., Osuna, D., Stowe, A., et al. (2007). Church-based breast cancer screening education: Impact of two approaches on Latinas enrolled in public and private health insurance plans. *Preventing Chronic Disease, 4*(4), A99.

Schumann, A., John, U., Ulbricht, S., Ruge, J., Bischof, G., & Meyer, C. (2008). Computer-generated tailored feedback letters for smoking cessation: Theoretical and empirical variability of tailoring. *International Journal of Medical Informatics, 77*(11), 715–722.

Shavers, V. L., Harlan, L. C., & Stevens, J. L. (2003). Racial/ethnic variation in clinical presentation, treatment, and survival among breast cancer patients under age 35. *Cancer, 97*(1), 134–147.

Sidani, S., & Braden, C. J. (1998). *Evaluating nursing interventions: A theory-driven approach.* Thousand Oaks, CA: Sage.

Smigal, C., Jemal, A., Ward, E., Cokkinides, V., Smith, R., Howe, H. L., et al. (2006). Trends in breast cancer by race and ethnicity: Update 2006. *CA: A Cancer Journal for Clinicians, 56*(3), 168–183.

Smith-Bindman, R., Miglioretti, D. L., Lurie, N., Abraham, L., Barbash, R. B., Strzelczyk, J., et al. (2006). Does utilization of screening mammography explain racial and ethnic differences in breast cancer? *Annals of Internal Medicine, 144*(8), 541–553.

Soeken, K. L., Lee, W. L., Bausell, R. B., Agelli, M., & Berman, B. M. (2002). Safety and efficacy of S-adenosylmethionine (SAMe) for osteoarthritis. *Journal of Family Practice, 51*(5), 425–430.

Sohl, S. J., & Moyer, A. (2007). Tailored interventions to promote mammography screening: A meta-analytic review. *Preventive Medicine, 45*(4), 252–261.

StataCorp. (2005). *Stata statistical software: Release 9.* College Station, TX: Author.

Suarez, L., Roche, R. A., Pulley, L. V., Weiss, N. S., Goldman, D., & Simpson, D. M. (1997). Why a peer intervention program for Mexican-American women failed to modify the secular trend in cancer screening. *American Journal of Preventive Medicine, 13*(6), 411–417.

Taylor, V. M., Jackson, J. C., Yasui, Y., Kuniyuki, A., Acorda, E., Marchand, A., et al. (2002). Evaluation of an outreach intervention to promote cervical cancer screening among Cambodian American women. *Cancer Detection and Prevention, 26*(4), 320–327.

Town, R. J., Wholey, D. R., Feldman, R. D., & Burns, L. R. (2007). Hospital consolidation and racial/income disparities in health insurance coverage. *Health Affairs, 26*(4), 1170–1180.

U.S. Preventive Services Task Force. (2002). *Screening for breast cancer: Recommendations and rationale.* Retrieved May 8, 2008, from http://www.ahcpr.gov/clinic/3rduspstf/breastcancer/brcanrr.htm

Wasserman, M., Bender, D., & Lee, S. Y. (2007). Use of preventive maternal and child health services by Latina women: A review of published intervention studies. *Medical Care Research and Review, 64*(1), 4–45.

*Welsh, A. L., Sauaia, A., Jacobellis, J., Min, S. J., & Byers, T. (2005). The effect of two church-based interventions on breast cancer screening rates among Medicaid-insured Latinas. *Preventing Chronic Disease, 2*(4), A07.

*Wood, R. Y., & Duffy, M. E. (2004). Video breast health kits: Testing a cancer education innovation in older high-risk populations. *Journal of Cancer Education, 19*(2), 98–104.

Yabroff, K. R., & Mandelblatt, J. S. (1999). Interventions targeted toward patients to increase mammography use. *Cancer Epidemiology, Biomarkers & Prevention, 8*(9), 749–757.

*Young, R. F., Waller, J. B. Jr., & Smitherman, H. (2002). A breast cancer education and on-site screening intervention for unscreened African American women. *Journal of Cancer Education, 17*(4), 231–236.

*Indicates studies included in this meta-analysis.*

*Supplemental digital content is available for this article. Direct URL citations appear in the printed text and are provided in the HTML and PDF versions of this article on the journal's Web site: www.nursingresearchonline.com*

**Editor's note**: Additional information provided by the authors expanding this article is on the Editor's Web site at http://www.nursing-research-editor.com

**Acknowledgments**: This study was supported by a grant from the National Cancer Institute (R01 CA129060). Editorial support was provided by the Johns Hopkins University School of Nursing Center for Collaborative Intervention Research. Funding for the Center is provided by the National Institute of Nursing Research (P30 NRO 8995). The content is solely the responsibility of the authors and does not necessarily represent the official views of the National Institute of Nursing Research or the National Institutes of Health.

**Address correspondence to**: Hae-Ra Han, PhD, RN, School of Nursing, The Johns Hopkins University, 525 North Wolfe Street, Room 448, Baltimore, MD 21205-2110. E-mail: hhan@son.jhmi.edu

# Exercise for Article 39

## Factual Questions

1. What is the explicitly stated *purpose* of this meta-analysis?

2. Why were international studies not included?

3. Of the 749 studies that were identified, how many were excluded?

4. How many quality rating points were awarded to a study for being a randomized experiment?

5. Of the 23 studies included in the analysis, how many had participants that were predominantly African American?

6. What was the overall effect size for the 23 studies?

## Questions for Discussion

7. Is it important for the reader of this research to know the key word phrases used in the literature search? (See lines 125–130.)

8. Do you think this meta-analysis was worth doing given that only 23 studies qualified for inclusion? Explain. (See lines 163–165 and Table 2.)

9. In your opinion, was the classification of the studies as being of either low quality or high quality an important feature of this study? Explain. (See lines 195–205, 355–360, and Table 1.)

10. In your opinion, how important is the limitation that the researchers describe in lines 493–502? Explain.

11. In your opinion, are the results of this meta-analysis important? Do the results have practical implications? Explain.

## Quality Ratings

Directions: Indicate your level of agreement with each of the following statements by circling a number from 5 for strongly agree (SA) to 1 for strongly disagree (SD). If you believe an item is not applicable to this research article, leave it blank. Be prepared to explain your ratings. When responding to criteria A and B, keep in mind that brief titles and abstracts are conventional in published research.

A.  The title of the article is appropriate.

SA   5   4   3   2   1   SD

B.  The abstract provides an effective overview of the research article.

SA   5   4   3   2   1   SD

C.  The introduction establishes the importance of the study.

SA   5   4   3   2   1   SD

D.  The literature review establishes the context for the study.

SA   5   4   3   2   1   SD

E.  The research purpose, question, or hypothesis is clearly stated.

SA   5   4   3   2   1   SD

F.  The method of sampling is sound.

SA   5   4   3   2   1   SD

G.  Relevant demographics (for example, age, gender, and ethnicity) are described.

SA   5   4   3   2   1   SD

H.  Measurement procedures are adequate.

SA   5   4   3   2   1   SD

I.  All procedures have been described in sufficient detail to permit a replication of the study.

SA   5   4   3   2   1   SD

J.  The participants have been adequately protected from potential harm.

SA   5   4   3   2   1   SD

K.  The results are clearly described.

SA   5   4   3   2   1   SD

L.  The discussion/conclusion is appropriate.

SA   5   4   3   2   1   SD

M.  Despite any flaws, the report is worthy of publication.

SA   5   4   3   2   1   SD

# Notes

# Notes